REPLACEMENT CARDIAC

VALVES

Titles of Related Interest

Macfarlane COMPREHENSIVE ELECTROCARDIOLOGY
Singh SILENT MYOCARDIAL ISCHEMIA AND ANGINA
Cheng COMPREHENSIVE CARDIOLOGY
Norman RAPID ECG INTERPRETATION

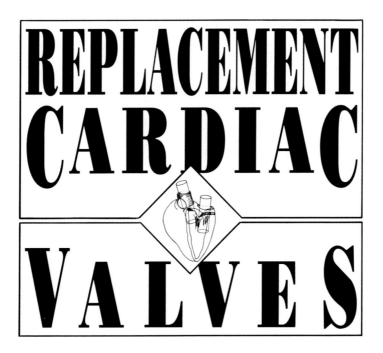

REPLACEMENT CARDIAC VALVES

Edited by

Endre Bodnar, M.D.
Middlesex, England
United Kingdom

Robert Frater, M.D.
Department of Surgery
Montefiore Medical Center
Bronx, New York

PERGAMON PRESS
Member of Maxwell Macmillan Pergamon Publishing Corporation
New York • Oxford • Beijing • Frankfurt
São Paulo • Sydney • Tokyo • Toronto

Pergamon Press Offices:

U.S.A.	Pergamon Press, Inc., Maxwell House, Fairview Park, Elmsford, New York 10523, U.S.A.
U.K.	Pergamon Press plc, Headington Hill Hall, Oxford OX3 0BW, England
PEOPLE'S REPUBLIC OF CHINA	Pergamon Press, Xizhimenwai Dajie, Beijing Exhibition Centre, Beijing 100044, People's Republic of China
GERMANY	Pergamon Press GmbH, Hammerweg 6, D-6242 Kronberg, Germany
BRAZIL	Pergamon Editora Ltda, Rua Eça de Queiros, 346, CEP 04011, Paraiso, São Paulo, Brazil
AUSTRALIA	Pergamon Press Australia Pty Ltd., P.O. Box 544, Potts Point, NSW 2011, Australia
JAPAN	Pergamon Press, 8th Floor, Matsuoka Central Building, 1-7-1 Nishishinjuku, Shinjuku-ku, Tokyo 160, Japan
CANADA	Pergamon Press Canada Ltd., Suite 271, 253 College Street, Toronto, Ontario M5T 1R5, Canada

Library of Congress Cataloging-in-Publication Data

Replacement cardiac valves / edited by Endre Bodnar and Robert Frater
    p. cm.
    Includes bibliographical references and index.
    ISBN 0-08-035773-3 (hard) :
    1. Heart valve prosthesis. I. Bodnar, Endre. II. Frater, Robert
William Mayo.
    [DNLM: 1. Heart Valve Prosthesis. WG 169 R424]
    RD598.35.H42R46 1991
    617.4'120592--dc20
    DNLM/DLC
    for Library of Congress
                       90-14314
                         CIP

Printing: 1 2 3 4 5 6 7 8 9 10   Year: 1 2 3 4 5 6 7 8 9 0

Printed in the United States of America

CONTENTS

LIST OF CONTRIBUTORS

Robert J. Akins
Carbon Implants
Austin, Texas

William H. Bain, MD, FRCS
Cardiac Department, Western Infirmary
Glasgow, United Kingdom

Martin M. Black, PhD
Department of Medical Physics and Clinical
  Engineering
Royal Hallamshire Hospital
Sheffield, United Kingdom

Eugene H. Blackstone, MD
Division of Cardiothoracic Surgery,
  Department of Surgery
The University of Alabama at Birmingham
Birmingham, Alabama

Endre Bodnar, MD
Pinner
Middlesex, United Kingdom

Jack C. Bokros, PhD
Carbon Implants
Austin, Texas

Uberto Bortolotti, MD
University of Padova
Padova, Italy

Eric G. Butchart, FRCS
Department of Cardiac Surgery
University Hospital of Wales
Cardiff, United Kingdom; and
University of Wales College of Medicine
Cardiff, United Kingdom

L. Andy Campbell
CarboMedics, Inc.
Austin, Texas

Grant W. Christie, PhD
Systematic Solutions Ltd.
Auckland, New Zealand

Thomas Cochrane, PhD
Department of Medical Physics and Clinical
  Engineering
Royal Hallamshire Hospital
Sheffield, United Kingdom

Carlos G. Duran, MD
Department of Cardiovascular Diseases
King Faisal Specialist Hospital and Research
  Center
Riyadh, Saudi Arabia

James I. Fann, MD
Department of Cardiovascular Surgery
Stanford University School of Medicine
Stanford, California

Victor J. Ferrans, MD, PhD
Ultrastructure Section, Pathology Branch
National Heart, Lung and Blood Institute
National Institutes of Health
Bethesda, Maryland

Robert W. M. Frater, MD
Division of Cardiothoracic Surgery
Albert Einstein College of Medicine
Bronx, New York

Vincenzo Gallucci, MD
University of Padova
Padova, Italy

Alfred N. Gerein, MD
University of British Columbia
Vancouver, Canada

Charles D. Griffin
CarboMedics, Inc.
Austin, Texas

Axel D. Haubold
Carbon Implants
Austin, Texas

Stephen L. Hilbert, PhD
Center for Devices and Radiological Health
Food and Drug Administration
Rockville, Maryland

Dieter Horstkotte, MD
Department of Cardiology, Pneumology, and
  Angiology
Heinrich-Heine University of Düsseldorf
Düsseldorf, Federal Republic of Germany

W. R. Eric Jamieson, MD
Division of Cardiovascular and Thoracic
  Surgery
Department of Surgery
University of British Columbia
Vancouver, British Columbia

Michael T. Janusz, MD
University of British Columbia
Vancouver, Canada

Michael Jones, MD
Surgery Branch
National Heart, Lung and Blood Institute
National Institutes of Health
Bethesda, Maryland

Ernest Lane
Lane Laboratories
Garden Grove, California

Patricia V. Lawford, PhD
Institute for Biomedical Equipment
  Evaluation and Services (IBEES)
Lodge Moor Hospital
Sheffield, United Kingdom

Michael D. Lelah, PhD
Materials and Membrane Technology Center
Baxter Healthcare Corporation
Round Lake, Illinois

Robert J. Levy, MD
Department of Pediatrics and
  Communicable Diseases
University of Michigan Medical Center
Ann Arbor, Michigan

A. Milano, MD
University of Padova
Padova, Italy

D. Craig Miller, MD
Department of Cardiovascular Surgery
Stanford University School of Medicine
Stanford, California

R. T. Miyagishima, MD
University of British Columbia
Vancouver, Canada

Carlos E. Moreno-Cabral, MD
Department of Cardiovascular Surgery
Stanford University School of Medicine
Stanford, California

Samer A. M. Nashef, FRCS
Cardiac Department, Western Infirmary
Glasgow, United Kingdom

Buddy D. Ratner, PhD
Center for Bioengineering and Department
  of Chemical Engineering
University of Washington
Seattle, Washington

Helmut Reul, PhD
Helmholtz–Institute for Biomedical
  Engineering
Aachen University of Technology
Aachen, Federal Republic of Germany

Francis Robicsek, MD
Institute of the Carolinas
Charlotte, North Carolina

Susanne Robicsek, JD
Winston-Salem, North Carolina

Benson B. Roe, MD
Department of Surgery
University of California San Francisco
School of Medicine
San Francisco, California

Donald N. Ross, DSc, FRCS
National Heart Hospital
London, United Kingdom

Frederick J. Schoen, MD, PhD
Department of Pathology
Brigham and Women's Hospital and
  Harvard Medical School
Boston, Massachusetts

Gaetano Thiene, MD
University of Padova
Padova, Italy

Agit Yoganathan, PhD
Georgia Institute of Technology
School of Chemical Engineering
Atlanta, Georgia

PREFACE

The evolution of surgery for heart valve disease is still in progress, with the number of questions awaiting an answer multiplying by the day. There are, however, a few conclusions deduced from past experience which offer themselves to be carved onto tablets, the chance of any modification being so remote.

First is the fact that heart valve disease is an operable disorder. Second is the overwhelming evidence that successful surgery extends life expectancy and improves the quality of life. Third is the recognition that surgical treatment of heart valve disease remains palliative in nature. Fourth and final is the inevitability that the patient's condition at the time of surgery and the performance of the implanted prosthesis will jointly decide the eventual outcome and long-term prognosis.

This book concentrates only on the last mentioned contributing factor: the replacement devices. The basic intention has not been to produce new and original information, but rather to gather existing knowledge from all relevant disciplines, and present it in a single, concise, and comprehensive volume. As it would fall far beyond human competence and capability to try to achieve this goal by relying on the expertise of only one or two authors, the best scientists in each discipline were asked for a contribution.

It is the editors' privilege to acknowledge and to thank all contributing authors sincerely for providing the scientific material for this book. They all understood the importance of the subject and the significance of the timing of this publication.

Reaching to poetry and literature for a simile, the pilgrim's progress springs immediately to mind. Even the most dedicated pilgrim would halt the voyage for a while and look back as well as ahead when a vantage point presents a panoramic view. Such a vantage point seems to be with us regarding the development of replacement heart valves.

It appears that basic design features have crystallized over the past two decades and a spectacular breakthrough is very unlikely to revolutionize this particular area. It also appears, however, that the same is not exactly true for the materials aspects of replacement valves, but that the future progress in materials is expected to be slow and tedious.

As the good performance of the currently available replacement valves is proved, so much so that in a way they are taken for granted, the safety of their use has become the primary concern for physicians, patients, and for the entire society in general. One has only to refer to recent newspaper articles and television programs addressing valve safety. This book intends to contribute in particular to this important facet of the complex issues pertaining to replacement valves.

The initiative for this volume came from the publishers, Pergamon Press, USA. They provided every possible help, supplemented sometimes by the impossible, and it is felt appropriate to acknowledge them formally.

It is hoped that the reader will benefit from this joint effort.

ENDRE BODNAR
ROBERT W.M. FRATER

Bodnar, E. and Frater, R. W. M., editors
(1991) *Replacement Cardiac Valves,*
Pergamon Press, Inc. (New York), pp. 1–20
Printed in the United States of America

CHAPTER 1

DESIGN AND FLOW CHARACTERISTICS

Martin M. Black, Thomas Cochrane, Patricia V. Lawford, Helmut Reul, and Agit Yoganathan

The replacement of diseased and malfunctioning heart valves has been a routine procedure for almost three decades. During this time there have been many developments in both surgical techniques and prosthetic valve design. Notwithstanding the advances that have been made, there is no ideal manufactured valve. The two major types of replacement valves, namely, mechanical or tissue (bioprosthetic), have their own particular advantages and disadvantages as listed in Table 1–1.

From both a manufacturing and a surgical point of view, the design and use of manufactured valves in the heart is, in many respects, a compromise between the ideal and what is practicable. All current valve designs involve the use of flow occluder systems (including flexible leaflets) housed in a frame or ring that is fitted with an appropriate sewing cuff. In the case of mechanical valves the ring is rigid. Frames for tissue valves are usually flexible in the axial direction but effectively rigid in the plane of the sewing ring. Consequently both valve types produce an orifice pressure drop effect as illustrated in the constricted tube in Fig. 1–1. Such changes in pressure produce short-term increases in kinetic energy just downstream of the valve. This is particularly true when one considers the presence of an occluder system that can also cause blood damage. This increased kinetic energy gives rise to flow conditions that in some circumstances can damage red blood cells.

The situation just described does not obtain in the normal healthy heart. In systole the normal aortic valve opens fully to provide an unobstructed flow tube from the left ventricle to the ascending aorta with no significant orifice effect at the level of the valve. In diastole the mitral valve retracts fully to provide a similar tube effect from the atrium through the mitral valve ring to the ventricle. These flow tubes are shown diagrammatically in Fig. 1–2. The insertion of any manufactured valve will inevitably inhibit the development of unconstricted tube flow paths by producing orifice effects at the valve position.

The rigid base rings of manufactured valves are particularly significant when the mitral valve is replaced. In a normal healthy heart the mitral annulus varies from an approximate D shape in systole to a circular form in diastole as illustrated diagrammatically in Fig. 1–3. The D shape in systole is necessary to accommodate the fully open aortic valve and concomitant systolic tubular flow passage. If the mitral valve replacement has a rigid base ring, the normal systolic–diastolic configurations of the left side of the heart cannot obtain.

It is clear from the above that current manufactured heart valves do not provide ideal replacements when compared with those of a normal healthy heart. They are, however, a reasonable compromise between the ideal and what is technologically practicable.

1

TABLE 1–1. *Advantages and Disadvantages of Mechanical and Tissue Valves*

Valve type	Advantages	Disadvantages
Mechanical	Long-term durability Consistency of manufacture	Unnatural form Patient usually requires long-term anticoagulant therapy
Tissue	More natural form and function Less need for long-term anticoagulant therapy	Unproven long-term durability Consistency of manufacture is more difficult In vivo calcification

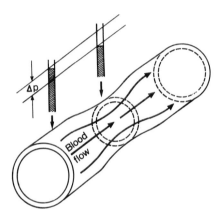

FIG. 1–1. Pressure drop ($\triangle$p) occurring through an orifice.

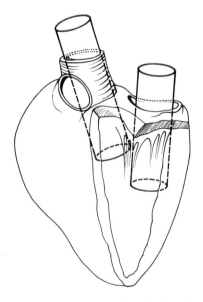

FIG. 1–2. Idealized flow tubes in systole and diastole through aortic and mitral valves, respectively.

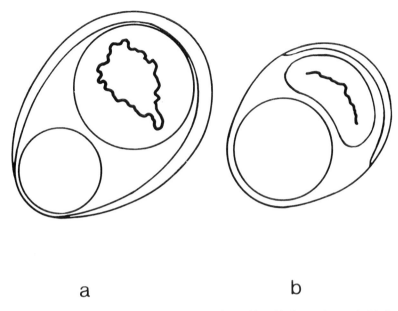

a   b

Fɪɢ. 1–3. The shape of the mitral annulus and its relationship with the aortic root in (a) diastole, and (b) systole.

Many different designs are available, and these will be discussed in the following section. Thereafter, details will be given of the laboratory testing of these prostheses and the limitations of such tests when predicting in vivo behavior.

VALVE CONFIGURATIONS

Three major criteria must be considered when assessing the hemodynamic performance of a particular valve design. The valve

1. Should function efficiently and present the minimum load to the heart.
2. Should be durable and maintain its efficiency for the life span of the patient.
3. Should *not* cause damage to molecular or cellular blood components or stimulate thrombus formation.

No current valve design completely meets these criteria. However, with these principles in mind it is possible to make a qualitative prediction as to the likely success of a particular valve design.

A valve with less than perfect hemodynamic function will cause energy dissipation, resulting in decreased efficiency and an increased workload for the heart. Obstructions in the flow pathway and flow disturbances or backflow during valve closure (closing regurgitation) and through the closed valve (leakage regurgitation) all contribute to energy losses. The magnitude of energy losses is dependent on valve design, with the size and shape of the occluder mechanism and supporting struts all having a significant effect on valve performance.

In addition, flow abnormalities may result in damage to blood components; this is the major cause of hemolysis and thromboembolism associated with prosthetic valves (1–4).

Blood components may also be damaged by contact with materials with poor blood compatibility; this and the important subject of durability are considered in subsequent chapters.

Currently, five basic configurations of heart valve substitutes are produced commercially. Three of these are mechanical prostheses: the caged-ball, tilting disk, and hinged bileaflet valves. The remaining two, the porcine aortic and bovine pericardial valves, are frame-mounted bioprostheses.

Mechanical Valves

All mechanical valves have an occluder mechanism around which the blood must flow. The size, geometric shape, degree of opening, and mass of the occluder, and the relationship between the external dimensions of the valve, tissue annulus diameter, (TAD) and the internal orifice all contribute to the degree of stenosis presented by the prosthesis. The volume of closing regurgitation is related to occluder size, travel, and speed of closure, while the leakage regurgitation depends on the size of the potential leakage gap between the occluder and the rim of the housing. Some manufacturers claim that they include a specific allowance for backflow in order to facilitate washout of the hinge mechanism.

Caged-Ball Valves

The long-established Starr-Edwards caged-ball valve (Fig. 1–4a) is by far the most commonly used example of its type. The valve comprises a polished stellite alloy orifice and cage that entraps a spherical silicone rubber occluder. The occluder seats directly onto the orifice ring, minimizing leakage through the closed valve. Flow through the open valve is obstructed by the presence of the silicone ball, which remains in the center of the flow pathway, leaving an annular area available for flow and causing regions of flow reversal and disturbance. The presence of the cage is also likely to increase flow abnormalities leading to turbulence (Fig. 1–5a) during the forward flow phase.

In addition, the high profile of this valve is particularly significant in large sizes. With mitral prostheses the cage may contact the ventricular wall during systole, particularly

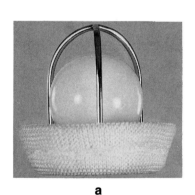 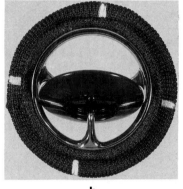 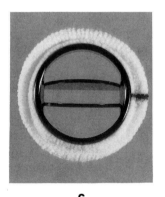

| a | b | c |

Fig. 1–4. Mechanical valves. (a) The Starr-Edwards caged-ball valve. (b) The Björk-Shiley monostrut tilting disk valve (outflow aspect). (c) The St. Jude Medical bileaflet valve (outflow aspect).

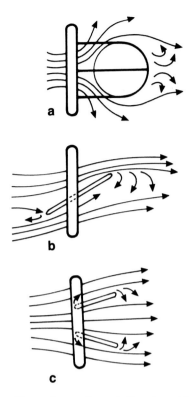

FIG. 1–5. Flow patterns for different forms of prosthetic valves. (a) Caged-ball valve. (b) Tilting disk valve. (c) Bileaflet valve.

in the case of a small left ventricle. This may ultimately lead to myocardial conduction disturbances or ventricular rupture. In the aortic position, size discrepancies may lead to secondary stenosis caused by the ball itself.

Tilting Disk Valves

The tilting disk valve has the advantages of a significantly lower profile and quasi-central flow. Several models of this type are currently available. These vary in terms of the design of the disk entrapment mechanism, disk shape, and the opening angle, which varies from 60 to 85°. An example of a disk configuration, the Björk-Shiley monostrut valve, is illustrated in Fig. 1–4b. This valve has a concavoconvex pyrolytic carbon disk that is supported within a stellite orifice ring, where it is captured between a U-shaped outlet strut and a single projecting inlet strut—the monostrut. The disk, which is free to rotate, opens to an angle of 70 degrees, dividing the valve into a major and a minor orifice. In the closed position, the disk sits within the valve orifice supported by the outlet strut. Flow through the valve is distorted by the presence of the occluder and supporting struts; however, the disturbance is significantly less than that observed for a caged-ball valve (Fig. 1–5b). This has been substantiated qualitatively by flow visualization studies. The circular gap between the occluder and the valve ring may facilitate washing out of the valve and reduce the risk of thrombus formation. However, flow through narrow gaps can lead to high shear stresses. Such stresses can result in blood cell damage and hemolysis.

Bileaflet Valves

Bileaflet valves represent the latest development in mechanical valve design. The occluder remains disk-shaped but is split into two parts that pivot in the center of the valve ring. Once again, several models are available, varying in disk shape and opening angle. An example of this type of design, the St. Jude Medical valve, is illustrated in Fig. 1–4c. In this model, the leaflets are flat and, together with the valve housing, are coated with pyrolytic carbon. When open, the valve is divided into one minor and two major orifices. The wide opening angle and thin cross-sectional area presented by the open leaflets present minimal disturbance to flow (Fig. 1–5c). Closing regurgitation is also minimized by the size and shape of the leaflets; however, the additional central gap between the leaflets will contribute to the leakage regurgitation.

Bioprostheses

Bioprostheses have the advantage of an unobstructed central orifice and are thus not likely to cause severe disturbance to flow. However, the presence of bulky, covered, supporting struts tends to reduce the ratio of tissue to orifice diameter and can significantly reduce the effective orifice area for any particular orifice diameter.

Porcine Aortic Valves

Figure 1–6a shows the flow pattern of the Carpentier-Edwards supraannular bioprosthesis. The valve is constructed from a single porcine aortic valve. This is treated with buffered glutaraldehyde at low pressure to maintain leaflet structure and pliability. The valve is mounted on a flexible Elgiloy wire frame that is designed to give a prosthesis with a minimum profile height.

The valve opens into an irregular cone shape, allowing central, unimpeded flow. However, flow disturbances may be introduced by the projection of the stent posts into the flow field and by buckling of the leaflet free edges, which produce an irregular outflow orifice. Leakage through the closed valve is minimal as the leaflets are forced together tightly under back pressure.

An equation by Gorlin and Gorlin has been used by some investigators to evaluate the effective orifice area of a valve from recorded pressure drops. These valves may then be compared with the actual orifice area calculated from the valve. However, the clinical significance of such analysis is not clear.

Pericardial Valves

At present, pericardial valves provide the best hemodynamic solution to the problem of valve design. The first examples of this type were constructed from glutaraldehyde-stabilized strips of bovine pericardium that were mounted on the outside of a supporting frame. This technique makes maximum use of the available flow area and results in a valve with a minimum resistance to flow. In addition, the cone shape of the open valve and smooth circular orifice minimize flow disturbances (Fig. 1–6b).

Recently, the popularity of pericardial valves has declined following increasing reports of poor durability. The major cause for concern, leaflet tearing, has been shown to be

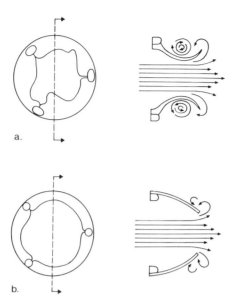

FIG. 1–6. Flow patterns for bioprosthetic valves. (a) Porcine bioprosthesis. (b) Pericardial bioprosthesis.

related to the method of valve construction and has led to the introduction of significant design modifications. In later models, for example the Edwards and Pericarbon valves, the tissue is mounted *within* the frame, resulting in a small reduction in orifice area. It is not clear to what extent this affects valve performance, but the consequent loss in hemodynamic efficiency is likely to be insignificant and a small price to pay for increased durability.

Although it may be possible to make a qualitative judgment as to the relative hemodynamic performance of the different valve types by simple visual assessment, quantitative information is required in order to establish the significance of minor differences in design. The ultimate evaluation of any replacement heart valve design can only be made after long-term clinical implantation. Nevertheless, some initial evaluation can be obtained from laboratory tests.

LABORATORY TESTING

There are three types of testing that yield information for both the cardiac surgeon and the valve designer—steady flow testing, pulsatile flow testing, and wear testing. The limitations of each test method must be considered before extrapolating results to the situation in vivo.

Steady Flow Testing

Apart from visual inspection, the steady flow test is the simplest method of obtaining first-line information on valve performance. In its basic form, the pressure drop across a valve and valve orifice is measured for a range of flow rates. In early studies, valves to be tested were simply placed in cylindrical tubes that were attached to a steady flow pump.

However, it was soon realized that the method of valve mounting and the geometric configurations of the flow passages have a strong influence on a valve's performance (5). The mounting arrangement should not impede proper valve opening, and the geometry of the flow section should approximate to the cardiovascular anatomy. In addition, if measurements obtained in different laboratories are to be compared, it should be recognized that the choice of downstream pressure measurement site is important if it is not to influence the measured pressure drop. Because of the phenomenon of pressure recovery, selection of standard pressure measurement sites is difficult (6, 7); also, with some valve designs, there may be a significant dynamic component to the measured pressure drop.

A good example of a steady flow apparatus for replacement aortic valve testing is that used in the Helmholtz Institute at Aachen (8) (Fig. 1–7). The information that can be obtained from steady flow measurements includes pressure drop across the valve (Fig. 1–8), effective orifice area, and pressure recovery at different flow rates (Fig. 1–9). Recently, several groups have introduced the use of the laser Doppler technique for the evaluation of heart valve function (4, 9, 10). This technique yields detailed data on flow velocities and turbulence intensities. This in turn allows estimation of shear rates and turbulent shear stresses, which provides information on the likelihood of damage to blood cells or tissue. In general, the method is only applied to the region immediately downstream of the valve because of the difficulty of beam access to other regions. Furthermore, laser Doppler technology is expensive, and it is tedious to chart velocity and turbulence fields point by point. Hence it is unlikely that the method will be of use for routine valve assessment. Rather, it should be available in only a few centers and should be used to answer specific design questions.

Flow visualization may also be used in conjunction with steady flow measurements to produce flow patterns at different flow rates (Figs. 1–10 and 1–11). These provide a useful

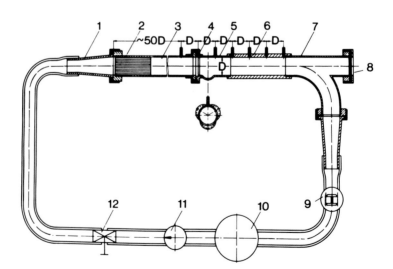

FIG. 1–7. Aachen steady flow system. (1) Flow inlet diffuser, (2) honeycomb, (3) inlet tube, (4) heart valve mounting ring, (5) model aortic root, (6) downstream measuring section, (7) bifurcation with optical observation window, (8) viewport allowing observation and recording of valve opening characteristics, (9) rotameter, (10) fluid reservoir, (11) centrifugal pump, and (12) throttle valve.

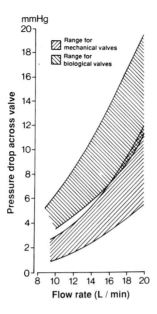

Fɪɢ. 1–8. Pressure drop–flow characteristics for mechanical and biological valves measured under steady flow conditions (all measurements are made 200 mm from the valve ring).

qualitative picture of the flow distribution and highlight regions of stagnation, recirculation, or turbulence, where cell damage or cell–cell interactions may occur.

Pressure drop, pressure recovery, and orifice area measurements relate to the obstructive properties of the valve. Laser Doppler and flow visualization studies tell us about flow, shear, and shear stress fields, which clearly have an important bearing on valve

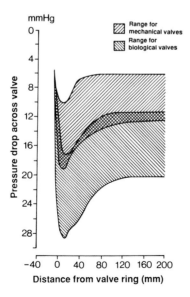

Fɪɢ. 1–9. Pressure recovery for mechanical and biological valves at a steady flow rate of 20 L/min.

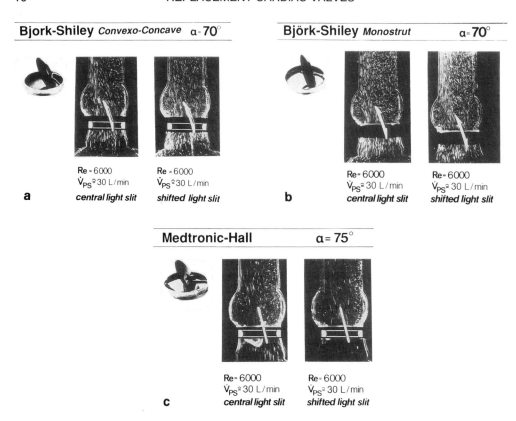

Fig. 1–10. Flow through these models of tilting-disk valves: (a) Björk-Shiley convexo-concave, (b) Björk-Shiley monostrut, and (c) Medtronic-Hall: (Left side) Central light plane; (right side) shifted light plane.

performance. However, the results of steady flow testing are not readily extrapolated to the clinical situation since they do not consider the dynamic operation of the valve or permit the assessment of valvular regurgitation. In order to investigate valve performance in greater depth, it is necessary to employ pulsatile flow testing at different rate–stroke volume combinations.

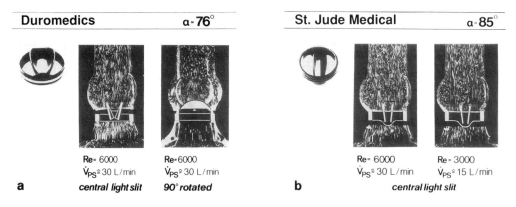

Fig. 1–11. Flow through two bileaflet valves. (a) Duromedics; (b) St. Jude Medical.

Pulsatile Flow Testing

Over the last 30 years many different pulse duplicators have been developed (4, 10–17). In each case, the design inevitably involves a compromise between the need to simulate the behavior and flow characteristics pertaining in vivo and the requirement of a system that is practicable for routine laboratory use. We briefly describe here three systems that are routinely used to assess prosthetic heart valves. The pulse duplicator used by Dr. Yoganathan, which also forms the basis of the Food and Drug Administration heart valve testing facility (11), is shown schematically in Fig. 1–12. It has a linear configuration, and, except for the geometry of mitral and aortic flow chambers, no attempt is made to simulate the anatomy of the left heart. Pumping action is achieved using a rubber bulb, contained inside a sealed plastic cylinder, which is air pressurized by means of electronically controlled solenoid valves. Timing parameters are selected using thumbwheel switches, and volume flow is controlled by regulating the solenoid valves.

The gemotric configuration used in Professor Reul's laboratory in Aachen (Fig. 1–13) approximates cardiac anatomy much more closely. In this case, the heart and connecting tubes are arranged vertically and the valves are mounted in their correct anatomic positions in a specially molded flexible ventricle. Flow is driven by an electrohydraulic piston drive unit that compresses the ventricle to simulate the systolic stroke. The drive control signal is generated on a digital computer using a digital-to-analogue converter to produce the output.

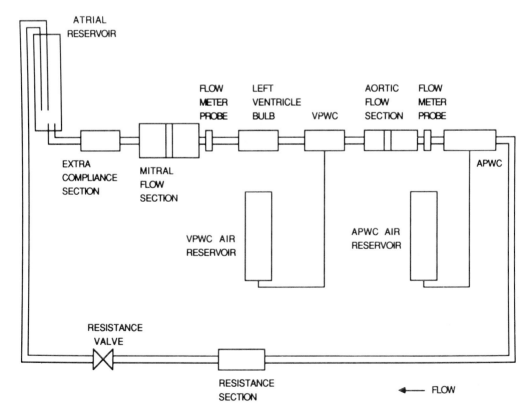

FIG. 1–12. Schematic diagram of the Yoganathan–FDA facility for pulsatile flow testing. The system is shown with the flow meter in place for aortic valve tests.

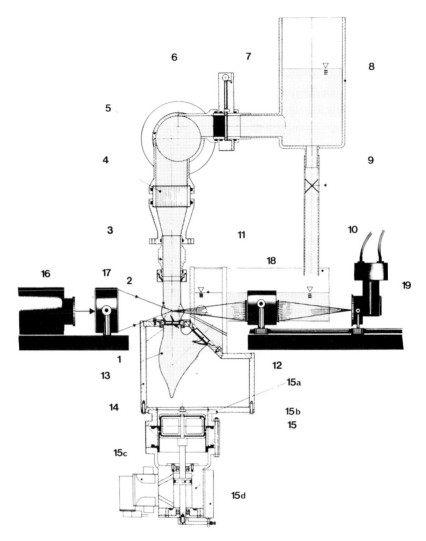

FIG. 1–13. Schematic diagram of the Aachen pulse duplicator. (1) Aortic valve, (2) elastic aortic root, (3) electromagnetic flow probe, (4) characteristic resistance, (5) adjustable compliance, (6) peripheral resistance, (7) adjusting mechanism for 6, (8) fluid reservoir, (9) adjusting throttle, (10) atrial reservoir, (11) left atrium (the atrial housing has a central slit in order to provide a free laser beam path), (12) mitral tilting disk–type valve, (13) elastic ventricular sac, (14) rigid Plexiglass housing, (15) hydraulic pumps, (15a) low-pressure piston, (15b) high-pressure piston, (15c) electromagnetic servovalve, (15d) displacement transducer, (16) He-Ne laser, (17) transmitting optics, (18) receiving optics, and (19) photomultiplier.

The design of the configuration used in Professor Black's laboratory in Sheffield (Fig. 1–14) lies somewhere between that of Dr. Yoganathan and that of Professor Reul. It is primarily designed for rapid testing of a range of valve sizes, in both mitral and aortic positions, over a wide range of rate–stroke volume combinations (40–140 cycles per minute, 20–150 ml).

Aortic and mitral valves are mounted in separate sections, the mitral valve in a chamber-to-chamber configuration and the aortic valve in a chamber-to-tube (with sinuses)

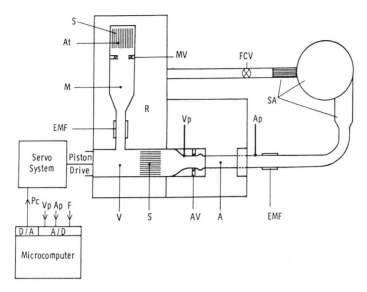

Fig. 1–14. Schematic diagrams of the Sheffield pulse duplicator. The diagram shows the system configured for aortic testing. (R) Fluid reservoir, (S) flow straighteners, (At) model atrium, (MV) mitral valve mounting, (V) model ventricle, (EMF) electromagnetic flow meter, (In) aortic inflow section, (AV) aortic valve mounting, (Vp) ventricular pressure transducer, (Ap) aortic pressure transducer, (A) model aorta, (SA) model systemic circulation, (FCV) flow control valve, (D/A) digital to analog converter, (Pc) position control signal, (A/D) analog-to-digital converter, (Vp) ventricular pressure signal, (Ap) aortic pressure signal, and (F) flow signal.

configuration. Flow is driven by the movement of a piston in a rigid cylindrical ventricular chamber. The piston is mounted on a ball screw that is driven by a DC motor and servo amplifier. The complete system, including drive, data collection, and analysis, is controlled by a microcomputer. Ventricular flow waveforms are generated automatically by the software once a rate, stroke volume, or cardiac output combination has been selected.

The parameters most commonly used to characterize valve performance in pulse duplicator studies are pressure drop (Fig. 1–15) and regurgitation. The latter is usually broken up into the backflow through the valve as it closes, and the leakage (Fig. 1–16).

Pressure drop and flow curves may also be used to derive work or energy loss parameters characterizing valve function (18–20). These are usually divided into systolic (or diastolic), closure, and leakage energy losses (18). These parameters indicate the work done during these phases of the "cardiac" cycle. They provide useful information for the valve designer, but their clinical significance is, as yet, unclear.

Flow visualization may also be employed in pulsatile flow studies. In this case it is usually necessary to record dynamic flow patterns using high-speed cine or video. Video recording can also capture valve opening and closing action throughout the cardiac cycle. This simple technique can often immediately show faults in valve design.

The laser Doppler method is also applicable to pulsatile studies and yields detailed information on flow velocities (Fig. 1–17), turbulence intensities (Fig. 1–18), shear rates, and shear stresses. The limitations that apply to steady flow testing also apply to pulsatile studies, perhaps even more so because of the additional temporal dimension.

A major problem, as yet unresolved, for those involved in the design, manufacture,

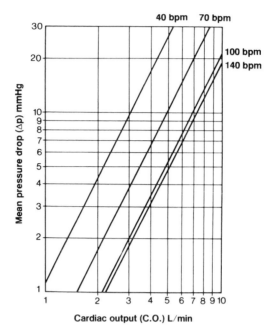

Fig. 1–15. Variation of mean pressure drop with cardiac output at different heart rates for a 23-mm Björk-Shiley monostrut valve.

and evaluation of heart valve substitutes is to decide which parameters are most relevant to the surgeon. Most replacement heart valves have acceptable pressure drop and regurgitation characteristics; nevertheless, some valves perform better than others. No one index can adequately describe all the characteristics of a valve. Problems of wear and tear are at least as important as the obstructive and regurgitation properties. A great deal of

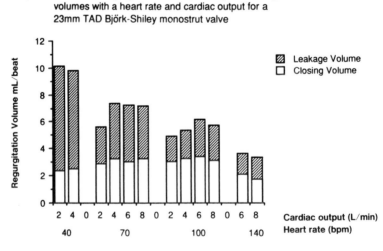

Fig. 1–16. Variation of total regurgitation, closing, and leakage volumes with cardiac output and heart rate for a 23-mm Björk-Shiley monostrut valve.

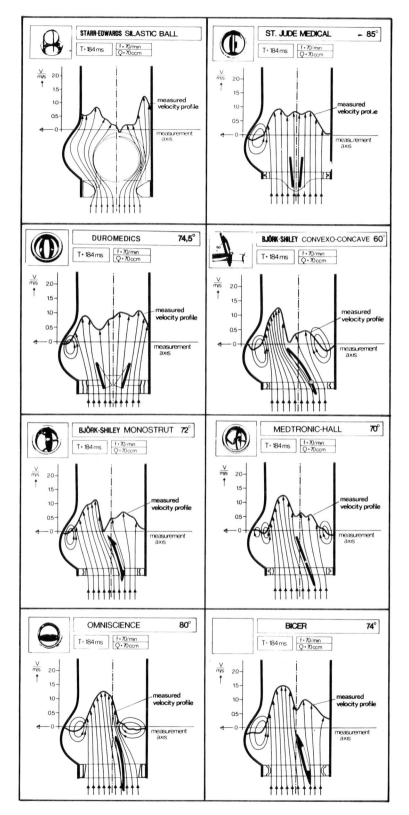

FIG. 1–17. Laser Doppler analysis of flow fields at peak systole for 10 mechanical valves.

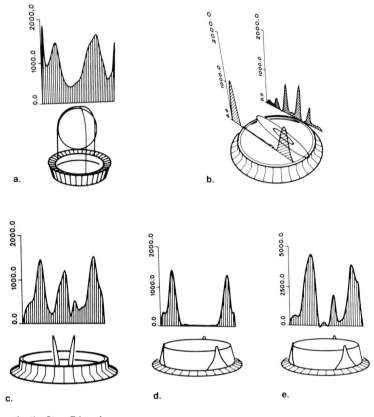

a. Aortic: Starr-Edwards
b. Aortic: Björk-Shiley *Monostrut*
c. Aortic: St. Jude
d. Aortic: I-S Pericardial
e. Aortic: C-E 2625 Porcine

FIG. 1–18. Turbulent shear-stress profiles at peak systole for three mechanical and two bioprosthetic valves. Shear stress is given in dyn/cm^2. (a) Starr-Edwards aortic valve turbulent shear-stress profile 30 mm downstream on the centerline. (b) Björk-Shiley monostrut valve turbulent shear-stress profile 17 mm downstream in the major and minor orifices. (c) St. Jude Medical valve turbulent shear-stress profile 13 mm downstream on the centerline. (d) Ionescu-Shiley pericardial valve turbulent shear-stress profile 27 mm downstream on the centerline. (e) Carpentier-Edwards 2625 porcine valve turbulent shear-stress profile 15 mm downstream on the centerline.

information is generated during testing of heart valves. All too often the results are presented in a form that is not easily assimilated by the surgeon. Still more needs to be done to improve the standardization of valve evaluation and to ensure that proper valve comparisons are made and that the results are effectively communicated to those who use them, be they designers, manufacturers, or clinicians.

Comparison of the Valves

No in-depth comparison of all the valve types across a range of heart rates and stroke volumes and across the range of valve sizes has been carried out. However, several limited studies have been performed, and these enable some general conclusions to be drawn

TABLE 1–2. *Valve Test Protocols at Three Test Centers*

Reference	Valve type studied*	Valve size & position*	Cardiac output (L/min)	Heart rate (bpm)	Stroke volume (mL)
Knott et al. (18, 20)	BC, TD, BL	27 (A)	3.0, 4.5, 6.5, 8.0	70	43, 64, 93, 114
Scotten et al. (24)	Po, Pe	19 (A)	1.8, 3.6, 7.3, 4.3	60, 80, 120, 200	35, 55, 70, 30
Black et al. (22)	BC, TD, BL, Pe	17, 19, 21, 23, 25, 27, 29, 31, 33 (M) (A)	2.0, 4.0, 6.0, 8.0	40, 70, 100, 120	50, 100, 28.6, 57.1, 85.7, 114.3, 20, 40, 60, 80, 42.9, 57.1

*BC = ball and cage; TD = tilting disk; BL = bileaflet; Po = porcine; Pe = pericardial; M = mitral; A = aortic; N/A = data not available.

about valve behavior in vitro (18, 21–25). The types and sizes of valves tested, and combinations of cardiac output, heart rate, and stroke volume used in three such studies are given in Table 1–2. The range of results obtained in these studies in terms of mean pressure difference, regurgitation, and energy losses are summarized in Table 1–3. Direct comparisons made between results obtained by different research groups must be made with caution as differences in test equipment and methodology influence the absolute values of any measurements made.

ANALYSIS OF THE RESULTS

The two most common parameters used in defining the performance of a valve are pressure drop and regurgitation since these relate most directly to the behavior of a diseased valve whether it is stenotic or incompetent. More recently, studies by Scotten (13),

TABLE 1–3. *Variation In Test Results Obtained at the Three Test Centers*

Reference	Valve type*	Mean pressure difference (mmHg)	Regurgitation Closing (mL/beat)	Leakage	E_C	Energy loss‡ E_L	E_S
Knott et al. (18, 20)	BC	8.5–32	4–1.5†	0–0.3†	1–0.3	0	10–22.5
	TD	2.0–6.5	7–2.5†	3–0.6†	1–0.6	2–0.5	2.5–5.5
	BL	1.5–5.5	6.5–2.5†	8.5–1.5†	1.5–0.7	4.5–0.7	2.5–5.5
Scotten et al. (24)	Po	5–24	0.6–0.15	0.4–0.8	1.5–0	0.7–1.5	5–21
	Pe	2–12	1.2–0.4	0.8–1.2	2.5–1	0.6–1.5	3.5–13
Black et al. (22)	BC	1.0–53	2.5–0.2	6.0–0	N/A	N/A	N/A
	TD	1.0–42	7.5–0.5	10.0–0.2	N/A	N/A	N/A
	BL	1.0–42	7.5–0.5	7.5–0.8	N/A	N/A	N/A
	Pe	1.0–28	1.5–0.1	5.0–0.2	N/A	N/A	N/A

*BC = ball and cage; TD = tilting disk; BL = bileaflet; Po = porcine; Pe = pericardial; M = mitral; A = aortic; N/A = data not available.

†Results for regurgitation presented in this group are given as a percentage of the stroke volume.

‡Energy losses are expressed as percentages of the mean aortic flow energy per beat. E_C = energy loss due to valve closure; E_L = energy loss due to valve leakage; E_S = energy loss due to pressure drop across valve during systole.

Knott (18), and Swanson (19) have introduced the concepts of energy loss and performance indices in an attempt to obtain a single parameter to aid comparison among the various prosthetic valves. At this stage it is not clear how these factors relate to overall heart valve performance, particularly when biological phenomena such as hemolysis and thromboembolism are considered. However, they do give a measure of the work required from the heart if any particular valve is implanted and in this sense complement in vitro measurements obtained from pulse duplicators. As the in vivo performance of a valve is ultimately dependent on both physical and biological factors, in this sense it is unlikely that a single parameter that can adequately predict long-term in vivo performance will be found.

At present, pulse duplicators provide the only means of initial assessment of the likely hemodynamic performance of a prosthetic valve. Laboratory testing using rigid-walled test chambers with no *vessel compliance* is bound to limit the validity of in vitro models particularly in relation to pulsatile flow conditions.

In addition, reference has been made to the phenomenon of pressure recovery and the concomitant exchanges between kinetic and potential energies. These hemodynamic aspects appear to be significant in laboratory testing but may not be of equal importance in vivo. Flow conditions induced by the shape of the open configuration of the occluder may be more significant in terms of energy loss than those relating to pressure recovery. This implies that part of the heart's work is dissipated in energy losses due to disturbed flow.

The problems produced by the use of inflexible valve frames, particularly in the plane of the orifice, have already been referred to. The significance of this phenomenon has never been assessed in vitro. This is because no pulse duplicator has adequately catered for the precise anatomic juxtaposition of the aortic and mitral valves, nor do pulse duplicators allow for precise myocardial and major vessel compliance obtaining in the heart.

Many of the above analyses can be enhanced by the use of computerized studies of both the hemodynamics and the mechanical behavior of the myocardium and major blood vessels. Studies by McQueen and Peskin (26) and by Mazumdar (27) provide interesting examples of computerized hemodynamic analysis. Such studies tend to be limited by being in only two dimensions and also by ignoring the deformability of the myocardium. On the other hand, a number of researchers have investigated stress analysis of the myocardium in general and valve leaflets in particular. The former has been studied in some depth by Yettram (28), and the latter work on valves has been undertaken on tissue valve leaflets (29). Little has been done by way of combining these two aspects as an aid to valve design.

Within the constraints of existing valve designs, simulated computer studies of a tilting disk valve by McQueen and Peskin have indicated optimum configurations for such valves. These studies indicate the value of computer simulations of the hemodynamics associated with heart valve design. However, once again it is not clear at this stage how significant such analyses are in relation to the clinical performance of the valves.

CONCLUSIONS

This chapter has discussed some of the basic concepts associated with the design, development, and laboratory testing of artificial heart valves. It must be noted that, as yet, there is no ideal replacement valve and all those currently implanted involve some degree of compromise between optimum hemodynamics and cardiac function.

Manufactured valves inevitably involve some degree of resistance to flow. Such resistance can, along with other performance parameters, be measured in the laboratory. There are no standard test systems, and individual researchers have designed their own unique experimental equipment. As a result, it is often difficult to compare the results of one investigator with those of any other. Furthermore, in vitro testing can only simulate the in vivo situation to a limited extent, and care must be taken when laboratory results are extrapolated to the in vivo situation. Notwithstanding these difficulties, laboratory investigations are of considerable value when comparing the hydrodynamic performance of various valve configurations.

REFERENCES

1. Yoganathan AP, Reamer HH, Corcoran WH, Harrison EC, Shulman IA, Parnassus W: The Starr-Edwards aortic ball valve. Flow characteristics, thrombus formation and tissue overgrowth. Artif Organs 1980;5:6–17.
2. Yoganathan AP, Corcoran WH, Harrison EC, Carl JR: The Bjork-Shiley Aortic Prosthesis. Flow characteristics, thrombus formation and tissue overgrowth. Circulation 1978;58:70–76.
3. Gabbay S, Kresh JY: Bioengineering of mechanical and biologic heart valve substitutes. In Morse D, Steiner RM, Fernandez J (eds): Guide to Prosthetic Cardiac Valves. New York, Springer-Verlag, 1985, chap 9.
4. Bruss K-H, Reul H, Van Gilse J, Knott E: Pressure drop and velocity fields at four mechanical heart valve prostheses: Bjork-Shiley standard, Bjork-Shiley Concave-Convex, Hall Kaster and St Jude Medical. Life Supp Syst 1983;1:3–22.
5. Bellhouse B, Bellhouse F: Fluid mechanics of model normal and stenosed aortic valves. Circ Res 1969;25:693–704.
6. Clark C: The fluid mechanics of aortic stenosis: I. Theory and steady flow experiments. J Biomech 1976;9:521–528.
7. Tindale WB, Trowbridge EA: Evaluation in vitro of prosthetic heart valves: Pulsatile flow through a compliant aorta. Life Supp Syst 1983;1:173–185.
8. Reul H, Black MM: The design, development and assessment of heart valve substitutes. In Bajzer Z, Baxa P, Franconi C (eds): Proceedings of the 2nd International Conference on Application of Physics to Medicine and Biology. Singapore, World Scientific Publishing, 1984, p 99.
9. Yoganathan AP, Corcoran WH, Harrison EC: In vitro velocity measurements in the vicinity of aortic prostheses. J Biomech 1979;12:135–152.
10. Yoganathan AP, Corcoran WH, Harrison EC: Pressure drops across prosthetic heart valves under steady and pulsatile flow—in vitro measurements. J Biomech 1979;12:153–164.
11. Simenauer PA: Test protocol: Interlaboratory comparison of prosthetic heart valve performance testing. Rockville, Md, US Food and Drug Administration, 1986.
12. Martin TRP, Palmer JA, Black MM: A new apparatus for the in vitro study of aortic valve mechanics. Eng Med 1978;7:229–230.
13. Walker DK, Scotten LN, Modi VJ, Brownlee RT: In vitro assessment of mitral valve prostheses. J Thorac Cardiovasc Surg 1980;79:680–688.
14. Gabbay S, McQueen DH, Yellin EL, Frater RWM: In vitro hydrodynamic comparison of mitral valve prostheses at high flow rates. J Thorac Cardiovasc Surg 1978;76:771–787.
15. Swanson WM, Clark RE: A simple cardiovascular system simulator: Design and performance. J Bioeng 1982;1:135–145.
16. Wieting DW: Dynamic flow characteristics of heart valves. Doctoral Dissertation, University of Texas, Austin, 1969.
17. Chandran KB: Pulsatile flow past St Jude Medical bi-leaflet valve: An in vitro study. J Thorac Cardiovasc Surg 1985;89:743–749.
18. Knott E, Reul H, Steinseifer U: Pressure drop, energy loss and closure volume of prosthetic heart valves in aortic and mitral position under pulsatile flow conditions. Life Supp Syst 1986;4(suppl 2):139–141.
19. Swanson WM: Relative performance of prosthetic heart valves based on power measurements. Med Instrum 1984;18:318–325.
20. Knott E, Reul H, Knoch M, Steinseifer U, Rau G: In vitro comparison of aortic valve prostheses: I. mechanical valves. J Thorac Cardiovasc Surg, 1988;96:952–961.
21. Dellsperger KC, Wieting DW, Baehr DA, Band RJ, Brugger J-P, Harrison EC: Regurgitation of prosthetic heart valves: Dependence on heart rate and cardiac output. Am J Cardiol 1983;51:321–328.
22. Black MM, Lawford PV, Cochrane T: Health Equipment Information Bulletin, 1990. In Press.

23. Chandran KB, Cabell GN, Kahalighi B, Chen CJ: Pulsatile flow past aortic valve bioprostheses in a model human aorta. J Biomech 1984;17:609–619.
24. Scotten LN, Walker DK, Brownlee RT: The in vitro function of size 19 mm bioprosthetic heart valves in the aortic position. Science and Engineering Research Council (SERC) report, 1989 (unpublished).
25. Yoganathan AP, Wou Y-R, Sung H-W, Williams FP, Franch RH, Jones M: In vitro hemodynamic characteristics of tissue bioprostheses in the aortic position. J Thorac Cardiovasc Surg 1986;92:198–209.
26. McQueen DM, Peskin CS: Computer assisted design of pivoting disk prosthetic mitral valves. J Thorac Cardiovasc Surg 1983;86:126–135.
27. Mazumdar J, Thalassoudis K: A mathematical model for the study of flow through disk-type prosthetic heart valves. Med Biol Eng Comput 1983;21:400–409.
28. Yettram AL, Vinson CA, Gibson DG: Influence of the distribution of stiffness in the human left ventricular myocardium on shape change in diastole. Med Biol Eng Comput 1979;17:553–562.
29. Black MM, Patterson EA, Howard ICH, Wang XW: The stress analysis of bicuspid bioprosthetic heart valves using finite element analysis. Science and Engineering Research Council (SERC) report, 1988 (unpublished).

Bodnar, E. and Frater, R. W. M., editors
(1991) *Replacement Cardiac Valves,*
Pergamon Press, Inc. (New York), pp. 21–48
Printed in the United States of America

CHAPTER 2

THE DURABILITY OF MECHANICAL HEART VALVE REPLACEMENTS: PAST EXPERIENCE AND CURRENT TRENDS

Jack C. Bokros, Axel D. Haubold, Robert J. Akins, L. Andy Campbell, Charles D. Griffin, and Ernest Lane

HISTORICAL ASPECTS

The challenge of replacing the natural heart valve with a prosthetic device continues to be a formidable one. Materials do not exist that can duplicate the flexibility of natural valves in which the orifice and leaflets can deform in harmony with myocardial action. Nor is it possible for man to match nature's ability to remodel and heal in order to maintain and preserve the function of an artificial device.

In spite of the magnitude of the challenge, the replacement of a diseased valve with a rigid prosthetic contrivance offers a better prognosis than today's medical treatments. For example, when aortic stenosis becomes symptomatic, mortality exceeds 90% within a few years (1). Early replacement of the diseased valve can extend life beyond a decade (Figs. 1–4 in Ref. 2), and patients with valve replacements generally do substantially better than those treated medically (3–7).

In the mid 1940s Hufnagel replaced the thoracic aorta of animals with an acrylic prosthesis without thrombosis. This provided the impetus for him to develop and then implant in 1952 the first prosthetic heart valve in the descending aorta of a human (8, 9). This pivotal event, together with the development of the technique of extracorporeal circulation three years later (10), provided the stimulus for Harken on March 10, 1960, to replace the diseased aortic valve of a human with a ball valve at the anatomical site (11). One of Hufnagel's early patients survived over two decades with a rigid methylmethacrylate aortic valve with no evidence of wear, thrombosis, or embolism (12).

Even though the first prosthetic valves that were implanted were ingenious mechanical devices, they did not come close to duplicating either the form or function of the normal valves. Following the first implantations, the major developmental thrust sprang from the idea that better valves would have to closely duplicate the flexible form and function of natural valves. Accordingly, the criteria listed by early researchers to specify the design and materials needed were both extensive and individually demanding (13–27).

Efforts to mimic the flexibility of the natural orifice and leaflets, using flexible synthetic materials, so that the prostheses could deform naturally with the heart (sometimes even incorporating prosthetic chordae tendineae) were soon abandoned. Synthetic flexible materials with the required durability remain an unrealized dream.

The shift in developmental emphasis is evidenced by comparing the published contents of the First and Second National Conferences on Prosthetic Heart Valves. The proceedings of the First Conference, held in 1960 (28), eight years after the first valve was implanted by Hufnagel, contained only two out of 29 chapters that were directed at the development of rigid mechanical heart valve prostheses (29, 30). In contrast, at the Second Conference, held in 1968, developmental reports of replacement valves were directed exclusively at rigid mechanical devices that included the Starr-Edwards, Smeloff-Cutter, Lillehei-Kaster, Cross-Jones, Kay-Shiley, Beall, Cooley-Cutter, Magovern-Cromie, Wada-Cutter, Gott and DeBakey designs.

In summarizing the Second Conference (31), the Journal of the American Medical Association (JAMA) (32) made reference only to the Starr (33), Kay (34), Cross (35), Beall (36), Magovern (37), toroidal (38) and Wada (39) valves—all mechanical. It was noted parenthetically that, although there was no report at the conference, the Hufnagel (40) flexible trileaflet valve, fabricated from synthetic cloth, was looking good; the hoped for longevity, however, was never realized. Someday perhaps a clever researcher will devise a means to couple a rigid prosthesis within the heart in such a way that the normal myocardial motion is not impaired. Such a compromise might prove better than forcing a rigid ring into the naturally flexible mitral orifice, so that there is serious reduction in myocardial contractibility.

The Second National Conference on Prosthetic Heart Valves coincidentally marked the start of an identifiable third stage of valve development. The third period was initiated by two important materials developments. First, the discovery of the remarkable blood compatibility of pyrolytic carbon (pyc) (41) which, when its ultimate wear and fatigue resistance had been determined, was to solve the durability problems plaguing mechanical valves. Second was the identification of glutaraldehyde as a tissue fixative, which was to improve the potential of heterographs as acceptable clinical alternatives.

Pyc, referenced only incidentally in 1968 as a new material having excellent thromboresistance (42) and possibly useful as an occluder material (42, 43) with the potential to decrease embolism (44), had yet to be used clinically. The first bileaflet concept from which the St. Jude Medical prosthesis evolved was presented at the 1968 conference (45); the identification of glutaraldehyde as a superior fixative was to follow shortly thereafter (46).

The decade of the 1970s was a period of important progress in prosthetic heart valve development. The use of pyc reduced the durability problems of mechanical valves. Devices fabricated entirely of pyc, even with focused wear in fixed pivots, were not expected to fail due to fatigue or by wearing out during the normal lifetime of any patient. The introduction of biological valves fixed with glutaraldehyde solved the problems with tissues fixed with, for example, formalin (47, 48).

Even though many modern mechanical valves are accepted as having long-term durability (49), the question of wear and fatigue remains a pertinent issue. Using demanding hinge concepts that prevent hemostasis by washing but require fixed pivots with focused wear, valve designers strive to improve both the micro and macro quality of flow in order to reduce the blood trauma that leads to clotting. Their aim is to eliminate the need for anticoagulants through improved microhemodynamics within the hinge mechanism, an objective that is yet to be realized. Consequently, for patients in whom anticoagulation therapy is contraindicated and who thus must have a bioprosthesis, there is the added risk of reoperation due to the limited durability of such prostheses (50–52).

The popularity of bioprostheses peaked in the mid to late 1970s and then decreased, so that the ratio of mechanical to bioprostheses in use now favors mechanical devices (53). The decrease in the use of bioprostheses is probably due to the fact that in the mid 1970s it was thought that their failure would be gradual and replacement surgery could be elective, carrying no greater risk than that of the first operation. As the reoperation rate increased in the late 1970s (for example, the Mayo Clinic reports the reoperation rates to be 3, 7.6, and 13% for the years 1965, 1979, and 1987, respectively (54)) and with longer follow-up with more patients, it was found that there was a disproportionately large percentage of patients experiencing sudden valve disruption which required emergency reoperation with associated higher surgical risk (55). Recent reviews (53–63) of this complex subject reflect current thinking and contrast with earlier reports (64–72).

Obviously, a major advance that increases the durability of bioprostheses could tip the balance of usage back toward such devices. On the other hand, a major improvement in the thromboresistance of mechanical valves could increase their usage even more.

FAILURE MODES

The way valves can fail have been grouped into two categories, intrinsic and extrinsic mechanisms. Failures by *intrinsic* mechanisms are inherently related to design and material properties. Examples are mechanical degradation caused by fatigue fracture, and abrasive wear or biochemical attack that causes, for example, polymers to crack, wear, or distort. *Extrinsic* mechanisms are externally generated interferences with the motion of a valve's occluding mechanism. Examples include massive thrombotic obstruction caused by thrombus formation in the left atrium that subsequently becomes lodged in a prosthesis causing impingement of occluders on adjacent anatomy, or lockup.

Lockup is the immobilization of occluders by a force acting in a direction perpendicular to the valve axis and caused by the wedging of material between the occluder and the occluder retention mechanism; it should not be confused with impingement. The wedging material can be overhanging or unraveling sutures, unresected valve leaflets or chordae, or an atrial monitoring catheter (Fig. 2–1).

Extrinsic Mechanisms

Thrombotic Obstruction

All prosthetic valves can thrombose and malfunction. Some of the causes may be patient-related and are distinctly extrinsic—others can be valve-related and caused by poor hemodynamic design or the use of thrombogenic materials in the construction of the valve (13, 73–77) and are, therefore, called intrinsic. Since the origin of thrombotic obstructions is not usually ascertainable, all such occurrences are arbitrarily included in this section.

Prostheses most prone to thrombosis are those that produce turbulence (with associated high shear stresses), and stasis in close proximity to thrombogenic surfaces (75). Conversely, those designs that produce little or no turbulence and low levels of shearing stresses with no persistent regions of stagnation and which employ thromboresistant materials are the least likely to cause thrombosis. Thrombosis is often secondary to impingement. Hylen reviewed the subject in 1972 (77); more recent experience has been reported (49, 78–95).

Impingement

Impingement is defined as the interference with the operation of the occluder mechanism of a prosthesis caused by adjacent anatomic obstruction and excludes the interference that causes lockup. Impingement can impair the hemodynamics of a device and lead to thrombotic and other complications (96–98). Early valves that use a nontilting

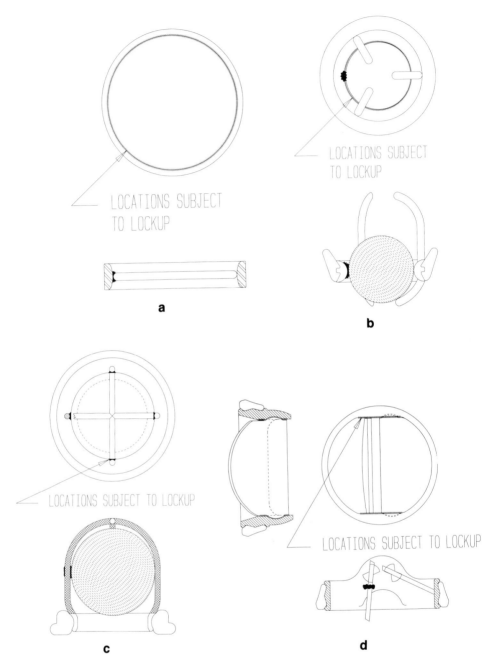

FIG. 2–1. Schematic diagram illustrating lock-up. (a) Full orifice tilting disk valve. (b) Full orifice ball valve. (c) Close-clearance cloth covered ball valve. (d) Bileaflet valve. The locking mechanism is caused by the jamming of material between the occluder and the valve support structure such that a force acting perpendicular to the valve axis immobilizes the occluder.

disk, such as the Kay-Shiley (34), as well as the modern tilting variety, are susceptible. Oversizing of modern tilting disk valves has often been cited as a cause (99–108).

Whether or not the chordae tendineae should be preserved was a question in 1961 (109). Since then, it has been shown that the separation of the continuity between the mitral annulus and the papillary muscles results in decreased left ventricular ejection fraction (110–112). Accordingly there has been an increased effort to preserve the posterior leaflet and its apparatus (113–116) as well as chordae tendineae to the anterior leaflet (117). In such situations, there is increased danger of impingement with mechanical mitral prostheses (118), especially those with occluders that extend into the left ventricle during diastole. The leaflets of the St. Jude valve are well protected in the orifice ring so that its use has been favored in this situation.

Kanting

The intentional implantation of valves that use tilting disks so that the orifice is not oriented with its axis parallel to flow (119–121), can cause regurgitation or failure to close (122–125). The greater the opening angle, the higher the propensity for such behavior. For example, the leaflets of the St. Jude prosthesis open to 85°, only 5° off the orifice axis. Tilting the orifice axis by only 5° in the plane that contains the normal to the plane of the leaflets causes one of the leaflets to be parallel to the normal flow. It has been suggested that kanting may contribute to asynchronous leaflet closure (125–130) and can cause inordinate retrograde flow. Chandran (131) has taken issue with intentional kanting carried out only in order to use an oversized valve.

Lockup

Lockup, when it occurs in full orifice tilting disk or ball valves, causes the occluder to be immobilized in the closed position. Lockup of the Björk-Shiley valve caused by the wedging of chordae, suture material, a thrombus, and catheters between the closed disk and the orifice ring has been reported (128–146), as has lockup caused by the swelling of Delrin (147).

Lockup of the Medtronic-Hall valve caused by suture material and chordae has been reported (141, 142, 148–153; and Ref. 96 in Chapter 15), as has lockup of the full orifice Bicer-Val prosthesis and a Russian version of the Björk-Shiley monostrut prosthesis (154–155). The latter two reports do not cite the wedging material.

The full orifice Smeloff-Cutter ball valve has been reported to lock up in the closed position due to thrombus (77, 156, 157). The ball of the cloth-covered, close-clearance Starr-Edwards valve has been reported to lock up in the open position (77, 158–161) due to thrombus. Other valves that are full orifice but on which reports of lockup were not found are the Sorin (162), Shanghai (163, 164), and Jatene (56).

Starek (165) studied the lockup of disks in five tilting disk type valves including the Björk-Shiley and Hall-Kaster (current name Medtronic-Hall) full orifice valves, the Omniscience and Lillehei-Kaster tilting disk valves with disks that overlap the orifice and are not full orifice, and the St. Jude valve. He found that the full orifice valves could be locked by sutures prolapsing at any point around the orifice circumference. The Lillehei-Kaster and Omniscience valves could be immobilized by prolapsing sutures only at termination points of the disk diameter that are perdendicular to the pivot axis. Similarly, the St. Jude valve can only be locked up at the points where the plane of the leaflet meets the flats of the orifice (Fig. 2–1d).

At the time of Starek's paper (1980), there was only one citable instance of lockup in a clinical case. Later reports indicated that occurrences of lockup caused by the wedging mechanism are not infrequent (77, 132–161).

The lockup mechanism is characterized by forces acting perpendicular to the valve axis and caused by entrapment of thrombotic material, suture, or tissue between the valve orifice structure and the occluder, or by a slight swelling of polymer occluders in full orifice devices. It can also be caused by a change in clearances in full orifice valves due to elastic distortion of the orifice in situ. The latter situation was cited by Ziemer (166) as the cause of a leaflet sticking in the St. Jude valve, and may also have been operative in the sticking reported in Ref. 75, Chapter 15. A number of cases of leaflet lockup in the St. Jude valve caused by the wedging action of thrombus and/or pannus have been reported (88, 89, 95, 108, 167; and Refs. 29, 76–79, 81, 82, and 91–94 in Chapter 15). It should be noted that lockup is peculiar to any design in which perpendicularity between the major plane of the occluder and the retaining mechanism exists together with close clearances; in such cases, lockup is possible. Full orifice devices are by design most susceptible. Since the perpendicularity is inherent to the design, lockup could be categorized as intrinsic—although without qualification, this may be too simplistic.

Other Extrinsic Mechanisms

Mechanical abuse of prosthetic heart valves prior to or at implantation can cause damage that ultimately leads to failure in vivo. Contemporary prosthetic mechanical valves, although they look like simple devices, are precision mechanisms. Their proper function depends on close clearances that must be maintained, for example, clearances between 25 and 75 μm and that must survive hundreds of millions of stress cycles without failing. For some materials, fatigue can be accelerated by a tiny crack, nick, or scratch; such failures have been called extrinsic.

Damage by mechanical overload can occur by attempting to rotate a valve not designed to be rotated, or by using an improper method to rotate a valve designed for rotation. The worst case is the unknowing introduction of a small flaw that remains undetected intraoperatively but later propagates in the patient causing sudden valve failure and death.

The failures of the Beall model 105 mitral valve prosthesis are examples of mechanical abuse. This model used pyc-coated metal (molybdemun-rhenium alloy) struts and a pyc-coated graphite disk (168). Four cases of strut failure were reported in the early 1970s (169–171). A field investigation of prostheses in hospital inventories found 11 (2.6%) damaged valves. All, with one possible exception, had been removed from their original container or were in original containers that showed gross external damage.

Studies of the damaged valves revealed that the carbon coating (the coating measured 0.4 mm thick on a 0.8 mm diameter metal substrate—see Figs. 15 and 16 in Ref. 172) could be cracked by applying lateral force on the strut during preoperative handling or at implantation. The hairline cracks were stress risers acting on the underlying metal struts at their points of termination on the carbon/metal interface. In service, the fluctuating stress at these points exceeded the endurance limit and caused fatigue failure of the metal.

There have been other reports of strut fractures and fractured carbon disks. Some may have been the consequence of attempts at improper rotation of valves during implantation (132, 173, 174). Reports of leaflet escapement from the St. Jude valve (175–179) include cases that are thought to be of extrinsic origin (177–179), as was an instance of disk embolization from an early model of the Björk-Shiley valve (180, 181) and escapement of leaflets from the Duromedics valve (Ref. 114 in Chapter 15). Cutting needles biting too close to the orifice ring of some valves can cut the sewing ring retention sutures and cause separation of the sewing ring from the valve.

Bacterial endocarditis with vegetations has also been cited as an extrinsic factor that can cause malfunction of mechanical valves (182–184).

Intrinsic Mechanisms

Intrinsic failure mechanisms of prosthetic heart valves are those that are inherently related to the design or to the materials used in their construction. Failure due to wear is clearly dependent on the design of a valve and the materials used in its construction and is therefore intrinsic.

Durability of Polymers

Degradation of synthetic materials in the body is a major limitation faced by valve designers. The natural valve can remodel and heal itself; the degradation of a manufactured device must remain insignificant throughout the life of the patient as no healing or remodeling is possible.

As previously mentioned, early ideas that the ideal valve must be flexible have been modified because flexible materials with the required durability simply did not and do not currently exist. Many of the rigid devices that evolved during the 1960s were accepted for clinical use because they offered a better course than any alternative. Nevertheless, they are fraught with problems.

Because of wear, design alternatives were severely limited; thus occluders fabricated from polymers had to be designed to rotate and distribute the wear. An exception that serves as an example is the Wada-Cutter valve (39).

Although silicone rubber balls, when properly cured, worked well, a crisis of major proportions arose in the 1960s due to the inadvertent distribution of prostheses that contained improperly cured balls (at that time there was no evidence to indicate the curing cycle being used was improper). These balls were degraded by the absorption of lipids and resulted in valve failure (33, 77, 185–187). In contrast, prostheses with properly cured silicone poppets have demonstrated good longevity (188–192).

Experience with silicone rubber lenticular shaped, nontilting disks that functioned in prostheses as a poppet whose axis remained roughly parallel to the valve orifice axis was not good. Malfunctions of the Cross-Jones (35) and Kay-Shiley (34) valves were caused by disk notching at the edges. The notching allowed the disk to cock and this, in turn, was responsible for thromboses, hemolysis, and other complications (193–196). Valves of this sort are considered obsolete.

If early valve designers had been aware of Charnley's (197) disastrous experience with the use of Teflon® in prosthetic hip joints and other early work (198, 199), it might not have been selected for use in artificial heart valves.

Although Teflon® exhibits a low coefficient of friction and a low surface energy, its lack of resistance to abrasive wear has been dramatically demonstrated by its poor performance in the Beall model 103 and 104 (200–206), and the Wada-Cutter (207–209) and DeBakey prostheses (210). Björk tested both Teflon® and Delrin® in vitro as candidates for use in the Björk-Shiley prosthesis. He reported that Teflon® wore seven times faster than Delrin® (211). Teflon® is no longer considered for use as a bearing surface in prosthetic cardiac valves.

In an effort to increase the thromboresistance of ball type prosthetic valves, the metal cage was covered with cloth. Severe complications secondary to cloth wear (212–221) caused this approach to be abandoned.

Of all the polymers considered for use as an occluder for the Björk-Shiley valve, Delrin® has exhibited the best abrasion resistance (222). Recent reports from long-term follow up by Björk (223, 224) and others (225) have not indicated any malfunction caused by the abrasive wear of the Delrin® disk. Björk estimated from studies of valves explanted after 12 years, that Delrin® would have a useful life of about 30 years in a patient (224).

However, there have been other problems with Delrin®. Delrin® expands during heat sterilization (226, 227). If a valve with such a disk is autoclaved in the closed position, the disk is restrained in the metal seat and buckles under the stress generated as it expands.

Larmi and Karkola (228) reported a death caused by the shrinkage of a Delrin® occluder in an aortic replacement. On inspection of their unused valves, they found that all the disks had shrunk and that some (the larger sizes) were distorted. They concluded that Delrin® may be a dangerous occluder material and should be discarded regardless of the cause of the shrinkage.

DeWall (147) reported that two Björk-Shiley valves with Delrin® disks "froze up" causing the death of two patients. Messmer, Rothlin, and Senning (180) reported early dislodgement of a Delrin® disk caused by its dimensional instability.

Results from in vitro tests reported by Clark (229, 230) showed wear and fracture of Delrin® disks. After implantation, results reported by Amstutz (231, 232) from in vitro tests showed that Delrin® absorbed water during in vivo implantation; the material was rejected for orthopedic use because of excessively high wear rates.

In 1971, the Delrin® disk in the Björk-Shiley valve was replaced with pyc.

Pyc–Metal Wear Couples

The remarkable blood compatibility of pyc (233–235) was responsible for its first recognition as a potential candidate to be used in the construction of an artificial heart. But if it had not been for its equally remarkable durability, its usage in prosthetic cardiac valves would have been limited.

Shim and Schoen (236) were the first to measure the wear characteristics of various combinations of pyc and metals (titanium and chromium-cobalt alloy). They found that the volume of wear for a given combination increased linearly with sliding distance so that volume wear rate, expressed as, for example, mm^3 per meter sliding distance, is a constant. In vitro tests of prosthetic valves (reported in the next section) have verified this relationship, which makes it convenient to extrapolate wear results to long times.

The data from Shim and Schoen are summarized in Fig. 2–2. The data are for a special form of pcy co-deposited with silicon at a nominal concentration of 10 wt% and present in the structure as a fine dispersion of silicon carbide. It is available under the trademark Pyrolite® carbon (PYC)* from CarboMedics, Inc., Austin, TX, and is the form of pyc

*Uppercase PYC refers to trademark Pyrolite® carbon, lowercase pyc refers to generic pyrolitic carbon.

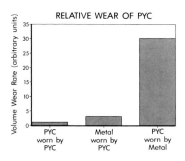

Fig. 2–2. Relative wear of PYC caused by PYC, of metal caused by PYC, of PYC caused by metal (data from Ref. 236).

that has been used in cardiac valve replacements. The data show that while the wear of PYC caused by PYC and the wear of titanium and chromium-cobalt alloy by PYC is very low, the wear of PYC caused by abrasion against either metal was more than an order of magnitude faster. This means that for a tilting disk valve with an orifice made from either titanium or chromium-cobalt alloy and PYC disk, the highest wear would be the wear of PYC caused by the metal, and not the wear of the metal caused by PYC. Accordingly, a tilting disk valve, like that of the Wada concept where a PYC disk is used with a metal orifice and a fixed pivot, would probably experience a high rate of wear of the PYC caused by the metal at the pivots. But a tilting disk valve with a circular PYC disk free to rotate about its own axis during function in order to distribute the wear, as in the Lillehei-Kaster valve, would be viable from a wear standpoint. Further, if the Wada design had used an orifice and disk both coated with PYC, the durability would probably have been exceptional.

There have been a number of reports of the wear actually realized in patients for valves that use metallic orifices and PYC coated disks. The DeBakey aortic valve prosthesis was the first valve prosthesis to use PYC. The earliest model used a hollow PYC coated graphite ball—a later version also used a PYC coated graphite orifice ring (Figs. 7, 8, 11, 12, and 13 in Ref. 172). During the period 1969 to 1972, about 3300 DeBakey aortic valves were implanted.

There have been a number of reports on valves removed from patients (237–242). No evidence of wear of the carbon components was found in these explants, but significant wear of the titanium struts (titanium, A70 grade) from a valve implanted in a patient for about four years was reported by Paton and Pine (237). In the fourth year, the patient developed an exceptionally loud, vibrant murmur and thrill, and the valve was replaced. It was found that an obstruction caused by the impingement of the cage against the aortic wall prevented full excursion of the ball and this, in turn, resulted in excessive lateral and rotary movement of the ball against the cage. Accordingly, the excessive wear was interpreted to be secondary to the anatomical obstruction of the ball motion. The appearance of a ball valve explanted from another patient (238) suggests that a similar mechanism may have caused excessive wear of the titanium cage. Another DeBakey aortic valve exhibited wear at the apex of the cage but no details were reported (239).

A report (240) of two DeBakey aortic ball valves, implanted for 48 and 85 months, respectively, indicated detectable wear on the titanium struts. Even at about seven years the wear in these struts was minimal. In comparison Paton and Pine (237) reported severe strut wear due to unusual anatomic constraints that prevented complete excursion of the ball; such wear was extrinsic since it was secondary to impingement.

It has been 18 years since the first DeBakey valve was implanted. Since that time the only reports of wear were those experienced by the titanium cage. It is worth noting that in vitro tests carried out in 1968 showed minimal wear of the titanium and a useful life of the ball that exceeded 200 years (for the test conditions, an estimate of 250 years would be required to wear halfway through the coating on the ball).

The Lillehei-Kaster cardiac valve has been in clinical use since mid 1970, so the first surviving implants have been in place for about 17 years. Extrapolation of data from in vitro preclinical testing indicated that the time to wear halfway through the carbon coating would be in excess of 200 years (243).

Lillehei (244) reported results from measurements of disks recovered from patients for implant times ranging from 46 to 80 months; these indicated a maximum linear penetration of 26 μm per year. Because of the constancy of the volumetric rate wear and the increasing bearing area as the depth increases, the penetration rate must decrease with time, so the extrapolation underestimates the time required for the disk to wear out. In fact, a parabolic extrapolation shows a time longer than 200 years is required to penetrate halfway through the PYC coating. Data for a disk recovered after 2.5 years showed wear penetration of less than about 0.2 μm (240), again much less than that predicted by in vitro tests.

There have been two reports of wear of the titanium cage caused by the PYC coated disk in Lillehei-Kaster valves recovered from patients (245, 246). A study of 10 valves in place for up to 10 years indicated that the maximum wear penetration of the titanium by the carbon disk was 1.1 and 2.5 μm for 8-year mitral and 10-year aortic implants, respectively, and this was judged to be insignificant to clinical function (245). From these data, Reif et al. (246), estimated that it would take 300 years and 90 years for mitral and aortic valves, respectively, to remove one-tenth of the titanium-carbon interference that retains the disk in the cage. These in vivo results indicate that the wear either of the titanium caused by the PYC or of the PYC by the titanium should not be a clinical problem for the Lillehei-Kaster prosthesis.

PYC-coated disks have been in use in the Björk-Shiley cardiac valve prosthesis since 1971. In this prosthesis, the PYC disk is captured between two chromium-cobalt alloy (trade name, Haynes 25 Stellite®) struts and is free to rotate about its own axis during function.

Björk (247) reported a wear track 5 μm deep worn into a pyc disk after 457 million cycles in vitro. A linear extrapolation by Björk gave an estimated 400 years to wear through the coating. Because the volume wear rate is constant and the linear penetration rate is not, the extrapolated time to penetrate the coating would be much greater than 400 years.

Clark and co-workers (230) tested a Björk-Shiley prosthesis until the major strut broke at the weld after 973 million cycles. The PYC did not rotate and an imprint of the strut was worn into the disk. In vitro tests of a Björk-Shiley prosthesis with a convexoconcave disk produced a wear track 11 μm deep in a simulated nine year test (230).

Subsequently, results from in vitro wear tests of many disk materials in the Björk-Shiley valve were reported (222). These data indicated that PYC-coated disks exhibited the lowest level of wear for any of the materials tested. After over one billion cycles, the wear track was only 2 μm deep, or less than 1% of the thickness of the carbon coating.

Results from in vitro tests of a Russian valve with a configuration similar to that of the Björk-Shiley monostrut, but using a titanium cage rather than chromium-cobalt alloy, indicated a wear mark depth of 8 μm in 400 million cycles (248).

Silver (249) examined wear on 13 Björk-Shiley valves recovered from patients up to 27 months after implantation. He reported wear comparable to that seen following accelerated cycle testing in vitro (222, 247), and concluded that wear was unlikely to seriously affect prosthesis function in the normal lifetime of an individual; however, he speculated that metal wear might cause the disk to flutter. Wear data (222) for PYC disks from Björk-Shiley prostheses is plotted in Fig. 2–3 together with in vitro data (247) and in vivo data from explanted Björk-Shiley valves (249, 250).

The Medtronic-Hall valve uses a PYC coated tilting disk occluder contained within a titanium cage. Details of the construction and function have been summarized by Morse et al. (251, pp 306–307). Extensive, accelerated dynamic wear test data submitted to the United States Food and Drug Administration (FDA) in support of a premarket approval application for the Medtronic-Hall valve are available (252) and include data for Lillehei-Kaster and Björk-Shiley control valves. The data showed that even in worst case situations (i.e., intermittent occluder rotation) the maximum depth of wear tracks observed for the occluders of all the valves, including the controls, was less than 25 μm in depth after 357 million cycles. Using a linear rate of penetration, which is incorrect (but conservative) because it is the volume wear rate that is constant rather than linear penetration rate, they estimated 50 years to be the minimum time to penetrate the coating. If a volume wear rate situation was assumed with a parabolic dependence, a minimum time of 80 years would be projected to wear halfway through the coating in the worst case. The wear of titanium, in all cases, was significantly less than the wear of the carbon, and this is consistent with the data in Fig. 2–2.

The Omniscience cardiac valve prosthesis uses a PYC-coated disk captured in a titanium cage. Details of its construction have been published (251, pp 304–305). Results from 20 Omniscience valves tested for an equivalent of 9.4 years were reported to the FDA in support of a premarket approval application and are available (253).

After 355 million cycles with the disk functioning with free rotation about its axis, the maximum depth of wear measured on the occluder outflow surface was about 1 μm, or approximately 0.5% of the coating thickness. In the worst case, that is, interrupted occluder rotation, the maximum localized wear depth measured 10 μm deep (5% of the coating thickness).

The maximum wear of the occluder edge where it abraded against the titanium retaining surface was 5 μm and the wear on the corresponding titanium surface was 2 μm. The

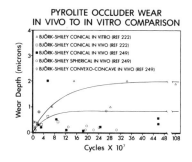

FIG. 2–3. Wear penetration versus number of cycles for valves retrieved from patients and for valve tested in vitro (data from 222, 247, 249, 250).

data are consistent with the relative rates reported by Shim and Schoen (236), as well as others (245), and indicate that failure by wear in any patient should never occur.

For comparison, the wear of chromium-cobalt caused by chromium-cobalt in one of the Starr-Edwards valves that used metallic wear tracks and studs abrading against a hollow metal ball (251, pp 278–280) has been reported (254). Prostheses in patients for 50 to 144 months exhibited severe stud erosion and erosion of the metallic ring itself with complete destruction of the cloth, causing hemolytic anemia and other thrombotic complications. Needless to say, metal-on-metal bearing situations are no longer considered for use in prosthetic heart valves.

PYC–PYC Wear Couples

Of all wear couples so far considered, the one that gives the best wear resistance is the one that uses the PYC–PYC couple. For the reader unfamiliar with carbon technology, it is worth noting that the term pyc is a generic term that applies to a large number of carbon materials that make up a family whose members include crystalline structure and morphologies together with their properties that can vary over wide ranges. The interested reader is referred to reviews of the subject (255, 256, 257).

The first heart valve prosthesis to be completely coated with PYC on all of its rigid members exposed to flowing blood was the Beall model 105 mitral valve prosthesis (168). The valve used a PYC-coated graphite lenticular disk. The disk was free to rotate about its axis but was the nontilting type, which maintained its axis more or less parallel to the orifice axis. The disk was contained in a cage fabricated from a refractory molybdenum-rhenium alloy and coated with PYC. The orifice was coated with Dacron® velour. The severest wear was that caused by the edge of the carbon disk abrading against the four legs of the cage.

In vitro wear data together with wear data from two valves explanted from calves after about one year (168) and data for another valve retrieved from patients after 48 months (240), are plotted in Fig. 2–4. The data demonstrate the good resistance to abrasion of the PYC–PYC wear couple. The wear actually observed on valves retrieved from patients is considerably less than that obtained from in vitro test data and from data obtained with tests in calves for up to one year. The data from calves show a higher wear rate, most likely because in the calf the valve becomes stenotic as the calf grows, imposing forces on the valve well above those ever experienced in a human.

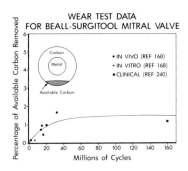

FIG. 2–4. Wear penetration versus number of cycles for explanted Beall model 105 valves retrieved from patients (data from Ref. 240) and for valves tested in vivo and in vitro in calves (data from Ref. 168).

The first valve to use the PYC–PYC wear couple in a design that used fixed pivots with focused wear was the St. Jude Medical cardiac valve prosthesis (251, pp 134–138, 312–313; Fig. 3 in Ref. 258). Gombrich and co-workers (258) reported that extrapolation of in vitro wear data from accelerated tests indicated that wear halfway through the PYC coating on a leaflet pivot point should occur in well over 200 years. They confirmed that such wear would not cause the valve to malfunction or break.

Data submitted to the FDA in support of a premarket approval application are available (259) and contain results from 17 valves tested in vitro for an equivalent of 0.24 to 10.61 years (based on 40 million cycles per year). The maximum wear depth reported was always observed on the inflow side of the leaflet ear. The wear from four valves tested for the equivalent of 10.6 years was 2 to 12.5% of the minimum coating thickness. This rate is low enough that no valve is expected to wear out in the normal lifetime of a patient.

The Omnicarbon prosthetic heart valve is similar to the Omniscience prosthesis but uses an orifice ring made of PYC-coated graphite rather than titanium (for example see Fig. 17 in Ref. 260). This valve uses the ideal wearing situation, that is, one in which the PYC-coated disk is free to rotate and distribute the wear circumferentially as it functions. On closing, when the pressure differential across the valve peaks, the disk separates from the pivot and comes to rest on a PYC seating lip, thereby transferring the load to a large surface area and distributing the wear. Wear data submitted to the FDA in support of a premarket approval application are available (261). The equivalent of 10 years of testing in water at accelerated rates indicated that the wear of titanium cages caused by PYC disks and that of PYC cages caused by PYC disks were both less than 5 μm (for example, see Fig. 2–5). Wear rates for accelerated tests carried out in blood analog (glycerol/water) solution were all lower than corresponding tests carried out in water and in all cases the penetration was less than 1 μm after the equivalent of 10 years of testing. Data include comparative results from tests of Medtronic-Hall control valves.

In the Duromedics bileaflet valve prosthesis, as for the St. Jude valve, all the rigid components that interface directly with blood are either coated with PYC or are PYC monoliths. Details of its construction and performance characteristics have been published (251, pp 298–300).

The Duromedics valve, like the Omnicarbon and St. Jude prostheses, are assembled by elastically deforming the orifice ring until the leaflets (or disk) can be inserted. The Duromedics valve, unlike the Omnicarbon and St. Jude valve, uses a monolithic PYC orifice that is stiffened after assembly by shrinking a metallic (chromium-cobalt alloy)

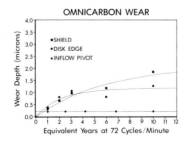

FIG. 2–5. Wear penetration versus number of cycles for Omnicarbon PYC cages worn by PYC disk, for PYC disk edges worn by PYC cages, and for PYC disks worn by PYC in-flow pivots, all tested in water (data from Ref. 261).

onto its circumference. This stabilizes the dimensions so that the precise clearances associated with the pivoting mechanism are maintained.

It should be noted that experience with in vitro testing of bileaflet tilting disk prosthetic heart valves has shown that the highest wear rates are those that occur in the mitral position on the inlet faces that carry the pressure load at closure. This is the time in the cardiac cycle when the transvalvular pressures are at a maximum and the leaflets shift into their final seating positions. The pressure load is further magnified in the mitral position because mitral prostheses are the largest.

For the St. Jude valve, the peaking transvalvular pressure at closure, which imposes maximum load on the leaflets, is localized on and borne by the leaflet tabs. In contrast, the loads imposed on the Duromedics leaflet are distributed in a fashion more similar to those in the Omnicarbon valve. To accomplish this, the Duromedics design uses a ball on the leaflet that engages an elongated slot in the orifice; the leaflet seats on a lip at closure so that the peak closure loads are transferred from the pivot onto the seating lip. In vitro testing to 400 million cycles indicates that the wear is indeed distributed over the large seating area; projected minimum wear lives are over several hundred years (262, 263).

The CarboMedics valve (CMI) incorporates some of the same features as the St. Jude and Duromedics designs. Like the Duromedics valve, the CarboMedics design uses a monolithic, solid PYC orifice ring with a metallic (titanium) stiffener ring and a Biolite® carbon coated sewing ring. The latter material has been discussed (235); it is incorporated to improve the biocompatibility of the sewing ring surfaces that interface directly with flowing blood in order to reduce pannus proliferation that could, in turn, cause impingement.

The pivots of the CarboMedics valve are generically like those of the St. Jude valve but have been modified to increase efficiency of back flushing when the valve is closed, and to allow the leaflets to rotate freely around the pivot on closure until they mate with one another along their straight seating surface (264). The benefits of these modifications have not been proved clinically. The radiographs in Fig. 2–6 compare the two configurations. The PYC coating in the St. Jude pivots is visible in the radiograph shown in Fig. 2–6a; no coating is visible on the radiograph shown in Fig. 2–6b because the orifice is a monolith of PYC.

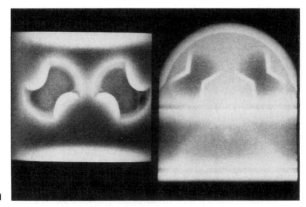

a   b

FIG. 2–6. Radiographs comparing pivot configurations. (a) St. Jude. (b) CarboMedics.

Because of these modifications, the wear is more localized on the CMI leaflet tabs than it is on the St. Jude tabs (for example, compare the wear tracks in Fig. 2–7), and this more focused wear must be compensated for through design. Since the orifice of the CMI valve is a PYC monolith and the specified leaflet tabs are also monoliths (Fig. 2–8), the wear life is not limited by penetrating a relatively thin coating on a graphite substrate; rather the valve is worn out when the magnitude of the wear impairs hemodynamic function, allows the leaflet to escape, or reduces the mechanical strength to the point that fracture is possible. From in vitro accelerated wear testing to 600 million cycles, it is estimated that it will take 100 years to wear 32% of the way through the tab. It has been demonstrated that this wear does not impair the hemodynamic function, cause the leaflet to escape, or cause the leaflet to fracture (265).

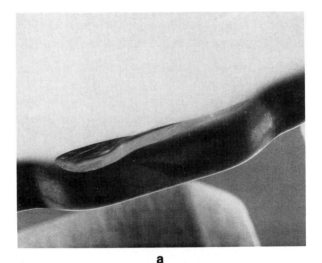

a

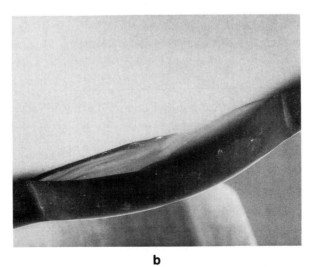

b

FIG. 2–7. Wear marks on pivot tabs after 400 million cycles of accelerated testing. (a) Carbo-Medics. (b) St. Jude.

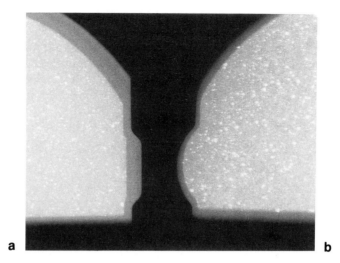

a   b

FIG. 2–8. Radiographs of pivot tabs. (a) St. Jude. (b) CarboMedics.

In the wear tests described above, St. Jude valves were used as controls. These tests confirm the fact that the volumetric wear rate is a constant. The results indicate that after 600 million cycles the volume of PYC worn from the CMI leaflets was 6.7×10^{-4} mm^3 and that worn from the St. Jude leaflets was 5.7×10^{-4} mm^3, a difference which was not statistically significant. This is a very useful result, because using the same test conditions one can estimate the change in wear rate if changes are made in the bearing configuration.

The Tascon bileaflet prosthetic valve, currently in preclinical testing, uses a pivot configuration that follows the Carpentier concept (266). The pivot, depicted in Fig. 2–9, uses no socket in the orifice. Instead, the leaflet is captured between two protrusions that extend about a half millimeter out from the orifice and are spaced so as to capture the leaflets at regions of localized thinning, that is, the depressions in the leaflet outlet plane.

Another valve in preclinical trials features a novel closing mechanism (267) together with a pivot design (268) that, like the Duromedics concept, is unloaded in the final phase of closure so that the bearing loads are optimally distributed over a large area (Fig. 2–10).

The condition for lockup with this novel design, that is, full orifice perpendicularity with close clearance, only exists at a point where the major diameter of the conical occluder is parallel to the pivot axis when the valve is closed. If the propensity for lockup is taken to be a linear function of the fraction of the occluder perimeter in which the

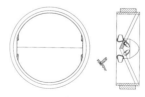

FIG. 2–9. Diagram showing pivot mechanism of the Tascon bileaflet prosthetic valve.

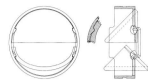

FIG. 2–10. Diagram showing pivot mechanism of the Sorensen-Woien bileaflet valve.

close-clearance perpendicularity occurs, the propensity for lockup would be, in decreasing order:

1. Full-orifice disk or ball in which the entire perimeter is susceptible (Fig. 2–1).

2. Bileaflet valves that use flats perpendicular to the pivot axis, in which only the fraction of the perimeter that is common with the flat is susceptible (Fig. 2–1).

3. Tilting disk valves that are not full orifice but are close-clearance at any segment of the locus of points swept out by the end points of the occluder diameter that is parallel to the pivot axis during the excursion of the occluder in the heart cycle (Fig. 2–1).

4. Bileaflet valves that do not have flats and are close-clearance only at the points where the major diameter of the conical occluder is parallel with the pivot axis when the valve is closed.

Fatigue Failure

Metals are polycrystalline solids that contain defects called dislocations. These can move under stress to cause plastic deformation at stress levels much lower than would be predicted from the atomic bond theory (269). Under cyclic loading, dislocations move to internal crystalline barriers such as intercrystalline boundaries, where they become stuck and accumulate to form complex arrays. Their coalescence utlimately leads to the formation of microfissures. These fissures can grow slowly in size under continued cyclic loading until they reach a critical size that can propagate and cause fracture. The degradation of strength under cyclic loading can be augmented and accelerated by the presence of existing internal flaws, surface defects that can act as stress risers, or crystalline morphologies such as those peculiar to welds that can increase the propensity for fatigue failure (270, 271).

Although there have been a number of reports of fatigue failures of valve replacements that use titanium (239, 241, 242, 272), the biggest single problem has been fatigue failures of chrome-cobalt alloy (Haynes 25 Stellite®) in the Björk-Shiley prosthesis.

There have been many case reports of Björk-Shiley valves, some of which have been discussed and summarized (273, 274); the details of the exact loading that caused fatigue failure remain undetermined (273). Other case reports for the fatigue failure of chrome-cobalt prosthetic valves (275–278) include a rare failure of the strut of a Starr-Edwards mitral prosthesis (278). Details of the fatigue problem with the Björk-Shiley valve together with analysis and correction has been reported by Björk, Lindblom, and Henze (279).

PYC has a turbostatic structure that has no crystalline order between the atomic layers in the lattice so mobile dislocation cannot exist (280, 281). Accordingly, there is no mechanism for the initiation of a fatigue crack and PYC has an endurance limit equal to its single cycle fracture stress.

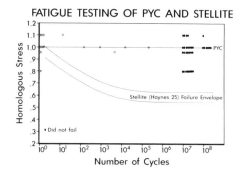

FIG. 2–11. Normalized cyclic stress versus number of cycles for PYC and Haynes 25 Stellite®.

Fatigue tests of pyc, which include PYC data reported by Schoen (282), Shim (283), and more recent data (284), are plotted in Fig. 2–11 together with data (279) for Haynes 25 Stellite®. The early data for PYC were obtained using a cantilever type specimen; the more recent data are from conventional rotating beam type tests using larger specimens.

The fact that PYC does not exhibit the degradation by cyclic loading that typifies metals, greatly simplifies the in vitro testing of PYC heart valves. One need only carry out stress analysis and apply a suitable safety margin. It is not necessary to deal with fatigue processes that degrade the strength of the valve over time. Thus the wear resistance, biocompatibility, and lack of fatigue are a fortunate combination that makes PYC uniquely suited for the construction of mechanical cardiac valve replacements.

It has been 39 years since the first mechanical valve was implanted and there has been considerable progress. The challenge that remains is to improve through design, the hemocompatibility of mechanical valves so that the need for anticoagulants with their associated bleeding problem is eliminated. Chapter 15 addresses this problem.

REFERENCES

1. Gaasch WH: Aortic valve disease: timing of valve replacement surgery. In Starek JKP (ed): Heart Valve Replacement and Reconstruction. Chicago, Year Book Medical Publishers, 1987, pp 21–29.
2. Lund O, Vaeth M: Prediction of late results following valve replacement in aortic valve stenosis. Thorac Cardiovasc Surgeon 1987;135:295–303.
3. Barratt-Boyes BG: The timing of operation in valvular insufficiency. J Cardiac Surgery 1987;12:435–452.
4. Kirklin JW, Barratt-Boyes BG: Surgical concepts, research methods, and data analysis and use. Cardiac Surgery: Morphology, Diagnostic Criteria, Natural History, Techniques, Results, and Indications. New York, John Wiley & Sons, 1986, pp 177–204.
5. Blackstone EH, Kirklin JW: Death and other time related events after valve replacement. Circulation 1985;72:753–767.
6. Munoz S, Gallardo J, Diaz-Gorrin JR, Medina O: Influence of surgery on the natural history of rheumatic mitral and aortic disease. Am J Cardiol 1975;35:234–242.
7. Rapaport E: Natural history of aortic and mitral valve disease. Am J Cardiol 1975;35:221–227.
8. Hufnagel CA: Permanent intubation of the thoracic aorta. Arch Surg 1947;54:382–389.
9. Hufnagel CA, Harvey WP: The surgical correction of aortic regurgitation. Bull Georgetown Univ Med Center 1953;6:60–61.
10. Gibbon JH: Application of a mechanical heart and lung apparatus to cardiac surgery. Minn Med 1954;37:171–185.
11. Harken DE, Soroff HS, Taylor WJ, LeFemine AA, Gupta SK, Lunzer S: Partial and complete prosthesis in aortic insufficiency. J Thorac Cardiovasc Surg 1960;40:744–762.
12. Hufnagel CA, Gomes MN: Late follow-up of ball-valve prostheses in the descending thoracic aorta. J Thorac Cardiovasc Surg 1976;72:900–909.
13. Davila JC: The mechanics of the cardiac valves—considerations pertinent to the design and construction

of prostheses. In Merendino KA, Morrow AG, Lillehei CW, Muller WH (eds): Prosthetic Heart Valves for Cardiac Surgery. Springfield IL, Charles C Thomas, 1961, pp 3–47.

14. Kolff WJ, Seidel W, Akutsu T, Mirkovitch V, Hindberg J: Studies of thrombosis on artificial heart valves. In Merendino KA, Morrow AG, Lillehei CW, Muller WH (eds): Prosthetic Heart Valves for Cardiac Surgery. Springfield IL, Charles C Thomas, 1961, pp 199–211.

15. Litwak RS, Norman MK, Meyer WH, Gadboys HL, Allen AC: Function and morphologic changes in monocusp prostheses after implantation in the dog. In Merendino KA, Morrow AG, Lillehei CW, Muller WH (eds): Prosthetic Heart Valves for Cardiac Surgery. Springfield IL, Charles C Thomas, 1961, pp 286–306.

16. Braumwald NS, Cooper T, Morrow AG: Clinical and experimental replacement of the mitral valve—experience with the use of a flexible polyurethane prosthesis. In Merendino KA, Morrow AG, Lillehei CW, Muller WH (eds): Prosthetic Heart Valves for Cardiac Surgery. Springfield IL, Charles C Thomas, 1961, pp 307–339.

17. Esmond WG, Attar S, Braley S, McGragor RR, Cowley RA: Design and implantation trials of prosthetic Silastic®-Dacron® (or Teflon®)-Ivalon® mitral heart valves. In Merendino KA, Morrow AG, Lillehei CW, Muller WH (eds): Prosthetic Heart Valves for Cardiac Surgery. Springfield IL, Charles C Thomas, 1961, pp 340–367.

18. Schimert G, Sellers RD, Lee CB, Bilgutay AM, Lillehei CW: Fabrication of mitral leaflet and aortic cusps from Silastic® rubber-coated Teflon® felt. In Merendino KA, Morrow AG, Lillehei CW, Muller WH (eds): Prosthetic Heart Valves for Cardiac Surgery. Springfield IL, Charles C Thomas, 1961, pp 368–384.

19. Long DM, Gott VL, Sterns LP, Finsterbusch W, Meyne N, Varco RL, Lillehei CW: Reconstruction and replacement of the mitral valve with plastic prostheses. In Merendino KA, Morrow AG, Lillehei CW, Muller WH (eds): Prosthetic Heart Valves for Cardiac Surgery. Springfield IL, Charles C Thomas, 1961, pp 385–401.

20. Kay EB, Suzuki A, Postigo J, Nogueira C: Prosthetic replacement of the mitral valve. In Merendino KA, Morrow AG, Lillehei CW, Muller WH (eds): Prosthetic Heart Valves for Cardiac Surgery. Springfield IL, Charles C Thomas, 1961, pp 402–425.

21. Cross FS, Jones RD, Gerein AN: The design, function and technical aspects of placement of single aortic valve leaflets. In Merendino KA, Morrow AG, Lillehei CW, Muller WH (eds): Prosthetic Heart Valves for Cardiac Surgery. Springfield IL, Charles C Thomas, 1961, pp 426–439.

22. Bahnson HT, Spencer FC, Jeckel NC: Experience with replacement of individual cusps of the aortic valve. In Merendino KA, Morrow AG, Lillehei CW, Muller WH (eds): Prosthetic Heart Valves for Cardiac Surgery. Springfield IL, Charles C Thomas, 1961, pp 440–450.

23. Hufnagel CA, Conrad PW: Prostheses for aortic valve replacement. In Merendino KA, Morrow AG, Lillehei CW, Muller WH (eds): Prosthetic Heart Valves for Cardiac Surgery. Springfield IL, Charles C Thomas, 1961, pp 451–461.

24. Roe BB, Moore D: A satisfactory flexible tricuspid elastomer prosthetic valve: problems of design and implantation. In Merendino KA, Morrow AG, Lillehei CW, Muller WH (eds): Prosthetic Heart Valves for Cardiac Surgery. Springfield IL, Charles C Thomas, 1961, pp 462–482.

25. Kay EB, Mendelsohn D, Nogueira C, Suzuki A, Zimmerman HA: Surgical treatment of aortic valvular disease. In Merendino KA, Morrow AG, Lillehei CW, Muller WH (eds): Prosthetic Heart Valves for Cardiac Surgery. Springfield IL, Charles C Thomas, 1961, pp 483–492.

26. Muller WH, Littlefield JB, Dammann JF: Subcoronary prosthetic replacement of the aortic valve. In Merendino KA, Morrow AG, Lillehei CW, Muller WH (eds): Prosthetic Heart Valves for Cardiac Surgery. Springfield IL, Charles C Thomas, 1961, pp 493–507.

27. Lillehei CW, Barnard CN, Long DM, Sellers RD, Schimert G, Varco RL: Aortic valve reconstruction and replacement by total valve replacement. In Merendino KA, Morrow AG, Lillehei CW, Muller WH (eds): Prosthetic Heart Valves for Cardiac Surgery. Springfield IL, Charles C Thomas, 1961, pp 527–586.

28. Merendino RA, Morrow AG, Lillehei CW, Muller WH (eds): Prosthetic Heart Valves for Cardiac Surgery. Springfield IL, Charles C Thomas, 1961.

29. Stuckey JH, Newman MM, Berg E, Goodman S, Dennis C: Design and placement of prosthetic valve to fit in the mitral ring of the dog after excision of the leaflets. In Merendino KA, Morrow AG, Lillehei CW, Muller WH (eds): Prosthetic Heart Valves for Cardiac Surgery. Springfield IL, Charles C Thomas, 1961, pp 266–285.

30. Harken DE, Soroff HS, Taylor WJ, Lefemine AA, Gupta SK, Lunzer S, Low HB: Aortic valve replacement. In Merendino KA, Morrow AG, Lillehei CW, Muller WH (eds): Prosthetic Heart Valves for Cardiac Surgery. Springfield IL, Charles C Thomas, 1961, pp 508–526.

31. Brewer LA, Cooley DA, Davila JC, Merendino KA, Sirak HD (eds): Prosthetic Heart Valves. Springfield IL, Charles C Thomas, 1969.

32. Outlook on prosthetic heart valves patient improves. JAMA 1968;205:28–30. Editorial.

33. Starr A, Herr R, Wood JA: Accumulated experience with the Starr-Edwards prosthesis 1960–1968. In Brewer LA, Cooley DA, Davila JC, Merendino KA, Sirak HD (eds): Prosthetic Heart Valves. Springfield IL, Charles C Thomas, 1969, pp 468–483.

34. Kay JH, Tsuji HK, Redington JV, Mendez A, Saji K, Kamatak M, Yokoyama T, Magidson O, Bernard K: Experience with the Kay-Shiley disk valve. In Brewer LA, Cooley DA, Davila JC, Merendino KA, Sirak HD (eds): Prosthetic Heart Valves. Springfield IL, Charles C Thomas, 1969, pp 609–621.
35. Cross FS, Akao M, Jones RD: Three years clinical experience with the lens mitral valve. In Brewer LA, Cooley DA, Davila JC, Merendino KA, Sirak HD (eds): Prosthetic Heart Valves. Springfield IL, Charles C Thomas, 1969, pp 579–586.
36. Cooley DA, Bloodwell RD, Okies JE, Bricker DL, Hallman GL, Beall AC, DeBakey ME: Long term results after cardiac valve replacement: clinical experience with 2,097 patients. In Brewer LA, Cooley DA, Davila JC, Merendino KA, Sirak HD (eds): Prosthetic Heart Valves. Springfield IL, Charles C Thomas, 1969, pp 530–540.
37. Magovern GJ, Kent EM: Sutureless mechanical fixation of aortic and mitral valves: a review of five years' experience. In Brewer LA, Cooley DA, Davila JC, Merendino KA, Sirak HD (eds): Prosthetic Heart Valves. Springfield IL, Charles C Thomas, 1969, pp 566–576.
38. Lillehei CW, Nakib A, Kaster RL, Ferlic RM: The toroidal heart valve. In Brewer LA, Cooley DA, Davila JC, Merendino KA, Sirak HD (eds): Prosthetic Heart Valves. Springfield IL, Charles C Thomas, 1969, pp 278–284.
39. Wada J, Komatsu S, Ikeda K, Kitaya T, Tanaka N, Yamada H: A new hingeless valve. In Brewer LA, Cooley DA, Davila JC, Merendino KA, Sirak HD (eds): Prosthetic Heart Valves. Springfield IL, Charles C. Thomas, 1969, pp 304–318.
40. Hufnagel CA, Conrad PW, Gillespie JF, Pifarre R, Ilana A, Yokoyama T: Comparative study of cardiac and vascular implants in relation to thrombosis. Surgery 1967;61:11–16.
41. Young WP, Daggett RL, Gott VL: Long-term follow-up of patients with a hinged leaflet prosthetic heart valve. In Brewer LA, Cooley DA, Davila JC, Merendino KA, Sirak HD (eds): Prosthetic Heart Valves. Springfield IL, Charles C Thomas, 1969, pp 622–632.
42. Gott VL, Dutton RL, Fadali AM, Ramos MD, Steig PD: The role of material surfaces in blood coagulation. In Brewer LA, Cooley DA, Davila JC, Merendino KA, Sirak HD (eds): Prosthetic Heart Valves. Springfield IL, Charles C Thomas, 1969, pp 178–197, and Discussion by Magovern GJ, p 197.
43. Wieting DW. In discussion: Sanvage LR, Berger K, Wood SJ, Viggers RF, Robel SB. In vivo testing of prosthetic heart valves and criteria for specimen evaluation. In Brewer LA, Cooley DA, Davila JC, Merendino KA, Sirak HD (eds): Prosthetic Heart Valves. Springfield IL, Charles C Thomas, 1969, pp 243–259.
44. Brewer, LA III: Epilogue. In Brewer LA, Cooley DA, Davila JC, Merendino KA, Sirak HD (eds): Prosthetic Heart Valves. Springfield IL, Charles C Thomas, 1969, pp 874–881.
45. Kalke BR, Lillehei CW, Kaster RL: Evaluation of a double-leaflet prosthetic heart valve of new design for clinical use. In Brewer LA, Cooley DA, Davila JC, Merendino KA, Sirak HD (eds): Prosthetic Heart Valves. Springfield IL, Charles C Thomas, 1969, pp 285–302.
46. Carpentier A, Lemaigre G, Robert L, Carpentier S, Dubost C: Biological factors affecting long-term results of valvular heterografts. J Thorac Cardiovasc Surg 1969;58:467–483.
47. Richardson JP, Clarebrough JK, Simpson WL: Heterologous aortic valves for mitral replacement: method of preparation and preservation and operative technique. J Thorac Cardiovasc Surg 1970;59:489–495.
48. Buch WS, Kosek JC, Angell WW: Deterioration of formalin-treated aortic valve heterografts. J Thorac Cardiovasc Surg 1970;60:673–682.
49. Silver MD, Butany J: Complications of mechanical heart valve prostheses. Cardiovasc Clin 1988;18:273–288.
50. Magilligan DJ Jr: Choice of heart valves. Trans Am Soc Artif Intern Organs 1987;33:90–95.
51. Schoen FJ, Clage HGP, Hill JD, Chenoweth DE, Anderson JM, Eberhart RC: The biocompatibility of artificial organs. Trans Am Soc Artif Intern Organs 1987;33:824–833.
52. Schoen FJ, Hobson CE: Anatomic analysis of removed prosthetic heart valves: cause of failure of 33 mechanical valves and 58 bioprostheses 1980 to 1983. Human Path 1985;16:549–559.
53. Rabago G: A worldwide overview of valve usage. In Rabago G, Cooley DA (eds): Heart Valve Replacement, Mount Kisco NY, Futura Publishing, 1987, pp 3–9.
54. Pluth JR: Reoperation on prosthetic heart valves. In Rabago G, Cooley DA (eds): Heart Valve Replacement, Mount Kisco NY, Futura Publishing, 1987, pp 421–433.
55. Odell JA, Mitha AS, Vankes EA, Whitton ID: Experience with tissue and mechanical valves in the pediatric group. In Rabago G, Cooley DA (eds): Heart Valve Replacement, Mount Kisco NY, Futura Publishing, 1987, pp 185–208.
56. Jatene AD: Reoperation on mechanical heart valves. In Rabago G, Cooley DA (eds): Heart Valve Replacement, Mount Kisco NY, Futura Publishing, 1987, pp 435–442.
57. Magilligan DJ Jr: Reoperation for primary tissue failure of porcine bioprosthetic heart valves. In Rabago G, Cooley DA (eds): Heart Valve Replacement, Mount Kisco NY, Futura Publishing, 1987, pp 443–451.
58. Fraile J, Martinell J, Cortina J, Artiz V, Rabago G: Early risk of reoperation for prosthetic valve replacement. In Rabago G, Cooley DA (eds): Heart Valve Replacement, Mount Kisco NY, Futura Publishing, 1987, pp 453–469.

59. Butchart EG, Breckenridge IM: Prosthetic valve reoperations. In Starek PJK (ed): Heart Valve Replacement and Reconstruction. Chicago, Year Book Medical Publishers, 1987, pp 293–303.
60. Geha AS: Long-term outcome of cardiac valve substitutes. Ann Thorac Surg 1987;44:566–567.
61. Foster AH, Greenberg GJ, Underhill DJ, McIntosh CL, Clark RE: Intrinsic failure of Hancock mitral bioprostheses: 10 to 15 year experience. Ann Thorac Surg 1987;44:568–577.
62. Antunes MJ: Isolated replacement of a prosthesis or a bioprosthesis in the aortic valve position. Am J Cardiol 1987;59:350–352.
63. Antunes MJ, Magalhaes MP: Isolated replacement of a prosthesis or bioprosthesis in the mitral position. Am J Cardiol 1987;59:346–349.
64. Magilligan DJ Jr, Lam CR, Lewis JW, Davila JC: Mitral valve the third time around. Circulation 1978;58(suppl 1):I36–I38.
65. Sandza JG Jr, Clark RE, Ferguson TB, Connors JP, Weldon CS: Replacement of prosthetic heart valve: a fifteen year experience. J Thorac Cardiovasc Surg 1977;74:864–874.
66. Rossiter SJ, Craig-Miller D, Stinson EB, Oyer PE, Reitz BA, Shumway NE: Aortic and mitral prosthetic valve reoperation. Early and late results. Arch Surg 1979;114:1279–1283.
67. Wisheart JD, Ross DN, Ross JK: A review of the effect of previous operation on the results of open heart surgery. Thorax 1972;27:137–142.
68. English TAH, Milstein BB: Repeat open mitracardiac operation: analyses of 50 operations. J Thorac Cardiovasc Surg 1978;76:56–60.
69. Lorde S, Sugg WL: The challenge of reoperation in cardiac surgery. Ann Thorac Surg 1974;17:152–162.
70. Parr GVS, Kirklin JW, Blackstone E: The early risk of re-replacement of aortic valves. Ann Thorac Surg 1977;23:319–325.
71. Husebye DG, Pluth JR, Piehler JM, Schaff HV, Orzalak TA, Puga FJ, Danielson GK: Reoperation on prosthetic heart valves. An analysis of risk factors in 525 patients. J Thorac Cardiovasc Surg 1983;86:543–552.
72. Bosch X, Pomar JL, Pelletier LC: Early and late prognosis after reoperation for prosthetic valve replacement. J Thorac Cardiovasc Surg 1984;88:567–572.
73. Davila JC, Palmer TE, Sethi RS, DeLaurentis DA, Enriquez F, Rincon NL, Lautsch EV: The problem of thrombosis in artificial cardiac valves. In Brest A (ed): Heart Substitutes. Springfield IL, Charles C Thomas, 1965, pp 25–53.
74. Davila JC, Lautsch EV, Weber KT, Sunmarco ME, Wilcox O: Prosthetic cardiac valves: principles and problems. In Segal BL, Kilpatrick DG (eds): Engineering in the Practice of Medicine. Baltimore, William & Wilkins, 1967, pp 267–277.
75. Davila JC, Amongero F, Sethi RS, Pincon NL, Palmer TE, Lautsch EV: The prevention of thrombosis in artificial cardiac valves. Ann Thorac Surg 1966;2:714–741.
76. Davila JC: The development of artificial heart valves. In Special Technical Publication No 386: Plastics in Surgical Implants. Philadelphia, American Society for Testing and Materials, 1965, pp 1–16.
77. Hylen JC: Mechanical malfunction and thrombosis of prosthetic heart valves. Am J Cardiol 1972;30:396–404.
78. Lindblom D: Long-term clinical results after mitral valve replacement with the Björk-Shiley prosthesis. J Thorac Cardiovasc Surg 1988;95:321–333.
79. Borkon AM, Soule L, Baughman KL, Aoun H, Gardner TJ, Watkins L Jr, Baumgartner WA, Gott VL, Reitz BA: Ten year analysis of the Björk-Shiley standard aortic valve. Ann Thorac Surg 1987;43:39–51.
80. Sethia B, Turner MA, Lewis S, Rodger RA, Bain WH: Fourteen years experience with the Björk-Shiley tilting disk prosthesis. J Thorac Cardiovasc Surg 1986;91:350–361.
81. Venugopal P, Kaul U, Izer KS, Rao MI, Balram A, Das B, Sampathkumar A, Mukherjee S, Rajani M, Wasir HS, Bhatin ML, Raghavan V, Reddy KS, Gopinath N: Fate of thrombectomized Björk-Shiley valves. J Thorac Cardiovasc Surg 1986;91:168–173.
82. Boskovic D, Elezovic I, Simin N, Rolovic Z, Josipovic V: Late thrombosis of Björk-Shiley tilting disk valve in the tricuspid position. J Thorac Cardiovasc Surg 1986;91:1–8.
83. DeWall RA, Schuster B, Hicks G Jr, Pelletier C, Bonan R, Martineau JP, Panebianco A, Yip L: Seventy-six month experience with the Omniscience cardiac valve. J Thorac Cardiovasc Surg 1987;28:328–332.
84. Callaghan JC, Coles J, Damle A: Six year clinical study of use of the Omniscience valve prosthesis in 2219 patients. J Am Coll Cardiol 1987;9:240–246.
85. Carrier M, Matineou JP, Bonan R, Pelletier LC: Clinical and hemodynamic assessment of the Omniscience prosthetic heart valve. J Thorac Cardiovasc Surg 1987;93:300–307.
86. Hall KV, Nittor-Hauze S, Abdelnoor M: Seven and one-half years experience with the Medtronic-Hall valve. J Am Coll Cardiol 1985;6:1417–1421.
87. Matsunaga H, Asano KI, Furuse A, Maku-Vohi H, Takayama T, Yagyu K: Clinical experience of Hall-Kaster valve. J Cardiovasc Surg 1984;25:138–144.
88. Deuvaert FE, LeClerc JL, Primo G, Wellens F, DePaepe J, Nooten GV, Dumont N: Thrombosis of the Saint Jude valve prosthesis in the aortic position. J Cardiovasc Surg 1986;27:622–624.
89. Prabhu S, Friday KJ, Reynolds D, Elkins R, Lazzara R: Thrombosis of aortic St. Jude valve. Ann Thorac Surg 1986;41:332–333.

90. Baudet EM, Oco CC, Roquec XF, Laborde MN, Hafez AS, Collot MA, Ghidoni IM: A 5½ year experience with the St. Jude Medical cardiac valve prosthesis. J Thorac Cardiovasc Surg 1985;90:137–144.
91. Douglas PS, Hirshfield JW Jr, Edie RN, Harken AH, Stephenson LW, Edmunds LH Jr: Clinical comparison of St. Jude and porcine aortic valve prostheses. Circulation 1985;72(suppl 2):135–139.
92. Czer LSC, Matloff JM, Chaux A, DeRobertis MA, Gray RJ: Comparative clinical experience with porcine bioprosthetic and St. Jude valve replacement. Chest 1987;91:503–514.
93. Kinsley RH, Autunes MJ, Colsen PR: St. Jude Medical valve replacement. J Thorac Cardiovasc Surg 1986;92:349–360.
94. Duncan JM, Cooley DA, Reul GH, Oh DA, Hallman GL, Frazier OH, Livesoy JJ, Walker WE, Adams PR: Durability and low thrombogenicity of the St. Jude Medical valve at 5 year follow-up. Ann Thorac Surg 1986;42:500–505.
95. Hartz RS, LoCicero J, Kucich V, DeBoer A, O'Mara S, Mezers SN, Michaelis LL: Comparative study of warfarin versus antiplatelet therapy in patients with St. Jude Medical valve in aortic position. J Thorac Cardiovasc Surg 1986;92:684–690.
96. Jarviner A, Virtanen K, Peltola K, Maamies T, Ketonen P, Mannikko A: Post operative disk entrapment following cardiac valve replacement. Thorac Cardiovasc Surgeon 1984;32:152–156.
97. Harjula A, Mattila S, Maamies T, Mattila I, Mattilu P, Skytta J, Pekka T: Long-term follow-up of Björk-Shiley mitral valve replacement. Scand J Thorac Cardiovasc Surg 1986;20:79–84.
98. Robert WC, Hammer WJ: Cardiac pathology after valve replacement with a tilting disk (Björk-Shiley) type. Am J Cardiol 1976;37:1024–1033.
99. McGoon DC: Editor's addendum. J Thorac Cardiovasc Surg 1984;88:308.
100. DeWall R: Omniscience valves. J Thorac Cardiovasc Surg 1984;87:1040.
101. Panebianco AC: Results of valve replacement with Omniscience prostheses. J Thorac Cardiovasc Surg 1984;87:939–947.
102. DeWall R: Reflections on the Omniscience heart valve. J Thorac Cardiovasc Surg 1984;87:941.
103. Mitha AS, Matisonn RE, Le Roux BT, Chesler E: Clinical experience with the Lillehei-Kaster cardiac valve prosthesis. J Thorac Cardiovasc Surg 1976;72:401–407.
104. Thulin LI, Bain WH, Huysmans HH, van Ingen G, Prieto I, Basile F, Lindbom DA, Olin CL: Heart valve replacement with the Björk-Shiley monostrut valve: early results of a multicenter clinical investigation. Ann Thorac Surg 1988;45:164–170.
105. Waller BF, Jones M, Roberts WC: Postoperative aortic regurgitation from incomplete seating of tilting disk occluders due to overhanging knots or long sutures. Chest 1980;78:565–568.
106. Jackson GM, Wolf PL, Bloor CM: Malfunction of mitral Björk-Shiley prosthetic valve due to septal interference. Am Heart J 1982;104:158–159.
107. Cleveland JC, Levenson IM, Dague JR: Early postoperative development of aortic regurgitation related to pannus ingrowth causing incomplete disk seating of Björk-Shiley prosthesis. Ann Thorac Surg 1981;33:497–498.
108. Kafka H, Parker JO, Charrette EJP, Salerno TA: Malfunction in a St. Jude Medical mitral valve prosthesis: a clinical diagnostic dilemma. Can J Surg 1983;26:84–86.
109. Long DM Jr: In discussion: Kay EB, Suzuki A, Postigo J, Nogueira C: Prosthetic replacement of the mitral valve. In Merendino KA, Morrow AG, Lillehei CW, Muller WH (eds): Prosthetic Heart Valves for Cardiac Surgery. Springfield IL, Charles C Thomas, 1961, p 422.
110. Kennedy JW, Doces JG, Stewart DK: Left ventricular function before and following surgical treatment of mitral valve disease. Am Heart J 1979;97:592–595.
111. Boucher CA, Bingham JB, Osbakken MD: Early changes in left ventricular size and function after correction of left ventricular volume overload. Am J Cardiol 1981;47:991–993.
112. Huikuri HV: Effect of mitral valve replacement on the left ventricular function in mitral regurgitation. Br Heart J 1983;49:328–331.
113. Lillehei CW, Levy MJ, Bonnabeau RC: Mitral valve replacement with preservation of papillary muscles and chordae tendineae. J Thorac Cardiovasc Surg 1964;47:532–535.
114. Hetzer R, Bougioukas G, Franz M, Borst HG: Mitral valve replacement with preservation of papillary muscles and chordae tendineae: revival of a seemingly forgotten concept, I: preliminary clinical report. Thorac Cardiovasc Surgeon 1983;31:291–294.
115. David TE: Left ventricular function after mitral valve replacement with preservation of chordae tendineae. In Starek PJK (ed): Heart Valve Replacement and Reconstruction. Chicago, Year Book Medical Publishers, 1987, pp 273–277.
116. Asano K: Mitral valve replacement by mechanical valves with preservation of chordae tendineae and papillary muscles. In Starek PJK (ed): Heart Valve Replacement and Reconstruction. Chicago, Year Book Medical Publishers, 1987, pp 27–31.
117. Miki S, Kusuhara K, Veda Y, Komeda M, Ohkita Y, Tahata T: Mitral valve replacement with preservation of chordae tendineae and papillary muscles. Ann Thorac Surg 1988;45:28–34.
118. Come PC, Riley ME, Weintaub RM: Dynamic left ventricular outflow track obstruction when the anterior leaflet is retained at prosthetic mitral valve replacements. Ann Thorac Surg 1987;43:561–564.

119. Olin CL, Bomfirn V, Halvazulis V, Holmgren AG, Lamke BJ: Optimal insertion technique for the Björk-Shiley valve in the narrow aortic astium. Ann Thorac Surg 1983;36:567–576.
120. Kinsley RH: The narrow aortic annulus. A technique for inserting a longer prosthesis. Am Heart J 1977;93:759–761.
121. Kinsley RH: Valve prosthesis-patient mismatch. Circulation 1979;59:418–419.
122. Aldrete V: Intermittent aortic regurgitation with tilting disk valves. J Thorac Cardiovasc Surg 1984;88:458–459.
123. Kugelberg J: In discussion: Sethia B, Turner MA, Lewis S, Rodger RA, Bain WH: Fourteen years experience with the Björk-Shiley tilting disk prosthesis. J Thorac Cardiovasc Surg 1986;91:350–361.
124. Antunes MJ, Colsen PR, Kinsley RH: Intermittent aortic regurgitation following aortic valve replacement with the Hall-Kaster prosthesis. J Thorac Cardiovasc Surg 1982;84:751–754.
125. Beaudet RL: The Hall-Kaster aortic valve. J Thorac Cardiovasc Surg 1983;86:456.
126. Rainer WG: Reply to letter to the editor: St. Jude Medical valve prosthesis. J Thorac Cardiovasc Surg 1981;82:462–463.
127. Antoniucci D, Paolini G, Salvatore L, Zerauschek M: Echocardiographic features of the St. Jude Medical valve prosthesis. Giorn Ital Cardiol 1981;11:2039–2047.
128. Chaux A, Gray RJ, Matloff JM, Feldman H, Sustaita H: An appreciation of the new St. Jude valvular prosthesis. J Thorac Cardiovasc Surg 1981;81:202–211.
129. Feldman HJ, Gray RJ, Chaux A: Noninvasive in vivo and in vitro study of the St. Jude valve prosthesis. Am J Cardiol 1982;49:1101.
130. Casteneda-Zuniga W, Nicoloff D, Jorgensen C: In vivo radiographic appearance of the St. Jude valve prosthesis. Radiology 1980;134:775–776.
131. Chandran KB, Fatemi R, Hiratzka LF, Harris C: Effect of wedging on the flow characteristics past tilting disk aortic valve prosthesis. J Biomechanics 1986;19:181–186.
132. Björk VO: Metallurgical and design development in response to mechanical dysfunction of Björk-Shiley heart valves. Scand J Thor Cardiovasc Surg 1985;19:1–12.
133. Harjula A, Mattila S, Maamie T, Mattila I, Mattila P, Skytta J, Talo P: Long-term follow-up of Björk-Shiley mitral valve replacement. Scand J Thorac Cardiovasc Surg 1986;20:79–84.
134. Kazama S, Kim K, Sato K, Moriya H, Kamijima J, Tominaga S, Ishihara A: Malfunction of Björk-Shiley mitral valve prosthesis due to excessive platelet-fibrin deposition on its sewing cuff. Jap Heart J 1980;21:429–433.
135. Raychaudhury T, Faichney A, Walbaum PR: Obstruction of a Björk-Shiley mitral prosthesis in a patient with idiopathic hypertrophic subaortic stenosis. Thorax 1983;38:388–389.
136. Williams DB, Pluth JR, Orszulak TA: Extrinsic obstruction of the Björk-Shiley valve in the mitral position. Ann Thorac Surg 1981;32:58–62.
137. Blasko EC, Plzak LF, Sohn M, Marion WL: Acute, complete extrinsic obstruction of the Björk-Shiley valve in the immediate post operative period. J Thorac Cardiovasc Surg 1983;88:630–631.
138. Solem JO, Kugelberg J, Stahl E: Immobilization of Björk-Shiley disk valve. Scand J Thorac Cardiovasc Surg 1983;17:217–219.
139. Kober G, Hilgermann R: Catheter entrapment in a Björk-Shiley prosthesis in aortic position. Cath Cardiovasc Diag 1987;13:262–265.
140. Horstkotte D, Jehle J, Loogen F: Death due to transprosthetic catheterization of Björk-Shiley prosthesis in aortic position. Am J Cardiol 1986;58:566–567.
141. Pai GP, Ellison RG, Rubin JW, Moore HV, Kamath MV: Disk immobilization of Björk-Shiley and Medtronic-Hall valves during and immediately after valve replacement. Ann Thorac Surg 1987;44:73–76.
142. Jarvinen A, Virtanen K, Peltola K, Maamies T, Ketonen P, Mannikko A: Post operative disk entrapment following cardiac valve replacement—a report of ten cases. Thorac Cardiovasc Surgeon 1984;32:152–156.
143. Saunders CR, Ross NP, Rittenhouse EA: Failure of a Björk-Shiley mitral valve prosthesis to open. J Cardiovasc Surg 1972;13:281.
144. Browdie DA, Agnew RF, Hamilton CS Jr: Poppet jamming during mitral valve replacement. Ann Thorac Surg 1978;26:591.
145. Jones A, Otis JB, Fletcher GF, Robert WC: A hitherto undescribed cause of prosthetic valve obstruction. J Thorac Cardiovasc Surg 1977;74:116.
146. Salem JO, Kugelberg J, Stahl E: Acute immobilization of the disk in a Björk-Shiley aortic tilting disk prosthesis. Scand J Thorac Cardiovasc Surg 1983;17:217.
147. DeWall R: Discussion to Björk VO, Henze A: Ten years' experience with the Björk-Shiley tilt disk valve. J Thorac Cardiovasc Surg 1979;78:341.
148. Masters RG, Keon WJ: Extrinsic obstruction of the Medtronic-Hall disk valve in the mitral position. Ann Thorac Surg 1988;45:210–212.
149. Trites PN, Kiser JC, Johnson C, Tycast FJ, Gobel FL: Occlusion of Medtronic-Hall mitral valve prosthesis by ruptured papillary muscle and chordae tendineae. J Thorac Cardiovasc Surg 1984;88:301–306.
150. Sakurada T, Okubo T, Atsumi H, Sekine S, Ishii M, Saito S, Abe T: Clinical evaluation of Bicer-Val prosthetic valve. Jinkozoki 1984;13:300.

151. Effler DB: Valve sticking: complication of the Medtronic-Hall prosthesis. Thai J Surg 1987;8:41–45.
152. Baeza O: Potential for immobilization of the valve occluder in various prostheses. In Matloff JM (ed): Cardiac Valve Replacement. Boston, Martinus Nijhoff Publishing, 1985, pp 281–284.
153. Mok CK, Cheung DLC, Chiu CSW, Aung-Khin M: An unusual lethal complication of preservation of chordae tendineae in mitral valve replacement. J Thorac Cardiovasc Surg 1988;95:534–536.
154. Tomizawa Y, Kitamura N, Minoji T, Irie T, Yamaguchi A, Ootaki M, Tamura H, Atobe M: Stuck prosthetic valve caused by pyrolytic carbon disk wear. Chest 1987;91:798.
155. Kardash AN, Iofis NA, Khurtsilava SG, Ryazantsev YS, Machulin AV, Yurechko VN, Grishkevich AM, Bukatov AS, Orlov AI: Causes and prevention of wedging of the OMHKC heart valve prosthesis. Grudn Khir 1986;1:15–18.
156. Pfeifer J, Goldschlazer N, Sweatman T, Gerbade F, Selzer A: Malfunction of mitral ball valve prosthesis due to thrombus. Am J Cardiol 1972;29:95–99.
157. Behi F, Chang S, Welch T: Malfunction of Cutter-Smeloff mitral prosthesis. J Thorac Cardiovasc Surg 1978;75:313–316.
158. Resnicoff SA, DeWeese JA: Acute aortic insufficiency due to ball impaction on a close clearance Starr-Edwards aortic prosthesis. Ann Thorac Surg 1971;12:660.
159. Mullin MJ, Muth WF, McNamara JJ: Sticking aortic valve. J Thorac Cardiovasc Surg 1972;63:215–217.
160. Mond HG, Clarebrough JK, Dawling JT, Sloman G, Westlake G: Entrapment of the mitral ball in series 6310 and 2310 Starr-Edwards prosthetic valves. J Thorac Cardiovasc Surg 1972;64:186–192.
161. Kahn DR, Willis PW III, Reynolds EW Jr, Sloan H: Swollen strut syndrome. Circulation 1968;37,38(suppl 6):109. Abstract.
162. Colombo T, Donatelli F, Quaini E, Vitali E, Pellegrini A: Results of heart valve replacement with the Sorin prosthesis. Tex Heart J 1987;14:77–87.
163. Cai Y, Zhang B, Chen R, Zhu J, Hao J, Geng Z: Experience with 124 consecutive elective mitral valve replacements with the Shanghai-made tilting disk prosthesis. Chinese Med J 1985;98:299–304.
164. Cai Y, Zhang B, Chen R, Zhu J, Hao J, Geng Z: Chinese J Cardiol 1985;13:81–83.
165. Starek PJK: Immobilization of disk heart valves by unraveled sutures. Ann Thorac Surg 1981;31:66–69.
166. Ziemer G, Luhmer I, Oelert H, Borst HG: Malfunction of a St. Jude Medical heart valve in the mitral position. Ann Thorac Surg 1982;33:391–395.
167. Nunez L, Iglesias A, Sotillo J: Entrapment of leaflet of St. Jude Medical cardiac valve prosthesis by minuscule thrombosis: report of two cases. Ann Thorac Surg 1980;29:567–569.
168. Beall AC Jr, Morris GC Jr, Noon GP, Guinn GA, Reul GJ, Letrak EA, Greenberg SD: An improved mitral valve prosthesis. Ann Thorac Surg 1973;15:25–34.
169. Beall AC Jr, Morris GC Jr, Howell JF Jr, Guinn GA, Noon GP, Reul GJ Jr, Greenberg JS, Ankeney JL: Clinical experience with an improved mitral valve prosthesis. Ann Thorac Surg 1973;15:601–606.
170. Nathan MJ: Strut fracture. Ann Thorac Surg 1973;16:610–612.
171. Gold H, Hertz L: Death caused by fracture of Beall mitral prosthesis. Am J Cardiol 1974;34:371–374.
172. Bokros JC, Akins RJ: Application of pyrolytic carbon in artificial heart valves. In Shaw MC (ed): Proceedings of the 4th Buhl Conference on Materials. Pittsburgh, Carnegie Press, 1971, pp 243–299.
173. Pilichowski P, Gandin P, Brichon PY, Neron L, Wolf JE, Machecount J, Latreille R: Fracture and embolization of a Lillehei-Kaster mitral valve prosthesis disk. Thorac Cardiovasc Surgeon 1987;35:385–386.
174. Norenberg DD, Evans RW, Gundersen AE, Abellera RM: Fracture and embolization of a Björk-Shiley disk. J Thorac Cardiovasc. Surg 1977;74:925–927.
175. Hasse J: Escaped leaflet in a Saint Jude Medical mitral prosthesis. In DeBakey ME (ed): Advances in Cardiac Valves: Clinical Perspective. New York, Yorke, 1983, pp 115–123.
176. Hjelms E: Escape of a leaflet from a St. Jude Medical prosthesis in the mitral position. Thorac Cardiovasc Surgeon 1983;31:310–312.
177. Burckhardt D, Hoffman A, Vogt S, Pfisterer M, Hasse J, Gradel E: Clinical evaluation of the St. Jude Medical heart valve prosthesis. J Thorac Cardiovasc Surg 1984;88:432–438.
178. Odell JA, Durandt J, Shama DM, Vythilingum S: Spontaneous embolization of a St. Jude mitral valve leaflet. Ann Thorac Surg 1985;39:569–572.
179. Thomas D: Discussion. In Matloff JM (ed): Cardiac Valve Replacement. Boston, Martinus Nijhoff Publishing, 1985, pp 296–297.
180. Messmer BJ, Rothlin M, Senning A: Early disk dislodgement: an unusual complication after insertion of a Björk-Shiley mitral valve prosthesis. J Thorac Cardiovasc Surg 1973;65:386–390.
181. Tellez G, Maronas JM, Iglesias A: Expulsion of a disk of a Björk-Shiley aortic prosthesis after temporary removal. Chest 1978;73:124.
182. Joassin A, Edwards JE: Late cause of death after mitral valve replacement. J Thorac Cardiovasc Surg 1973;65:255.
183. Killen DA, Collins HA, Koenig MG, Goodman JS: Prosthetic cardiac valves and bacterial endocarditis. Ann Thorac Surg 1970;9:238.
184. Roberts WC, Morrow AG: Late post operative pathology after valve replacement. Circulation 1967;35,36(suppl 1):48.

185. Hylen JC, Kloster FE, Starr A, Griswold HE: Aortic ball variance: diagnosis and treatment. Ann Intern Med 1970;72:1–8.
186. Joyce LD, Emery RW, Nicoloff M: Ball variance and fracture of mitral valve prosthesis causing recurrent thrombolmboli. J Thorac Cardiovasc Surg 1978;75:309–312.
187. Grunkemeier GL, Starr A: Late ball variance with the model 1000 Starr-Edwards aortic valve prosthesis. J Thorac Cardiovasc Surg 1986;91:918–923.
188. Miller DC, Oyer PE, Stinson EB, Reitz BA, Jamieson SW, Baumgartner WA, Mitchell RS, Shumway NE: Ten to fifteen year reassessment of the performance of the Starr-Edwards model 6120 mitral valve prosthesis. J Thorac Cardiovasc Surg 1983;85:1–20.
189. Cobanoghu A, Grunkemeier GL, Aru AM, McKinley CL, Starr A: Mitral replacement: clinical experience with a ball-valve prosthesis: twenty-five years later. Ann Surg 1985;202:376–383.
190. Miller DC, Oyer PE, Mitchell RS, Stinson EB, Jamieson SW, Baldwin JC, Shumway NE: Performance characteristics of the Starr-Edwards model 1260 aortic valve prosthesis beyond ten years. J Thorac Cardiovasc Surg 1984;88:193–207.
191. Fessatidis I, Hackett D, Oakley CM, Sapsford RN, Bentall HH: Ten year clinical evaluation of isolated mitral valve and double valve replacement with the Starr-Edwards prostheses. Ann Thorac Surg 1987;43:368–372.
192. Cobanoglu A, Fessler CL, Guvendik L, Grunkemeier G, Starr A: Aortic valve replacement with the Starr-Edwards prosthesis: a comparison of the first and second decades of followup. Ann Thorac Surg 1988;45:248–252.
193. Hammer WJ, Hearne MJ, Roberts WC: Cocking of a poppet-disk prosthesis in the aortic position. J Thorac Cardiovasc Surg 1976;71:259–261.
194. Hopeman AR, Treasure RL, Hall RJ: Mechanical dysfunction in caged-lens prostheses. J Thorac Cardiovasc Surg 1970;60:51–53.
195. Boretos JW, Petmer DE, Braumiould NS: Factors influencing longevity of low-profile prosthetic heart valves. J Biomed Mat Res 1972;6:185–192.
196. Bowen TE, Zajtehuk R, Brott WH, deCastro CM: Isolated mitral valve replacement with the Kay-Shiley prosthesis. J Thorac Cardiovasc Surg 1980;80:45–49.
197. Charnley J: Factors in the design of an artificial hip joint, II: lubrication and wear in living and artificial human joints. Proc Inst Mech Eng 1966–67;181, pt.3J, 104–111.
198. Lancaster JK: Abrasive wear of polymers. Wear 1969;14:223.
199. Vetz H, Breckel H: Reibungs and Verschleissversuche mit PTFE. Wear 1967;10:185.
200. Montoya A, Sullivan HJ, Pifarre R: Disk variance: a potentially lethal complication of the Beall valve prosthesis. J Thorac Cardiovasc Surg 1976;71:904–906.
201. Jost GR, McKnight RC, Roper CL: Failure of Beall mitral valve prosthesis. J Thorac Cardiovasc Surg 1975;70:163.
202. Clark RE, Grubbs FL, McKnight RC, Ferguson TD, Roper CL, Weldon CS: Late clinical problems with Beall model 103 and 104 mitral valve prosthesis: hemolysis and wear. Ann Thorac Surg 1976;21:475–482.
203. Evangelista-Masip A, Batlle-Diaz J, Garcia-Del-Castillo H, Galve-Basilio E, Soler-Soler J: Phonoechographic findings in disk variance of a Beall mitral prosthesis. Am Heart J 1984;108:178–180.
204. Berroya RB, Escano FB Jr: Mitral disk-valve variance. Thorax 1972;27:87–89.
205. Robinson MJ, Hildner FJ, Greenberg JJ: Disk variance of Beall mitral valve. Ann Thorac Surg 1971;11:11–17.
206. Silver MD, Wilson GJ: The pathology of wear in the Beall model 104 heart valve prosthesis. Circulation 1977;56:617–622.
207. Björk VO: Experience with the Wada-Cutter valve prosthesis in the aortic area. J Thorac Cardiovasc Surg 1970;60:26–33.
208. duPriest RW, Semler HJ, Oyama AA, Nohlgren JE: Sudden death due to dislodgement of disk occluder of Wada-Cutter prosthesis. J Thorac Cardiovasc Surg 1973;66:93–95.
209. Hughes DA, Leatherman LL, Norman JC, Cooley DA: Late embolization of prosthetic mitral valve occluder with survival following reoperation. Ann Thorac Surg 1975;19:212–215.
210. Schoen FJ, Titus JL, Lawrie GM: Bioengineering aspects of cardiac valve replacement. Ann Biomed Eng 1982;10:97–128.
211. Björk VO: A new tilting disk prosthesis. Scand J Thorac Cardiovasc Surg 1969;3:1–10.
212. Blackstone EH, Kirklin JW, Pluth JR, Turner ME, Parr VS: The performance of the Braumwald-Cutter aortic prosthetic valve. Ann Thorac Surg 1977;23:302–318.
213. Schoen FJ, Goodenough SH, Ionescu MI, Braumwald NS: Implications of late morphology of Braumwald-Cutter mitral heart valve prosthesis. J Thorac Cardiovasc Surg 1984;88:208–216.
214. Dumanian GA, Dumanian AV: Late embolic phenomena associated with cloth-covered Starr-Edwards aortic valve prostheses. Am J Cardiol 1987;60:914–915.
215. Angelini GD, Kulatilake ENP, Armistead SH: Right coronary artery occlusion by cloth from a Starr-Edwards aortic valve prosthesis. Thorac Cardiovasc Surgeon 1984;32:379–380.

216. Thormac CS Jr, Duncan AK, Alford WC, Burruc GR, Stoney WS: Cloth disruption in the Starr-Edwards composite mitral valve prosthesis. Ann Thorac Surg 1973;15:434–438.
217. Cieland J, Molloy PJ: Thrombo-embolic complications of the cloth-covered Starr-Edwards prostheses no. 2300 aortic and no. 6300 mitral. Thorax 1973;28:41–47.
218. Crawford FA, Sethi GK, Scott SM, Takaro T: Systemic emboli due to cloth wear in a Starr-Edwards model 2320 aortic prosthesis. Ann Thorac Surg 1973;16:614–619.
219. Reis RL, Glancy DL, O'Brien K, Epstein S, Morrow AG: Clinical and hemodynamic assessment of fabric covered Starr-Edwards prosthetic valve. J Thorac Cardiovasc Surg 1970;59:84–91.
220. Ablaza SG, Blanco G, Javan MB, Maranharo V, Goldberg H: Cloth cover wear of struts of Starr-Edwards prosthesis. J Thorac Cardiovasc Surg 1971;61:315–318.
221. Boruchow I, Ramsey HW, Wheat MW Jr: Complications following destruction of cloth covering of a Starr-Edwards aortic valve prosthesis. J Thorac Cardiovasc Surg 1971;62:290–292.
222. Fettel BE, Johnston DR, Morris PE: Accelerated life testing of prosthetic heart valves. Med Instrument 1980;14:161–164.
223. Björk VO, Lindblom D, Lindblom U: The Delrin aortic Björk-Shiley valve 15 years followup. J Am Coll Cardiol 1985;6:1142–1147.
224. Björk VO: The Björk-Shiley tilting disk valve: past, present and future: Cardiac Surgery: State of the Art Reviews. Philadelphia, Hanley & Belfus, 1987, pp 183–202.
225. Montero CG, Rofilanchas JJ, Juffe A, Burgos R, Ugarte J, Figuera D: Long-term results of cardiac valve replacement with the Delrin-disk model of the Björk-Shiley valve prosthesis. Ann Thorac Surg 1984;37:328–336.
226. Björk VO: Delrin as implant material for occluders. Scand J Thorac Cardiovasc Surg 1972;6:103–107.
227. Björk VO, Henze A, Holmgren A: Five years experience with the Björk-Shiley tilting disk valve in isolated aortic valvular disease. J Thorac Cardiovasc Surg 1974;68:393–404.
228. Larmi TKI, Karkola P: Shrinkage and degradation of the Delrin occluder in the tilting disk valve prosthesis. J Thorac Cardiovasc Surg 1974;68:66–69.
229. Clark RE, Hagen RW, Siegfried BA, Schier JJ, Rusche JM: Accelerated fatigue testing of prosthetic heart valves. Surg Forum 1975;26:242–251.
230. Clark RE, Swanson WM, Kardos JL, Hagen RW, Beauchamp RA: Durability of prosthetic heart valves. Ann Thorac Surg 1978;26:323–335.
231. Amstutz HC, Lodwig M: War of polymeric bearing materials: the effect of in vivo implantation. J Biomed Mat Res 1976;10:25–31.
232. McKellop HA, Clark IC, Markolf KL, Amstutz HC: High wear rates with Delrin 150—a clinical hazard? Final Program of the 24th Annual Orthopedic Research Society, Dallas TX, February 21–23, 1978.
233. Bokros JC, LaGrange LD, Schoen FJ: Control of the structure of carbon for use in bioengineering. In Walker PL Jr (ed): Chemistry and Physics of Carbon. New York, Marcel Dekker, 1972, vol 9, pp 103–171.
234. Bokros JC: Carbon in biomedical devices. Carbon 1977;15:355–371.
235. Haubold AD, Shim HS, Bokros JC: Carbon in medical devices. In Williams DF (ed): Biocompatibility of Clinical Implant Materials. Boca Raton FL, CRC Press, 1981, vol 2, pp 3–42.
236. Shim HS, Schoen FJ: The wear resistance of pure and silicon alloyed isotropic carbons. Biomat Med Dev Art Org 1974;2:103–118.
237. Paton BC, Pine MB: Aortic valve replacement with DeBakey valve. J Thorac Cardiovasc Surg 1976;72:652–656.
238. Jacovella G, Milazzoto F, Giovannini E, Costantini A, Marsocci G, Rabitti G, Masini V: Sindrome da malfunzione delle valvole artificiali intracardiache. Giorn Ital Cardiol 1972;2:993–1009.
239. Scott SM, Sethi GK, Paulson DM, Takaro T: Insidious strut failure in a DeBakey-Surgitool aortic valve prosthesis. Ann Thorac Surg 1978;25:382–384.
240. Schoen FJ, Titus JL, Lawrie GM: Durability of pyrolytic carbon-containing heart valve prostheses. J Biomed Mat Res 1982;16:559–570.
241. Pettersson GD, Sudow G, Scholossman D: Strut fractures in DeBakey aortic valves. Scand J Thorac Cardiovasc Surg 1983;17:89–92.
242. Zumbro GL Jr, Cundey PE, Fishback ME: Strut-fracture in DeBakey valve. Successful reoperation and valve replacement. J Thorac Cardiovasc Surg 1977;74:469–470.
243. Lillehei CW, Kaster RL, Bloch JH: Clinical experience with the new central flow pivoting disk aortic and mitral prosthesis. Chest 1971;60:298.
244. Lillehei CW: Heart valve replacement with the pivoting disk prosthesis: appraisal of results and description of a new all-carbon model. Med Instrument 1977;11:85–94.
245. Silver MD, Koppenhoefer H, Heggtveil HA, Reif TH: Wear in Lillehei-Kaster heart valve prostheses. Artif Organs 1985;9:270–275.
246. Reif TH, Silver MD, Koppenhoefer H, Huffstutler MC Jr: Estimation of the abrasive wear coefficient in Lillehei-Kaster cardiac valve prostheses. J Biomechanics 1986;19:93–101.
247. Björk VO: The pyrolytic carbon occluder for the Björk-Shiley tilting disk valve prosthesis. Scand J Thorac Cardiovasc Surg 1972;6:109–113.

248. Dobrova NB, Iofis NA, Kozyrkin BI, Agafonov AV, Zaretskii YV, Kevovkova RA: Analysis of cause for wear and breakdown elements in artificial valves of tilting disk types. Meditsin Tekhn 1987;2:8–12.
249. Silver MD: Wear in Björk-Shiley heart valve prostheses recovered at necropsy or operation. J Thorac Cardiovasc Surg 1980;79:693–699.
250. More RB, Silver MD: Pyrolytic carbon prosthetic heart valve occluder wear: in vivo vs. in vitro results for the Björk-Shiley prosthesis. J Applied Biomaterials 1990;1:267–278.
251. Morse D, Steiner RM, Fernandez J (eds): Guide to Prosthetic Heart Valves. New York, Springer-Verlag, 1985.
252. Summary of safety and effectiveness of the Hall-Kaster prosthetic heart valve prosthesis. Submitted to the United States Food and Drug Administration, PMA No P790018, Silver Springs MD, June 29, 1979.
253. Summary of safety and effectiveness of the Omniscience® cardiac valve prosthesis. Submitted to the United States Food and Drug Administration, PMA No P830039, Silver Springs MD, November 5, 1984.
254. Warner CA, McIntosh CL, Roberts WC: Wear of the metallic studs on the composite seat of the 2320 Starr-Edwards aortic valve and its clinical consequences. Am J Cardiol 1983;52:1062–1065.
255. Bokros JC: Deposition, structure, and properties of pyrolytic carbon, in Walker PL (ed): Chemistry and Physics of Carbon. New York, Marcel Dekker, 1969, vol 5, pp 1–117.
256. Kaae JL, Gulden TD: Structure and mechanical properties of codeposited pyrolytic C-SiC alloys. J Am Ceram Soc 1971;54:605–609.
257. Kaae JL: Structure and properties of isotropic pyrolytic carbons deposited below 1600°C. J Nucl Mat 1971;38:42–50.
258. Gombrich PP, Villafana MA, Palmquist WE: From concept to clinical—the St. Jude Medical bileaflet pyrolytic carbon cardiac valve. Presented at Association for the Advancement of Medical Instrumentation, 14th Annual Meeting; May 20–24, 1979; Las Vegas NV.
259. Summary of safety and effectiveness of the St. Jude Medical replacement heart valve. Submitted to the United States Food and Drug Administration, PMA No 810002, Silver Springs MD, October 23, 1981.
260. Schoen FJ: Carbon in heart valve prostheses: foundations and clinical performance. In Szycher ML (ed): Biocompatible Polymers, Metals and Ceramics: Science and Technology. Westport CT, Technomic Publishing 1983, pp 239–261.
261. Omnicarbon® cardiac valve prosthesis. Premarket approval application (PMAA) to the Food and Drug Administration (FDA), PMA No P860039, Silver Springs MD, June 17, 1986.
262. Klawitter JJ: Preclinical in vitro testing of a new carbon bileaflet heart valve. In Proceedings of the International Symposium on Acquired Cardiac Valvular Diseases, Catania, Italy, June 20–23, 1983, Italy, Acta Cardiologica Mediterranea, 1983;1(suppl 3):1113–1117.
263. Summary of safety and effectiveness of the Duromedics cardiac valve prosthesis. Submitted to the United States Food and Drug Administration, PMA No P850006, Silver Springs MD, January 29, 1986.
264. Bokros JC: Heart valve prosthesis. US Patent No 4,692,165, 1987.
265. Beavan A: Accelerated durability tests of the CarboMedics prosthetic heart valve (unpublished data).
266. Carpentier A: Artificial cardiac valve with active opening. US Patent No 4,605,408, 1986.
267. Sorensen HR, Woien A: Heart valve. US Patent No 4,676,789, 1987.
268. Johnson K: Prosthetic Heart Valve. US Patent No 4,808,180, February 28, 1989.
269. Weertman J, Weertman JR: Elementary Dislocation Theory. New York, MacMillan, 1964, pp 1–4.
270. Boyd GM: From Griffith to COD and beyond. Engineering Fracture Mechanics. Oxford UK, Pergamon Press, 1972, vol 4, pp 459–482.
271. Gurney TR: Fatigue of Welded Structures. London, Cambridge University Press, 1968, pp 196–212.
272. Ansbro J, Clark R, Gerbode F: Successful surgical correction of an embolized prosthetic valve poppet. J Thorac Cardiovasc Surg 1976;72:130–131.
273. Lindblom D, Björk VO, Semb KH: Mechanical failure of the Björk-Shiley valve. J Thorac Cardiovasc Surg 1986;92:894–907.
274. Ostermeyer J, Horskotte D, Bennett J, Huysmans H, Lindblom D, Olin C, Orinivs E, Semb G: The Björk-Shiley 70° convexo-concave prosthesis strut fracture problem. Thorac Cardiovasc Surgeon 1987;35:71–77.
275. Garcia-del-Castillo H, Larrousse-Perez E, Murtra-Ferre M, Soler-Soler J: Strut fracture and disk embolization of a Björk-Shiley mitral valve prosthesis. Am J Cardiol 1985;55:597–598.
276. Chandra R, Bilsker M, Myerberg RJ, Kessler KM: Echocardiographic diagnosis of outlet strut fracture of a Björk-Shiley prosthesis in the mitral position. Am J Cardiol 1986;58:1117–1118.
277. Scalia D, Giacomin A, Dalol U, Valfre C: Successful treatment of a patient after sudden loss of the disk in a Björk-Shiley convexo-concave mitral prosthesis. Thorac Cardiovasc Surgeon 1987;35:318–320.
278. Criswell CB, Schuchmann GF, Acker JJ: Strut fracture of a Starr-Edwards mitral valve prosthesis. Am J Cardiol 1987;60:916–917.
279. Björk VO, Lindblom D, Henze A: The monostrut strength. Scand J Thor Cardiovasc Surg 1985;19:13–19.
280. Tzuzuku T: Mechanical energy losses due to motions of dislocations in graphite and carbons. Carbon 1963;1:25–31.
281. Tzuzuku T: Mechanical damping in carbon and graphite at low temperatures. Carbon 1964;1:511–517.

282. Schoen FJ: On the fatigue behavior of pyrolytic carbon. Carbon 1973;11:413–414.
283. Shim HS: The behavior of isotropic pyrolytic carbon under cyclic loading. Biomat Med Dev Art Org 1974;2:55–65.
284. Kepner J, Haubold AD, Beavan LA: "Cyclic Fatigue Testing of Pyrolitic Carbon," presented at the 41st Pacific Coast Regional Meeting of the American Chemical Society, San Francisco, October 26, 1990.

Bodnar, E. and Frater, R. W. M., editors
(1991) *Replacement Cardiac Valves,*
Pergamon Press, Inc. (New York), pp. 49–76
Printed in the United States of America

CHAPTER 3

BIOMATERIALS

VICTOR J. FERRANS, STEPHEN L. HILBERT, AND MICHAEL JONES

This chapter presents a survey of the morphology of biomaterials used in the fabrication of bioprosthetic cardiac valves. The basic cellular and extracellular components are described first, followed by a review of the morphologic features of biomaterials, and by a description of the changes that occur in these biomaterials as a result of various pre-implantation processes.

COMPONENTS OF BIOMATERIALS

Extracellular Elements of Connective Tissue

Collagens

The heterogeneous group of proteins collectively known as collagens are the major structural fibrous proteins of the body (1, 2). At least 12 different types of collagen are known to occur (3). These types differ in the biochemical and polypeptide chain composition and in the ability of these chains to aggregate into filaments or fibrils with or without a cross-banded appearance indicative of periodic subunits. Types I and III have certain structural similarities. They are the most abundant types of collagen in the body and are responsible for the tensile properties of tissues. Types I and III collagens form cross-banded fibrils that are visible on electron microscopic examination of the extracellular matrix in tissue sections and are responsible for the tensile properties of tissues. Types II, IX, X, and XI are found exclusively in cartilaginous tissues. Type IV collagen is present in basement membranes, in which it forms filaments that lack cross-banding and constitute the major structural scaffold. Types V and VI have been found in valves, blood vessels, and other tissues. The function of these types is unknown, although it has been suggested that type V either forms small fibrils or can be incorporated into larger fibrils of type I collagen (4, 5). Type VI is involved in the formation of small fibrils that differ from the microfibrils associated with elastic fibers. Type VII is present in the form of *anchoring fibrils,* structures that are located just beneath the epithelial cells in a variety of tissues (6). Type VIII is associated with vascular endothelium and with cornea. Types I and III constitute the most important types of collagens present in native cardiac valves and in the parietal pericardial tissue used in the fabrication of pericardial bioprosthetic valves. Type V collagen has also been identified in bovine heart valves (7). In addition,

The opinions or assertions about specific products identified by brand name contained herein are the private views of the authors and are not to be construed as conveying either an official endorsement or criticism by the U.S. Department of Health and Human Services, the National Institutes of Health, or the Food and Drug Administration.

porcine and bovine cardiac valves contain highly insoluble collagens that have not been fully characterized.

It was initially thought that type I and type III collagens formed different types of fibrils of homogeneous compositions, with those of type I being larger (from 50 to more than 100 nm in diameter) and those of type III being smaller (25 to 40 nm) (1, 2). The latter fibrils were believed to correspond to the reticular fibers that are demonstrable by silver staining methods used in light microscopy. However, recent data show that mixed fibrils containing both types of collagens can occur, and that the relative content of type III collagen determines the diameter of the resulting fibrils (8). Types II, V, IX, and XI collagen also have been reported to form mixed fibrils (4, 9). Therefore, the identification of collagen types in tissue sections depends on immunohistochemical methods rather than on measurements of the sizes of the fibrils. The collagen fibrils are associated with other proteins and with proteoglycans, which participate in the aggregation of collagen molecules into fibrils and also form interconnections between adjacent collagen fibrils. Thus, all these components are integrated into a complex network of connective tissue that provides tensile strength and maintains the shape of the tissue in which it occurs.

Each collagen fibril is composed of three precursor pro-α chains that are about 1000 amino acids long and are wound into a characteristic left-handed triple helix (2). The helical configuration of the chains gives the collagen molecule its highly stable, rigid, rodlike shape. The three polypeptide chains may be similar or different, depending on the type of collagen. A total of more than 20 different types of α chains have been identified among the various types of collagens. The amino acid glycine (Gly) is present at every third residue in the α chains, with a repeating Gly-X-Y sequence in which X and Y can be any amino acid, but most frequently proline and hydroxyproline, respectively. The two latter amino acids are present in large amounts in all collagen types and account for about 20% of their total amino acid composition. Hydroxyproline occurs in noncollagenous proteins to a very limited extent, and for this reason measurements of this amino acid can be used as an index of the collagen content of tissues. Most collagens also contain hydroxylysine, which is of importance in the formation of intramolecular and intermolecular cross-links of collagen, especially those induced by treatment with aldehyde fixatives used in the preparation of bioprosthetic valves (10). The hydroxylysine content of valvular collagen is higher than that of collagen in other vascular tissues or in the skin (7).

Collagen is synthesized in a precursor form known as protocollagen, which is composed of three precursor pro-α chains. Between the synthesis of the precursor pro-α chains and the formation of the mature collagen fibrils, a complex series of events must take place, including

1. hydroxylation of prolyl and lysyl residues,

2. glycosylation,

3. alignment of component α chains and triple-helix formation,

4. secretion from the cell into the extracellular environment in a nonfibrillar form,

5. selected proteolytic digestion of the procollagen molecule (this step requires at least two different enzymes and is a necessary prerequisite for the polymerization of procollagen fibrils),

6. fibril formation, and

7. cross-linking of fibrils, which gives them additional mechanical strength (2).

Types I and III collagen fibrils have typical cross-banding, which is due to the quarter-stagger arrangement of their individual collagen subunits. Collagen fibrils form parallel arrays, which usually are referred to as *collagen fibers* or *collagen bundles.* In most tissues, including heart valves, pericardium, and dura mater, the collagen fibrils and bundles are not completely straight but follow undulating or wavy courses. This arrangement, usually referred to as crimping, allows the tension-induced changes in the geometry of collagen-containing structures. Once this waviness is fully straightened out, however, the collagen fibrils are very intensible (11). Collagen fibers are strongly birefringent, due to their highly organized, periodic substructure, and can be visualized, even in intact valvular cusps, by polarized light microscopy (12).

Elastic Fibers

Elastic fibers are largely responsible for the elasticity of tissues. They have two biochemically and structurally distinct components: elastin and microfibrils (13, 14). The elastin forms the core of each elastic fiber, is structurally amorphous in conventional electron microscopic preparations, for which reason it is referred to as the *amorphous component,* and is responsible for the staining pattern seen on histologic study of tissue sections treated with selective stains for elastic fibers, such as the Weigert, Verhoeff, and Gomori methods. In electron micrographs of tissues fixed with glutaraldehyde, postfixed with osmium tetroxide, and stained with uranyl acetate and lead citrate, the elastin cores of elastic fibers usually appear either unstained or very lightly stained; however, these cores can be stained very darkly by other methods such as the tannic acid method, which has proved extremely useful for the study of bioprosthetic valvular tissue (15). The elastic fibers actually vary in shape from true cylindrical fibers, which measure less than 3 μm in diameter and are present in most tissues, to greatly flattened lamellae, which are usually fenestrated and are interconnected with adjacent lamellae, forming a continuous, tridimensional network.

The microfibrils surround the elastin cores and are well stained with uranyl acetate and lead citrate. They measure about 10 to 15 nm in diameter and often have clear, lucent centers that give them a tubular appearance. The microfibrils tend to decrease in number with increasing age and maturity of the elastic fibers, but they are not precursors of the elastin cores (14).

The elastin component of elastic fibers is a highly insoluble polymer of tropoelastin, a protein that is synthesized in the endoplasmic reticulum of various types of mesenchymal cells and is secreted into the extracellular space, where it undergoes polymerization. Tropoelastin differs markedly from collagen in its amino acid composition. It contains a high proportion of branched amino acids, including desmosine and isodesmosine, which appear to contribute to its property of elasticity. It also contains a number of lysyl residues that become converted into covalent cross-links when tropoelastin is polymerized in the extracellular space. The microfibrils contain large amounts of carbohydrate components, while elastin does not. The composition of microfibrils is uncertain. It is very difficult to distinguish morphologically between the microfibrillar component of elastic fibers and certain types of collagens (13, 14).

Proteoglycans

Proteoglycans are composed of glycosaminoglycans and proteins. The glycosaminoglycans are complex mucopolysaccharides (acid mucopolysaccharides) and are covalently linked to the protein portion by serine or threonine ester bonds. At least seven types of proteoglycans occur in mammalian tissues: hyaluronic acid, chondroitin-4-sulfate, chondroitin-6-sulfate, heparin, heparin sulfate, dermatan sulfate, and keratin sulfate. Each of these compounds is composed of repeating dissaccharide units, which contain one amino sugar (hexosamine) and one uronic acid sugar. The number of repeating disaccharide units in each chain of glycosaminoglycan varies from 10 to 60, except in hyaluronic acid, which may have as many as 2500 units. Because of these branched and elongated chains, the proteoglycans have a high viscosity in solution. They are important components of the extracellular matrix (ground substance). The acid residues in proteoglycans serve as the basis for their histochemical identification at the light microscopic level, using stains such as the colloidal iron and Alcian blue methods and various metachromatic dyes. In electron microscopic preparations many proteoglycans appear as star-shaped granules that measure from 20 to 50 nm in diameter. Many proteoglycans are highly soluble and are not retained in tissues prepared using routine fixation procedures. Similarly, they are largely lost during the manufacturing process of bioprosthetic heart valves. Because proteoglycans are closely associated with collagen fibrils, with which they are normally complexed, it is thought that the loss of proteoglycans predisposes bioprosthetic tissues to calcification after implantation. Furthermore, some proteoglycans, especially chondroitin sulfate, function naturally as inhibitors of calcification in connective tissue (16, 17).

Cellular Components of Biomaterials

The cellular components found in biomaterials used in the fabrication of prosthetic heart valves can be classified into two categories: lining cells and connective tissue cells. Lining cells are either endothelial cells, as in porcine aortic valves and in aortic and pulmonary allografts, or mesothelial cells, as in parietal pericardium. As discussed below, dura mater and fascia lata do not have a layer of lining cells. Both the mesothelial and endothelial lining cells play important roles as permeability barriers in living tissues; however, such cells are either lost by abrasion and autolysis or killed by chemical treatment during preimplantation processing. Thus, a continuous lining layer of cells is not present in most unimplanted biomaterials. Connective tissue cells present in biomaterials include fibroblasts, myofibroblasts, smooth muscle cells, and possibly undifferentiated mesenchymal cells, all of which represent normal tissue components responsible for the synthesis and turnover of connective tissue proteins. A well-developed layer of cardiac muscle cells is found in the right coronary cusp of the porcine aortic valve. These cells are an extension of ventricular septal muscle and are usually collectively referred to as the *muscle shelf*. In addition to the cells of graft origin that have just been mentioned, explanted biomaterials often contain cells of host origin that have infiltrated or relined the prosthetic tissue. Such cells include macrophages, platelets, leukocytes, and erythrocytes that become adherent to the surfaces of the graft, and connective tissue cells and endothelial cells that may form a distinct layer (fibrous sheath or fibrous peel) over the original surface of the implanted tissue (18).

STRUCTURE OF BIOMATERIALS

Aortic Valves

Porcine Aortic Valve

The most commonly used bioprosthetic valves (BPs) at the present time are porcine aortic valves (PAVs) that have been treated with low concentrations of glutaraldehyde to increase their durability, reduce their antigenicity, and ensure sterility. The PAV is composed of three cusps—namely, the left, the right, and the noncoronary cusp—the aortic valve annulus, and the aortic sinuses of Valsalva. The right coronary cusp is the largest and contains a layer of cardiac myocytes (muscle shelf). This layer, which represents an extension of ventricular septal muscle, may also be present in the left coronary cusp, but to a much smaller extent. Because of this muscle shelf, the right coronary cusp of the PAV tends to have a delayed or incomplete opening, particularly at low rates of flow. In addition, the cardiac myocytes in this cusp can become calcified after PAV implantation (18).

On histologic examination, three regions are identified in the PAV: the ventricularis, which faces the inflow surface (i.e., the ventricular side) of the valve; the spongiosa, which occupies the central region; and the fibrosa, which faces the outflow surface (i.e., the aortic side) (Fig. 3–1). The ventricularis contains collagen and much more abundant elastic fibers than do the other two layers. Most of the elastic fibers are oriented perpendicular to the free edge of the cusp. The collagen in the ventricularis has a multidirectional orientation. The spongiosa contains loosely arranged collagen and large amounts of proteoglycans. The spongiosa is thickest in the basal third of the valve; however, this layer disappears almost completely in the area near the free edge. The fibrosa contains densely packed collagen, much of which is arranged parallel to the free edge of the cusp, particularly in the form of prominent bundles (collagen chords). The chords progressively thicken as they approach the commissures and become anchored to the aortic root. The collagen fibrils in porcine aortic valves are relatively small in diameter (about 50 nm). In addition, small fibrils with poorly defined banding patterns and small diameters (10–20 nm) have been observed in aortic valves. These fibrils may represent unusual types of collagen (18).

The morphology of the bundles of collagen in the fibrosa varies according to the amount of pressure applied to the valve at the time of fixation. As expected, the cusps of PAVs fixed under conditions of low pressure are thicker and retain much more crimping, and their surfaces appear much more irregular and have more prominent chords (Figs. 3–1 and 3–2). The cuspal thickness and the prominence of the chords are reduced in PAVs that have undergone high-pressure fixation. This was the case with many models of PAVs that were fixed at a pressure of 60 to 80 mmHg to maintain the cusps in a fully closed configuration and to preserve the natural anatomic configuration of the aortic

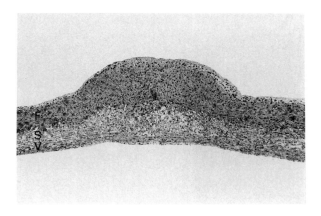

FIG. 3–1. Histologic section of an unimplanted low-pressure-fixed PAV bioprosthesis. Note the prominent collagen chord present on the outflow surface. Glycol methacrylate–embedded tissue, alkaline toluidine blue stain. (V) Ventricularis, (S) spongiosa, (F) fibrosa.

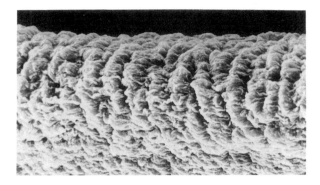

Fɪɢ. 3–2. Scanning electron micrograph of the free edge of a low-pressure-fixed PAV bioprosthesis. Note the retention of wavy, or crimped, collagen.

root. This largely eliminated the crimping of collagen (Fig. 3–3). Subsequently, it was
suggested, but not proved, that the durability of PAVs would be increased if they were
fixed at a pressure of just a few mmHg (low-pressure fixation) to maintain the crimping
of collagen. This crimping is thought to distribute the mechanical forces associated with
valvular opening and closure more evenly, thus minimizing the breakage of collagen
fibrils associated with repetitive bending forces (11, 18).

Both surfaces of the PAV are lined by a continuous layer of endothelial cells (Fig. 3–
4). On scanning electron microscopic study the surface features of these cells are readily
recognizable and include intercellular junctions, surface microvilli, single cilia, and
nuclear outlines. However, the endothelial cell layer becomes denuded as a result of preimplantation processing. The basement membrane of the endothelial lining is redupli-
cated in the outflow surface. The various layers of the PAV contain fibroblasts, undifferentiated mesenchymal cells, adipose tissue cells, myofibroblasts, and smooth muscle
cells, all of which can serve as loci in which calcification is initiated after implantation.
The connective tissue cells in cardiac valves form an interconnected network in which

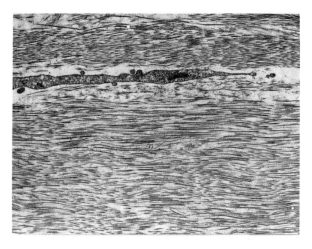

Fɪɢ. 3–3. Transmission electron micrograph depicting the loss of collagen crimp in the fibrosa of
a high-pressure-fixed PAV bioprosthesis. Uranyl acetate and lead citrate stain.

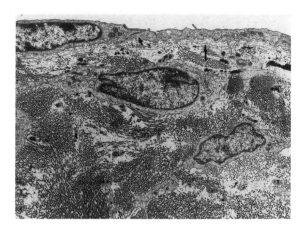

Fig. 3–4. Transmission electron micrograph of the outflow surface of a native PAV. Note the presence of an intact endothelial cell layer, a cell–cell junctional complex (arrowhead), and reduplication of basement membrane (arrow). Fibroblasts, collagen fibrils, and elastic fibers (stained black) are also present. Kajikawa stain.

the individual cells make intercellular contacts in the form of nexuses (gap junctions) located at the tips of their elongated cytoplasmic processes (19). The ability of connective tissue cells to produce extracellular proteins has been demonstrated by autoradiographic studies of amino acid incorporation (20).

Human Aortic Valve and Pulmonary Valve

The human pulmonary valve is thinner and more delicate than the human aortic valve, but histologic differences between these two valves are minimal. Both valves have the same three layers (ventricularis, spongiosa, and fibrosa) found in porcine aortic valves. The ventricularis (inflow side), which may be regarded as an extension of the ventricular endocardium, has prominent elastic fibers oriented perpendicular to the free edge of the cusp. It is thickened along the coaptation surface, forming a fibroelastic nodule in the center of the free edge (nodulus Arantii and nodulus Morgagni, aortic and pulmonary valves, respectively). The spongiosa consists of a matrix with loosely organized collagen fibers and abundant proteoglycans, in which fibroblasts, myofibroblasts, and poorly differentiated mesenchymal cells are embedded. The fibrosa is composed of collagen bundles oriented parallel to the free edge, fibroblasts, and a small number of elastic fibers. These elastic fibers may appear as a distinct layer, known as the arterialis, near the outflow surface in the basal region of the cusp. The cuspal surfaces are covered by a layer of endothelial cells. The human aortic and pulmonary valves do not contain a muscle shelf such as that present in procine aortic valves (21, 22).

Progressive morphologic changes occur in human aortic valves with increasing age. These changes are more common in men than in women and include degeneration of collagen fibers, the formation of a fibroelastic "spur" along the coaptation surface, a decrease in the numbers of fibroblasts and in proteoglycan content, and accumulation of lipid and calcific deposits (22, 23). For these reasons, donor criteria for allograft heart valves usually include an age restriction (<50 years) and lack of a medical history of previous cardiac surgery, uncontrolled hypertension, significant murmurs, rheumatic fever, malignant disease, and autoimmune or vascular diseases (24, 25) (Virginia Tissue Bank, Virginia Beach, Virginia, personal communication).

Parietal Pericardium

The majority of pericardial BPs are fabricated from bovine parietal pericardium, with the exception of the Polystan valve, in which porcine parietal pericardium is used (26). Pericardial BPs are most frequently configured into trileaflet valves; however, monocusp and bicuspid valves have also been designed (27–32).

Parietal pericardium is composed of three layers: a serosal layer, which consists of mesothelial cells, their basement membrane, and a narrow submesothelial space; the fibrosa, which contains collagen bundles, elastic fibers, nerves, blood vessels, and lymphatics; and the epipericardial connective tissue, which is composed of loosely arranged collagen and elastic fibers. Fibroblasts are present in the fibrosa and epipericardial connective tissue; a few histiocytes and mast cells are also seen. Clusters of adipose tissue cells are found, especially in the epipericardial connective tissue layer. In pericardial BPs the epipericardial tissue layer corresponds in orientation to the inflow surface, and the serosal layer to the outflow surface (Fig. 3–5). The epipericardial surface is extremely rough because of its content of large, coarse bundles of collagen (Fig. 3–6). At least some of these bundles represent transected fibers of the pericardiosternal ligament. The serosal surface is lined by mesothelial cells with numerous microvilli, which characteristically are much longer and numerous than those present in valvular endothelial cells. During preimplantation processing, the mesothelial cells are largely lost, and then the serosal surface appears smooth because it is composed of exposed basement membrane and underlying collagen fibrils (Fig. 3–7). Lastly, the free edge of the pericardial valve is formed by cutting the tissue (Fig. 3–8) (33). The collagen bundles in parietal pericardium are overlapping and multidirectional rather than highly oriented and layered. The waviness, or crimp, of the collagen bundles is more pronounced, and the mean diameter of the collagen fibrils is larger in parietal pericardium (about 100 nm) than in porcine aortic valves. Elastic fibers in pericardium are larger but less numerous than those in any of the

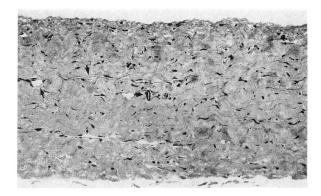

FIG. 3–5. Histologic section of an unimplanted bovine pericardial bioprosthetic leaflet. Note the rough inflow surface (bottom), the smooth outflow surface (top), and the presence of blood vessels (arrows). Compare with Fig. 3–1, unimplanted PAV bioprosthesis. Glycol methacrylate-embedded tissue, alkaline toluidine blue stain.

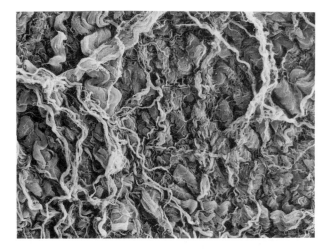

Fɪɢ. 3–6. Scanning electron micrograph of the rough inflow surface of an unimplanted bovine pericardial BP.

layers of porcine aortic valves (18). Biochemical studies have shown that 90% of the protein in bovine pericardium is collagen, mostly type I (34).

Dura Mater

Normal human dura mater is composed of two layers of fibrous tissue: an outer, or endosteal, layer, and an inner, or meningeal, layer. The outer layer contains large bundles of collagen and constitutes about two-thirds of the total thickness of the dura mater. About 50% of the bundles of collagen are oriented in the same direction; the other 50% are multidirectional. The inner layer is thinner and has smaller bundles of collagen.

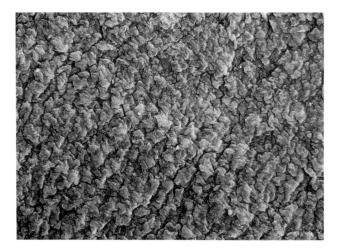

Fɪɢ. 3–7. Scanning electron micrograph of the smooth outflow surface of an unimplanted bovine pericardial BP.

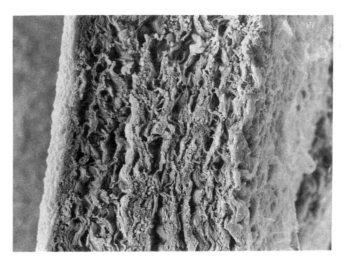

Fig. 3–8. Scanning electron micrograph of the free edge of an unimplanted bovine pericardial BP. Note that the free edge is composed of transected collagen bundles.

Many of these are arranged irregularly, often obliquely or at right angles to the main direction of the collagen fibers in the outer layer. In some areas, the two layers of dura mater are closely apposed; in other areas, they are separated by spaces of variable width. Some of these spaces are occupied by blood vessels or lymphatics; others are empty and represent areas of separation of adjacent collagen bundles. The collagen in both layers shows a considerable amount of waviness. Elastic fibers are small and few in both layers. As estimated by staining with Alcian blue, the content of proteoglycan material is very low in each of the two layers of dura mater. Cellular elements in dura mater are scarce and consist of elongated fibroblasts with spindle-shaped nuclei and scanty cytoplasm. Minute calcific deposits are occasionally present in the meningeal layer of the dura mater from older patients (our own unpublished observations).

On scanning electron microscopic examination, the endosteal (outer) surface of the dura mater differs from the meningeal (inner) surface with respect to the arrangement of the collagen fibrils. In the endosteal surface, the collagen fibrils are larger and wavier than those in the meningeal surface. In addition, the endosteal surface shows a pattern of ridges and grooves that correspond to the presence of vascular elements. The meningeal surface appears much flatter and smoother, and its collagen fibrils are less wavy and more parallel.

Transmission electron microscopic study confirms that collagen fibrils are the major component of both layers of dura mater. The diameters of these fibrils are large, ranging from 20 to 180 nm (average, 110 nm). The fibrils show the usual periodicity of collagen and are associated with only small amounts of filamentous material, which probably represents proteoglycans. Elastic fibers are roughly cylindrical and consist mainly of the amorphous (elastin) component, with few associated microfibrils. Elongated fibroblast-like cells that are rich in rough-surfaced endoplasmic reticulum and lack basement membranes are present in the dura mater connective tissue.

The calcific deposits in dura mater are composed of granular masses of electron-dense crystals that measure up to 70 nm in length and 20 nm in width. Some of these deposits are surrounded by single limiting membranes. The individual granules measure up to 3 μm in diameter and are present in extracellular locations, usually between normal-appearing collagen bundles, without any apparent relationship to other cellular or extracellular structures. We are not aware of studies on the biochemical characterization of the types of collagen in dura mater.

PREIMPLANTATION PROCESSING

Some type of preimplantation processing is given to all biomaterials used for fabrication of bioprosthetic heart valves and for implantation of allografts, as mentioned above. Such processing is necessary to reduce the antigenicity of the biomaterials, increase their durability, achieve sterility or disinfection, and reduce the rate of calcification. Three major types of technology have been independently developed for these purposes: aldehyde fixation, which is used for porcine aortic valves and for pericardial tissue; treatment with glycerol, which has been used only for dura mater valves, and various methods for sterilization, disinfection, and storage of allografts.

Aldehyde Fixation

Preimplantation processing of porcine valves and bovine parietal pericardium is initiated by rinsing the harvested tissues in saline, followed by fixation either of large pieces of parietal pericardium or of the entire porcine aortic root with a buffered glutaraldehyde solution. Glutaraldehyde, a dialdehyde, is used extensively as a primary fixative to prepare tissues for electron microscopic examination because of its ability to cross-link proteins. After fixation of the PAV, the aortic root is trimmed and the valve is mounted on a stent. As mentioned previously, the PAV can be fixed at low or high pressure. The pericardial tissue is fixed by immersion, without pressure or stretching. After fixation, pericardial tissue leaflets are cut and mounted on a stent. The prepared valves are then stored in formaldehyde solution until they are ready for use, when they are rinsed carefully to remove residual aldehydes, as these have been thought to induce tissue necrosis resulting in the production of a perivalvular leak in the valvular annulus in which the BP is implanted.

The shape of pericardial tissue as leaflets is maintained by packing cotton balls against the surfaces of the cusps, particularly the outflow surfaces. This procedure results in characteristic indentations on the cuspal surfaces and in adherence of cotton fibers to the pericardial surfaces, with entanglement of these fibers with the collagen bundles on the surfaces. After implantation, this leads to the eventual formation of minute foreign body granulomas on the surfaces of the BPs (33).

Glutaraldehyde and Its Reactions

The concentration of glutaraldehyde used for the processing of valves ranges from 0.2 to 0.6%; lower concentrations are ineffective sterilants, particularly against certain types of mycobacteria, and higher concentrations result in excessive stiffness of the tissue, as is the case with the 2.5% or higher concentrations of glutaraldehyde used for fixation for electron microscopy. The chemical aspects of fixation with glutaraldehyde solutions are complex (10, 35, 36). The conditions of fixation, including purity, concentration, temperature, and pH of the glutaraldehyde solution, and the time of exposure to this reagent, determine the type and extent of the resulting protein cross-links. Furthermore, at neutral pH, the molecules of glutaraldehyde in aqueous solutions tend to undergo a series of spontaneously occurring reactions involving changes in hydration of the glutaraldehyde as well as formation of several types of glutaraldehyde polymers. Thus, aqueous solutions of glutaraldehyde are complex, variable mixtures of free aldehyde, mono- and dehydrated monomeric glutaraldehyde, monomeric and polymeric cyclic hemiacetals formed by cyclization of dehydrated glutaraldehyde molecules, and various α,β-unsaturated polymers. In concentrated solutions (>25%) of glutaraldehyde, the hemiacetal component is the predominant form and can undergo polymerization; however, upon dilution these polymers revert to an equilibrium mixture of monomeric glutaraldehyde. Free glutaraldehyde can also polymerize to form α,β-unsaturated dimers, trimers, or larger polymers by aldol condensation reactions. These reactions increase with increasing time, pH, and concentration of the glutaraldehyde, and high-molecular-weight polymers of this type become insoluble in aqueous solutions. All these reactions that glutaraldehyde can undergo in solution may contribute to variations in the quality of the fixation. Monomeric glutaraldehyde can be separated from glutaraldehyde polymers by distillation or by purification with activated charcoal, but this has not been shown to result in clearly improved tissue fixation.

Glutaraldehyde reacts with amino groups, such as those in lysine, hydroxylysine, and NH_2-terminal amino acid residues in collagen, forming Schiff base, unsaturated addition reaction, and pyridinium types of products (cross-links) (10). It has been suggested that the type of cross-linking that occurs is dependent upon the glutaraldehyde concentration (35). Fixation of pericardial tissue with glutaraldehyde (0.05 to 5%, 15 min to 48 h exposure) results in a time-dependent intermolecular cross-linking requiring more time than would be expected if only the rate of penetration of glutaraldehyde was involved. As the glutaraldehyde concentration is increased, additional intermolecular cross-linking does not occur, but high-molecular-weight aldehyde polymers are formed on the surfaces of collagen fibers, at the initial lysyl reaction sites (36). The presence of a highly polymerized glutaraldehyde matrix on the surface of the collagen fiber may explain the slow penetration of this agent.

Collagen in glutaraldehyde-treated biomaterials is altered in comparison with that in the correspondent native tissues, as demonstrated by a reduction in tissue compliance, increased thermal stability (measured by the "shrinkage temperature"), and increased resistance to proteolytic enzyme digestion (10, 35–38). The number of demonstrable lysine and hydroxylysine residues is also decreased, as the result of irreversible reactions of many of these residues with glutaraldehyde.

Formaldehyde and Its Reactions

Formaldehyde is less effective than glutaraldehyde as a cross-linking agent. It reacts with primary amines in proteins to form hydroxymethyl-secondary amines. These can react with free amides to form cross-links that are unstable and capable of undergoing dissociation (10). Studies of the thermal stability of formaldehyde- versus glutaraldehyde-fixed PAVs indicate that formaldehyde-induced cross-links are initially stable but steadily dissociate following storage at 37°C in normal saline over a period of 10 months; however, glutaraldehyde-induced cross-links remain stable under these conditions (10). This may account for the increased durability of glutaraldehyde-treated BPs compared with formaldehyde-treated ones (39–44). The stability of glutaraldehyde-induced cross-links is not compromised by storage of the bioprostheses in formaldehyde.

Autolytic Changes Preceding Fixation

The fixation of pericardial and PAV tissue usually begins only several hours after the death of the animal at a slaughterhouse. The exact duration of this period of prefixation autolysis varies considerably, and its effects on the development of dehiscences or calcific deposits are unknown. In PAVs, it results in a variable, but usually considerable, degree of autolytic change, which is manifested by loss of proteoglycan material from the fibrosa and the ventricularis, partial or complete detachment of the endothelial cell layer (due to the fixation, this layer no longer has a function as a permeability barrier), and damage to organelles of the connective tissue cells (clumping of nuclear chromatin, cytoplasmic swelling, and formation of intramitochondrial amorphous inclusions). Comparable changes occur in pericardial tissue.

Glycerol Treatment

For the preparation of valves, the dura mater tissue is removed at necropsy, up to 20 h after death, from 10- to 50-year-old individuals. The tissue is then washed in water for 1 to 2 h and placed in 98% glycerol at room temperature for 10 to 20 days. The dura mater is then rehydrated in sterile saline for 5 to 10 min and cut into leaflets. These are mounted on the stent, and the valve is stored in glycerol. One day before use, the valves are placed at 4°C in a physiological electrolyte solution containing cephalothin, rifampin, and amphotericin B (45). Glycerol-treated dura mater is almost transparent but becomes opaque white when rehydrated.

The changes induced in the collagen in dura mater by glycerol treatment probably involve a combination of effects, including dehydration, extraction of tissue components, chemical denaturation by glycerol, and fixation by aldehydes present as impurities. Glycerol treatment results in increased durability of dura mater valves, in contrast to that of untreated dura mater valves (45). Nevertheless, implanted dura mater valves develop tears and calcific deposits (44) that resemble those observed in PAVs and pericardial BPs, and their use has decreased sharply (46, 47). The transmission of Creutzfeldt-Jakob disease has also been implicated with the use of cadaveric human dura mater (48). The potential for the transmission of this and other virus-related neurologic disorders may further limit the use of dura mater in BPs.

Anticalcification Treatments

The cusps of porcine, pericardial, and dura mater BPs develop calcific deposits after implantation as substitute cardiac valves in animals (34, 49–53) and patients (17, 54–56). Calcific deposits are the most important single factor resulting in altered hemodynamic performance of BPs (57, 58) because of their tendency to produce cuspal stenosis as well as cuspal tears. Calcification mainly involves devitalized cells, collagen fibrils, and microthrombi (53, 59). The calcification of BPs initially involves the devitalized organelles, such as mitochondria and nuclei, of connective tissue cells (60), and it has been suggested that the phospholipids in the membranes of these structures serve as nucleation

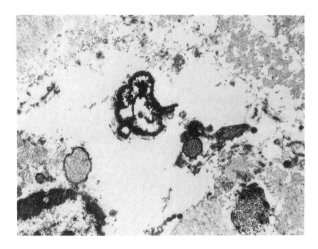

Fɪɢ. 3–9. Transmission electron micrograph illustrating membrane-associated calcification occurring in a devitalized cell. Uranyl acetate and lead citrate.

sites for calcification (Fig. 3–9). However, collagen fibrils rapidly become the most important sites of calcification of BPs. Ultrastructural studies have disclosed three distinct patterns of collagen fibril calcification: calcification of the fibrils, calcification restricted to the surfaces of the fibrils, and calcification limited to the space between the fibrils (Fig. 3–10) (59). The significance of these patterns is unclear.

Pathogenesis of Calcific Deposits

A high risk of developing calcification of implanted BPs has been found in children and young adults, patients with chronic renal disease or hyperparathyroidism (complex metabolic factors in these groups favor deposition of calcium and phosphates in tissues),

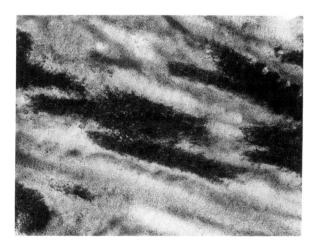

Fɪɢ. 3–10. Transmission electron micrograph showing collagen fibril calcification, which is frequently observed in explanted PAV and bovine pericardial BPs. Uranyl acetate and lead citrate stain.

and patients with infected BPs (both the vegetations and the bacteria themselves calcify rapidly) (61–72). Tissue-related factors are also thought to be of importance in the pathogenesis of BP calcification. Included among these are (1) preimplantation treatment of biomaterials with aldehyde fixatives, (2) the use of phosphate buffer in preimplantation solutions, (3) the loss of proteoglycans during preparation of the tissues, (4) the presence of free hydroxyl groups and of calcium-binding carboxylated amino acids in tissues, and (5) the amount of time elapsed between the initial aldehyde fixation and the actual implantation of the BP. It is not known whether autolysis caused by delays in harvesting and fixing tissues has an influence on the development of calcification, or whether inadequate fixation is the cause of immune reactions against the implanted material.

Subcutaneous implantation studies showed that type I collagen sponges that had been either untreated or exposed briefly (15 min) to formaldehyde vapor did not calcify and were resorbed, while sponges fixed by immersion in glutaraldehyde did calcify and were not resorbed (73). These studies were interpreted as indicating that aldehyde fixation increases the tendency of biomaterials to calcify. Other subcutaneous implantation studies also showed that glutaraldehyde-treated pericardium calcified more than did untreated pieces of pericardium (74, 75); however, the degree of cross-linking induced by glutaraldehyde fixation did not have a clear relationship to the extent of calcification. Furthermore, glutaraldehyde fixation did not increase the amount of calcification of pieces of human dura mater implanted subcutaneously in rats (75). Thus, the relationship of glutaraldehyde cross-linking to calcification of collagen remains unclear, particularly because the reabsorption of unfixed tissues, but not of fixed tissues, tends to make comparisons between the two situations very difficult. The use of HEPES buffer instead of phosphate buffer in preimplantation processing has been recommended to reduce calcification, on the assumption that phosphate can become bound to the tissue and then promote calcium binding. Similarly, the loss of collagen-associated proteoglycans is thought to lead to uncovering of sites that could bind first phosphate and then calcium to the collagen molecules. It is for this reason that a preimplantation procedure involving an esterification reaction to block these residues was suggested as a means of mitigating calcification of BPs.

Another factor that must be considered in the pathogenesis of calcific deposits in biomaterials is the presence of calcium-binding proteins in tissues, including BPs, that are undergoing calcification (52, 53, 76–81). These proteins are probably derived from plasma and penetrate into the valvular biomaterials. The affinity of these proteins for calcium is due to their content of carboxylated amino acids such as γ-carboxyglutamic acid and aminomalonic acid. Both these have been detected in high amounts in extracts of calcified PAVs and in human aortic valves with dystrophic calcification, compared with noncalcified BPs (76–81). These amino acids are formed by posttranslational or postribosomal carboxylation involving a vitamin K–dependent reaction (82) after the proteins are synthesized in the endoplasmic reticulum. It is not known whether these proteins initiate calcification (by binding to tissue and then trapping calcium) or only increase it (by binding to calcium already present in the tissue and then trapping more calcium). Because this reaction is vitamin K–dependent, it has been suggested that BP calcification may be decreased by the administration of vitamin K antagonists (coumarin anticoagulants) (83, 84). Recently, subcutaneous implantation studies in rats were reported to show that PAVs stored in 0.2% glutaraldehyde for 12 to 40 months developed less calcification than did PAVs stored for shorter periods of time (85). This study concluded that the time elapsed (shelf life) between initial tissue fixation and BP implantation influences the extent of calcification; however, review of the results of intracardiac implantation in sheep indicated that the degree of calcification of PAVs and pericardial BPs is not influenced by the shelf-life of the BP (51).

Mitigation of Calcification by Surfactants

The clinical importance of the calcific deposits developing in BPs has served as a stimulus for research on methods to minimize this complication. Experimental studies, based on the work by Urist and colleagues in the 1950s on the inhibition of calcification of bone and cartilage, have shown that preimplantation treatment with surfactants, such as polysorbate and sodium dodecyl sulfate, decreases the calcification of BP leaflets implanted subcutaneously (84, 86) and of BPs used as substitute cardiac valves in experimental animals (50, 51, 86). These compounds are applied to the biomaterials after glutaraldehyde fixation, usually in association with treatment with ethanol and propanol.

In subcutaneous and intramuscular implantation studies, other anionic surfactants, such as decane sulfonic acid, dodecylbenzene sulfonic acid, maypon, N-lauroyl sarcosine, and deoxycholic acid, also mitigated calcification of PAVs and pericardial BPs, as did Triton X-100, a neutral surfactant. Cationic surfactants such as decyltrimethyl ammonium bromide, hexadecyltrimethyl ammonium bromide, and trimethylphenyl ammonium bromide had no effect. These agents retard the time course of the calcification process (which seems to eventually reach a certain point of saturation), so that at a few weeks after implantation the total amount of calcium is reduced in the treated implants. However, in the case of all agents except Triton X-100, the amount of calcium rises gradually, and several months after implantation it reaches levels comparable to those found at a few weeks in control (untreated) tissues. In valves implanted in the mitral and tricuspid positions of sheep for 10 to 52 weeks, the polysorbate and sodium dodecyl sulfate processes reduce the calcification that develops in PAVs, but not in pericardial BPs (50, 51, 87) (Table 3–1). The reason for this difference is unknown.

The mechanism by which preimplantation surfactant treatment of PAVs reduces cal-

TABLE 3–1. *Calcium Content of Valves Treated with Anticalcification Agents*

Valve type*	n	mg Ca/g tissue dry weight, (mean ± SEM)
Standard PAVs (controls for polysorbate-80 and Triton X-100 + N-lauryl sarcosine)	22	99.8 ± 11.1
Polysorbate-80-treated PAVs	15	7.6 ± 2.6 ($P < .001$)
Triton X-100 plus N-lauryl sarcosine–treated PAVs	14	12.7 ± 3.8 ($P < .001$)
Standard BPVs (controls for polysorbate-80)	18	73.1 ± 10.3
Polysorbate-80-treated BPVs	11	55.2 ± 12.7
Standard BPVs (polyacrylamide controls)†	10	66.1 ± 15.5
Polyacrylamide-treated BPVs†	8	112.9 ± 15.3 ($P < .05$)
Standard PAVs (sodium dodecyl sulfate controls)	28	64.7 ± 9.6
Sodium doecyl sulfate–treated BPVs	24	117.7 ± 5.3
Standard BPVs (diphosphonate controls)	17	104.3 ± 9.1
Diphosphonate (ADP)–treated BPVs	12	126.6 ± 7.3 ($P < .07$)
Standard PAVs (toluidine blue controls)	17	139.3 ± 14.7
Toluidine blue–treated PAVs	21	81.6 ± 12.0 ($P < .05$)

*PAVs = porcine aortic valves; BPVs = bovine pericardial valves.

†Implanted in the tricuspid position; all other valves implanted in the mitral position.

cification is unclear; however, promoters of calcification such as phospholipids and proteins containing carboxylated amino acids may be affected by these processes (84, 88), resulting in a decrease of calcium-binding constituents within the cusps. It has been suggested that surfactants affect the membrane surface charge, the ground substance, or the collagen fibrils (86); that they extract phospholipids from valvular tissue (50); and that they form a hydrophobic barrier to the penetration of phospholipids from the blood into valvular tissue (84). Although there is no direct evidence to support these hypotheses at the present time, morphologic studies have shown that decreased calcification of collagen fibrils is the major change observed in explanted PAVs that had undergone preimplantation surfactant treatments (50, 51).

Alterations Induced in Bioprosthetic Tissues by Surfactants

In addition to their anticalcification effects, surfactants can alter the properties of bioprosthetic tissues, perhaps by extracting some tissue components and thereby compromising their durability. Bodnar et al. showed that sodium dodecyl sulfate produced severe alterations in the morphology of collagen in unfixed valvular tissue, in that it caused unraveling of the fibrils, although this effect was not evident in glutaraldehyde-fixed collagen (88a). This effect was similar to that produced by treatment of unfixed collagen with highly concentrated solutions of urea or guanidine, agents that disturb the tertiary structure of proteins. In our experience, polysorbate and sodium dodecyl sulfate treatments do not alter the durability of BPs implanted in the mitral position in sheep for 20 weeks. However, PAVs treated with Triton X-100 and N-lauroyl sarcosine and implanted in the sheep model for 20 weeks showed frequent cuspal tears and perforations (Fig. 3–11) (87). These results are in contrast with those of "in vitro stability tests" (84), which gave normal results in tissues treated with these agents. Thus, because of the powerful effects of surfactants on protein structure, it is necessary to evaluate the effects of these agents not only on the process of calcification, but also on the long-term mainte-

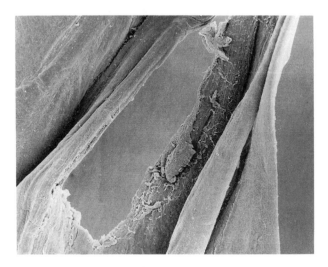

FIG. 3–11. Scanning electron micrograph of a PAV cuspal perforation that was observed in a BP that had undergone anticalcification treatment with Triton X-100 plus N-lauryl sarcosine following 20 weeks of implantation (mitral position) in sheep.

nance of normal cuspal structure. It appears inadvisable to apply these reagents to unfixed tissues.

Diphosphonates

The systemic administration of diphosphonates (pyrophosphate analogs) reduces the amount of calcification that occurs in BP leaflets implanted subcutaneously in animals (89, 90). Diphosphonates form complexes with calcium, resulting in a localized reduction in extracellular calcium, and also interfere with the formation of hydroxyapatite crystals (91–93). However, the systemic use of diphosphonates is severely limited by their adverse effects on growth and calcification of bone (89, 94). These effects have been minimized by local administration of the diphosphonate in close proximity to the subcutaneously implanted tissue (94–96). Encouraging initial results have been obtained by the cardiac implantation of valves in which slow-release pellets of diphosphonates have been placed in the sewing ring (97). No anticalcification benefit could be demonstrated in sheep after intracardiac implantation of pericardial BPs in which aminohydroxypropane diphosphonic acid had been covalently bound to the tissue (87). It is possible that these results are a consequence of an instability of the covalent bonding of the diphosphonates to the tissues.

Other Anticalcification Treatments

A number of other anticalcification treatments have been developed, including blocking potential calcium-binding sites in collagen with compounds such as magnesium chloride, toluidine blue, and leuco toluidine blue (84, 86, 98, 99); chemical modification by means of esterification (100); charge modification using protamine sulfate (101); formation of a copolymer of collagen and polyacrylamide (which was thought to prevent phospholipid penetration into the PAV cusp) (84); and decreasing the available calcium by local administration of phosphocitrate (102). All these treatments have been effective following subcutaneous or intramuscular implantation in small animals; however, only the toluidine blue and polyacrylamide incorporation methods have been tested in large-animal models.

Polyacrylamide incorporation into leaflets was found to mitigate BP calcification when evaluated by subcutaneous implantation in rabbits; however, this effect was lost if the treated BPs were mechanically cycled (i.e., pulse duplicator performance testing) before implantation (84). A protective effect of polyacrylamide could not be demonstrated after intracardiac implantation in calves or sheep (84, 87).

Toluidine blue treatment also resulted in a reduction in leaflet calcification following intramuscular implantation in rats (86), but not after intracardiac implantation in calves (86) or sheep (87). However toluidine blue lost its effectiveness as an anticalcification agent after 12 weeks of intramuscular implantation. It would appear that the binding of toluidine blue to glutaraldehyde-treated tissues is reversible, as is the staining of tissues with this dye (86).

The discrepancies in the results obtained when BP anticalcification treatments are evaluated by subcutaneous implantation in small animals and by intracardiac implantation in sheep may be related to long-term instability of the interaction between glutaraldehyde-treated tissue and the anticalcification agent, to the presence or absence of direct contact between the BP and the blood, and to the physiologic and mechanical differences associated with intracardiac versus subcutaneous or intramuscular implantation. Therefore, data from subcutaneous implantation experiments should be regarded only as general screening results and should not be extrapolated to predict the effectiveness of anticalcification treatments following cardiac valve replacement.

Preimplantation Processing of Human Aortic and Pulmonary Valve Allografts

Human aortic and pulmonary valve allografts are not usually treated with aldehyde fixatives or with anticalcification agents. Instead, they undergo sterilization or disinfection, and in some instances cryopreservation, to maintain the viability of the cells in the grafts. The long-term clinical performance of allografts is influenced by the methods used for preimplantation processing and storage (24, 103–117).

Allograft Sterilization

Allograft disinfection or sterilization has been accomplished by exposure to ethylene oxide gas; immersion in solutions containing glutaraldehyde, formaldehyde, β-propiolactone or antibiotics; and γ or electron beam irradiation. Ideally, the method selected for sterilization should not alter the morphology or the mechanical properties of the allograft. The mechanical properties of the valves are altered by aldehydes, ethylene oxide, and β-propiolactone, but not by low levels of γ or electron beam irradiation or by antibiotics (112, 118). An increased rate of cusp rupture has been reported to occur in allografts treated with ethylene oxide or β-propiolactone (23, 119). In addition to a reduction in tensile strength, β-propiolactone sterilization induces cuspal thickening and shrinkage (118), thus predisposing allografts to regurgitation. β-Propiolactone and ethylene oxide are carcinogenic (120). Sterilization methods using exposure to low doses of radiation or high concentrations of antibiotics do not alter the geometry of the cusps but result in loss of cell viability. This loss is minimized by treatment with low concentrations of several antibiotics, such as gentamicin, lincomycin, colistimethate, kanamycin, cefoxitin, vancomycin, polymyxin B, and amphotericin.

It is necessary to point out that the "sterilization" of bioprosthetic heart valves either with aldehydes or with antibiotics actually consists of a high-level disinfection process, and that the effectiveness of such treatments against viral agents, e.g., retroviruses, slow viruses, has not been established (121). This is a particular concern with dura mater tissue, which has been suspected of being involved in the transmission of Creutzfeldt-Jakob disease, a slow virus infection of the central nervous system.

Allograft Storage

Lyophilization (freeze-drying), immersion in antibiotic-containing solutions, and freezing have all been employed as methods of allograft storage (104, 115, 116, 122–125). The results of short-term implantation in animals suggest that the performance of fresh and lyophilized valves is comparable (104, 121); however, the mechanical durability of collagen seems to be decreased by the lyophilization process. This would account for the cuspal ruptures that have been reported to occur in regions of high bending stress, either at the cusp–aortic wall junction or at the free edge near a commissure, in lyophilized allografts implanted for long times in patients (104, 118, 126). Lyophilized allografts have also been reported to be more susceptible to calcification, although great variability has been observed in this regard (127). The majority of the allografts currently in clinical use are either stored in nutrient solutions with antibiotics at 4°C or are cryopreserved, frozen, and subsequently stored in liquid nitrogen vapor (24, 111, 114, 116).

Cellular Viability in Allografts

Storage in antibiotics is effective and does not affect the mechanical properties or the morphology of collagen or elastin (109, 128); however, whether the allograft is stored in antibiotics, Hanks' balanced salt solution, or nutrient media, the number of viable cells decreases markedly as the storage time increases from 1 to 4 weeks (108). Recent studies of explanted valves (24, 114) have concluded that cell viability is retained after implantation in allografts prepared using contemporary techniques of cryopreservation (prompt harvesting, exposure to less toxic antibiotics, reduced storage time in nutrient media); however, this is in contrast to previous investigations (109, 116) that concluded that allograft viability was lost under different conditions of harvesting and storage (including exposure to high concentrations of antibiotics and prolonged storage in media).

A detailed assessment has not yet been made of the extent of the distribution and biosynthetic activity of viable cells within explanted allografts that have undergone pre-implantation processing by new cryopreservation methods that maximize cell survival. As the initial step in this evaluation, we have examined preimplantation changes in human pulmonary valves that were harvested within 24 h of death, stored in tissue culture media on ice for <32 h, sterilized with antibiotics (24 h at 37°C or 48 h at 4°C), placed in nutrient media containing 10% dimethyl sulfoxide, control-rate frozen (1°C/min) to −40°C, and stored in liquid nitrogen vapor (−150 to −190°C). In these valves, we observed a normal extent and magnitude of collagen crimping within the fibrosa and collagen chords of the cusps. At less than 9 h postmortem, there was patchy loss of endothelial cells on the cuspal surfaces of unprocessed valves. Additional losses of endothelial cells followed antibiotic treatment, cryopreservation, and freezing and thawing. Remaining endothelial cells often assumed a plump appearance. Proteoglycans were also progressively lost during preimplantation processing. During collection and processing, the cuspal connective tissue cells developed a spectrum of alterations, including cellular and mitochondrial swelling; dilation of endoplasmic reticulum; degranulation of rough endoplasmic reticulum; mitochondrial flocculent densities; autophagic and hydropic vacuoles; nuclear pyknosis, karyorrhexis, and karyolysis; lipid accumulation; and disruption of organelle and plasma membranes. The longer the time elapsed before preimplantation processing was initiated, the greater the extent of cellular injury observed in the allograft. Alterations such as cellular and mitochondrial swelling, dilation of the endoplasmic reticulum, hydropic vacuoles, and lipid accumulation are considered to be reversible changes, but damage to membranes and nuclear alterations are indicative of irreversible damage (129). Factors such as cell type, degree of differentiation, and level of metabolic activity have been reported to predispose cells to cellular injury (129), and our study suggests that metabolically active cells, such as endothelial cells and cardiac myocytes, are more sensitive to irreversible cellular injury resulting from allograft preimplantation processing than are connective tissue cells and macrophages. Although variable degrees of cell damage and death are found in cryopreserved pulmonary allografts, some cells appear to survive preimplantation processing and may remain viable following implantation of these valves (Fig. 3–12). It is not known whether the denuded surfaces of cryopreserved

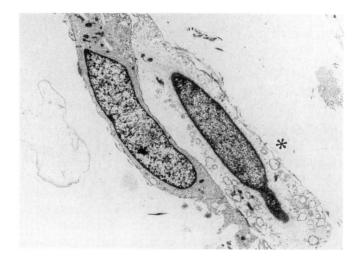

Fɪɢ. 3–12. Transmission electron micrograph depicting two fibroblasts in a cryopreserved pulmonary valve allograft. One of the cells (asterisk) has undergone irreversible cell injury. Uranyl acetate and lead citrate stain.

allografts are relined by surviving endothelial cells of donor origin or by cells of host origin (as are xenografts).

Mounting

The mounting of bioprosthetic tissues on supporting structures, known as *stents,* constitutes a most important aspect of the technology of prosthetic heart valves. All currently available BPs are mounted on either rigid or flexible stents. The flexibility of different types of "flexible" stents varies greatly. The main advantage of flexible stents is their contribution to the dissipation of mechanical forces that can lead to leaflet damage.

Stents

Stents are composed of an outer sewing ring; a ringlike structural frame with three stent posts or struts, which provide anchoring for the commissures; and a covering layer of cloth (usually Dacron or Teflon). In rigid stents the frame is composed of metal; in flexible stents it is made of synthetic polymer or thin metal wire that allows for a slight bending motion of the stent posts during cuspal opening and closing. Practically all BPs are trileaflet valves, regardless of the position in which they are implanted. Thus, they correspond anatomically to semilunar valves, rather than to atrioventricular valves. However, the sewing rings usually vary in shape and size according to whether the BP is to be implanted in the semilunar or the atrioventricular position, to conform to the different techniques of surgical insertion (i.e., from the outflow or the inflow side, respectively) in these two positions.

The stents of BPs are not expansile, as are the native valve annuli. Therefore, stented BPs do not undergo the same cyclic changes (systolic expansion, diastolic contraction, and a systolic outward deflection of the commissures) as do the annulus and cusps of native aortic valves. Because of this, the mechanical forces exerted on the leaflets during opening and closing are greater and less evenly distributed in BPs than in native valves (130–134).

Stents for PAVs

When the *native* PAV is completely open, the valvular ring expands, its orifice is circular in shape and the cusps are flat, under tension, and at constant length (132, 134). When the *mounted* PAV opens, the shape of its orifice may be circular or some variation of a circular form, depending upon specific conditions of pressure and flow (132). These shapes result from a reversal of curvature of the cusps as they open and close in a nonexpansile stent (131). The mechanical forces associated with this reversal of curvature lead to gradual mechanical breakage of the collagen fibrils in the cusps. This mechanical fragmentation may also predispose the collagen to hydrolytic breakdown. Since the cusps of BPs do not have any mechanisms of tissue repair (their cells having been killed by preimplantation processing), this breakage of collagen fibrils can eventually cause tissue dehiscence and tears (135). These were relatively frequent in early models of PAVs, which were mounted on rigid stents (41–43). To dissipate the stresses associated with cuspal motion, particularly during cuspal closure, flexible stents were introduced, and a cloth bias strip (buttress) is sewn over the PAV–stent interface to reduce the stresses that would otherwise be applied to the tissue at this site (136, 137).

Continuing modifications have been made in the design of stents for PAVs, including changes in the technique of mounting tissue on the stent (e.g., mounting the PAV higher on the stent increases the effective orifice size), the configuration of the metal or plastic stent material, the height of the stent posts, and the materials contained within the sewing ring (138, 139). To increase the effective orifice area of the PAV, a modified orifice valve has been fabricated (140) by removing the right coronary cusp (which contains the muscle shelf) and replacing it by a non–muscle shelf cusp from another aortic valve. This BP has had limited clinical use (140). Effective orifice size is also increased by curetting part of the muscle shelf and incorporating the remainder into the sewing ring. Supraannular valves have also been fabricated with a sewing ring that has a scalloped configuration resembling that of the native aortic root (141).

Flexible Stents

Two general types of flexible stents have been designed. Of these, the most commonly used is a stent with a rigid inlet and with posts that undergo some degree of outward motion during valve opening and inward motion during valve closure (136, 138). The second type is a stent made of thin wire configured such that it allows for expansion and contraction of the inflow orifice as well as for radial deflections of the stent posts (139). The long-term durability of BPs with the latter stent design has not been assessed.

The materials used to fabricate flexible stents range from polypropylene and polyacetal resin to metal wire. Ideally, the stent material should be resistant to fatigue induced by cyclic bending (to avoid stent fracture) and should undergo minimal plastic deformation (creep). Progressive inward deflection of polypropylene stent posts has resulted from creep, external compression of oversized valves, and tissue ingrowth into the stent cloth (142–145).

Stents for Pericardial Valves

Pericardial valves have been constructed with rigid and with flexible stents (146). Considerations of stent design for pericardial valves have been complicated by the difficulties encountered in the attachment of the pericardial tissue leaflets to the stent posts. In some pericardial valves this attachment is accomplished by an alignment suture placed near the top of the stent posts. This creates an area of localized high mechanical stress (as well as a hole in the tissue) that leads to tissue tears near the commissures of pericardial BPs (147–149). These tears are relatively frequent in pericardial BPs, particularly in those implanted in the mitral position (150–155). Pericardial BPs have also developed perforations secondary to abrasions caused by contact, during leaflet opening and closing, between pericardial tissue and either the cloth covering the stent rail (i.e., the portion of the stent between two stent posts) or a fabric buttress placed on the outside of the stent post (148).

REFERENCES

1. Miller EJ, Gray S: The collagens: An overview and update. Meth Enzymol. 1987;144:3–41.
2. Nimini ME, Harkness RD: Molecular structure and functions of collagen. In Nimini N (ed): Collagen: Biochemistry, Biotechnology and Molecular Biology. Boca Raton FL, CRC Press, 1988, pp 1–77.
3. Dublet B, van der Rest M: Type XII collagen is expressed in embryonic chick tendons. J Biol Chem 1987;262:17724–17727.
4. Birk DE, Fitch JM, Babiarz JP, Linsenmayer TF: Collagen type I and type V are present in the same fibril in the avian corneal stroma. J Cell Biol 1988;106:999–1008.
5. Linsenmayer TF, Fitch JM, Schmid TM, Zak NB, Gibney E, Sanderson RD, Mayne R: Monoclonal antibodies against chicken type V collagen: Production, specificity, and use for immunocytochemical localization in embryonic cornea and other organs. J Cell Biol 1983;96:124–132.
6. Burgeson RE, Morris NP, Murray LW, Duncan KG, Keene DR, Sakai LY: The structure of type VII collagen. In Fleischmajer R, Olsen BR, Kuhn K (eds): Biology, Chemistry and Pathology of Collagen. Ann NY Acad Sci 1985;460:47–57.
7. Bashey RI, Jimenez SA: Collagen in heart valves. In Nimni N (ed): Collagen: Biochemistry, Biotechnology and Molecular Biology. Boca Raton, CRC Press, 1988, pp 257–274.
8. Keene DR, Sakai LY, Bachinger HP, Burgeson RE: Type III collagen can be present on banded collagen fibrils regardless of fibril diameter. J Cell Biol 1987;105:2393–2402.
9. Mendler M, Eich-Bender SG, Vaughan L, Winterhalter KH, Bruckner P: Cartilage contains mixed fibrils of collagen II, IX, and XI. J Cell Biol 1989;108:191–197.
10. Woodroof EA: The chemistry and biology of aldehyde treated tissue heart valve xenografts. In Ionescu MI (ed): London, Butterworths, 1979, pp 347–362.
11. Broom ND, Thomson FJ: Influence of fixation conditions on the performance of glutaraldehyde-treated porcine aortic valves: Towards a more scientific basis. Thorax 1979;34:166–176.
12. Hilbert SL, Ferrans VJ, Swanson WM: Optical methods for the nondestructive evaluation of collagen morphology in bioprosthetic heart valves. J Biomed Mater Res 1986;20:1411–1421.
13. Rosenbloom J: Elastin: An overview. Meth Enzymol 1987;144:172–196.
14. Pasquali-Ronchetti I, Formieri C: The ultrastructural organization of the elastic fibre. In Ruggeri A, Motta PM (eds): Ultrastructure the connective tissue matrix. Boston, Nijhoff, 1984, pp 126–139.
15. Kajikawa K, Yamaguchi T, Katsuda S, Miwa A: An improved electron stain for elastic fibers using tannic acid. J Electron Microsc 1975;24:287–289.
16. Thyberg CJO: Electron microscopy of proteoglycans. In Ruggeri A, Motta PM (eds): Ultrastructure of the Connective Tissue Matrix. Boston, Nijhoff, 1984, pp 95–112.
17. Ferrans VJ, Spray TL, Billingham ME, Roberts WC: Structural changes in glutaraldehyde-treated porcine heterografts used as substitute cardiac valves. Transmission and scanning electron microscopic observations in 12 patients. Am J Cardiol 1978;41:1159–1184.
18. Ferrans VJ, Hilbert SL, Tomita Y, Jones M, Roberts WC: Morphology of collagen in bioprosthetic heart valves. In Nimni M (ed): Collagen. Boca Raton FL, CRC Press, 1988, vol. 3, pp 145–189.
19. Filip DA, Radu A, Simionescu M: Interstitial cells of the heart valve possess characteristics similar to smooth muscle. Circ Res 1986;59:310–320.
20. Deck JD, Thubrikar WJ, Schneider PJ, Nolan SP: Structure, stress and tissue repair in aortic valve leaflets. Cardiovasc Res 1988;22:7–16.

21. Ferrans VJ, Thiedemann KU: Ultrastructure of the normal heart. In Silver MD (ed): Cardiovascular Pathology. New York, Churchill Livingston, 1983, pp 31–86.
22. Gross L, Kugel MA: Topographic anatomy and histology of the valves in the human heart. Am J Pathol 1931;7:445–473.
23. Smith JC: The pathology of human aortic valve homografts. Thorax 1967;22:114–138.
24. O'Brien MF, Strafford EG, Gardner MAH, Pohler PG, McGiffin DC: A comparison of aortic valve replacement with viable cryopreserved and fresh allograft valves, with a note on chromosomal studies. J Thorac Cardiovasc Surg 1987;94:812–823.
25. Sell S, Scully RE: Aging changes in the aortic and mitral valves. Histologic and histochemical studies, with observations on the pathogenesis of calcific aortic stenosis and calcification of the mitral annulus. Ann J Pathol 1965;46:345–365.
26. Polystan Bioprostheses Information Bulletins BPA, BPC, BPD, BPE, BPF, and BP1. Copenhagen, Polystan A/S, 1980.
27. Ionescu MI (ed): Tissue Heart Valves. London, Butterworths, 1979.
28. Cohn LH, Gallucci V (eds): Cardiac Bioprostheses. New York, Yorke, 1982.
29. Bodnar E, Yacoub M (eds): Biologic and Bioprosthetic Valves. New York, Yorke, 1986.
30. Gabbay S, Frater RWM: The unileaflet heart valve bioprosthesis: New concept. In Cohn LH, Gallucci V (eds): Cardiac Bioprostheses. New York, Yorke, 1982, pp 411–424.
31. Bodnar E, Bowden NL, Drury PJ, Olsen EGJ, Durmaz I, Ross DN: Biscuspid mitral bioprosthesis. Thorax 1981;36:45–51.
32. Black MM, Drury PJ, Tindale WB, Lawford PV: The Sheffield bicuspid valve: Concept, design and in vitro and in vivo assessment. In Bodnar E, Yacoub M (eds): Biologic and Bioprosthetic Valves. New York, Yorke, 1986, pp 709–717.
33. Ishihara T, Ferrans VJ, Jones M, Boyce SW, Roberts WC: Structure of bovine parietal pericardium and of unimplanted Ionescu-Shiley pericardial valvular bioprostheses. J Thorac Cardiovasc Surg 1981;81:747–757.
34. Schoen FJ, Tsao JW, Levy RJ: Calcification of bovine pericardium used in cardiac valve bioprostheses: Implicated for the mechanism of bioprosthetic tissue mineralization. Am J Pathol 1986;123:134–145.
35. Cheung DT, Perelman N, Ko EC, Nimni ME: Mechanism of crosslinking of proteins by glutaraldehyde: III. Reaction with collagen in tissues. Connect Tissue Res 1985;13:109–115.
36. Cheung DT, Nimni ME: Mechanism of crosslinking of proteins by glutaraldehyde: II. Reaction with monomeric and polymeric collagen. Connect Tissue Res 1982;10:201–216.
37. Broom ND: Simultaneous morphologic and stress-strain studies of fibrous components in wet heart valve leaflet tissue. Connect Tissue Res 1978;6:37–50.
38. Broom N, Christie GW: The structure/function relationship of fresh and glutaraldehyde-fixed aortic valve leaflets. In Cohn LH, Gallucci V (eds): Cardiac Bioprostheses. New York, Yorke, 1982, pp 476–491.
39. Sade RM, Greene WB, Kurtz SM: Structural changes in a porcine xenograft after implantation for 105 months. Am J Cardiol 1979;44:761–766.
40. O'Brien MF: Heterologous replacement of the aortic valve. In Ionescu MI, Ross DN, Woller GH (eds): Biological Tissue and Heart Valve Replacement. London, Butterworths, 1972, pp 445–466.
41. Buch WS, Kosek JC, Angell WW, Shumway SE: Deterioration of formalin-treated aortic valve heterograft. J Thorac Cardovasc Surg 1970;60:673–682.
42. Dubiel WT, Johansson L, Willen R: Late changes in formalin-treated porcine aortic heterografts replacing human mitral valves. Scand J Thorac Cardiovasc Surg 1975;9:16–26.
43. Bortolotti V, Milano A, Mazzucco A, Valfre C, Fasoli G, Valente M, Thiene G, Gallucci V: Longevity of the formaldehyde-preserved Hancock porcine heterograft. J Thorac Cardiovasc Surg 1982;84:451–453.
44. Yarbrough JW, Roberts WC, Reis RL: Structural alterations in tissue cardiac valves implanted in patients and in calves. J Thorac Cardiovasc Surg 1973;65:364–375.
45. Zerbini EJ, Puig LB: The dura mater allograft valve. In Ionescu MI (ed): Tissue Heart Valves. London, Butterworths, 1979, pp 253–301.
46. Puig LB, Verginelli G, Iryia K, Kawabe L, Belotti G, Sosa E, Pilleggi F, Zerbini EJ: Homologous dura mater cardiac valves. Study of 533 surgical cases. J Thorac Cardiovasc Surg 1975;69:722–728.
47. Bodnar E, Ross DN: Mode of failure in 226 explanted biologic and bioprosthetic valves. In Cohn LH, Gallucci V (eds): Cardiac Bioprostheses. New York, Yorke, 1982, pp 401–407.
48. Centers for Disease Control: Rapidly progressive dementia in a patient who received a cadaveric dura mater graft. MMWR 1984;36:49–50.
49. Barnhart GR, Jones M, Ishihara T, Rose DM, Chavez AM, Ferrans VJ: Degeneration and calcification of bioprosthetic cardiac valves. Bioprosthetic tricuspid valve implantation in sheep. Am J Pathol 1982;106:136–139.
50. Arbustini E, Jones M, Moses RD, Eidbo EE, Carroll JR, Ferrans VJ: Modification by the Hancock T6 process of calcification of bioprosthetic cardiac valve implanted in sheep. Am J Cardiol 1984;53:1388–1396.
51. Jones M, Eidbo EE, Walters SM, Ferrans VJ, Clark RE: Effects of two types of preimplantation processes

on calcification of bioprosthetic valves. In Bodnar E, Yacoub M (eds): New York, Yorke, 1986, pp 451–459.

52. Fishbein MC, Levy RJ, Ferrans VJ, Dearden LC, Nashef A, Goodman AP, Carpentier A: Calcification of cardiac valve bioprostheses. Biochemical, histologic and ultrastructural observations in a subcutaneous implantation model system. J Thorac Cardiovasc Surg 1982;83:602–609.

53. Schoen FJ, Levy RJ, Nelson AC, Bernhard WF, Nashef A, Hawley M: Onset and progression of experimental bioprosthetic heart valve calcification. Lab Invest 1985;52:523–532.

54. Thiene G, Arbustini E, Bortolotti V, Talenti E, Milano A, Valente M, Molin G, Gallucci V: Pathologic substrates of porcine valve dysfunction. In Cohn LH, Gallucci V (eds): Cardiac Bioprostheses. New York, Yorke, 1982, pp 378–400.

55. Schoen FJ, Hobsen CE: Anatomic analysis of removed prosthetic heart valves: Causes of failure in 33 mechanical valves and 58 bioprostheses, 1980 to 1983. Hum Pathol 1985;16:549–559.

56. Schoen FJ, Kujovich JL, Levy RJ, St. John Sutton M: Bioprosthetic valve failure. Cardiovasc Clin 1987;18:289–317.

57. Gallucci V, Bortolotti U, Milano A, Mazzucco A, Valfre C, Guerra F, Faggian G, Theine G: The Hancock porcine valve 15 years later: An analysis of 575 patients. In Bodnar E, Yacoub M (eds): Biologic and Bioprosthetic Valves. New York, Yorke, 1986, pp 91–97.

58. Milano A, Bortolotti V, Talenti E, Valfre C, Arbustini E, Valente M, Mazzucco A, Gallucci V, Thiene G: Calcific degeneration as the main course of porcine bioprosthetic valve failure. Am J Cardiol 1984;53:1066–1070.

59. Ferrans VJ, Boyce SW, Billingham ME, Jones M, Ishihara T, Roberts WC: Calcific deposits in porcine bioprostheses: Structure and pathogenesis. Am J Cardiol 1980;46:721–734.

60. Valente M, Bortolotti U, Theine G: Ultrastructural substrates of dystrophic calcification in porcine bioprosthetic valve failure. Am J Pathol 1985;119:12–21.

61. Carpentier A, Lemaigre G, Robert L, Carpentier S, Dubost C: Biological factors affecting long-term results of valvular heterografts. J Thorac Cardiovasc Surg 1969;58:467–483.

62. Dunn JM, Marmon L: Mechanisms of calcification of tissue valves. Cardiol Clin 1985;3(3):385–396.

63. Sanders SP, Levy RJ, Freed MD, Norwood WI, Castaneda AR: Use of Hancock porcine xenografts in children and adolescents. Am J Cardiol 1984;46:429–438.

64. Silver MS, Pollock J, Silver MD, Williams WG, Trusler GH: Calcification in porcine xenograft valves in children. Am J Cardiol 1980;45:685–689.

65. Gallucci V, Bortolotti U, Milano A, Valfre C, Mazzucco A, Thiene G: Isolated mitral valve replacement with the Hancock bioprosthesis: A 13-year appraisal. Ann Thorac Surg 1984;38:571–577.

66. Oyer PE, Miller DC, Stinson EB, Jamieson SW, Shumway NE: The performance of the Hancock bioprosthetic valve over an 11½ year follow-up period: A preliminary report. In Duran C, Angell WW, Johnson AD, Oury JH (eds): Recent Progress in Mitral Valve Disease. London, Butterworths, 1984, pp 244–251.

67. Magilligan DJ Jr, Lewis JW Jr, Tilley B, Peterson E: The porcine bioprosthetic valve: Twelve years later. J Thorac Cardiovasc Surg 1985;89:499–507.

68. Gallo I, Nistal F, Artinano E: Six- to ten-year follow-up of patients with the Hancock cardiac bioprosthesis: Incidence of primary tissue failure. J Thorac Cardiovasc Surg 1986;92:14–20.

69. Foster AH, Greenberg GJ, Underhill DJ, McIntosh CL, Clark RE: Intrinsic failure of Hancock mitral bioprostheses: 10- to 15-year experience. Ann Thorac Surg 1987;44:568–577.

70. Brofman PR, Carvalho RG, Ribeiro EJ, Almeida RS, Coelho A, Loures DRR: Dura mater bioprostheses in young patients. In Cohn LH, Gallucci V (eds): Cardiac Bioprostheses. New York, Yorke, 1982, pp 265–272.

71. Ferrans VJ, Boyce SW, Billingham ME, Spray TL, Robert WC: Infection of glutaraldehyde-preserved porcine valve heterografts. Am J Cardiol 1979;43:1123–1136.

72. Ferrans VJ, Ishihara T, Jones M, Barnhart GR, Boyce SW, Kravitz AB, Roberts WC: Pathogenesis and stages of bioprosthetic infection. In Cohn LH, Gallucci V (eds): Cardiac Bioprostheses. New York, Yorke, 1982, pp 346–361.

73. Levy RJ, Schoen FJ, Sherman FS, Nichols J, Hawley MA, Lund SA: Calcification of subcutaneously implanted type I collagen sponges. Am J Pathol 1986;122:71–82.

74. Golomb G, Schoen FJ, Smith MS, Linden S, Dixon M, Levy RJ: The role of glutaraldehyde-induced cross-links in calcification of bovine pericardium used in cardiac valve bioprostheses. Am J Pathol 1987;127:122–130.

75. Harasaki H, Nose Y, McMahon JT, Kiraly RJ, Uchida N, Smith WA, Kambic H, Murabayashi S, Richards T: Calcification in blood pumps. In Program, Devices and Technology Branch Contractors Meeting 1987. Division of Heart and Vascular Diseases, National Heart, Lung and Blood Institute, National Institutes of Health, U.S. Department of Health and Human Services, Bethesda, Md, 1987.

76. Van Buskirk JJ, Kirsch WM, Kleyer DL, Barkley RM, Koch TD: Aminomalonic acid: Identification in E. coli and atherosclerotic plaque. Proc Natl Acad Sci USA 1984;81:722–725.

77. Koch TH, Bohemier D, Wheelan P, Delos S, Gaudiano G, Kirsch W, van Buskirk J, Becker K, Sillerud

L: Aminomalonic acid and the calcification of protein. In Program, Devices and Technology Branch Contractors Meeting 1987. Division of Heart and Vascular Diseases, National Heart, Lung and Blood Institute, National Institutes of Health, U.S. Department of Health and Human Services, Bethesda, 1987.

78. Lian JB, Skinner M, Glimcher MJ, Gallop P: The presence of gamma-carboxyglutamic acid in the proteins associated with ectopic calcification. Biochem Biophys Res Commun. 1976;73:349–355.

79. Levy RJ, Schoen FJ, Levy JT, Nelson AC, Howard SL, Oshry LJ: Biologic determinants of dystrophic calcification and osteocalcin deposition in glutaraldehyde-preserved porcine aortic valve leaflets implanted subcutaneously in rats. Am J Pathol 1983;113:143–155.

80. Levy RJ, Zenker JA, Lian JB: Vitamin K-dependent calcium binding proteins in aortic valve calcification. J Clin Invest 1980;65:563–566.

81. Levy RJ, Zenker JA, Bernhard WF: Porcine bioprosthetic valve calcification in bovine left ventricle-aorta shunts: Studies of the deposition of vitamin K-dependent proteins. Ann Thorac Surg 1983;36:187–192.

82. Bick RL: Anticoagulant and antiplatelet therapy. In Murano G, Bick RL (eds): Basic Concepts of Hemostasis and Thrombosis. Boca Raton FL, CRC Press, 1980, pp 245–258.

83. Stein PD, Riddle JM, Kemp SR, Lee MV, Lewis JW, Magilligan DJ Jr: Effect of warfarin on calcification of spontaneously degenerated porcine bioprosthetic valves. J Thorac Cardiovasc Surg 1985;90:119–125.

84. Carpentier A, Nashef A, Carpentier S, Ahmed A, Goussef N: Techniques for prevention of calcification of valvular bioprostheses. Circulation 1984;70(suppl I):I-165–I-168.

85. Schryer PJ, Tomasek FR, Starr JA, Wright JTM: Anticalcification effect of glutaraldehyde-preserved valve tissue stored for increasing time in glutaraldehyde. In Bodnar E, Yacoub M (eds): New York, Yorke, 1986, pp 471–477.

86. Lentz DJ, Pollock EM, Olsen DB, Andrews EJ, Murashita J, Hastings WL: Inhibition of mineralization of glutaraldehyde-fixed Hancock bioprosthetic heart valves. In Cohn LH, Gallucci V (eds): Cardiac Bioprostheses. New York, Yorke, 1982, pp 306–319.

87. Jones M, Eidbo EE, Hilbert SL, Ferrans VJ, Clark RE: Anticalcification treatments of bioprosthetic heart valves: In vivo, in situ studies in the sheep model. International Symposium on Cardiac Bioprostheses, Coronado, California, 1988. Abstract.

88. Dmitrovsky E, Boskey AL: Calcium-acidic phospholipid-phosphate complexes in human atherosclerotic aortas. Calcif Tissue Int 1985;37:121–125.

88a. Bodnar E, Olsen EJG, Dobrin J, Florio R: Damage of porcine valve tissue caused by the surfactant sodiumdodecylsulphate. Thorac Cardiovasc Surg 1986;34:287–290.

89. Levy RJ, Hawley MA, Schoen FJ, Lund SA, Liu PY: Inhibition by diphosphonate compounds of calcification of porcine bioprosthetic heart valve cusps implanted subcutaneously in rats. Circulation 1985;71:349–356.

90. Schoen FJ, Levy RJ: Pathophysiology of bioprosthetic heart valve calcification. In Bodnar E, Yacoub M (eds): Biologic and Bioprosthetic Valves. New York, Yorke, 1986, pp 418–441.

91. Gasser AB, Morgan DB, Fleisch HA, Richelle LJ: The influence of two diphosphonates on calcium metabolism in rats. Clin Sci 1972;43:31–45.

92. Meyer JL, Nancollas GH: The influence of multidentate organic diphosphonates on crystal growth of hydroxyapatite. Calcif Tissue Res 1973;13:265–303.

93. Lamson ML, Fox JL, Higuchi WJ: Calcium and 1-hydroxyethylidene-1, 1-diphosphonic acid: Polynuclear complex formation in physiological range of pH. Int J Pharm 1966;21:143–154.

94. Levy RJ, Schoen FJ, Lund SA, Smith MS: Prevention of leaflet calcification of bioprosthetic heart valves with diphosphonate injection therapy. Experimental studies of optimal dosages and therapeutic durations. J Thorac Cardiovasc Surg 1987;94:551–557.

95. Levy RJ, Wolfrum J, Schoen FJ, Hawley MA, Lund SA, Langer R: Inhibition of calcification of bioprosthetic heart valves by local controlled release diphosphonate. Science 1985;228:190–192.

96. Golomb G, Langer R, Schoen FJ, SMith MS, Choi YM, Levy RJ: Controlled release diphosphonate to inhibit bioprosthetic heart valve calcification: Dose response and mechanistic studies. J Contr Rel 1986;4:181–194.

97. Levy RJ, Amidon G, Johnston T, Schoen FJ: Cardiovascular calcification: Pathophysiology and treatment. In Program, Devices and Technology Branch Contractors Meeting, 1987. Division of Heart and Vascular Diseases, National Heart, Lung and Blood Institutes, National Institutes of Health, Department of Health and Human Services, Bethesda, Md, p 142.

98. Urist MR, Admas JM: Effects of various blocking agents upon local mechanisms and calcification. Arch Pathol 1966;81:325–342.

99. Carpentier A, Nashef A, Carpentier S, Goussef N, Relland J, Levy RJ, Fishbein MC, El Asmar B, Benmar M, El Sayed S, Donzeau-Gouge PG: Prevention of tissue valve calcification by chemical techniques. In Cohn LH, Gallucci V (eds): Cardiac Bioprostheses. New York, Yorke, 1982, pp 320–327.

100. Menasche P, Hue A, Lavergne A, Miravet L, Piwnica A: Selective blockade of collagen-calcium binding sites: New process to decrease bioprosthetic valvular calcification. In Bodnar E, Yacoub M (eds): Biologic and Bioprosthetic Valves. New York, Yorke, 1986, pp 478–483.

101. Golomb G, Levy RJ: Prevention of calcification of glutaraldehyde-treated biomaterials by charge modification. Trans Soc Biomater 1987, p 108.

102. Tsao JW, Schoen FJ, Shanker R, Sallis JD, Levy RJ: Retardation of bovine pericardial bioprosthetic tissue calcification by a physiologic mineralization inhibitor, phosphocitrate, administered locally. Trans Soc Biomater 1987, p 144.

103. Foster JH, Collins AH, Jacobs JK, Scott HW Jr: Long term follow-up of homografts used in the treatment of coarctation of the aorta. J Cardiovasc Surg 1965;6:111–120.

104. Ross D, Yacoub M: Homograft replacement of the aortic valve. A critical review. Prog Cardiovasc Dis 1969;11:275–293.

105. Davies H, Lessof MH, Robert CI, Ross DN: Homograft replacement of the aortic valve. Lancet 1965;1:926–929.

106. Barratt-Boyes BG, Roche HG, Brandt PWT, Smith JC, Lowe JB: Aortic homograft valve replacement: A long-term follow-up of an initial series of 101 patients. Circulation 1969;40:763–775.

107. Barratt-Boyes BG, Roche AHG, Whitlock RML: Six year review of the results of freehand aortic replacement using an antibiotic sterilized homograft valve. Circulation 1977;55:353–361.

108. Angell WW, Shumway NE, Kosek JC: A five year study of viable aortic valve homografts. J Thorac Cardiovasc Surg 1972;64:329–338.

109. Virdi IS, Monro JL, Ross JK: Eleven year experience of aortic valve homografts. J Thorac Cardiovasc Surg 1972;54:329–338.

110. Yacoub M, Kittle CF: Sterilization of valve homografts by antibiotic solution. Circulation 1970;41(suppl II):II-29–II-31.

111. Wain WH, Pearce HM, Riddell RW, Ross DN: A re-evaluation of antibiotic sterilization of heart valve allografts. Thorax 1977;32:740–742.

112. Malm JP, Bowman FO Jr, Harris PD, Kovalik ATW: An evaluation of aortic homografts sterilized by electron beam energy. J Thorac Cardiovasc Surg 1967;54:471–477.

113. Aparicio SR, Donnelly RJ, Dexter F, Watson DA: Light and electron microscopic studies on homograft and heterograft heart valves. J Pathol 1975;115:147–162.

114. Angell WW, Angell JD, Oury JH, Lamberti JJ, Grehl TM: Long-term follow-up of viable frozen aortic homografts. A viable homograft valve bank. J Thorac Cardiovasc 1987;93:815–822.

115. Bodnar E, Wain WH, Martelli V, Ross DN: Long term performance of 580 homograft and autograft valves used for aortic valve replacement. Thorac Cardiovasc Surg 1979;27:31–38.

116. Barratt-Boyes BG, Roche AHG, Subramanyan R, Pemberton JR, Whitlock RML: Long-term follow-up of patients with the antibiotic-sterilized aortic homograft valve inserted free-hand in the aortic position. Circulation 1987;75:768–777.

117. Wain WH, Greco R, Ingegneri A, Bodnar E, Ross DN: 15 years' experience with 615 homograft and autograft aortic valve replacements. Int J Artif Organs 1980;3:169–172.

118. Harris PD, Kovalik AJW, Marks JA, Malm JP: Factors modifying aortic homograft structure and function. Surgery 1968;63:45–59.

119. Hudson REB: Pathology of human aortic valve homografts. Thorax 1967;22:114–138.

120. Roe FJC, Glendenning OM: The carcinogenicity of beta-propiolactone for mouse skin. Br J Cancer 1956;10:357–362.

121. Dempsey DJ, Thirucote RR: Sterilization of medical devices: A review. J Biomater Appl 1989;3:454–522.

122. Kolman A, Naslund M, Calleman CJ: Genotoxic effects of ethylene oxide and the relevance to human cancer. Carcinogenesis 1986;7:1245–1250.

123. Davies H, Missen GAK, Blandford G, Roberts CJ, Lessof MH, Ross DN: Homograft replacement of the aortic valve. A clinical and pathologic study. Am J Cardiol 1968;22:195–217.

124. Barratt-Boyes BG: Long-term follow-up of aortic valve grafts. Br Heart J 1971;33(suppl):60–65.

125. Ingegneri A, Wain WH, Martelli V, Bodnar E, Ross D: An 11 year assessment of 93 flash frozen homograft valves in the aortic position. Thorac Cardiovasc Surg 1979;27:304–397.

126. Pat JW, Sawyer PN: Freeze dried aortic grafts: A preliminary report of experimental evaluation. Am J Surg 1953;86:3–13.

127. Reichenbach DD, Mohri H, Merendino KA: Pathological changes in human aortic valve homografts. Circulation 1969;39(suppl I):I-47–I-56.

128. Brock RC: Long-term degenerative changes in aortic segment homografts with particular reference to calcification. Thorax 1968;23:249–255.

129. Robbins SL: Cell injury and cell death. In: Pathologic Basis of Disease. Philadelphia, Saunders, 1974, pp 21–54.

130. Thubrikar MJ, Skinner JR, Eppink RT, Nolan SP: Stress analysis of porcine bioprosthetic heart valves in vivo. J Biomed Mater Res 1982;16:811–826.

131. Thubrikar M, Piegrass WC, Deck JD, Nolan SP: Stresses of natural versus prosthetic aortic valve leaflets in vivo. Ann Thorac Surg 1980;30:230–239.

132. Brewer RJ, Deck JD, Capati B, Nolan SP: The dynamic aortic root. Its role in aortic valve function. J Thorac Cardiovasc Surg 1976;72:413–417.

133. Thubrikar M, Piegrass, Bosher LP, Nolan SP: The elastic modulus of canine aortic valve leaflets in vivo and in vitro. Circ Res 1980;47:792–800.

134. Thubrikar M, Carabello BA, Aouad J, Nolan SP: Interpretation of aortic root angiography in dogs and in humans. Cardiovasc Res 1982;16:16–21.

135. Broom ND: An in vitro study of mechanical fatigue in glutaraldehyde-treated porcine aortic valve tissue. Biomaterials 1980;1:3–8.

136. Reis RL, Hancock WD, Yarbrough JW, Glancy DL, Morrow AG: The flexible stent. A new concept in the fabrication of tissue heart valve prostheses. J Thorac Cardiovasc Surg 1971;62:683–689.

137. Thomson FJ, Barratt-Boyes BG: The glutaraldehyde-treated heterograft valve. J Thorac Cardiovasc Surg 1977;74:317–321.

138. Wright JTM, Eberhart CE, Gibbs ML, Saul T, Gilpin CB: Hancock II—An improved bioprosthesis. In Cohn LH, Gallucci V (eds): Cardiac Bioprostheses. New York, Yorke, 1982, pp 425–444.

139. Carpentier AF, Lane E: Supported bioprosthetic heart valve with compliant orifice ring. US Patent 4,106,129, 1978.

140. Levine FH, Buckley MJ, Austen WG: Hemodynamic evaluation of the Hancock modified orifice bioprosthesis in the aortic position. Circulation 1978;58(suppl I):33–35.

141. Carpentier A, Dubost C, Lane E, Nashef A, Carpentier S, Relland J, Deloche A, Fabiani JN, Chaurand S, Perier P, Maxwell S: Continuing improvements in valvular bioprostheses. J Thorac Cardiovasc Surg 1982;83:27–42.

142. Borkon AM, McIntosh CL, Jones M, Roberts WC, Morrow AG: Inward stent-post bending of a porcine bioprosthesis in the mitral position. Cause of bioprosthetic dysfunction. J Thorac Cardiovasc Surg 1982;83:105–107.

143. Salomon NW, Copeland JG, Goldman S, Larson DF: Unusual complication of the Hancock porcine heterograft. Strut compression in the aortic root. J Thorac Cardiovasc Surg 1979;77:294–296.

144. Magilligan DJ, Fisher E, Alam M: Hemolytic anemia with porcine xenograft aortic and mitral valves. J Thorac Cardiovasc Surg 1980;79:628–631.

145. Schoen FJ, Schulman LJ, Cohn LH: Quantitative anatomic analysis of "stent creep" of explanted Hancock standard porcine bioprostheses used for cardiac valve replacement. Am J Cardiol 1985;56:110–114.

146. Wright JTM: Porcine or pericardial valves? Now and the future: Design and engineering considerations. In Bodnar E, Yacoub M (eds): Biologic and Bioprosthetic Valves. New York, Yorke, 1986, pp 567–579.

147. Schoen FJ, Fernandez J, Gonzalez-Lavin L, Cernaianu A: Causes of failure and pathologic findings in surgically removed Ionescu-Shiley standard bovine pericardial heart valve bioprostheses: Emphasis on progressive structural deterioration. Circulation 1987;76:618–627.

148. Wheatley DJ, Fisher J, Reece IJ, Spyt T, Breeze P: Primary tissue failure in pericardial heart valves. J Thorac Cardiovasc Surg 1987;94:367–374.

149. Walley VM, Keon WJ: Patterns of failure on Ionescu-Shiley bovine pericardial bioprosthetic valves. J Thorac Cardiovasc Surg 1987;93:925–933.

150. Gabbay S, Bortolotti U, Wasserman F, Tindel N, Factor SM, Frater RWM: Long-term follow-up of the Ionescu-Shiley mitral pericardial xenograft. J Thorac Cardiovasc Surg 1984;88:758–763.

151. Brais MP, Bedard JP, Goldstein W, Koshal A, Keon WJ: Ionescu-Shiley pericardial xenografts: Follow-up to 6 years. Ann Thorac Surg 1985;39:105–111.

152. Reul GJ, Cooley DA, Duncan JM, Frazier OH, Hallman GL, Livesay JJ, Ott DA, Walker WE: Valve failure with the Ionescu-Shiley bovine pericardial bioprosthesis: Analysis of 2680 patients. J Vasc Surg 1985;2:192–203.

153. Nistal F, Garcia-Satue E, Artinano E, Duran CMG, Gallo I: Comparative study of primary tissue valve failure between Ionescu-Shiley pericardial and Hancock porcine valves in the aortic position. Am J Cardiol 1986;57:161–164.

154. Cooley DA, Ott DA, Reul GJ, Duncan JM, Frazier OH, Livesay JJ: Ionescu-Shiley bovine pericardial bioprostheses: Clinical results in 2701 patients. In Bodnar E, Yacoub M (eds): Biologic and Bioprosthetic Valves. New York, Yorke, 1986, pp 177–198.

155. Bortolotti U, Milano A, Thiene G, Guerra F, Mazzucco A, Valente M, Talenti E, Gallucci V: Early mechanical failures of the Hancock pericardial xenograft. J Thorac Cardiovasc Surg 1987;94:200–207.

Bodnar, E. and Frater, R. W. M., editors
(1991) *Replacement Cardiac Valves,*
Pergamon Press, Inc. (New York), pp. 77–98
Printed in the United States of America

CHAPTER 4

THROMBOSIS, EMBOLISM, AND BLEEDING

ERIC G. BUTCHART

As prosthetic heart valve technology has advanced over the last three decades, most modern mechanical prostheses now offer good hemodynamic performance coupled with mechanical reliability and durability (1). The choice between prostheses of different design and manufacture has therefore often to be made on the basis of their thrombotic and embolic characteristics. It is thus important for the cardiac surgeon to have reliable information about individual prosthesis thrombogenicity in order to make a logical choice. Furthermore because prostheses differ in their thrombogenicity, optimum anticoagulation levels for each need to be defined in order to ensure maximum safety in long-term management.

Unfortunately, considerable confusion exists in the prosthetic heart valve literature on the subjects of valve thrombosis, embolism, and anticoagulant-related bleeding (2). Much of this confusion stems from lack of clear definitions and lack of standardization of anticoagulation practice (3, 4). Disappointingly, the recently published guidelines on the reporting of prosthetic heart valve complications continue to advocate the amalgamation of valve thrombosis and embolism under one heading (5). This ignores the fact that these two important complications may have different etiologies and incidences and are entirely different in terms of the magnitude or severity of their consequences. Embolism produces a complete spectrum of effects, ranging from the trivial to the fatal; valve thrombosis, in contrast, is always life-threatening. Although both are influenced by anticoagulation levels achieved, the incidence of embolism appears less dependent on the particular prosthesis used than the incidence of valve thrombosis, which is probably mainly influenced by the design and construction of the prosthesis. The reasons for this difference are central to the understanding of the subject and are discussed in detail below.

In 1856, the German pathologist Virchow emphasized the three important factors influencing abnormal blood clotting taking place within the vascular system: the surface in contact with the blood, blood flow, and the constituents of the blood (6). These factors subsequently became known as Virchow's triad and form the basis for the understanding of any intravascular thrombosis. Thrombus formation on prosthetic heart valves may thus be influenced by (1) the surface characteristics of the prosthesis, its sewing ring and its anchoring sutures and pledgets, (2) blood flow, both total (i.e., cardiac output) and local (turbulence, stagnation, etc.), and (3) alterations in the constituents of the circulating blood. Small thrombi, forming on or adjacent to the prosthesis, which subsequently break off and embolize to various parts of the body can justifiably be ascribed to the prosthesis. Thrombi that originate elsewhere cannot since they either result from pathologic processes associated with the original valve disease or form part of the "background" incidence of embolism and occlusive vascular disease endemic in the general population (7, 8) and associated with nonprosthetic risk factors.

Thus many of the factors that influence embolism are patient-related rather than prosthesis-related (9). Others may be surgeon-related or management-related (10). In trying to establish the thrombogenicity of a given prosthesis on the basis of embolism, it is therefore necessary to exclude, as far as possible, all "extraneous" factors that may cloud the issue before an evaluation of the prosthesis itself can be made. These factors include

1. The background incidence of embolism and occlusive vascular disease.
2. Risk factors that may predispose to embolism from background, cardiac, and prosthetic sources.
3. The influence of anticoagulation level and antiplatelet drugs.
4. The influence of temporal effects and statistical methods.
5. The influence of surgical technique.

THE EPIDEMIOLOGY OF BACKGROUND "EMBOLISM" AND OCCLUSIVE VASCULAR DISEASE

In discussing embolism in relation to prosthetic heart valves there is a tendency to attribute all emboli, or sudden events suspicious of embolism, to the prosthesis itself. However, this is clearly an oversimplification. One only has to take the example of sudden cerebrovascular events, which account for about 80% of all clinically diagnosed "emboli" in most prosthetic valve series (11), to understand the reason. Stroke is the third commonest cause of death in most western countries (7), after ischemic heart disease and cancer, and the commonest cause of death in Oriental persons (12). The general

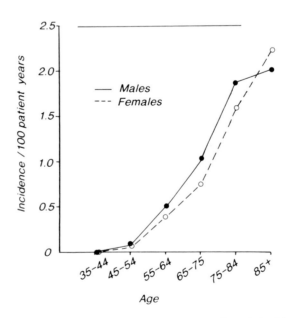

Fɪɢ. 4–1. Incidence of stroke and TIA according to age and sex. Data derived from Refs. 7 and 8.

population exhibits an incidence of stroke (7) and transient ischemic attacks (TIAs) (8) that gradually rises with age, reaching a combined rate of approximately 2 per 100 patient years over the age of 80 (Fig. 4–1). If one examines subgroups of the general population with particular risk factors for stroke, the rate is even higher and is not abolished by anticoagulation (7, 13).

Patients in atrial fibrillation *without valvular heart disease* have an incidence of stroke five times higher than patients in sinus rhythm (14) (see below). Both systemic hypertension (15–17) and heavy cigarette smoking (>40/day) (16) independently double the risk of stroke. Other factors that raise the incidence include diabetes (approximately three times), certain drugs, and various biochemical and hematologic abnormalities that are discussed below. The multiplicity of conditions associated with TIA alone are summarized in Table 4–1 (18).

This background incidence of stroke and TIA has two important implications with

TABLE 4–1. *Conditions Associated with Transient Cerebral Ischemic Attacks*

Abnormalities of Blood Vessels
Atherosclerosis of extracranial or intracranial arteries
Fibromuscular dysplasia
Inflammatory disorders
   Giant cell arteritis
   Systemic lupus erythematosus
   Polyarteritis nodosa
   Meningovascular syphilis
   Granulomatous angiitis
Dissection of extracranial arteries
   Spontaneous
   Traumatic
Multiple progressive intracranial arterial occlusions
   (Moya-moya)

Cardiac Abnormalities
Ischemic heart disease
   Myocardial infarct with mural thrombus
   Arrhythmia
Rheumatic heart disease
Infective endocarditis
Atrial myxoma
Mitral valve prolapse

Hematologic Abnormalities
Platelet abnormalities
Red blood cell abnormalities
Hyperviscosity
Sickle cell anemia

Altered Cerebral Circulation
Orthostatic hypotension
Cervical spondylosis with vertebral artery compression
Abnormal shunts

Miscellaneous Conditions
Migraine headache with transient ischemic accompaniments
Use of oral contraceptive agents
Hereditary hemorrhagic telangiectasis
   (Rendu-Weber-Osler)
Complications of cerebral angiography

Data from Ref. 18.

regard to the interpretation of reported series of prosthetic heart valves. First, any large series of prosthetic valves, mechanical or biological, that reports a zero incidence of embolism should be viewed with great suspicion, since it implies deficiencies in data acquisition or interpretation. One possible exception might be a series composed entirely of young patients. Second, unless sufficient information is given about patient characteristics, it is difficult to decide what influence the background incidence has had on the reported incidence. One striking difference between the incidence of cerebrovascular accidents in the general population and that seen in series of prosthetic valve patients is that in the general population the incidence of stroke is much higher than the incidence of TIA, whereas in most prosthetic valve series the reverse is true. This may be partly due to differences in data collection methods and analysis (8). Alternatively, it is perhaps more likely that a prosthetic valve acts as a source of predominantly very small emboli that only produce transient ischemic symptoms. Larger emboli leaving permanent neurologic deficits are probably more likely to have arisen from the left atrium (14).

Sufficient epidemiologic data are now available from many countries (7, 8, 12, 19–24) to allow an expected background incidence to be calculated and subtracted from the observed incidence in a prosthetic valve series. The residue would perhaps more accurately represent the series, although it would still be influenced by factors other than the prosthesis itself, for example, surgical technique and anticoagulation management.

FACTORS PREDISPOSING TO EMBOLISM FROM NONPROSTHETIC AND PROSTHETIC SOURCES

Although reported incidences of embolism following valve replacement probably underestimate the size of the problem because many small emboli go to clinically silent areas of the body (11), or even silent areas of the brain (25), the fact remains that the majority of patients appear to escape significant embolic complications. It is widely assumed that many patients who succumb to embolism have simply been inadequately anticoagulated (26). However, a recent review of our own data, using one type of mechanical valve and a standardized surgical technique, failed to show any relationship between embolism in individual patients and anticoagulation level, irrespective of the way this was characterized numerically (i.e., mean level, level immediately prior to an event, degree of variability of level, etc.) (4). This lack of correlation suggests that some patients may be inherently more susceptible to embolism or to cerebrovascular disease and that the factors responsible are little affected by anticoagulation. This accords with the finding of many series, that a history of preoperative embolism increases the risk of postoperative embolism (26).

The risk factors involved can be divided into three main groups: (1) those that predispose to atherosclerosis of the carotid, vertebral, and intracranial arteries, (2) those that provide a potential source of emboli other than the prosthesis itself, and (3) those that result in alterations of certain constituents of the circulating blood and favor thrombus formation at many sites, including the prosthesis.

The risk factors for cerebrovascular occlusive disease are now well established (27) and include hypertension (15–17), cigarette smoking (16), diabetes (28), hyperlipidemia (29), and raised fibrinogen levels (30, 31). Even mildly elevated blood glucose levels may increase risk (32). The role of alcohol intake remains controversial, but current epidemiologic evidence suggests that excessive alcohol consumption increases the risk of ischemic stroke, probably through several different pathophysiologic mechanisms, whereas moderate alcohol consumption may even have a protective role (33).

Potential nonprosthetic cardiac sources of embolism include the fibrillating left atrium (14), abnormalities of the remaining native cardiac valves (34, 35), and left ventricular mural thrombus following myocardial infarction (18). Atrial fibrillation (AF) is a common arrhythmia in most prosthetic valve series (26) and is undoubtedly the most important patient-related factor in embolism (14). In combination with untreated rheumatic heart disease, it has long been known to be associated with a linearized incidence of embolic events of about 7 per 100 patient years, falling only to about 4 per 100 patient years with anticoagulation (36). However, only in recent years have epidemiologic data shown that AF *without valve disease* (so-called nonvalvulopathic AF) is also associated with a high incidence of embolism. The statistics reveal the magnitude of the effect: nonvalvulopathic AF increases the risk of stroke approximately fivefold, more than one-third of ischemic strokes in the elderly are associated with AF, and approximately one in three patients with AF will experience a stroke during their lifetime (14). Congestive heart failure and sustained chronic AF as opposed to paroxysmal AF appear to increase risk (14).

Even these statistics may underestimate the size of the problem since a significant proportion of cerebral infarcts in patients with AF are clinically silent and only detected on computerized tomography scanning (25) and a significant proportion of stroke and TIA victims apparently in sinus rhythm reveal intermittent atrial arrhythmias on long-term ECG recording (37).

A summation of published data on stroke incidence in nonvalvulopathic AF yields an average rate of about 5 per 100 patient years (14), while the corresponding rate with anticoagulation has been reported to be about 3 per 100 patient years (38).

Even in the absence of valve disease, most emboli associated with AF probably originate in the left atrium (14), and increased left atrial size may be an additional risk factor (39). It follows that many emboli in patients with prosthetic valves in AF probably also originate from the left atrium rather than the prosthesis. Since AF and left atrial enlargement are more common in mitral than in aortic valve disease, a higher incidence of embolism is to be expected following mitral valve replacement (26). This effect may be accentuated by prosthetic mitral valves that fail to adequately relieve a transvalvular gradient. Because they are themselves intrinsically stenotic due to their design characteristics or because they fail to open completely due to surgical error (see below), they may also fail to reduce the risk of embolism from the left atrium below that associated with native mitral stenosis. This secondary thrombogenicity is discussed in detail later.

Many factors modify the coagulability of the blood, particularly when it comes into contact with abnormal (nonendothelialized) surfaces or encounters regions of abnormal flow. Artificial surfaces in contact with flowing blood induce a complex series of reactions involving platelets, leukocytes, and various blood proteins including fibrinogen and the complement system (40). The delicate balance of this series of reactions can be tipped in the direction of enhanced coagulability by factors that increase platelet adhesion, raise fibrinogen levels, or increase blood viscosity. Cigarette smoking, for example, in addition to its atherogenic potential, increases all three of these closely related thrombogenic effects (30, 41). Raised fibronogen levels are also found in diabetes, pregnancy, and inflammatory conditions and in response to endotoxins, stress, and high dietary fat intake (42). Many drugs also increase coagulability in various ways (43). Oral contraceptives increase platelet aggregation by enhancing platelet response to ADP, increase levels of many clotting factors (43) and fibrinogen (42), and decrease levels of antithrombin III, an important natural anticoagulant (43). The use of newer low-dose estrogen compounds reduces but does not eliminate the risk (44). Pertinent to this discussion is the increased risk of cerebrovascular accidents in women taking oral contraceptives (45, 46). Other drugs that have been implicated in enhanced coagulability include corticosteroids, adrenaline, chlorpromazine, and some cytotoxic drugs (43).

Many systemic diseases are associated with a hypercoagulable state. These include malignant disease, diabetes, nephrotic syndrome, hyperlipidemia, and various myeloproliferative disorders (47). Pregnancy is also associated with hypercoagulability. Apart from these secondary causes of increased susceptibility to intravascular clotting, an increasing number of inherited primary hypercoagulable states in which a physiologic anticoagulant mechanism is defective are now being recognized. However, most of these conditions predispose to venous thrombosis rather than arterial thrombosis (47).

The purpose of detailing these various disease conditions and external influences that can modify the incidence of "embolism" in a prosthetic valve series is to demonstrate the complexity of the subject and to point out the danger of adopting too simplistic an approach. These additional risk factors could be handled in one of two different ways in the analysis of a prosthetic valve series; either the background incidence of TIA and stroke for the general population (calculated from epidemiologic data by age and sex) could be subtracted from the observed incidence of "embolism," or patients with known risk factors could be excluded from the series. Clearly this latter approach would be of value only if all authors reporting valve series used the same exclusions. An obvious problem would arise in patients with atrial fibrillation since to exclude them would remove about half the patients from most series. A more sensible approach would be to report groups of patients in sinus rhythm and atrial fibrillation separately.

THE INFLUENCE OF ANTICOAGULATION AND ANTIPLATELET DRUGS

Many authors report "unsatisfactory" or "poorly controlled" anticoagulation as a risk factor for embolism, and some regard it as the most important risk factor (26). Yet in most reported series of prosthetic valves, it is difficult to determine the precise effect that anticoagulation level has had on the incidence of embolism or valve thrombosis. In many cases, this is simply because insufficient information is given about anticoagulation levels actually *achieved* as opposed to *recommended*. In others, a much more fundamental problem interferes with the comparability of anticoagulation information: the way that anticoagulation level is measured (3).

Anticoagulation Measurement

Warfarin, the most commonly used coumarin anticoagulant, acts by reducing the activity in blood coagulation of factors II (prothrombin), VII, IX, and X. Because the absorption and metabolism of vitamin K, warfarin, and the coagulation factors vary in different individuals and also with such factors as diet and concomitant drugs, it is necessary to adjust the dose of warfarin according to the results of laboratory tests. The most convenient test of the effect of warfarin is the prothrombin time (Fig. 4–2), in which a volume of tissue extract (thromboplastin) is added to plasma in a test tube and the time for clotting to occur after the addition of calcium is measured. The normal prothrombin time is between 12 and 15 s. This deceptively simple test is in fact subject to considerable variability in end point, particularly when the prothrombin time is prolonged, depending on which thromboplastin reagent is used for the test (3).

Rabbit brain extract has been used as a thromboplastin for many years in the United

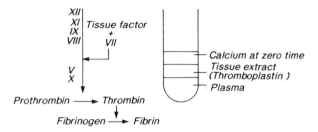

Fɪɢ. 4–2. Diagram of the prothrombin time test. Reproduced with permission from Bloom AL: The need for standardisation of anticoagulant management. In Rabago G and Cooley DA (eds): Heart Valve Replacement. New York, Futura, 1987, pp 319–333.

States, while human brain has been used in the United Kingdom until recently, and ox brain has been used in Europe. Even in the United States there has been no uniformity because different commercial preparations of rabbit brain may give different prothrombin times for the same sample (3). It is thus meaningless to express prothrombin time as "twice normal" or "1.5 times normal," as has been the practice in the United States for many years (11), unless the sensitivity index of the thromboplastin used is also given. In an effort to overcome this problem and to standardize anticoagulation measurement, the World Health Organization introduced reference thromboplastins, against which national reference thromboplastins could be calibrated, and a system of expressing the

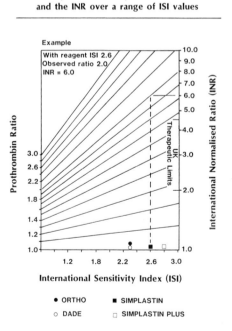

Fɪɢ. 4–3. Nomogram relating INR to measured prothrombin time according to the international sensitivity index (ISI) of available thromboplastins. Adapted with permission from Poller L: A simple nomogram for the derivation of international normalised ratios for the standardisation of prothrombin times. Throm Haemost 1988;60:18–20.

results taking into account the sensitivity index of each thromboplastin: the International Normalized Ratio, or INR. A nomogram relating INR to the measured prothrombin time, depending on the thromboplastin reagent used (48), is depicted in Fig. 4–3. It can be seen, for example, that a "raw" prothrombin time of "twice normal" as expressed in the United States is equivalent to an INR of between 5.0 and 7.0, according to which reagent is used. Although the INR has some imperfections, it provides consistent and reproducible results in the therapeutic range and has been adopted in the United Kingdom, Australasia, and parts of Europe. It has not yet been received enthusiastically in the United States.

Implications of Nonstandardized Anticoagulation Measurement

No apology is made for describing the prothrombin time test in so much detail, because knowledge of its inaccuracies and shortcomings is fundamental to the understanding of so much apparently conflicting information in the literature concerning the anticoagulation of prosthetic heart valves.

Despite recent attempts to introduce international standardization to anticoagulation management (49, 50), there has been resistance to change, and the proposed therapeutic range (INR 3.0–4.5) for prosthetic heart valves has not been widely implemented (4). Since it has been traditional in the past to maintain the anticoagulation level of patients with prosthetic heart valves at the equivalent of an INR of between 5.0 and 7.0 in the United States (11) and between 2.0 and 3.0 in the United Kingdom (4), no useful comparison can be made between past American and British series with respect to embolic, thrombotic, or anticoagulant-related complications (4). Furthermore, it is not surprising that most American prosthetic valve series report a higher incidence of anticoagulant-related bleeding than British series and greater anticoagulant risk in the elderly (26) in contrast to equal risk in the elderly when the INR is less than 3.0 (51, 52). Nor is it surprising that certain prostheses appear more prone to thrombotic obstruction in the United Kindgom (53) than they do in North America (54).

Such disparity between American and European series, and even between American series from different institutions, render invalid attempts to combine embolic, thrombotic, and bleeding complications as a summation of complications that can be attributable to a particular prosthesis. The widely quoted paper of Edmunds (26), entitled *Thrombotic and bleeding complications of prosthetic heart valves,* attempts to do this by analyzing 55 reported prosthetic valve series from many different countries. Not only are valve thrombosis and embolism combined under the one heading "thrombotic," but no account is taken of the level of anticoagulation achieved (even if stated) in each series when recording the complications. While it is of course true that the complications of both mechanical prostheses and bioprostheses in this context are inevitably the sum of the embolic, thrombotic, and bleeding complications and that a low embolic or thrombotic rate may in some instances be achieved only at the expense of a high bleeding rate, it is fundamental that bleeding rates are directly related to anticoagulation intensity (55) and have no association with individual prostheses. For example, some prostheses with inherently low thrombogenicity may have been anticoagulated at a level that was unnecessarily high and would not have significantly lowered the embolic rate, given the background incidence of TIA and stroke referred to earlier. Furthermore, the higher the level of anticoagulation, the greater the likelihood that some events ascribed to embolism are in fact due to cerebral hemorrhage (56). Finally, the reporting of a zero incidence of bleeding events, a feature of many nonanticoagulated bioprosthetic series, is no more believable than a zero incidence of embolism, since there is also a background incidence of bleeding events in the general population.

Choosing the Optimum Level of Anticoagulation

Given that it is probably impossible to eliminate embolism altogether, a balance has to be struck, minimizing the incidence of embolism, valve thrombosis, and bleeding events. Clearly this will be easier to achieve with a prosthesis of inherently low thrombogenicity. The problem is summarized in Fig. 4–4, a theoretical graph relating the incidence of embolism of three hypothetical prostheses to anticoagulation level and showing the effect of increasing anticoagulation level on the incidence of bleeding. The depiction of the "background incidence" of TIA and stroke as a straight line is probably an oversimplification, but insufficient data are available to draw it otherwise. In the case of prosthesis A (of low thrombogenicity) the incidence of embolism falls rapidly even with low levels of anticoagulation and approaches the background incidence. The embolic rate of prosthesis B (of medium thrombogenicity) only reaches a low figure with high levels of anticoagulation and a high incidence of bleeding, while prosthesis C (of high thrombogenicity) never attains a low embolic rate.

Application of this hypothesis to two comparable groups of patients who had undergone isolated mitral valve replacement (MVR) with a single type of prosthesis (Medtronic-Hall), but who had been anticoagulated at two different mean levels, confirmed for the first time that small measured differences in anticoagulation level could indeed influence the incidence of embolism (57). In this study, a modest increase in mean INR was associated with a fall in the risk of all grades of embolic events at the expense of a small increase in all grades of bleeding events (Fig. 4–5). However, most of these bleeding events were of a minor nature, and only one bleeding event resulted in death. Embolic deaths and events leaving a permanent deficit were totally eliminated in the group of patients with the slightly higher mean INR. Extrapolation from these data would suggest

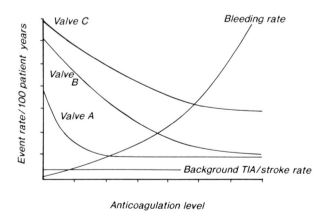

FIG. 4–4. Theoretical graph relating the incidence of thromboembolism of three hypothetical prostheses to anticoagulation. See text for explanation.

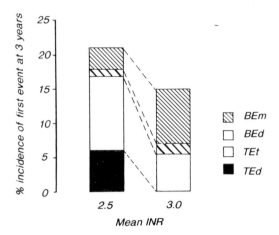

F<small>IG</small>. 4–5. Effect of two different anticoagulation levels on thromboembolic and bleeding events stratified by grade of severity. Actuarial analysis at 3 years following isolated MVR with Medtronic-Hall valve. Data from Ref. 57. BEm = minor bleeding event, requiring no treatment; BEd = bleeding event requiring transfusion or surgical treatment or causing death; TEt = transient thromboembolic event; and TEd = thromboembolic event causing permanent deficit or death.

that, for the Medtronic-Hall valve, a further increase in INR would be counterproductive since any further small decrease in an already low embolic rate could probably be achieved only at the expense of an unacceptable increase in the number and severity of bleeding events. The optimum INR for patients undergoing MVR with the Medtronic-Hall valve would appear to be in the region of 3.0 (57). Similar, as yet unpublished, data for the Medtronic-Hall valve in the aortic position suggest that the optimum INR following aortic valve replacement is between 2.0 and 2.5 (58).

It should be stressed that these recommendations apply only to the Medtronic-Hall valve, which appears to be a prosthesis of very low thrombogenicity (see below). Similar studies are required to establish optimum anticoagulation levels for other prostheses. It would appear that the recently recommended but not fully implemented anticoagulation level for "all prosthetic cardiac valves" (INR 3.0 to 4.5) (49, 50) is certainly too high for the Medtronic-Hall valve and perhaps also for some other modern prostheses of low thrombogenicity. It may be that certain categories of patients with particular risk factors for embolism will require a slightly higher INR, but insufficient data are currently available to make any firm recommendations. Matintaining the INR below 3.0 substantially reduces the incidence of anticoagulant-related death to around 0.1% per patient year (51, 52). Aiming for the lowest possible INR consistent with effective embolic and thrombotic prophylaxis is therefore eminently worthwhile.

Recent confirmatory evidence that excessively high levels of anticoagulation (INR 9.0) confer no advantage over moderate anticoagulation (INR 2.65), in terms of minimizing embolic risk, comes from a prospective randomized study carried out in Saudi Arabia in patients receiving five different mechanical prostheses and two different levels of anticoagulation (59). Overall, the embolic rate was quite high, perhaps in keeping with the predominantly first- and second-generation mechanical valves used in the series. The embolic incidence of such valves might thus be represented by the curve of valve C in Fig. 4–4.

The Effect of Antiplatelet Drugs

Since thrombi on artificial surfaces in contact with fast-flowing blood are initiated by platelets (40), there is clearly a logic in attempting to prevent platelet adhesion pharmacologically. An apparent basis for this approach was introduced by the finding in the late 1960s that the platelet consumption caused by mechanical valves in proportion to their surface area could be abolished by dipyridamole in a dose of 400 mg/day, even though no alteration in platelet function could be detected in response to the drug (60). Aspirin, in contrast, although producing easily measurable changes in platelet function, had little corrective effect on platelet survival.

These studies on platelet survival were performed on patients with ball valves (60), considered thrombogenic by modern standards, probably because their design produces considerable turbulence (61), which is known to increase platelet deposition through the induction of shear stresses (62). It is likely that ADP is the principal mediator of shear-induced platelet aggregation (63), following its release from damaged platelets and red blood cells (64). Dipyridamole appears to work at least in part by inhibiting ADP-induced platelet aggregation (65, 66). This may explain why its clinically useful effects appear limited to inhibition of platelet deposition on artificial surfaces when combined with anticoagulation. It has not been shown to have any effect in preventing arterial or venous thrombosis elsewhere in the body when used alone (67). In particular, it does not influence the incidence of TIA and stroke (68).

It is interesting and perhaps significant that all the studies that are reported to show an advantage from combining oral anticoagulation with dipyridamole (69) have involved the use of ball valves or caged-disk valves, both of which create massive turbulence. In most of these studies a very high embolic rate was reduced to a rate now commonly associated with modern third-generation valves with anticoagulation alone. One is therefore led to question the necessity of using dipyridamole in modern valves with low turbulence. Prospective randomized trials are clearly required to provide the answer, although if the embolic rate is already low, very large numbers of patients would be needed to detect any significant difference between groups.

In summary, in the search for a measure of thrombogenicity of a particular prosthesis, the interpretation of reported embolic data is further complicated by the use of antiplatelet drugs, which may introduce bias in favor of prostheses with high degrees of turbulence by making them appear more comparable with prostheses of low turbulence.

TEMPORAL EFFECTS AND THE INFLUENCE OF STATISTICAL METHODS

A feature of many prosthetic valve series is the occurrence of a higher number of embolic events in the first few months after implantation of the prosthesis (11). In the very early events this may be due to inadequate anticoagulation in the first few postoperative days, perhaps coupled with low cardiac output in some patients. However, the majority of early emboli probably arise from the sewing ring of the prosthesis with its attendant knots and pledgets and from exposed "raw" muscle, before these rough surfaces are covered by endothelium (70), a process that usually takes about 3 months. The incidence of bleeding may also show a temporal effect caused by anticoagulation unmasking preexisting occult pathologic lesions in other systems during the first few months of treatment, for example, duodenal ulcer, bladder papilloma, and so forth.

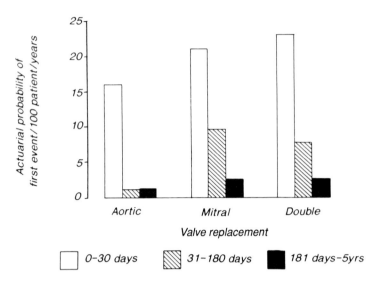

FIG. 4–6. Temporal effect on thromboembolism after valve replacement. Medtronic-Hall valve. Data from Ref. 4.

Our own results using the Medtronic-Hall valve show the temporal effect on embolism very clearly (Fig. 4–6) (4). The differences in risk of embolism in the various time periods are most striking in the mitral and double-valve patients. This is probably simply because embolism is more common after mitral valve replacement than after aortic valve replacement. However, part of the explanation may be that more exposed raw muscle remains following mitral valve replacement due to the amputation of papillary muscles. Beyond six months the risk of embolism falls to a long-term rate, which is probably more truly representative of the effect of the prosthesis itself.

The implications of this temporal effect are threefold. Firstly, the longer a series of prosthetic valve patients is followed, the lower the overall rate of embolism will become since the early high incidence will be diluted by time. Hence a series with long follow-up may appear to give better results than one with short follow-up, and the longer comparative valve series are followed, the more difficult it may be to distinguish between the prostheses in terms of embolism (71).

Secondly, the method of reporting embolic events must take the temporal effect into account. Linearized rates (the number of events divided by the number of patient years of follow-up, expressed as a percentage) are applicable only to events with constant temporal relationships and are thus inappropriate for the reporting of embolic events unless calculated for separate time periods (72). Linearized rates also include multiple events in the same patient; thus a few patients with particular risk factors for embolism may introduce bias into a whole series, the bias being greater the smaller the series. The risk of embolism with a particular prosthesis in a particular time frame is of more relevance to both surgeon and patient and has more meaning. For this reason actuarial analysis of embolic risk is more appropriate. (73, 74).

The third implication of the temporal effect concerns the comparability of embolism in valve series from different institutions. Comparability is very difficult for many reasons already discussed in this chapter, mainly lack of standardization of patient risk factors and anticoagulation measurement. Another step toward greater comparability might be to use only *long-term* (beyond six months) actuarial embolic risk for comparative purposes since this would exclude the early nonprosthetic factors that modify the risk.

Methods of data collection and interpretation also have important effects on subsequent analysis (75). Definition of what constitutes an embolic event, the completeness of follow-up and the means of classifying unexplained deaths all have an impact on the accuracy of the analysis. Similarly, the composition of many series renders them difficult to compare. For example, many European series of mitral valve replacement contain a preponderance of patients with rheumatic disease, and therefore stenotic lesions, whereas in most North American series the commonest indication for operation is mitral regurgitation of various etiologies. Since mitral stenosis is associated with a higher incidence of preoperative embolism than mitral regurgitation (76), and the need for smaller prostheses, the risk of embolism is likely to be higher in the European series, especially when different anticoagulation practice on the two sides of the Atlantic is also taken into account.

THE INFLUENCE OF SURGICAL TECHNIQUE

The sewing ring of the prosthesis and its associated suture knots and pledgets have already been mentioned as sites of known platelet deposition and possible sources of embolism (70). These rough surfaces should therefore be kept to a minimum. Historically, some early prostheses incorporated shields to cover the valve sutures (77), although in the case of early Starr-Edwards valves, these shields were limited to valves used for experimental animal implantation (78). In an approach to shorten operating time and reduce the thrombogenicity of the operative site, Wada devised an ingenious method of preventing knots coming into contact with the bloodstream by using continuous implantation sutures and bringing the suture ends to the external surface of the left atrium or aorta before tying them (79). This particular technique never enjoyed widespread popularity although the advantage of conventional continuous sutures in minimizing the number of knots on the sewing ring has been acknowledged (10).

The thrombogenicity of different suture materials varies considerably (80) and may have an impact on embolism until the sutures have been covered by endothelium. Prolene appears to be the least thrombogenic suture material and silk the most thrombogenic (80). The routine use of pledgeted sutures for valve implantation has been popular in the United States for many years in the belief that the incidence of valve dehiscence is thereby reduced, although this view has been challenged (81). To date, no studies have addressed the possible influence of multiple Teflon pledgets on embolism, although Starek has highlighted the danger of pledgets on the ventricular side of the mitral annulus in predisposing to valve thrombosis in tilting disk valves (82).

With all prosthetic valves, correct sizing is important in the prevention of complications. Oversizing a prosthesis, in addition to placing a strain on the annulus and predisposing to cardiac rupture (10), may, in the case of tilting disk or bileaflet valves, result in impingement of the disk or leaflet against an intracardiac structure, preventing full opening. In the case of ball valves, the combination of a large mitral prosthesis and a small left ventricle may prevent full ball travel. The associated turbulence or stagnation of flow may lead to thrombus formation either in the left atrium or on the prosthesis (83). Lack of care in orientation of tilting disk and bileaflet valves may lead to the same problem (10). Physiologic blood flow patterns should be interfered with as little as possible in valve orientation, given the primary objective of free occluder movement. In tilting disk valves in the mitral position for example, blood flow is most physiologic if the larger orifice of the prosthesis is orientated posteriorly (84). Although physiologic flow patterns should produce less turbulence and thereby reduce thrombotic and embolic risk, no prospective randomized studies have compared different valve orientations with this object in mind.

INDIVIDUAL PROSTHESIS THROMBOGENICITY

The thrombogenicity of a prosthesis may be defined as the propensity of that prosthesis to induce thrombus formation. It is probably a composite of two effects. The first is the susceptibility of the prosthesis to thrombus formation on any part of its mechanics as the result of its design characteristics and the materials used for its construction. The other is the secondary effect that it may have on thrombus formation in other sites, principally the left atrium, if its hemodynamic performance is suboptimal. This effect, which is difficult to quantify, is likely to be most marked in prostheses in the mitral position and may even be the predominant effect in particularly stenotic prostheses, generating an incidence of embolism from the left atrium little different to that seen in mitral stenosis. In this context it should be remembered that all mitral prostheses are "stenotic" to some extent (85) since even the prostheses with the best hemodynamic performance have an effective orifice area much smaller than that of a normal mitral valve (86). Some indication of the site of origin of an embolus may be obtained from its size; large emboli producing permanent neurologic deficits, for example, are more likely to have arisen from the left atrium than from the prosthesis (a possible exception might be ball valves—see below). This is a further argument for stratifying reported embolic events according to their severity (2).

The *measurement* of prosthesis thrombogenicity is difficult. Much of the earlier discussion in this chapter has highlighted the numerous factors that may confound an apparently simple embolic rate as expressed in many papers in the voluminous prosthetic heart valve literature. The reliability and value of such embolic rates have accordingly been questioned (2). Unless uniformity of reporting methods can be ensured in the future along the lines already discussed, embolic rates will be too insensitive to distinguish between prostheses of low or moderate thrombogenicity. Most presently available data are probably only useful in identifying prostheses whose embolic rate is well above the background incidence of TIA and stroke (Fig. 4–4).

The incidence of prosthetic valve thrombosis may be a more useful indication of the thrombogenicity of a prosthesis than the embolic rate (87). However, certain caveats need to be mentioned: (1) definitions of valve thrombosis, (2) the different mechanisms of valve thrombosis in different prostheses and their relation to embolism, and (3) the influence of anticoagulation. In *defining valve thrombosis,* it is important to distinguish between the type of major valve thrombosis that interferes with the mechanism of the prosthesis or liberates emboli and thereby produces symptoms, often of a catastrophic nature, and the type of "minor" thrombus formation sometimes seen as an incidental finding at reoperation or autopsy, which is very small, recent, and does not appear to have interfered with the function of the prosthesis. In this context, it should be remembered that most patients undergoing elective reoperation on mechanical prostheses will have had their anticoagulants discontinued preoperatively and their INR lowered below the usual therapeutic range, and many patients examined at autopsy will have had a prolonged period of low cardiac output prior to death. For these reasons, the incidental

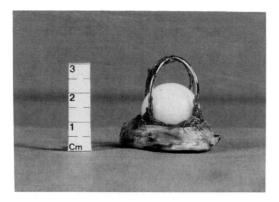

FIG. 4–7. Thrombosis of Starr-Edwards silastic ball mitral prosthesis showing typical pattern of thrombus formation on the struts.

finding of "minor" thrombi at reoperation or autopsy should not be included in valve thrombosis calculations.

The various types of mechanical prostheses show different patterns of thrombus formation. Caged-ball valves exhibit thrombus accumulation along the struts, particularly at the apex of the cage, and around the orifice (61) (Fig. 4–7). Initially this does not interfere with ball travel, but the repetitive movements of the ball are prone to dislodge emboli. Eventually, ball movement becomes increasingly restricted and progressive obstruction causes symptoms. Proponents of the ball valve claim this insidious development of thrombosis to be an advantage in that emergency reoperation is infrequently required and mortality from the complication is correspondingly low (88). The initial site of thrombus formation in *tilting disk valves* is usually in relation to the pivoting points (53) or at the minor orifice, areas of relative stagnation of blood flow in first- and second-generation disk valves (89). The low velocity of blood flow in the region of the minor orifice predisposes to tissue ingrowth, which further narrows the minor orifice and increases the risk of thrombosis (89). From this site, thrombus gradually spreads over the whole prosthesis, severely limiting its ability to open (Fig. 4–8). Although possibly occur-

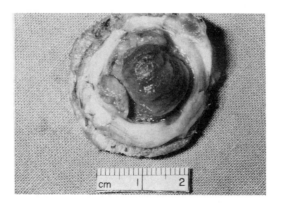

FIG. 4–8. Complete thrombosis of Björk-Shiley standard mitral prosthesis showing successive layers of thrombus formation and total immobolization of disk.

ring more rapidly than thrombosis in ball valves, disk valve thrombosis may develop gradually over several weeks as in the Björk-Shiley standard valve illustrated in Fig. 4–8, in which successive layers of thrombus deposition can be seen. Some third-generation tilting disk valves such as the Medtronic-Hall have endeavored to overcome the problem of stagnation by increasing the size of the minor orifice (90). Thrombus formation in *bileaflet valves* is most likely to begin in the region of the hinge pockets, and in this situation even a very small thrombus may completely immobilize one or both leaflets (91).

Thus the basic difference between these valves of different design is that in tilting disk and bileaflet valves, thrombus formation tends to immobilize or severely restrict the moving parts, whereas in the ball valve the moving part is able to repeatedly strike the surface covered by thrombus, thereby dislodging emboli. It is not surprising therefore to find that many patients with Starr-Edwards valves who have recurrent emboli are found to have significant thrombus on the prosthesis at reoperation or autopsy. (92, 93). In contrast, a recent study of tilting disk (Björk-Shiley standard) and bileaflet valves (Duromedics) showed no correlation between linearized incidence rates of embolism and thrombotic obstruction and found that valve thrombosis was never preceded by embolism in individual patients (71). It is probable therefore that embolism and valve thrombosis are closely related in ball valves but not in more modern prostheses of different design. This basic difference provides further fuel to the argument that the two complications should be reported separately.

Although it is probably a better and more sensitive index of prosthesis thrombogenicity than embolism, the incidence of valve thrombosis is also influenced by some of the same factors, particularly *anticoagulation and surgical technique.* For example, the Omniscience valve, a tilting disk valve with a small minor orifice, appears particularly prone to valve thrombosis, yet reported valve thrombosis rates in the mitral position vary from 0.4% per patient year in North America (54) to 9.4% per patient year in the United Kingdom (53). The difference is almost certainly mainly explained by the different levels of anticoagulation used (4), although patient characteristics and surgical technique may have differed also. Hence, if valve thrombosis rates are to be used as indices of prosthesis thrombogenicity, they must either be expressed in relation to anticoagulation levels achieved or sufficient numbers of series must be averaged in the analysis to take into account high and low anticoagulation levels. Valve thrombosis rates should only be used in this type of cumulative analysis if they can be extracted from a sufficient number of recent, large, well-documented series with worthwhile periods of follow-up and no unusual factors known to increase the incidence of valve thrombosis (87).

An example of this approach to quantifying the thrombogenicity of currently available prostheses according to their incidence of thrombotic obstruction is illustrated in Table 4–2, the data for which were obtained from 51 sources published between 1983 and 1987 (87). One problem with this approach is that it is necessary to wait until several reports have appeared in the literature before a worthwhile quantity of data is available for analysis. Newer prostheses with design or construction changes aimed at improved thrombogenicity cannot therefore be assessed until they have been in clinical use for some years. Nevertheless, there is no substitute for long-term follow-up in proper clinical evaluation of prostheses since excellent hydrodynamic performance in vitro does not guarantee good thromboembolic performance in vivo. At present, little published clinical information is available on the Omnicarbon tilting disk valve or the Carbomedics bileaflet valve. Preliminary results with the Björk-Shiley monostrut tilting disk valve are presented in Chapter 8.

TABLE 4–2. *Average Thrombosis Rates for Prosthetic Valves*

	Rate (%/yr)	Patient years of follow-up
AORTIC VALVE REPLACEMENT		
Medtronic-Hall	0.02	5,065
St. Jude Medical	0.09	5,772
Starr-Edwards*	0.15	23,039
Björk-Shiley standard	0.36	7,461
Omniscience	0.53	561
MITRAL VALVE REPLACEMENT		
Medtronic-Hall	0.11	3,620
Starr-Edwards*	0.32	19,949
St. Jude Medical	0.38	4,434
Björk-Shiley standard	0.55	9,707
Omniscience	2.85	1,017

*The rate for the Starr-Edwards valve may be an underestimate; see text for explanation.

Data derived from Ref. 87.

In view of the unique features of ball valve thrombosis referred to earlier, which might allow nonprogressive valve thrombosis to present only as recurrent embolism, the rates shown for the Starr-Edwards valve in Table 4–2 may underestimate the true thrombogenicity of this prosthesis. The disk valve data in Table 4–2 suggest that some currently available tilting disk valves (Medtronic-Hall) are considerably less thrombogenic than others (Björk-Shiley standard and Omniscience). It follows that it is inappropriate to aggregate mixed series of different tilting disk valves for the purpose of comparison with prostheses of other generic design. Similarly, data from first- and second-generation tilting disk valves should not be extrapolated to make unqualified statements about the thrombogenicity of "all tilting disk valves" (88), an oversimplification that has unfortunately been commonplace in the literature for some time. The practice of comparing embolic and bleeding complications between mixed series of mechanical valves and mixed series of bioprostheses is perhaps even more inappropriate and misleading.

Some authors have attempted to quantify the thrombogenicity of heart valve prostheses by various measurements of platelet consumption (60, 94) and platelet function (95). However, much of the data on platelet consumption relates to older prostheses, some of which are no longer in use, and currently available platelet function measurements are insufficiently sensitive to distinguish between prostheses of different thrombogenicity (95).

Most of this chapter has concentrated on mechanical valves, but it should not be forgotten that bioprostheses are also susceptible to embolism and even valve thrombosis. Many authors have documented similar incidences of embolism in bioprostheses without anticoagulation and third-generation mechanical valves with anticoagulation (26). Valve thrombosis is now rare in both these categories. Comparative risk between the best modern mechanical valves and bioprostheses is thus a balance between the risks of low-level anticoagulation in the former (51, 52, 57) and the risk of reoperation for valve failure in the latter (96). Unless current research can significantly extend the lifespan of bioprostheses, it is likely that long-term risk analysis will favor modern, low-thrombogenicity mechanical valves provided that they are anticoagulated at low levels. Prospective randomized trials are awaited with interest. Retrospective studies comparing older first- and second-generation mechanical prostheses with biological valves are of little relevance to present-day decision making (97).

SUMMARY, RECOMMENDATIONS, AND FUTURE TRENDS

Because they can be influenced by so many nonprosthetic factors, currently available embolic rates in the literature are of little guidance in assessing the thrombogenicity of a prosthesis. Only in ball valves does there appear to be any relationship between embolism and valve thrombosis. Therefore this relationship should not be extrapolated to other prostheses. If embolic rates are to be used in any meaningful way for prosthesis assessment in the future, it will be necessary to standardize the exclusion of many nonprosthetic risk factors and to take into account the influence of anticoagulation level measured in a standardized fashion. Actuarially calculated long-term rates beyond the first 6 postoperative months would help to eliminate the influence of perioperative factors.

Valve thrombosis rates are probably the most useful currently available parameter for assessing prosthesis thrombogenicity providing the caveats previously discussed are heeded; rates from as many large, recent, well-documented series as possible *employing low as well as high anticoagulation levels* should be averaged for each prosthesis. If series with high anticoagulation levels are the only ones available for a particular prosthesis, these should not be considered reliable for comparative purposes since they may underestimate the true thrombogenicity of that prosthesis.

Recommended anticoagulation levels in the future should be matched to individual prosthesis thrombogenicity. Detailed dose–response studies along the lines of that carried out for the Medtronic-Hall valve should provide an accurate indication of the optimum level for each prosthesis. The current blanket recommendation of an INR of 3.0 to 4.5 for all prosthetic heart valves is certainly too high for prostheses of low thrombogenicity, since it carries an unnecessarily high risk of bleeding.

Until dose–response studies are available for other prostheses, it may be possible to extrapolate to a limited extent from the data presented in Table 2 in choosing anticoagulation levels for individual prostheses. For example, the Omniscience valve clearly requires anticoagulation at a much higher level than the Medtronic-Hall valve if the risk of valve thrombosis is to be reduced. The value of adding dipyridamole to anticoagulation for all prostheses remains uncertain, although it appears to be useful in minimizing embolic risk in patients with ball valves (69).

The management of patients with recurrent embolism remains a problem. These patients require detailed investigation to identify underlying risk factors. Many will be found simply to have very poor anticoagulant control. In a few patients, recurrent emboli in a short time period may be the first indication of prosthetic endocarditis. In patients with ball valves it should be remembered that recurrent embolism may signify early valve thrombosis. This is supported by evidence that replacing Starr-Edwards valves associated with recurrent embolism with biological valves significantly reduces the incidence of embolism, despite other risk factors' remaining constant (92).

One of the goals in prosthetic heart valve design has always been the development of a prosthesis made from artificial materials that would not require anticoagulation. This goal has yet to be achieved, but research continues in that direction with the search for new designs and new materials (40, 98) and for means of coating artificial surfaces to make them more thromboresistant (99). Experimental evidence in animals suggests that coumarin anticoagulants may merely reduce the growth rate and tenacity of adhesion of thrombi on artificial surfaces, thereby causing a continuous liberation of microemboli too small to be detected clinically (100). If this is true of prosthetic valves in clinical use, worthwhile advances are more likely to be made by concentrating on rendering surfaces more thromboresistant.

In the meantime, research continues on newer antiplatelet drugs. Ticlopidine is one such agent that appears to show promise (67). It appears to work by a mechanism different from that of other antiplatelet agents, possibly by altering the reactivity of the platelet membrane to activating stimuli. The results of ongoing trials are awaited with interest. α-tocopherol, vitamin E, has also been shown to be an effective inhibitor of platelet adhesion (101). However, no information is yet available on its effects in patients with prosthetic heart valves.

Progress in the future will probably be achieved by a combination of new prosthetic designs and materials together with improved drug control to minimize embolism. Less thrombogenic prostheses with better hemodynamic performance might also justify surgical intervention earlier in the natural history of the disease process before the onset of atrial fibrillation, thereby avoiding the major nonprosthetic factor involved in embolism. Attention to other risk factors will continue to be important for patients with prosthetic heart valves, including strict control of hypertension and diabetes, the avoidance of cigarette smoking and oral contraceptives, and careful attention to diet.

REFERENCES

1. Gabbay S, Kresh JY: Bioengineering of mechanical and biologic heart valve substitutes. In Morse D, Steiner RM, Fernandez J (eds): Guide to Prosthetic Cardiac Valves. New York, Springer-Verlag, 1985, pp 239–256.
2. McGoon DC: The risk of thromboembolism following valvular operations: How does one know? J Thorac Cardiovasc Surg 1984;88:782–786.
3. Bloom AL: The need for standardisation of anticoagulation management. In Rabago G, Cooley DA (eds): Heart Valve Replacement. New York, Futura, 1987, pp 319–333.
4. Butchart EG, Lewis PA, Kulatilake ENP, Breckenridge IM: Anticoagulation variability between centres: Implications for comparative prosthetic valve assessment. Eur J Cardiothorac Surg 1988;2:72–81.
5. Clark RE, Edmunds LH Jr, Cohn LH, Miller DC, Weisel RD: Guidelines for reporting morbidity and mortality after cardiac valvular operations. Eur J Cardiothorac Surg 1988;2:293–295.
6. Virchow R: Gesammelte Abhandlungen zur wissenschaftlichen Medizin: IV. Thrombose und Embolie. Gefassentzundung und septische Infektion. Frankfurt, Meidinger, 1856.
7. Warlow CP: Antithrombotic drugs and the prevention of stroke (stroke incidence and outcome). In Verstraete M, Vermylen J, Lijnen HR, Arnout J (eds): Thrombosis and Haemostasis. Leuven, Holland, Leuven University Press, 1987, pp 301–324.
8. Dennis MS, Bamford JM, Sandercock PAG, Warlow CP. Incidence of transient ischaemic attacks in Oxfordshire, England. Stroke 1989;20:333–339.
9. Mitchell RS, Miller DC, Stinson EB, Oyer PE, Jamieson SW, Baldwin JC, Shumway NE: Significant patient-related determinants of prosthetic valve performance. J Thorac Cardiovasc Surg 1986;91:807–817.
10. Butchart EG: The potential complications of heart valve replacement and their prevention: Technical considerations. In Rabago G, Cooley DA (eds): Heart Valve Replacement. New York, Futura, 1987, pp 31–53.
11. Edmunds LH Jr: Thromboembolic complications of current cardiac valvular prostheses. Ann Thorac Surg 1982;34:96–106.
12. Shi F, Hart RG, Sherman DG, Tegeler CH: Stroke in the People's Republic of China. Stroke 1989;20:1581–1585.
13. Lodder J, Dennis MS, Van Raak L, Jones LN, Warlow CP: Cooperative study on the value of long-term anticoagulation in patients with stroke and non-rheumatic atrial fibrillation. Br Med J 1988;296:1435–1438.
14. Halperin JL, Hart RG: Atrial fibrillation and stroke: New ideas, persisting dilemmas. Stroke 1988;19:937–941.
15. Evans JG: Blood pressure and stroke in an elderly English population. J Epidemiol Community Health 1987;41:275–282.
16. Wolf PA, D'Agostino RB, Kannel WB, Bonita R, Belanger AJ: Cigarette smoking as a risk factor for stroke. The Framingham Study. JAMA 1988;259:1025–1029.

17. Salonen JT, Puska P, Tuomilehto J, Homan K: Relation of blood pressure, serum lipids and smoking to the risk of cerebral stroke. A longitudinal study in Eastern Finland. Stroke 1982;13:327–333.
18. Schmidley JW, Caronna JJ: Transient cerebral ischaemia: Pathophysiology. Prog Cardiovasc Dis 1980;22:325–342.
19. Marquardsen J: Stroke registration: Experiences from a WHO multicentre study. In Rose FC (ed): Clinical Neuroepidemiology. Tunbridge Wells, Pitman Medical, 1980, pp 105–111.
20. Whisnant JP: The decline of stroke. Stroke 1984;15:160–168.
21. Urakami K, Igo M, Takahashi K: An epidemiologic study of cerebrovascular disease in Western Japan with special reference to transient ischaemic attacks. Stroke 1987;18:396–401.
22. Boysen G, Nyboe J, Appleyard M, Sorensen PS: Stroke incidence and risk factors for stroke in Copenhagen, Denmark. Stroke 1988;19:1345–1353.
23. Fratiglioni L, Arfaioli C, Nencini P, Ginanneschi A: Transient ischemic attacks in the community: Occurrence and clinical characteristics. A population survey in the area of Florence, Italy. Neuroepidemiology 1989;8:87–96.
24. Stewart WE, Jamrozik K, Ward G: The Perth community stroke study: Attack rates for stroke and TIA in Western Australia. Clin Exp Neurol 1987;24:39–44.
25. Kempster PA, Gerraty RP, Gates PC: Asymptomatic cerebral infarction in patients with chronic atrial fibrillation. Stroke 1988;19:955–957.
26. Edmunds LH Jr: Thrombotic and bleeding complications of prosthetic heart valves. Ann Thorac Surg 1987;44:430–445.
27. WHO Task Force on Stroke and Other Cerebrovascular Disorders: Stroke 1989; recommendations on stroke prevention, diagnosis and therapy. Stroke 1989;20:1407–1431.
28. Kannel WB, McGee DL: Diabetes and cardiovascular disease: The Framingham Study. JAMA 1979;241:2035–2038.
29. Meyer JS, Rogers RL, Mortel KF, Judd BW: Hyperlipidaemia is a risk factor for decreased cerebral perfusion and stroke. Arch Neurol 1987;44:418–422.
30. Wilhelmsen L, Svarsudd K, Korsan-Bengtsen K, Larsson B, Welin L, Tibblin G: Fibrinogen as a risk factor for stroke and myocardial infarction. N Engl J Med 1984;311:501–505.
31. Kannel WB, D'Agostino RB, Belanger AJ: Fibrinogen, cigarette smoking and the risk of cardiovascular disease. Am Heart J 1987;113:1006–1010.
32. Riddle MC, Hart J: Hyperglycaemia, recognized and unrecognised, as a risk factor for stroke and transient ischemic attacks. Stroke 1982;13:356–359.
33. Gorelick PB: The status of alcohol as a risk factor for stroke. Stroke 1989;20:1607–1610.
34. Pleet AB, Massey EW, Vengrow ME: TIA, stroke and the bicuspid aortic valve. Neurology 1981;31:1540–1542.
35. Barnett HJM, Boughner DR, Taylor DW, Cooper PE, Kostuk WJ, Nichol PM: Further evidence relating mitral valve prolapse to cerebral ischaemic events. N Engl J Med 1980;302:139–144.
36. Szekely P: Systemic embolism and anticoagulant prophylaxis in rheumatic heart disease. Br Med J 1964;1:1209–1212.
37. Abdon NJ, Zetterval O, Carlson J, Berglund S: Is occult atrial disorder a frequent cause of non-haemorrhagic stroke? Long-term ECG in 86 patients. Stroke 1982;13:832–837.
38. Lundstrom T, Ryden L: Haemorrhagic and thromboembolic complications in patients with atrial fibrillation on anticoagulant prophylaxis. J Intern Med 1989;255:137–142.
39. Caplan LF, D'Crux I, Hier DB, Reddy H, Shah S: Atrial size, atrial fibrillation and stroke. Ann Neurol 1986;19:158–161.
40. Joist JH, Pennington DG: Platelet reactions with artificial surfaces. Trans Am Soc Artif Intern Organs 1987;33:341–344.
41. Meade TW, Imeson J, Stirling Y: Effect of changes in smoking and other characteristics on clotting factors and the risk of ischaemic heart disease. Lancet 1987;2:986–988.
42. Di Minno G, Cerbone AM: Fibrinogen: A coagulation protein in the cardiovascular risk factor profile. In Crepaldi G, Gotto AM, Manzato E, Baggio G (eds): Atherosclerosis VIII. Amsterdam, Elsevier, 1989, pp 469–474.
43. Zbinden G: Evaluation of thrombogenic effects of drugs. Annu Rev Pharmacol Toxicol 1976;16:177–188.
44. Stolley PD, Tonascia JA, Tockman MS, Sartwell PE, Rutledge AH, Jacobs MP: Thrombosis with low-estrogen oral contraceptives. Am J Epidemiol 1975;102:197–208.
45. Collaborative Group for the Study of Stroke in Young Women: Oral contraception and increased risk of cerebral ischemia or thrombosis. N Engl J Med 1973;288:871–878.
46. Collaborative Group for the Study of Stroke in Young Women: Oral contraceptives and stroke in young women; associated risk factors. JAMA 1975;231:718–722.
47. Schafer AI: The hypercoagulable states. Ann Intern Med 1985;102:814–828.
48. Poller L: A simple nomogram for the derivation of International Normalised Ratios for the standardisation of prothrombin times. Thromb Haemostasis 1988;60:18–20.

49. Loeliger EA: Laboratory control, optimal therapeutic ranges and therapeutic quality control in oral anti-coagulation. Acta Haematol 1985;74:125–131.
50. Hirsh J, Poller L, Deykin D, Levine M, Dalen JE: Optimal therapeutic range for oral anticoagulants. Chest 1989;95(suppl):5S–11S.
51. Forfar JC: A seven year analysis of haemorrhage in patients on long term anticoagulation treatment. Br Heart J 1979;42:128–132.
52. Second report of the Sixty Plus Reinfarction Study Group: Risks of long-term anticoagulant therapy in elderly patients after myocardial infarction. Lancet 1982;2:64–68.
53. Fanapazir L, Clarke DB, Dark JF, Lawson RAM, Mousalli H: Results of valve replacement with the Omniscience prosthesis. J Thorac Cardiovasc Surg 1983;86:621–625.
54. Callaghan JC, Coles J, Damle A: Six year clinical study of the Omniscience valve prosthesis in 219 patients. J Am Coll Cardiol 1987;9(suppl 1):240–246.
55. Levine MN, Raskob G, Hirsh J: Haemorrhagic complications of long-term anticoagulant therapy. Chest 1989;95(suppl):26S–36S.
56. Silverstein A: Neurological complications of anticoagulation therapy. Arch Intern Med 1979;139:217–220.
57. Butchart EG, Lewis PA, Coombes JA, Breckenridge IM: Moving towards prosthesis-specific anticoagulation. In Bodnar E (ed): Surgery for Heart Valve Disease. London, ICR Publishers, 1990, pp 174–183.
58. Butchart EG, Lewis PA: Tailoring anticoagulation levels to individual prosthesis thrombogenicity; recommendations for the Medtronic Hall valve in the aortic and mitral positions. Circulation: In press.
59. Saour JN, Sieck JO, Mamo LAR, Gallus AS: Trial of different intensities of anticoagulation in patients with prosthetic heart valves. N Engl J Med 1990;322:428–432.
60. Harker LA, Sherrill SJ: Studies of platelet and fibrinogen kinetics in patients with prosthetic heart valves. N Engl J Med 1970;283:1302–1305.
61. Yoganathan AP, Reamer HH, Corcoran WH, Harrison EC, Shulman IA, Parnassus W: The Starr-Edwards aortic ball valve: Flow characteristics, thrombus formation and tissue overgrowth. Artif Organs 1981;5:6–17.
62. Stein PD, Sabbah HN: Measured turbulence and its effect on thrombus formation. Circ Res 1974;35:608–614.
63. Moritz MW, Reimers RC, Baker RK, Sutera SP, Joist JH: Role of cytoplasmic and releasable ADP in platelet aggregation induced by laminar shear stress. J Lab Clin Med 1983;101:537–544.
64. Reimers RC, Sutera SP, Joist JH: Potentiation by red blood cells of shear-induced platelet aggregation: Relative importance of chemical and physical mechanisms. Blood 1984;64:1200–1206.
65. Emmons PR, Harrison MJG, Honour AJ: Effect of dipyridamole on human platelet behaviour. Lancet 1965;2:603–606.
66. Philp RB, Lemieux V: Comparison of some effects of dipyridamole and adenosine on thrombus formation, platelet adhesiveness and blood pressure in rabbits and rats. Nature 1968;218:1072–1074.
67. Harker LA, Gent M: The use of agents that modify platelet function in the management of thrombotic disorders. In Coleman RW, Hirsch J, Marder VJ, Salzman EW (eds): Hemostasis and Thrombosis. Philadelphia, JB Lippincott, 1987, pp 1438–1466.
68. Acheson J, Danta G, Hutchinson EC: Controlled trial of dipyridamole in cerebral vascular disease. Br Med J 1969;1:614–615.
69. Chesebro JH, Adams PC, Fuster V: Antithrombotic therapy in patients with valvular heart disease and prosthetic heart valves. J Am Coll Cardiol 1986;8:41B–56B.
70. Dewanjee MK, Kaye MP, Fuster V: Non-invasive radioisotopic techniques for detection of platelet deposition in mitral valve prosthesis and quantitation of cerebral, renal and pulmonary microembolism in dogs. Circulation 1980;62(suppl III):III-8.
71. Nashef SAM, Stewart M, Bain WH: Heart valve replacement: Thromboembolism or thrombosis and embolism? In Bodnar E (ed): Surgery for Heart Valve Disease. London, ICR Publishers, 1990, pp 159–170.
72. Grunkemeier GL: Statistical analysis of prosthetic valve series. In Rabago G, Cooley DA (eds): Heart Valve Replacement. New York, Futura, 1987, pp 11–26.
73. Grunkemeier GL, Lambert LE, Bonchek LI, Starr A: An improved statistical method for assessing the results of operation. Ann Thorac Surg 1975;20:289–298.
74. Bodnar E, Wain WH, Haberman S: Assessment and comparison of the performance of cardiac valves. Ann Thorac Surg 1982;34:146–156.
75. Grunkemeier GL, Starr A: Pitfalls in statistical analysis of heart valve prostheses. Ann Thorac Surg 1989;48(suppl):S14–S15.
76. Neilson GH, Galea EG, Hossack KF: Thromboembolic complications of mitral valve disease. Aust NZ J Med 1978;8:372–376.
77. Harken DE, Collins JJ Jr: Mitral and aortic valve surgery. In Cooper P (ed): The Craft of Surgery. Boston, Little, Brown, 1964, pp 620–644.

78. Lefrak EA, Starr A: Starr-Edwards ball valve. In Cardiac Valve Prostheses. New York, Appleton-Century-Crofts, 1979, pp 67–117.
79. Wada J: The knotless suture method for prosthetic valve fixation. Int Surg 1966;46:317–320.
80. Dahlke H, Dociu N, Thurau K: Thrombogenicity of different suture materials as revealed by scanning electron microscopy. J Biomed Mater Res 1980;14:251–268.
81. Dhasmana JP, Blackstone EH, Kirklin JW, Kouchoukos NT: Factors associated with periprosthetic leakage following primary mitral valve replacement, with special consideration of the suture technique. Ann Thorac Surg 1983;35:170–178.
82. Starek PJK: Technical aspects of uncomplicated valve replacement. In Starek PJK (ed): Heart Valve Replacement and Reconstruction. Chicago, Year Book Medical, 1987, pp 61–79.
83. Roberts WC, Morrow AG: Mechanisms of acute left atrial thrombosis after mitral valve replacement. Am J Cardiol 1966;18:497–503.
84. Jones M, Eidbo EE: Doppler color flow evaluation of prosthetic mitral valves: Experimental epicardial studies. J Am Coll Cardiol 1989;13:234–240.
85. Rahimtoola SH: The problem of valve prosthesis-patient mismatch. Circulation 1978;58:20–24.
86. Westaby S, Karp RB, Blackstone EH, Bishop SP: Adult human valve dimensions and their surgical significance. Am J Cardiol 1984;53:552–556.
87. Butchart EG, Lewis PA, Grunkemeier GL, Kulatilake ENP, Breckenridge IM: Low risk of thrombosis and serious embolic events despite low intensity anticoagulation. Experience with 1,004 Medtronic Hall valves. Circulation 1988;78(suppl I):I-66–I-77.
88. Metzdorff MT, Grunkemeier GL, Pinson CW, Starr A: Thrombosis of mechanical cardiac valves: A qualitative comparison of the silastic ball valve and the tilting disc valve. J Am Coll Cardiol 1984;4:50–53.
89. Yoganathan AP, Corcoran WH, Harrison EC, Carl JR: The Bjork-Shiley aortic prosthesis: Flow characteristics, thrombus formation and tissue overgrowth. Circulation 1978;58:70–76.
90. Hall KV, Kaster RL, Woien A: An improved pivotal disc type prosthetic heart valve. J Oslo City Hosp 1979;29:3–21.
91. Nunez L, Iglesias A, Sotillo J: Entrapment of leaflet of St Jude Medical cardiac valve prosthesis by miniscule thrombus: Report of two cases. Ann Thorac Surg 1980;29:567–569.
92. Reitz BA, Stinson EB, Griepp RB, Shumway NE: Tissue valve replacement of prosthetic heart valves for thromboembolism. Am J Cardiol 1978;41:512–515.
93. Acar J, Enriquez-Sarano M, Farah E, Kassab R, Tubiana P, Roger V: Recurrent systemic embolic events with valve prosthesis. Eur Heart J 1984;5(suppl D):33–38.
94. Rajah SM: Platelet survival in patients with homograft and prosthetic heart valves: Correlation with incidence of thromboembolism. Br J Haematol 1976;33:148.
95. Pumphrey CW, Davies J: The platelet release reaction in cardiovascular disease: Evaluation of plasma betathromboglobulin as a marker of a prothrombotic state. Eur Heart J 1984;5(suppl D):7–11.
96. Bortolotti U, Milan A, Mazzucco A, Valfre C, Talenti E, Guerra F, Thiene G, Gallucci V: Results of reoperation for primary tissue failure of porcine bioprostheses. J Thorac Cardiovasc Surg 1985;90:564–569.
97. Hammond GL, Geha AS, Kopf GS, Hashim SW: Biological versus mechanical valves: Analysis of 1,116 valves inserted in 1,012 adult patients with a 4,818 patient-year and a 5,327 valve year follow up. J Thorac Cardiovasc Surg 1987;93:182–198.
98. Vroman L: Problems in the development of materials that are compatible with blood. Biomat Med Dev Art Org 1984\5;12:307–323.
99. Joseph G, Sharma CP: Prostacyclin immobilised albuminated surfaces. J Biomed Mat Res 1987;21:937–945.
100. Madras PN, Thomson CL, Johnson WR: The effect of Coumadin upon thrombus forming on foreign surfaces. Artif Organs 1980;4:192–198.
101. Jandak J, Steiner M, Richardson PD: Alpha-tocopherol, an effective inhibitor of platelet adhesion. Blood 1989;73:141–149.

Bodnar, E. and Frater, R. W. M., editors
(1991) *Replacement Cardiac Valves,*
Pergamon Press, Inc. (New York), pp. 99–124
Printed in the United States of America

CHAPTER 5

MODES OF FAILURE AND OTHER PATHOLOGY OF MECHANICAL AND TISSUE HEART VALVE PROSTHESES

FREDERICK J. SCHOEN

This chapter summarizes a pathologist's view of cardiac valve prostheses. The significance, morphology, and pathogenesis of the observed major complications and other alterations during function of mechanical and bioprosthetic valves are reviewed. The reader is also referred to other recent discussions of various pathologic considerations in cardiac valve replacement (1–4).

ROLE OF PROSTHESIS-RELATED COMPLICATIONS IN THE OUTCOME OF CARDIAC VALVE REPLACEMENT

The long-term result of successful valve replacement is determined primarily by three factors: (1) irreversible structural alterations in the heart and lungs secondary to valvular disease (especially left ventricular myocardial hypertrophy and degeneration caused by chronic pressure and/or volume overload, and pulmonary vascular disease), (2) occlusive coronary artery disease, and (3) the mechanical reliability of the prosthesis and the consequences of thrombus formation and other prosthesis–host tissue interactions. For patients who undergo valve replacement sufficiently early in the course of their disease to benefit from hemodynamic adjustment, prosthesis-associated pathologic conditions are a major determinant of the long-term prognosis.

Valve-related complications have been frequent in large series with previously and currently used substitute valves. Less than 50% of patients with Starr-Edwards caged-ball aortic and mitral replacements were free of serious valve-related complications 10 years following surgery (5–7). With the more contemporary Björk-Shiley standard aortic valve, 54% of patients in one study had experienced at least one form of major valve-related complication by 10 years postoperatively, of which 16% were fatal (8); in another, freedom from all valve-related complications was 66% at 12 years (9). In a large comparative study, the freedom from all valve-related mortality and morbidity at 10 years was reported at 57% for various mechanical valves and 36% (58% at 8 years) for bioprostheses (10). The overall linearized rate of complications is 6 to 9% per patient year for contemporary mechanical and bioprosthetic valves (i.e., Björk-Shiley, St. Jude, Hancock porcine) (10–13). Reoperations on patients who have had valve replacement, which now probably account for at least 15% of all valve surgery, are almost always necessitated by prosthetic valve–related complications (14–17). Furthermore, many patients die of complications of the prosthesis (18). Clinical series suggest that approximately 20% of late deaths result from prosthesis-associated pathologic lesions (5–7). However, the cause of death of many patients described in clinical studies has not been verified by postmortem

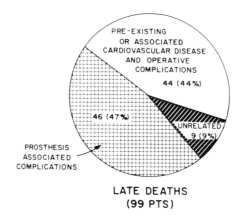

Fig. 5–1. Causes of late death following cardiac valve replacement. Reproduced with permission from Schoen FJ, Titus JL, Lawrie GM: Autopsy-determined causes of death after cardiac valve replacement. JAMA 1983;249:899–902. Copyright 1983, American Medical Association.

examination, and thus some sudden deaths attributed to arrhythmias or progressive congestive heart failure could be valve-related. Indeed, autopsy studies show that valve prosthesis pathologic conditions revealed by autopsy were not clinically appreciated in many cases, and that prosthesis-related events cause approximately half of late deaths (18) (Fig. 5–1).

In general, large studies show almost no differences in rates of valve-related complications between mechanical prostheses and bioprostheses 10 years postoperatively (10–12). However, since the major factor in the prognosis of patients with mechanical valves relates to thromboembolic problems, whose likelihood is not strongly dependent on postoperative interval, and because the most frequent complications of bioprosthetic valves only become statistically important approximately 5 years or more postoperatively (i.e., progressive degenerative dysfunction), comparative studies with lesser periods of follow-up often show bioprosthetic valves to be advantageous.

A comparison biased toward bioprostheses is based on the *treatment failure* concept (19). Treatment failure includes valve-related deaths or permanent disability; successful reoperations are excluded, while emboli with permanent residua are included. When this patient-oriented definition is applied, bioprosthetic valves in the mitral but not the aortic site retain a small advantage over mechanical valves at 10 years. This arises because there is a higher likelihood that a mechanical valve problem will have a catastrophic outcome or permanent consequence, relative to the usually progressive, recognizable, and treatable deterioration in patients who have bioprosthetic valve failure.

VALVE FAILURE AND OTHER VALVE-RELATED PATHOLOGIC CONDITIONS: MORPHOLOGY, SECONDARY EFFECTS, AND PATHOGENESIS

Although most comparisons between contemporary mechanical prostheses and bioprostheses yield similar overall complication rates, as discussed above, *the frequency and in some cases the nature of specific valve-related complications* vary with the type (and sometimes model) of replacement device (1–4, 20). Valve-related complications causing the ultimate failure of cardiac valve replacement are summarized in Table 5–1. The most

TABLE 5–1. *Prosthetic Heart Valve Failure*

Death caused by or reoperation necessitated by any of the following:
1. Occlusion or dysfunction by thrombus
2. Thromboembolism
3. Prosthetic valve endocarditis (active or inactive)
4. Anticoagulant-related hemorrhage
5. Hemodynamic prosthetic valve dysfunction (including structural failure of any valve component)
6. Occlusion or dysfunction by tissue overgrowth
7. Sterile periprosthetic leak
8. Reoperation for any other reason (e.g., hemolysis, extrinsic interference with normal function, noise)

commonly encountered valve-related complications in patients with mechanical or bio-prosthetic valves are thromboembolic problems, infective endocarditis, paravalvular leak, and degradative dysfunction (1–4, 20).

The causes of the removal of dysfunctional valves reflect the relative frequencies of specific indications for reoperation. For 112 consecutive porcine bioprostheses and 45 mechanical valve prostheses surgically removed at our hospital during a 66-month inter-val during 1980–1985, the causes of failure of all valves (including mechanical and bio-prosthetic replacements) included thrombosis (9%), tissue overgrowth (5%), endocarditis (16%), paravalvular leak (11%), and degenerative dysfunction (53%) (Fig. 5–2) (21). Thrombosis was a major cause of mechanical valve dysfunction (18% of failures) but was infrequent with bioprostheses. Degenerative dysfunction of mechanical valves was not encountered frequently, but sterile primary tissue degeneration was overwhelmingly the most frequent cause of bioprosthetic valve failure (74% of removed bioprostheses). Thus, it is not surprising that the major consideration in valve selection for an individual patient is generally the trade-off of the risks of thrombosis or thromboembolism despite

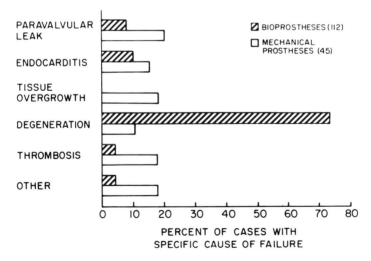

FIG. 5–2. Causes of failure of mechanical prosthetic and bioprosthetic heart valves, 1980–1985. Failure modes of mechanical valves are diverse; thromboembolic complications are most fre-quent. In contrast, the overwhelming cause of failure of bioprosthetic valves is degenerative pro-cesses. Reproduced with permission from Schoen FJ: Surgical pathology of removed natural and prosthetic heart valves. Hum Pathol 1987;18:558–567. Copyright 1987, WB Saunders.

anticoagulation, and anticoagulation hemorrhage, with mechanical prostheses, versus the limited long-term durability of bioprostheses. However, treatment of some patient subpopulations such as children (22, 23), women of child bearing age (24), adults with aortic stenosis and hemorrhagic colonic angiodysplasia (21), and individuals in socioeconomically underdeveloped regions (25) often necessitates more complex considerations.

Thromboembolic Complications

Thromboembolic complications (including thrombosis, thromboembolism, and anti-coagulation-related hemorrhage) are major causes of mortality and morbidity after cardiac valve replacement, accounting for 55 to 79% and 19 to 79% of valve-related complications in patients with mitral mechanical valves and bioprosthetic valves, respectively, and for 57 to 92% and 31 to 71% in patients with aortic mechanical valves and bioprostheses, respectively (26). Thrombotic occlusion and thromboemboli have been reported with all currently available types of prosthesis, and contemporary prostheses generally have thromboembolic rates of 1 to 4% per patient year (8–13, 26). In recent clinical studies from our institution, freedom from thrombosis or thromboembolism at 108 months for patients with porcine bioprostheses was 85% (mitral and aortic), compared with 77% (mitral) and 83% (aortic) with tilting disk prosthetic valves (11, 12), data consistent with those of other clinical series (27). Rates of thromboembolism depend on the specific prosthesis used, cardiac rhythm, anticoagulation regimen, and site of valve replaced. Moreover, the incidence of thromboembolic complications is greatest in the first postoperative year, probably due to early thrombogenicity of the valve sewing ring prior to its incorporation by tissue.

Role of Anticoagulation

The major factor controlling the risk of thromboembolism is the adequacy of anticoagulation (as assessed by prothrombin times within the therapeutic range), which overshadows the importance of other contributory factors including atrial fibrillation and left atrial thrombus, particularly with mechanical valves (26). However, the chronic oral anticoagulation required in many patients receiving prosthetic valves induces a risk of hemorrhage (5–7, 13, 26, 28). Indeed, patients receiving therapeutic long-term anticoagulation for any reason are susceptible to hemorrhage, particularly retroperitoneal, gastrointestinal, or cerebral. The frequency is approximately 4% per patient year (18). Fifteen to 25% of such events are fatal (26). In some clinical studies, decreases in thromboembolic risk have been accompanied by increases in anticoagulation-related hemorrhage (7). In a recent study of a large group of patients with the St. Jude valve, the most frequent complication was warfarin-related hemorrhage, at a rate of 2.6% per patient year (13). Death occurred in 23% of the hemorrhagic events. This exceeded the rates of both embolism (2.1% per patient year) and thromboembolic fatalities (4% of events).

Pathology of Valve Thrombosis and Thromboembolism

Both fibrin (red) thrombus and platelet (white) thrombus form in association with valve substitutes. Thrombotic deposits on prosthetic heart valves can interfere with function by partially or completely immobilizing the occluder, preventing full opening or closing, obstructing the valve orifice, or generating thromboemboli to distal arterial beds. Over 80% of clinically detectable thromboemboli involve the central nervous system (26).

As in the cardiovascular system in general, surface thrombogenicity, hypercoagulability, and locally static blood flow (Virchow's triad) (29) largely determine the relative propensity and sites of thrombus with specific valve prostheses. The surfaces of biomaterials used to construct valve prostheses have relatively good thromboresistance, but none presently used have the superior thromboresistance of properly functioning endothelium. Prosthetic surfaces not only potentiate coagulation protein contact activation and platelet adhesion, but also activate additional platelets, thereby producing conditions of local hypercoagulability.

Heart valve designs causing increased turbulence or regions of stasis have higher clinical rates of thromboembolic complications than those types with improved hemodynamics. Moreover, the sites where valve thrombi occur are associated with local hemodynamic disturbances. For example, in a caged-ball prosthesis, thromboemboli probably arise from minute, often locally inconsequential, thrombi that form at the apex of the cage, a region associated with considerable flow abnormality (30). In contrast, a tilting disk prosthesis is particularly susceptible to thrombus formation, occasionally progressive to total thrombotic occlusion, generally initiated in a stagnation zone in the minor orifice of the outflow region of the prosthesis (Fig. 5–3) (16, 27). Futhermore, early thrombosis, a rare occurrence possible with any valve, involves the host tissue–valve interface or a large left atrial cavity.

Thromboembolic complication rates are generally less with bioprostheses than with mechanical valves (3, 10–12, 19, 26). Patients with bioprostheses in normal sinus rhythm have very low rates of thromboembolism, but the risk increases with atrial fibrillation or heart block (11). Indeed, patients with atrial fibrillation of any cause have a substantially increased incidence of stroke, probably due to cerebrovascular emboli (31, 32). Therefore, since patients not in sinus rhythm would require chronic anticoagulation irrespective of valve prosthesis type, the major advantage of a bioprosthesis is negated in such patients. Late thrombosis of aortic or mitral bioprostheses occurs at the bioprosthetic cusps, with large thrombotic deposits usually present in one or more of the prosthetic

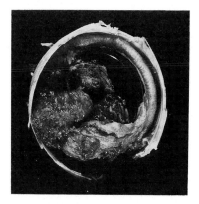

Fig. 5–3. Thrombosis of an aortic tilting disk valve prosthesis. Reproduced with permission from Schoen FJ: Surgical pathology of removed natural and prosthetic heart valves. Hum Pathol 1987;18:558–567. Copyright 1987, WB Saunders.

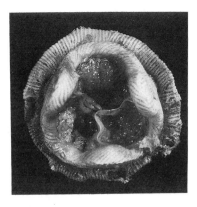

FIG. 5–4. Thrombosis of a porcine bioprosthesis. Reproduced with permission from Schoen FJ, Hobson CE: Anatomic analysis of removed prosthetic heart valves: Causes of failure of 33 mechanical valves and 58 bioprostheses, 1980–1983. Hum Pathol 1985;16:549–559. Copyright 1985, WB Saunders.

sinuses of Valsalva (Fig. 5–4); in most cases there is no demonstrable underlying cuspal pathologic lesion (16, 33).

The lack of vascularity adjacent to thrombi on bioprosthetic or mechanical valves retards the typical histologic progression of their organization, and such thrombi can be friable for extended periods. This not only suggests that embolic risk can persist long-term but also rationalizes fibrinolytic treatment with streptokinase and urokinase (34, 35) or surgical thrombectomy (36), despite temporal delay from onset of dysfunction. However, neither thrombolysis nor thrombectomy prevent recurrence of thrombosis and embolization (34–36); moreover, damage to the valve is an important potential hazard of surgical thrombectomy.

Role of Platelets in Valve Thromboembolism

Despite the importance of good anticoagulant control in preventing thromboembolism, platelet deposition dominates initial blood–surface interaction when valves and other devices with artificial surfaces are exposed to blood at high fluid shear stresses (37, 38). Deposition of radiolabeled platelets has been directly observed on mechanical and bioprosthetic valve surfaces, as well as on the immediately adjacent damaged vascular surfaces (39, 40). Platelet survival measurements and assays of circulating platelet release products indicate that platelets are activated by prosthetic heart valves (41–43). With mechanical prosthetic heart valves, thromboembolic risk is related, at least in part, to the amount of exposed surface area; as the prosthetic surface area increases, so do thromboembolic risk and platelet function abnormalities (41). Administration of platelet-suppressive drugs largely normalizes indices of platelet function and partially reduces the frequency of thromboembolic complications in patients with prosthetic valves (44–46). In contrast, there is insignificant shortening of platelet survival in patients with homograft cardiac valves, in whom there is a low frequency of thromboembolic events (43).

The risk of thromboembolic complications is particularly high during pregnancy, when there is a hypercoagulable state (24, 47, 48). The use of coumarin derivatives may present serious risks to the fetus, including major congenital abnormalities (*coumarin embryopathy*, the most important feature of which is hypoplastic nasal structures) or death, especially if the drugs are administered during the first trimester (49, 50). The most vulnerable period for coumarin embryopathy is the 6th through 12th weeks of gestation (48), but important anomalies can develop at any time during pregnancy.

Prosthetic Valve Endocarditis

Infective endocarditis is an infrequent but potentially serious complication of all valve replacements, occurring in 1 to 6% of patients (51–53). In two recent series that jointly encompassed more than 4000 patients at the University of Alabama and Massachusetts General Hospitals, the risk of developing prosthetic valve endocarditis was 4.1% at 48 months and 5.7% at 60 months after valve replacement (52, 53). Patients originally requiring valve replacement for endocarditis on their native valves develop prosthetic valve endocarditis at five times the overall rate, making them the highest-risk group. Frequently, the same organism that caused the initial infection is responsible for subsequent prosthetic valve endocarditis, suggesting failure to sterilize the original lesion. Secondary thrombotic or embolic complications occur in 13 to 40% of patients with bacterial and over 70% of patients with fungal prosthetic valve endocarditis (26). The rates of infection of mechanical valves and bioprostheses are approximately the same.

Pathology of Prosthetic Valve Endocarditis

Since the synthetic biomaterials used in mechanical prostheses, (e.g., plastics, metals, carbons) generally cannot support bacterial or fungal growth, infections are almost always localized to the prosthesis–tissue interface at the sewing ring, causing a *ring abscess* (Fig. 5–5) (54–56). The resultant tissue destruction may induce dehiscence of the prosthesis, with regurgitation of blood around the prosthesis (paravalvular or paraprosthetic leak), or cause complete or partial interference with atrioventricular conduction.

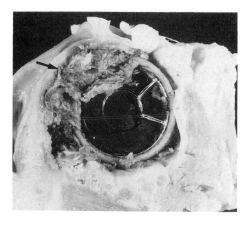

FIG. 5–5. Ventricular view of mitral tilting disk prosthesis in patient dying of infective endocarditis. Large bulky vegetations consisting of bacterial organisms and platelet/inflammatory cell/fibrin thrombus cover part of the sewing ring and form an abscess within tissue of the annulus (arrow). Reproduced with permission from Schoen FJ: Cardiac valve prostheses: Pathological and bioengineering considerations. J Cardiac Surg 1987;2:65–108. Copyright 1987, Futura Publishing Company.

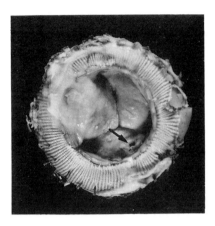

FIG. 5–6. Bioprosthetic bacterial endocarditis involving cusps, with secondary cuspal perforation (arrow). Reproduced with permission from Schoen FJ, Collins JJ, Cohn LH: Long-term failure rate and morphologic correlations in porcine bioprosthetic heart valves. Am J Cardiol 1983;51:957–964.

Rarely, the infection is confined to tissue associated with the valve superstructure or poppet (57). The complications of prosthetic valve endocarditis include embolization of vegetations, congestive heart failure secondary to valvular obstruction or regurgitation caused by bulky vegetations or paraprosthetic leaks, or the consequences of ring abscess. Due to the burrowing nature of the infection, prosthetic valve endocarditis infrequently responds to antibiotic therapy. Clinically complicated cases (generally considered to be those with a new or changing murmur, new or worsening heart failure, new or progressing cardiac conduction abnormalities, emboli, or prolonged fever despite therapy), carry an especially poor prognosis.

Bioprosthetic valve endocarditis, like mechanical prosthetic valve endocarditis, can be localized to the prosthesis sewing ring and complicated by ring abscess and its sequelae (56, 58, 59). Nevertheless, not infrequently, infections involve, and occasionally are confined to, the cuspal tissue (Fig. 5–6) (16, 58–60). Evidence suggests that cusp-limited infections are more readily sterilized by antibiotic therapy than those with a ring abscess (61). In some such cases, cuspal tearing, perforation, or destruction leads to valve incompetence. Histologic examination of the cusps of bioprosthetic valves with endocarditis often demonstrates deep clusters of organisms with few inflammatory cells. Degenerating bacteria (62) and inflammatory cells (59, 60) within cuspal vegetations of bioprosthetic valve endocarditis can undergo mineralization (extrinsic calcification).

Causes and Outcome of Prosthetic Valve Endocarditis

The mechanisms of potentiation of infection by a prosthetic heart valve or other implanted device, recently reviewed, are summarized in Table 5–2 (63, 64). Prosthetic valve endocarditis is generally classified as *early,* within 60 days of valve replacement, or *late,* after 60 days (51). The etiology, risk factors, causative microorganisms, and treatment are different in each of these time periods.

The risk of endocarditis is lifelong; we have encountered cases occurring at 19 and 22

TABLE 5–2. *Factors Contributing to Prosthetic Heart Valve Infection*

Preoperative contamination
Intraoperative contamination
Operative site hemorrhage and necrosis
Postoperative percutaneous lines and catheters
Postoperative bacteremia
Bacterial adhesion to prosthetic surface
Limited inflammatory cell access
Limited exposure to antibiotics
Local phagocytic defects

years postoperatively (56, 57). Prosthetic valve endocarditis occurs most frequently in the first several months postoperatively, reflecting the risk of perioperative valve seeding. The preponderance of organisms comprising normal skin flora in perioperative infections emphasizes the etiologic importance of both valve contamination during implantation and early postoperative surgical infection with concomitant bacteremia. Operative site tissue necrosis, hematoma, and early reoperation probably potentiate prosthetic valve endocarditis. Arterial and central venous lines, urinary catheters, pacing wires, chest tubes, and intracardiac lines are potential portals of organism entry. Antibiotic prophylaxis for patients undergoing valve replacement probably offsets the early risk, since the incidence was as high as 10% in the early days of cardiac surgery (65).

In contrast, late infections are more likely to be due to bacteremia associated with dental manipulation, surgical procedures, or extracardiac pyogenic infections (51). Should bacteremia occur, mechanical and bioprosthetic valves are more susceptible than natural valves to endocarditis. Prompt, appropriate antibiotic therapy for confirmed or suspected bacterial infections, and prophylactic antibiotic coverage for patients having dental, diagnostic, or surgical procedures associated with bacteremia diminishes late susceptibility.

Prosthetic valve endocarditis is relatively resistant to host defense mechanisms and antibiotics and therefore has a high mortality, approximately 60% overall, being significantly higher in cases occurring within the first 2 months postoperatively (51). The high frequency of staphylococcal infection *(Staphylococcus epidermidis, S. aureus)* with prosthetic valves, particularly in early cases, contrasts with the relatively low frequency of this organism in endocarditis on natural valves (51). Streptococci, gram-negative bacilli, and fungi are also prevalent organisms. In many cases, preoperative blood cultures will give a specific microbiological diagnosis. When identification of an organism is sought at reoperation, specimens for microbiological cultures obtained in the operating room, prior to sending the valve for pathologic study, have a high yield. Nevertheless, in about 15% of cases, a causative organism cannot be cultured (61). It is possible that some of these infections are caused by anaerobes (63). Dental infections, considered to be a major factor in prosthetic valve endocarditis, are frequently anaerobic and can generate blood-borne bacteria. Fortunately, anaerobes are generally susceptible to widely used antibiotics. Moreover, some cases of "culture-negative" prosthetic valve endocarditis have recently been related to either legionella (66) or Q fever (67), organisms not readily cultured by routine techniques.

Paravalvular Leak (Dehiscence, Paraprosthetic Leak)

Early dehiscence is usually the result of technical error or separation of sutures from a pathologic annulus when valve replacement was done for endocarditis with ring abscess, myxomatous valvular degeneration, or calcified aortic valve or mitral annulus (68). In contrast, late small paravalvular leaks are usually caused by tissue retraction from the sewing ring between sutures during healing. Small periprosthetic defects can be extremely difficult to detect, despite careful examination of the annulus. Although most such defects are clinically inconsequential, some can aggravate or cause hemolysis or heart failure.

The sewing ring is a major area of tissue–prosthesis interaction (69). In most cases, tissue from the adjacent myocardium or aortic wall grows into and over the fabric, covering the rough surface and partially anchoring the valve. Organization of thrombus probably contributes to the fibrous covering. Morphologic examination suggests that, although in most cases the tissue–valve interface is sealed by the adherent tissue, much of the strength of the valve–tissue bond is provided by the sutures. It is unclear why in some cases this tissue retracts unevenly, producing a paravalvular leak, while in others it grows exuberantly, compromising the orifice.

Durability Considerations

Failure of prosthetic valves is frequently due to the limited durability of the materials that compose them (1–4, 56). Durability considerations vary widely for mechanical valves and bioprostheses, and for the specific types of each. The frequency of complications can differ significantly for different models of a particular prosthesis (using different materials or design features) or for the same model prosthesis placed in the aortic rather than the mitral site (1–4, 56). For example, bare-caged and cloth-covered caged-ball prostheses have had different problems, and problems with susceptible valves in the aortic site have been uncommon in mitral replacements with these designs (70–72). Furthermore, isolated changes in either materials composition (73), materials preparation details (74, 75), or design (73, 76) have significantly either alleviated or altered complications with mechanical prosthetic and bioprosthetic valves. Since patients with valve types no longer implanted can have late problems that are potentially valve-related, major complications with models no longer used are described briefly below along with the pathology of contemporary prostheses.

Mechanical Prostheses

The silicone elastomeric ball occluders of early caged-ball prostheses absorbed blood lipids and almost uniformly subsequently developed swelling, distortion, grooving, cracking, embolization of poppet material or abnormal movement of the poppet due to sticking (ball variance) (Fig. 5–7) (70, 74, 77). A complex interplay of both mechanical and biochemical factors was responsible. Ball variance in the mitral site has been distinctly less common than in the aortic (70), and changes in elastomer fabrication in 1964, including more complete polymer curing, and more stringent poppet selection criteria virtually eliminated lipid-related ball variance in subsequently implanted valves (74).

Cloth-covered caged-ball valves suffered problems related to cloth abrasion by the occluder with fragmentation and sometimes embolism of pieces sufficiently large to

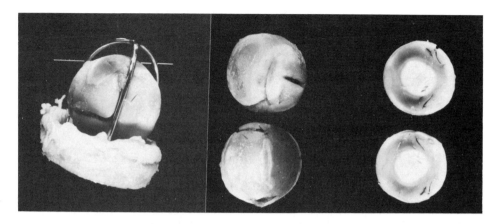

Fig. 5–7. Distortion and cracking of silicone poppet of caged-ball prosthesis due to lipid absorption causing sticking in cage (ball variance). Photos of ball cross-section reveal cracks and discoloration by deep lipid insudation. Reproduced with permission from Muller WA, Cohn LH, Schoen FJ: Infection within a degenerated Starr-Edwards silicone rubber poppet in the aortic valve position. Am J Cardiol 1984;54:1146.

cause arterial occlusion (71, 73), ball entrapment with thrombosis or fibrous overgrowth and resultant stenosis (those models with metal poppets) (78), or escape (in aortic but not mitral models with silicone occluders, due to mutual cloth–poppet abrasive wear) (72) (Fig. 5–8). Structural failure is exceedingly rare in the presently used caged-ball prostheses without cloth covering.

Since wear on a disk occluder is distributed over a much smaller area than that of a ball, caged-disk valves with plastic disks often developed disk wear with notching, reduction in diameter, and resultant valve incompetence (79, 80) (Fig. 5–9). Valves with plastic-coated stents usually also have stent wear (73, 80). Acute valvular dysfunction with

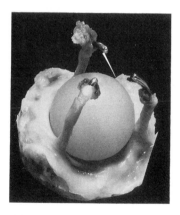

Fig. 5–8. Cloth-covered ball valve prosthesis with tearing and focal retraction of cloth covering at the distal aspect of the struts. Reproduced with permission from Schoen FJ, Goodenough SH, Ionescu MI, Braunwald NS: Implications of late morphology of Braunwald-Cutter mitral heart valve prosthesis. J Thorac Cardiovasc Surg 1984;88:208–216. Copyright 1984, CV Mosby Company.

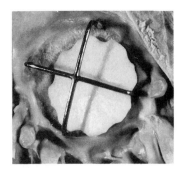

Fig. 5–9. Severe disk notching of caged-disk mitral prosthesis. The obvious mechanical degeneration in this prosthesis caused the disk to stick in the partially opened, partially closed position, causing fatal dysfunction. Reproduced with permission from Schoen FJ, Titus JL, Lawrie GM: Bioengineering aspects of heart valve replacement. Ann Biomed Engin 1982;10:97–128. Copyright 1983, Pergamon Press plc.

mixed obstruction and regurgitation can result from locking of a severely worn disk in an abnormal orientation (81). Previously used tilting disk valves with polymeric disks in which free rotation of the disk was not possible had severely limited durability because of concentrated wear on the disk (82). With abrasive wear of mechanical components, microfragments of nonphysiologic material may embolize throughout the body. One study suggested that liver biopsy may aid the recognition of ball or disk variance by revealing foreign body granulomas (83).

Contemporary tilting disk designs with pyrolytic carbon occluders, with or without carbon cage components, have generally demonstrated favorable durability (73, 84–86). Pyrolytic carbon has high strength and high wear resistance; its widespread use as an occluder and strut covering material for mechanical valve prostheses appears to have eliminated abrasive wear as a long-term complication of cardiac valve replacement (73, 84–86). Nevertheless, rare defects or fractures of metallic or carbon valve components and escape of parts from such valves have been reported (76, 87–92). Fractures are also a particularly troublesome feature of tilting disk valve prostheses used in mechanical circulatory support devices (93, 94), probably due to the hostile mechanical environment of such valves, due to high dp/dt of the prosthetic cardiac cycle and lack of normal annular cushioning mechanisms.

An unusual cluster of a frequently fatal complication of the widely used Björk-Shiley 60-degree and 70-degree convexoconcave (C-C) heart valves has been reported, in which the welded outlet strut has fractured and separated from the valve, leading to disk escape (2, 76, 90, 95) (Fig. 5–10). An actuarial incidence of mechanical failure at 5 years of 2.2% for the size 23-mm aortic 60-degree C-C valve and 8.3% for the 29- to 31-mm mitral 70-degree C-C valves has been reported (76). Survival following strut fracture depends on emergency reoperation permitted by rapid recognition of this complication. Standard chest roentgenography can often ascertain the diagnosis of strut fracture by revealing the broken wire and/or the absence of the radiopaque disk marker in the valve ring (90).

Although contemporary tilting disk valves allow free disk rotation, bileaflet disk valves have a relatively fixed pivot point at the periphery of each disk. The exact configuration of this pivot region varies with specific manufacturer and design; for example, the pivot

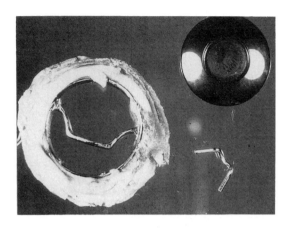

FIG. 5–10. Fractured lesser strut of a Björk-Shiley heart valve prosthesis. This model has the strut welded to the metal frame. Both the fractured strut and disk embolized to the bifurcation of the aorta. Reproduced with permission from Silver MD, Butany J: Mechanical heart valves: Methods of examination, complications and modes of failure. Human Pathol 1987;18:577–585. Copyright 1987, WB Saunders.

region of the St. Jude valve differs considerably from that of the Edwards-Duromedics valve (86). Despite favorable intermediate-term results with rigid bileaflet disk prostheses, disk escape is a potential complication, and continued surveillance for critical abrasive wear localized to vulnerable sites is important. Indeed, there have now been reported at least 17 cases of leaflet escape from the Edwards-Duromedics bileaflet valve (96). No single cause of leaflet escape is yet apparent. Moreover, cavitation, a mode of material degradation in which the bursting of air bubbles generated in a low-pressure area behind a rapidly moving part can chip out microscopic fragments, has been observed during in vitro valve testing (97), and has been hypothesized, but not substantiated, to occur in vivo. In this respect, detailed pathologic studies of valves removed following function may be useful in predicting long-term wear behavior, even when such valves have not suffered overt structural dysfunction (73, 84, 98).

Bioprostheses

Porcine aortic valve. Clinically significant deterioration of porcine bioprostheses is strongly time-dependent (1, 4, 95); this accounts for an accelerated rate of valve failure following 4 to 5 years of function. Although less than 1% of valves implanted for less than 5 years suffer structural dysfunction (59, 99), approximately 20 to 30% of glutaraldehyde-pretreated porcine aortic valves require replacement for sterile tissue degeneration *(primary tissue failure)* within 10 years following implantation in adults (1, 4, 11, 12, 100). Recent data suggest that more than half of porcine bioprostheses will fail by 15 years postoperatively (101–104).

Primary tissue failure, especially that related to cuspal mineralization, is the major cause of dysfunction of porcine bioprosthetic valves, (1, 3, 4, 11, 12, 100–107). Moreover, valve failure in general, and calcification in particular, is markedly accelerated in bioprostheses implanted in children, adolescents, and young adults (1, 103, 105–107). Fewer than 60% of valves implanted in the pulmonary circulation in this population

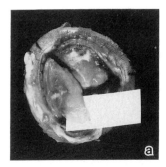 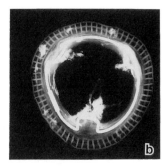

FIG. 5–11. Calcification with secondary tear of mitral bioprosthesis. (a) Gross photograph. (b) Specimen radiograph, same orientation. Reproduced with permission from Schoen FJ, Hobson CE: Anatomic analysis of removed prosthetic heart valves: Causes of failure of 33 mechanical valves and 58 bioprostheses, 1980–1983. Hum Pathol 1985;16:549–559. Copyright 1985, WB Saunders.

remain intact 3 to 5 years postoperatively (106); a recent study found that left-sided porcine valves in children, subjected to more rigorous mechanical loading, had a failure rate of 94% within 6 years (107). Regurgitation through tears forming secondary to calcific nodules is the most frequent failure mode (Fig. 5–11); pure stenosis due to calcific cuspal isolated stiffening and noncalcific cuspal tears or perforation are less frequent (1, 4, 16). Noncalcific tissue tears, revealed by scanning electron microscopy as fraying and disruption of collagen fibers (3, 108), usually reflect direct mechanical damage to collagen.

Calcification is noted in almost all porcine aortic valve bioprostheses implanted in adult recipients for at least 3 to 4 years, but the extent of calcification of removed valves varies widely among individuals after long-term implantation (Fig. 5–12) (109). In a recent study of 31 valves with calcific failure, the mean calcium content was 113 μg/mg; most valves with calcific failure had 34 μg/mg or greater (109). Nevertheless, bioprostheses with minimal or no radiographically demonstrable calcific deposits are occasionally encountered after extended implantation (>10 years) (16, 109). Degenerative cuspal calcific deposits, composed of calcium phosphate mineral, somewhat similar to physiologic bone mineral, generally predominating at the cuspal commissures and basal attachments, are grossly visible as nodular gray or white masses that often ulcerate through the cuspal tissue and are most extensive in the porcine valve spongiosa layer (1, 4, 16, 110). Ultrastructurally, calcific deposits are related to cuspal connective tissue cells and collagen (110, 111). The pathobiology and potential prevention of bioprosthetic valve calcification have been recently reviewed (1, 4, 112–114).

Primary tissue failure of porcine bioprostheses generally leads to gradually progressive dysfunction, allowing elective reoperation, which can be performed with an acceptable operative mortality risk. In some cases, however, primary tissue failure of such devices can cause precipitous deterioration, necessitating emergency reoperation. In one study, 6% of patients with failed porcine bioprostheses required emergency reoperation; their operative mortality was 44% (115). Most of the explanted valves had severe incompetence due to calcification-related cuspal tears; some had superimposed calcific stenosis.

Bovine pericardial valve. Despite favorable early clinical results with bovine pericardial bioprostheses, calcific and noncalcific degenerative failure are now encountered fre-

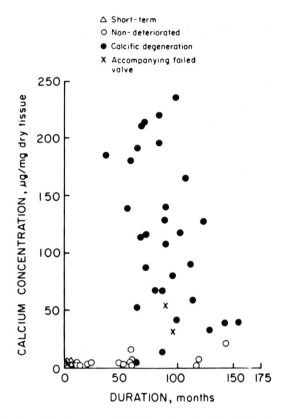

FIG. 5–12. Quantitative calcium in removed failed porcine valves functioning long term, compared with valves removed following short-term function and nonfailed, long-term valves. Reproduced with permission of the American Heart Association, Inc., from Schoen FJ, Kujovich JL, Webb CL, Levy RJ: Chemically-determined mineral content of explanted porcine aortic valve bioprostheses: Correlation with radiographic assessment of calcification and clinical data. Circulation 1987;76:1061–1066.

quently in both adults and children (116–122). Clinical studies have shown widely varying rates of failure of commercially prepared Ionescu-Shiley valves, with actuarially determined freedom from primary tissue failure of 60% at 6 years and 80% at 6 to 7 years, to 90% at 11 years (116–119, 122). Some comparative data suggest that bovine pericardial bioprostheses have an even greater propensity to late failure than porcine valves (122).

We recently analyzed 22 Ionescu-Shiley standard bovine pericardial bioprostheses removed at surgery from 21 adults, following function up to 84 months (121). Valve failure was due to endocarditis (10 cases), primary structural dysfunction (8 cases), bland paravalvular leak (2 cases), and other causes (2 cases). Valves with degenerative failure functioned for 32 to 84 months and had intrinsic cuspal calcification in 6 cases. The morphology of calcific deposits in pericardial valves was remarkably similar to those of failed porcine valves (Fig. 5–13). Seven degenerated valves had cuspal tears or perforations, or both.

The specific contribution to failure of complex mechanisms of noncalcific cuspal dam-

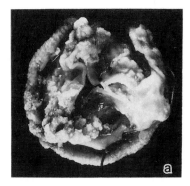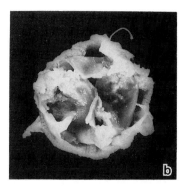

Fig. 5–13. Calcific failure of bovine pericardial valves. (a) Calcific stenosis. b) Calcification with tears. (a) Reproduced with permission from Schoen FJ: Cardiac valve prostheses: Pathological and bioengineering considerations. J Cardiac Surg 1987;2:65–108. Copyright 1987, Futura Publishing. (b) Reproduced with permission of the American Heart Association, Inc., from Schoen FJ, Fernandez J, Gonzalez-Lavin L, Cernaianu A: Causes of failure and pathologic findings in surgically removed Ionescu-Shiley standard bovine pericardial heart valve bioprostheses: Emphasis on progressive structural deterioration. Circulation 1987;76:618–627.

age, as shown in Fig. 5–14, is likely to be more important in clinical pericardial than in porcine bioprostheses. Cuspal perforations and tears frequently cause failure (117–123). Large defects are usually basal, probably related to continuous trauma of the tissue against the bare Dacron cloth. This failure mode often leads to sudden clinical deterioration (117), contrasting with the usually insidious deterioration in porcine valve recipients with primary tissue failure. Cuspal perforation and tears are also frequently associated with a commissural suture *(alignment stitch),* which holds cusps in apposition near the free edge of the leaflet, adjacent to the stent post (120, 121). This feature is unique to the Ionescu-Shiley standard design. In subsequent models (Ionescu-Shiley low-profile

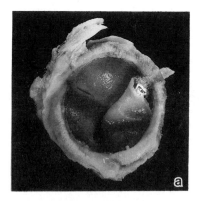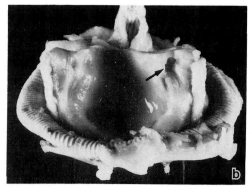

Fig. 5–14. Noncalcific failure of bovine pericardial valves. a) Large basal tear. (b) Alignment suture defect (arrow). (a) Reproduced with permission from Schoen FJ: Cardiac valve prostheses: Pathological and bioengineering considerations. J Cardiac Surg 1987;2:65–108. Copyright 1987, Futura Publishing Company.

pericardial bioprosthesis), this suture has been moved both away from the cuspal free edge and toward the stent. Nevertheless, failures of this model have also been reported, due to leaflet tears initiated in the area of the modified suture (123). The propensity to noncalcific tissue failure of pericardial valves is discussed in Chapter 11 (114).

Other Tissue Valves

Noncommercial, hospital-made autologous and homologous tissue valves, constructed from fascia lata and dura mater mounted on cloth-covered metal stents, have also been used. Clinical studies reveal extremely high failure rates. Removed valves had thick connective tissue overgrowth, stiffening, shrinkage, calcification, and tearing (124, 125). In contrast, unstented, cadaver-derived aortic homografts, used for selected patients with isolated aortic valve disease, pulmonary atresia, or complex congential malformations, have excellent function with a low rate of primary tissue failure (126–130). With homografts, the major problem relates to late degeneration with resultant insufficiency, largely from simple wear and tear, and to a lesser extent calcification (126–130). The most common cause of late valve incompetence is cuspal rupture. Rates of valve failure are thought to be the greatest in valves that had been either chemically sterilized or preserved by freeze-drying. Fresh, antibiotic-sterilized or cryopreserved valves seem to have the most favorable performance, and there is considerable interest in the expanded use of such valves (126, 127).

Miscellaneous Valve-Related Pathology

Obstruction to Flow

Although natural cardiac valves with normal anatomy permit low-resistance central flow when open and minimal regurgitation when closed, all prosthetic valves present some degree of obstruction to forward flow and variable regurgitant flow, often intentionally designed into the mechanism to enhance closing. Thus, the effective prosthetic valve orifice area of almost all types of devices is less than that of the properly functioning human heart valve, and postoperative hemodynamic gradients may be substantial (1, 131). The increased hemodynamic burden of the resultant chronic pressure overload probably contributes to postoperative progressive myocardial deterioration in some patients, but the extent is unknown. Of mechanical valves, tilting disk valves (especially the bileaflet types) have the most favorable ratio of orifice area to tissue annulus diameter, but hemodynamic obstruction is accentuated in small sizes, even in the most efficient designs (1, 81). Some functional prosthetic valve orifice areas, calculated at postoperative cardiac catheterization, approach those measured in patients with moderate to severe valve stenosis who have not had surgery. The relationship between valve orifice area and transvalvular pressure gradient at small valve sizes predicts a substantial increase in measured obstruction for small decreases in valve area. For example, the calculated functional valve orifice area for a 19-mm Lillehei-Kaster tilting disk aortic prosthesis is estimated to be approximately 2 cm^2, compared with a normal aortic valve area of 3 to 4 cm^2, which predicts a mean systolic pressure gradient of 10 to 20 mmHg (81). Occasionally, removal of an otherwise normally functioning valve is necessitated because it is too small for the patient (132).

The central flow pattern of bioprosthetic heart valves generally enhances hemody-

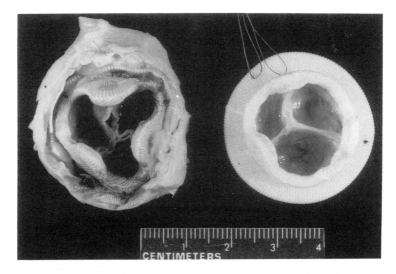

F<small>IG</small>. 5–15. Gross photograph of stent creep of porcine bioprosthesis. (Left) A 25-mm aortic prosthesis implanted for 36 months. The compromise of the outflow orifice is apparent. (Right) An unimplanted 25-mm prosthesis for comparison. Reproduced with permission from Schoen FJ, Schulman LJ, Cohn LH: Quantitative anatomic analysis of "stent creep" of explanted Hancock standard porcine bioprostheses used for cardiac valve replacement. Am J Cardiol 1985;56:110–114.

namic function relative to mechanical prostheses, but bioprostheses can cause significant obstruction, also particularly in small sizes, where the bulk of the supporting struts is not proportionally reduced. Furthermore, progressive inward deflection of the stent posts *(stent creep)* during function of some porcine bioprostheses with polypropylene stents (no longer used) may contribute to progessively increasing stenosis (Fig. 5–15) (133).

Prosthetic Disproportion and Extrinsic Factors

As large a prosthesis as possible is often implanted into a fixed annulus because of its perceived tendency to be less inherently obstructive than a smaller-sized prosthesis. However, prostheses inappropriately large for the anatomic site of implantation can either not function properly (because poppet motion is restricted), cause damage to surrounding structures (by impingement), or actually be severely obstructive (flow around the poppet may be impeded) (134). Mechanical prostheses too big for the ventricle or ascending aorta into which they are placed can have limited occluder motion with potential flow obstruction causing interference to left ventricular filling or emptying in the mitral position, and interference to left ventricular emptying in the aortic position. This problem, *prosthetic disproportion,* is most likely to occur in the mitral position (particularly when valve replacement is carried out for mitral stenosis with a small left ventricle) and in the aortic position when the aorta is small. Prosthetic disproportion was a major problem with large bulky caged-ball valves in the early years of valve replacement. Moreover, since chamber size and configuration are to some extent dynamic postoperatively, mitral prosthetic valve disproportion may become apparent in some cases only following regression of ventricular dilatation (1).

Anatomic and other factors extrinsic to a properly chosen and implanted valve pros

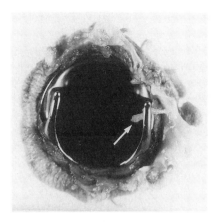

FIG. 5–16. Interference with tilting disk valve occluder motion by suture with long cut end. Reproduced with permission from Schoen FJ: Surgical pathology of removed natural and prosthetic heart valves. Human Pathol 1987;18:558–567. Copyright 1987, WB Saunders.

thesis may promote stenosis or regurgitation. For example, unraveled or excessively long ends of sutures or retained valve remnants may interfere with valve occluder motion (Fig. 5–16) (135–139). A large mitral annular calcific nodule or septal hypertrophy can prevent full excursion of a mitral tilting disk valve occluder (Fig. 5–17) (1, 138, 140). Like prosthetic disproportion, impingement effects sometimes become apparent only after a moderate postoperative interval (such as the case illustrated in Fig. 5–17). Exuberant overgrowth of fibrous tissue can obstruct the inflow orifice of any valve, prevent full mechanical valve occluder excursion, or cause stenosis or regurgitation of bioprostheses (16, 141). The frequency of this group of complications is unknown, but we found approximately 5% of all valve failures were in this spectrum of complications. Intermittent sticking of tilting disk prostheses has been recognized; since such valves may appear to function normally when removed, the cause of malfunction may be obscure

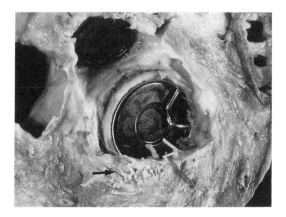

FIG. 5–17. Interference with mitral valve tilting disk valve occluder motion by left ventricular free wall calcific nodule (arrow) extending from calcified mitral annulus. Reproduced with permission from Schoen FJ: Cardiac valve prostheses: Pathological and bioengineering considerations. J Cardiac Surg 1987;2:65–108. Copyright 1987, Futura Publishing Company.

(142). Sutures may be looped around bioprosthetic valve stents, particularly with pericardial bioprostheses (1, 143), restricting cuspal motion, and suture ends cut too long may perforate a bioprosthetic valve cusp (1, 144). Specific details of valve orientation may be contributory in some cases to extrinsic interference (145–147). For example, in the aortic position, tilting disk valve closure may be hampered by wide opening in which the occluder slips beyond the axis of blood flow; this problem can be avoided by a different valve orientation (146); and an improperly oriented mitral bioprosthesis can obstruct left ventricular outflow (147).

Leaflet entrapment by extravalvular cardiac structures is more frequently reported after mitral than aortic valve replacement. This is probably due to the fact that there are more potential mechanisms of interference in this anatomic position. The probability and mechanisms of extrinsic interference may depend on valve type; for example, in bileaflet tilting disk valves, pivot mechanisms are close to one end of the leaflet at the level of the annulus, and the area susceptible to leaflet trapping by suture or tissue is reduced. Moreover, if a piece of foreign material migrates into the valve causing an extrinsic obstruction of one of the leaflets, the other would still be free to operate. Additionally, since the leaflets have a width only one-half of the annular diameter, they do not descend as far into the ventricle as a single disk and, in the mitral position, are less likely to "impinge" on surrounding tissue during closure. While a bileaflet valve with a single entrapped leaflet would be rather stenotic, it would be less likely than a single-disk valve to cause circulatory collapse. Nevertheless, the delicate hinge mechanism of bileaflet tilting disk valves is more likely to be disrupted by a strategically located small thrombus or other tissue fragment.

Hemolysis

Due in large part to turbulent flow, some destruction of red blood cells by prosthetic heart valves is common. Hemolysis is generally slight and well compensated, so that severe hemolytic anemia is unusual (148); however, many patients with older-model heart valve prostheses had renal tubular hemosiderosis or cholelithiasis (149), suggesting chronic hemolysis. Hemolysis is accentuated and can become decompensated when paravalvular leaks develop or dysfunction occurs as a result of materials degeneration, such as ball or disk variance (150), cloth wear (71), valvular thrombosis (151), or bioprosthesis dysfunction (152).

Nonspecific Changes of Uncertain Significance in Bioprosthetic Valves

Deep fluid insudation and loss of cuspal architectural definition are often prominent after long-term clinical function of bioprostheses (3, 116, 153). Intrinsic cuspal architecture is usually disrupted, with the large collagen bundles appearing separated and distorted (3, 16, 121, 153). Focal superficial microthrombi and attached macrophages are frequent (3, 16). Reendothelialization of porcine bioprosthetic valve cusps is minimal (154). Erythrocytes are commonly noted deep in the cuspal connective tissue of removed porcine bioprostheses, and in some cases, large accumulations of blood yield grossly visible hematomas. These have been postulated to stiffen the cusps or provide sites for mineralization in some cases (155–156). Intracuspal material with the staining qualities of amyloid, noted in some porcine bioprostheses implanted longer than several years, is of unknown significance (157). Moreover, systemic diseases may involve bioprostheses.

Whipple's disease involving the cusps of a porcine bioprosthesis has been reported (158). Plaque characteristic of carcinoid heart disease was noted on the atrial surface of a bioprosthetic tricuspid valve implanted 8 months previously for carcinoid heart disease due to a pancreatic carcinoid tumor with extensive liver metastases (159). These latter cases suggest that implantation of a mechanical rather than a tissue valve prosthesis may be preferable in systemic, nonthrombotic diseases.

REFERENCES

1. Schoen FJ: Cardiac valve prostheses: Pathological and bioengineering considerations. J Cardiac Surg 1987;2:65–108.
2. Silver MD, Butany J: Mechanical heart valves: Methods of examination, complications, and modes of failure. Human Pathol 1987;18:577–585.
3. Ferrans VJ, Tomita Y, Hilbert SL, Jones M, Roberts WC: Pathology of bioprosthetic cardiac valves. Human Pathol 1987;18:586–595.
4. Schoen FJ, Kujovich JL, Levy RJ, St. John Sutton M: Bioprosthetic valve failure. Cardiovasc Clin 1988;18/2:289–317.
5. Miller DC, Oyer PE, Stinson EB, Reitz BA, Jamieson SW, Baumgartner WA, Mitchell RS, Shumway NE: Ten to fifteen year reassessment of the performance characteristics of the Starr-Edwards Model 6120 mitral valve prosthesis. J Thorac Cardiovasc Surg 1983;85:1–20.
6. Miller DC, Oyer PE, Mitchell RS, Stinson EB, Jamieson SW, Baldwin JC, Shumway NE: Performance characteristics of the Starr-Edwards Model 1260 aortic valve prosthesis beyond ten years. J Thorac Cardiovasc Surg 1984;88:193–207.
7. Cobanoglu A, Grunemeier GL, Aru GM, McKinley CL, Starr A: Mitral replacement: Clinical experience with a ball-valve prosthesis. Twenty-five years later. Ann Surg 1986;202:376–383.
8. Borkon AM, Soule L, Baughman KL, Aoun H, Gardner TJ, Watkins L, Baumgartner WA, Gott VL, Reitz BA: Ten-year analysis of the Björk-Shiley standard aortic valve. Ann Thorac Surg 1987;43:39–51.
9. Sethia B, Turner MA, Lewis S, Rodger RA, Bain WH, Kouchoukos NT: Fourteen years' experience with the Björk-Shiley tilting disk prosthesis. J Thorac Cardiovasc Surg 1986;91:350–361.
10. Hammond GL, Geha AS, Kopf GS, Hashin SW: Biological versus mechanical valves. Analysis of 1,116 valves inserted in 1,012 adult patients with a 4,818 patient-year and a 5,327 valve-year follow-up. J Thorac Cardiovasc Surg 1987;93:182–198.
11. Cohn LH, Allred EN, DiSesa VJ, Sawtelle K, Shemin RJ, Collins JJ: Early and late risk of aortic valve replacement. A 12 year concomitant comparison of the porcine bioprosthetic and tilting disk prosthetic aortic valves. J Thorac Cardiovasc Surg 1984;88:695–705.
12. Cohn LH, Allred EN, Cohn LA, Austin JC, Sabik J, DiSesa VJ, Shemin RJ, Collins JJ: Early and late risk of mitral valve replacement. A 12 year concomitant comparison of the porcine bioprosthetic and prosthetic disk mitral valves. J Thorac Cardiovasc Surg 1985;90:872–881.
13. Czer LSC, Matloff JM, Chaux A, DeRobertis M, Stewart ME, Gray RJ: The St. Jude valve: Analysis of thromboembolism, warfarin-related hemorrhage, and survival. Am Heart J 1987;114:389–397.
14. Husebye DG, Pluth JR, Piehler JM, Schaff HV, Orszulak TA, Puga FJ, Danielson GK: Reoperation on prosthetic heart valves. J Thorac Cardiovasc Surg 1983;86:543–551.
15. Antunes MJ, Magalhaes MP: Isolated replacement of a prosthesis or a bioprosthesis in the mitral valve position. Am J Cardiol 1987;59:346–349.
16. Schoen FJ, Hobson CE: Anatomic analysis of removed prosthetic heart valves: Causes of failure of 33 mechanical valves and 58 bioprostheses, 1980 to 1983. Human Pathol 1985;16:549–559.
17. Bortolotti U, Milano A, Mazzucco A, Valfre C, Talenti E, Guerra F, Thiene G, Gallucci V: Results of reoperation for primary tissue failure of porcine bioprostheses. J Thorac Cardiovasc Surg 1985;90:564–569.
18. Schoen FJ, Titus JL, Lawrie GM: Autopsy-determined causes of death after cardiac valve replacement. JAMA 1983;249:899–902.
19. Cobanoglu A, Jamieson WRE, Miller DC, McKinley C, Grunkemeier GL, Floten HS, Miyagishima RT, Tyers GF, Shumway NE, Starr A: A tri-institutional comparison of tissue and mechanical valves using a patient-oriented definition of "treatment failure." Ann Thorac Surg 1987;43:245–253.
20. Schoen FJ: Surgical pathology of removed natural and prosthetic heart valves. Human Pathol 1987;18:558–567.
21. Scheffer SM, Leatherman LL: Resolution of Heyde's syndrome of aortic stenosis and gastrointestinal bleeding after aortic valve replacement. Ann Thorac Surg 1986;42:477–480.
22. Gardner TJ, Roland JMA, Neill CA, Donahoo JS: Valve replacement in children. A fifteen-year perspective. J Thorac Cardiovasc Surg 1982;83:178–185.

23. Sade RM, Crawford FA, Fyfe DA, Stroud MR: Valve prostheses in children: A reassessment of antico-agulation. J Thorac Cardiovasc Surg 1988;95:553–561.
24. Salazar E, Zajarias A, Gutierrez N, Iturbe I: The problem of cardiac valve prostheses, anticoagulants, and pregnancy. Circulation 1984;70(suppl I):I-169–I-177.
25. Antunes MDJ: Prosthetic heart replacement. Choice of prosthesis in a young, underdeveloped population group. S Afr Med J 1985;68:755–758.
26. Edmunds LH: Thrombotic and bleeding complications of prosthetic heart valves. Ann Thorac Surg 1987;44:430–445.
27. Yoganathan AP, Corcoran WH, Harrison EC, Carl JR: The Björk-Shiley aortic prosthesis: Flow charac-teristics, thrombus formation and tissue overgrowth. Circulation 1978;58:70–76.
28. Levine MN, Raskob G, Hirsh J: Risk of haemorrhage associated with long term anticoagulant therapy. Drugs 1985;30:444–460.
29. Wessler S, Thye Yin E: On the mechanism of thrombosis. Prog Hematol 1969;6:201–232.
30. Yoganathan AP, Reamer HH, Corcoran WH, Harrison EC, Shulman IA, Parnassus W: The Starr-Edwards aortic ball valve: Flow characteristics, thrombus formation, and tissue overgrowth. Artif Organs 1981;5:6–17.
31. Wolf PA, Dawber TR, Thomas E, Kannel WB: Epidemiologic assessment of chronic atrial fibrillation and risk of stroke: The Framingham study. Neurology 1978;28:973–977.
32. Gajewski J, Singer RB: Mortality in an insured population with atrial fibrillation. J Am Coll Cardiol 1981;245:1540–1544.
33. Thiene G, Bortolotti U, Panizzon G, Milano A, Gallucci V: Pathological substrates of thrombus forma-tion after heart valve replacement with the Hancock bioprosthesis. J Thorac Cardiovasc Surg 1980;80:414–423.
34. Ledain LD, Ohayon JP, Colle JP, Lorient-Roudaut FM, Roudaut RP, Besse PM: Acute thrombotic obstruction with disk valve prostheses: Diagnostic considerations and fibrinolytic treatment. J Am Coll Cardiol 1986;7:743–751.
35. Czer LS, Weiss M, Bateman TM, Pfaff JM, DeRobertis M, Eigler N, Vas R, Matloff JM, Gray RJ: Fibri-nolytic therapy of St. Jude valve thrombosis under guidance of digital cinefluoroscopy. J Am Coll Cardiol 1985;5:1244–1248.
36. Venugopal P, Kaul U, Iyer KS, Rao IM, Balram A, Das B, Sampathkumar A, Mukherjee S, Rajani M, Wasir HS: Fate of thromboectomized Björk-Shiley valve. A long-term cinefluoroscopic, echocardiographic, and hemodynamic evaluation. J Thorac Cardiovasc Surg 1986;91:168–173.
37. Fuster V, Chesboro JH: Antithrombotic therapy: Role of platelet-inhibitor drugs: I. Current concepts of thrombogenesis: Role of platelets. Mayo Clin Proc 1981;56:102–112.
38. Anderson JM, Kottke-Marchant K: Platelet interactions with biomaterials and artificial devices. CRC Crit Rev Biocompat 1985;1:111–204.
39. Dewanjee MK, Trastek VF, Tago M, Torianni M, Kay MP: Non-invasive radioisotopic technique for detection of platelet deposition on bovine pericardial mitral-valve prosthesis and in vitro quantification of visceral microembolism in dogs. Trans Am Soc Artif Intern Organs 1983;29:188–193.
40. Dewanjee MK, Solis E, Lenker J, Tidwell C, Mackey S, Didisheim P, Kay MP: Quantitation of platelet and fibrinogen-fibrin deposition on components of tissue valves (Ionescu-Shiley) in calves. Trans Am Soc Artif Intern Organs 1986;32:591–594.
41. Harker LA, Slichter SJ: Studies of platelet and fibrinogen kinetics in patients with prosthetic heart valves. N Engl J Med 1970;283:1302–1305.
42. Pumphrey CW, Dawes J: Elevation of plasma B-thromboglobulin in patients with prosthetic cardiac valves. Thromb Res 1981;22:147–155.
43. Weily HS, Steele PP, Davies H, Pappas G, Genton E: Platelet survival in patients with substitute heart valves. N Engl J Med 1974;290:534–537.
44. Steele P, Rainwater J, Vogel R: Platelet suppressant therapy in patients with prosthetic cardiac valves. Relationship of clinical effectiveness to alteration of platelet survival time. Circulation 1979;60:910–913.
45. Harker LA: Antiplatelet drugs in the management of patients with thrombotic disorders. Semin Thromb Hemost 1986;12:134–155.
46. Harker LA: Clinical trials evaluating platelet-modifying drugs in patients with atherosclerotic cardiovas-cular disease and thrombosis. Circulation 1986;73:206–223.
47. Schafer AI: The hypercoagulable states. Ann Intern Med 1985;102:814–828.
48. Iturbe-Alessio I, Fonseca MC, Mutchinik O, Santos MA, Zajaria A, Salazar E: Risks of anticoagulant therapy in pregnant women with artificial heart valves. N Engl J Med 1986;315:1390–1393.
49. Hall JG, Pauli RM, Wilson KM: Maternal and fetal sequelae of anticoagulation during pregnancy. Am J Med 1980;68;122–140.
50. Warkany J: Warfarin embryopathy. In Sever JL, Brent RL (eds): Teratogen Update. Environmentally Induced Birth Defects. New York, Alan R Liss, 1986, pp 23–27.
51. Wilson WR, Danielson GK, Giuliani ER, Geraci JE: Prosthetic valve endocarditis. Mayo Clin Proc 1982;57:155–161.
52. Ivert TSA, Dismukes WE, Cobbs CG, Blackstone EH, Kirklin JW, Bergdahl LA: Prosthetic valve endo-carditis. Circulation 1984;69:223–232.

53. Calderwood SB, Swinski LA, Waternaux CM, et al: Risk factors for the development of prosthetic valve endocarditis. Circulation 1985;72:31–37.
54. Arnett EN, Roberts WC: Prosthetic valve endocarditis. Clinicopathologic analysis of 22 necropsy patients with comparison of observations in 74 necropsy patients with active infective endocarditis involving natural left-sided cardiac valves. Am J Cardiol 1976;38:281–292.
55. Anderson DJ, Bulkley BH, Hutchins GM: A clinicopathologic study of prosthetic valve endocarditis in 22 patients: Morphologic basis for diagnosis and therapy. Am Heart J 1977, 94:324–332.
56. Schoen FJ: Pathology of cardiac valve replacement. In Morse D, Steiner RM, Fernandez J (eds): Guide to Prosthetic Cardiac Valves. New York, Springer-Verlag, 1985, pp 209–238.
57. Muller WA, Cohn LH, Schoen FJ: Infection within a degenerated Starr-Edwards silicone rubber poppet in the aortic valve position. Am J Cardiol 1984;54:1146.
58. Bortolotti U, Thiene G, Milano A, Panizzon G, Valente M, Gallucci V: Pathological study of infective endocarditis on Hancock porcine bioprostheses. J Thorac Cardiovasc Surg 1981;81:934–942.
59. Schoen FJ, Collins JJ, Cohn LH: Long-term failure rate and morphologic correlations in porcine bioprosthetic heart valves. Am J Cardiol 1983;51:957–964.
60. Ferrans VJ, Boyce SW, Billingham ME, Spray TL, Roberts WC: Infection of glutaraldehyde-preserved porcine valve heterografts. Am J Cardiol 1979;43:1123–1136.
61. Baumgartner WA, Miller DC, Reitz BA, Oyer PE, Jamieson SW, Stinson EB, Shumway NE: Surgical treatment of prosthetic valve endocarditis. Ann Thorac Surg 1983;35:87–104.
62. Knight JP, Torell JA, Hunter RE: Bacterial associated porcine heterograft heart valve calcification. Am J Cardiol 1984;53:370–372.
63. Schoen FJ: Biomaterials-associated infection, neoplasia and calcification: Clinicopathologic features and pathophysiologic concepts. Trans Am Soc Artif Intern Organs 1987;33:8–18.
64. Gristina AG: Biomaterial-centered infection: Microbial adhesion versus tissue integration. Science 1987;237:1588–1595.
65. Geraci JE, Dale AJD, McGoon DC: Bacterial endocarditis and endarteritis following cardiac operations. Wis Med J 1963;62:302–315.
66. Tompkins LS, Roessler BJ, Redd SC, Markowitz LE, Cohen ML: Legionella prosthetic-valve endocarditis. N Engl J Med 1988;318:530–535.
67. Fernandez-Guerrero ML, Muelas JM, Aguado JM, Renedo G, Fraile J, Soriano F, De-Villalobos E: Q fever endocarditis on porcine bioprosthetic valves. Clinicopathologic features and microbiologic findings in three patients treated with doxycycline, cotrimoxazole, and valve replacement. Ann Intern Med 1988;108:209–213.
68. Dhasmana JP, Blackstone EH, Kirklin JW, Kouchoukos NT: Factors associated with periprosthetic leakage following primary mitral valve replacement: With special consideration of the suture technique. Ann Thorac Surg 1983;35:170–178.
69. Berger K, Sauvage LR, Wood SJ, Wesolowski SA: Sewing ring healing of cardiac valve prostheses. Surgery 1967;61:102–117.
70. Hylen JC, Kloster FE, Starr A, Griswold HE: Aortic ball variance: Diagnosis and treatment. Ann Intern Med 1970;72:1–8.
71. Shah A, Dolgin AM, Tice DA, Trehan N: Complications due to cloth wear in cloth-covered Starr-Edwards aortic and mitral valve prosthesis—and their management. Am Heart J 1978;96:407–414.
72. Schoen FJ, Goodenough SH, Inoescu MI, Braunwald NS: Implications of late morphology of Braunwald-Cutter mitral heart valve prostheses. J Thorac Cardiovasc Surg 1984;88:208–216.
73. Schoen FJ, Titus JL, Lawrie GM: Durability of pyrolytic carbon-containing heart valve prostheses. J Biomed Mater Res 1982;16:559–570.
74. Hylen JC, Hodam RP, Kloster FE: Changes in the durability of silicone rubber in ball-valve prostheses. Ann Thorac Surg 1972;13:324–329.
75. Bortolotti U, Talenti E, Milano A, Thiene G, Gallucci V: Formaldehyde- versus glutaraldehyde-processed porcine bioprostheses in the aortic valve position: Long-term follow-up. Am J Cardiol 1984;54:681–682.
76. Lindblom D, Bjork VO, Semb BKH: Mechanical failure of the Björk-Shiley valve. Incidence, clinical presentation, and management. J Thorac Cardiovasc Surg 1986;92:894–907.
77. Chin HP, Harrison EC, Blankenhorn DH, Moacanin J: Lipids in silicone rubber valve prostheses after human implantation. Circulation 1971;43/44(suppl I):I-51–I-56.
78. Huber S, Burckhardt D, Raeder EA, Follath F, Hasse J, Gradel E: Complications in patients with cloth-covered Starr-Edwards prostheses. J Cardiovasc Surg 1980;21:19–29.
79. Roberts WC, Fishbein MC, Golden A: Cardiac pathology after valve replacement by disk prosthesis. A study of 61 necropsy patients. Am J Cardiol 1975;35:740–760.
80. Silver MD, Wilson GJ: The pathology of wear in the Beall model 104 heart valve prosthesis. Circulation 1977;56:617–622.
81. Schoen FJ, Titus JL, Lawrie GM: Bioengineering aspects of heart valve replacement. Ann Biomed Eng 1982;10:97–128.
82. Roe BB, Fishman NH, Hutchins JC, Goodenough SH: Occluder disruption of Wada-Cutter valve prostheses. Ann Thorac Surg 1975;20:256–264.

83. Ridolfi RL, Hutchins GM: Detection of ball variance in prosthetic heart valves by liver biopsy. Johns Hopkins Med J 1974;134:131–140.

84. Silver MD: Wear in Björk-Shiley heart valve prostheses recovered at necropsy or operation. J Thorac Cardiovasc Surg 1980, 79:693–699.

85. Schoen FJ: Carbon in heart valve prostheses: Foundations and clinical performance. In Szycher ML (ed): Biocompatible Polymers, Metals and Ceramics, Science and Technology. Westport, Technomic Publishing, 1983, pp 239–261.

86. Bokros JC, Haubold A, Akins R, Campbell LA, Griffin CD, Lane E: The durability of mechanical heart valve replacements: Past experience and current trends. In Bodnar E, Frater R (eds): Replacement Cardiac Valves, Chapter 2. Elmsford, NY, Pergamon Press, 1991.

87. Norenberg DD, Evans RW, Gunderson AE, Abellera RM: Fatal failure of a prosthetic mitral valve. J Thorac Cardiovasc Surg 1977;74:924–927.

88. Kabbani SS, Bashour TT, Elolertson DG, Crew JR, Hanna ES: Mechanical valve occluder dislodgment. Am Heart J 1984;108:1374–1377.

89. Odell JA, Durandt J, Shama DM, Vythilingum S: Spontaneous embolization of a St. Jude prosthetic mitral valve leaflet. Ann Thorac Surg 1985;39:569–572.

90. Davis PK, Myers JL, Pennock JL, Thiele BL: Strut fracture and disk embolization in Björk-Shiley mitral valve prostheses: Diagnosis and management. Ann Thorac Surg 1985;40:65–68.

91. Hjelms E: Escape of a leaflet from a St. Jude Medical prosthesis in the mitral position. Thorac Cardiovasc Surg 1983;31:310–312.

92. Tomizawa Y, Kitamura N, Minoji T, Irie T, Yamaguchi A, Oataki M, Tamura H, Atobe M: Stuck prosthetic valve caused by pyrolytic carbon disk wear. Chest 1987;91:798.

93. Dew PA, Olsen DB, Kessler TR, Coleman DL, Kolff WJ: Mechanical failures in in-vivo and in-vitro studies of pneumatic total artificial hearts. Trans Am Soc Artif Intern Organs 1984;30:112–116.

94. DeVries WC, Anderson JL, Joyce LD, Anderson FL, Hammond EH, Jarvik RK, Kolff WJ: Clinical use of the total artifical heart. N Engl J Med 1984;310:273–278.

95. Sack SH, Harrison M, Bischler PJE, Martin JW, Watkins J, Gunning A: Metallurgical analysis of failed Björk-Shiley cardiac valve prostheses. Thorax 1986;41:142–147.

96. A discussion of leaflet escape from the Edwards-Duromedics bileaflet valve. Clinical Data Report 14, Edwards CVS Division. Santa Ana, CA, Baxter Healthcare Corporation, January 1988.

97. Schoen FJ: Surface studies of carbons for prosthetic application. Scan Electron Microsc 1971;part 1:385–392.

98. Silver MD, Koppenhoefer H, Heggtveit HA, Reif TH: Metal wear in Lillehei-Kaster heart valve prostheses. Artif Organs 1985;9:270–275.

99. Blackstone EH, Kirklin JW: Death and other time-related events after valve replacement. Circulation 1985;72:753–767.

100. Oyer PE, Stinson EB, Miller DC, Jamieson SW, Mitchell RS, Shumway NE: Thromboembolic risk and durability of the Hancock bioprosthetic cardiac valve. Eur Heart J 1984;5:81–85.

101. Foster AH, Greenberg GJ, Underhill DJ, McIntosh CL, Clark RE: Intrinsic failure of Hancock mitral bioprostheses: 10- to 15-year experience. Ann Thorac Surg 1987;44:568–577.

102. Gallo I, Nistal F, Blasquez R, Arbe E. Artinano E: Incidence of primary tissue valve failure in porcine bioprosthetic heart valves. Ann Thorac Surg 1988;45:66–70.

103. Jamieson WRE, Rosado LJ, Munro AI, Gerein AN, Burr LH, Miyagishima RT, Janusz MT, Tyers GFO: Carpentier-Edwards standard porcine bioprosthesis: Primary tissue failure (structural valve deterioration) by age groups. Ann Thorac Surg 1988;46:155–162.

104. Milano AD, Bortolotti U, Mazzucco A, Guerra F, Stellin G, Talenti E, Thiene G, Gallucci V: Performance of the Hancock porcine bioprosthesis following aortic valve replacement: Considerations based on a 15-year experience. Ann Thorac Surg 1988;46:216–222.

105. Sanders SP, Levy RJ, Freed MD, Norwood WI, Castaneda AR: Use of Hancock porcine xenografts in children and adolescents. Am J Cardiol 1980;46:429–438.

106. Miller DC, Stinson EB, Oyer PE, Billingham ME, Pitlick PT, Reitz BA, Jamieson SW, Baumgartner WA, Shumway NE: The durability of porcine xenograft valves and conduits in children. Circulation 1982;(suppl I)66:I-172–I-185.

107. Kopf GS, Geha AS, Hellenbrand WE, Kleinman CS: Fate of left-sided cardiac bioprosthesis valves in children. Arch Surg 1986;121:488–490.

108. Ishihara T, Ferrans VJ, Boyce SW, Jones M, Roberts WC: Structure and classification of cuspal tears and perforations in porcine bioprosthetic cardiac valves implanted in patients. Am J Cardiol 1981;48:665–678.

109. Schoen FJ, Kujovich JL, Webb CL, Levy RJ: Chemically determined mineral content of explanted porcine aortic valve bioprostheses: Correlation with radiographic assessment of calcification and clinical data. Circulation 1987;76:1061–1066.

110. Ferrans VJ, Boyce SW, Billingham ME, Jones J, Ishihara T, Roberts WC: Calcific deposits in porcine bioprostheses: Structure and pathogenesis. Am J Cardiol 1980;46:721–734.

111. Valente M, Bortolotti U, Thiene G: Ultrastructural substrates of dystrophic calcification in porcine bio-prosthetic valve failure. Am J Pathol 1985;119:12–21.
112. Schoen FJ, Harasaki H, Kim KM, Anderson HC, Levy RJ: Biomaterial-associated calcification: Pathology, mechanisms and strategies for prevention. J Biomed Mater Res: Appl Biomater 1988;22(A1):11–36.
113. Schoen FJ, Levy RJ: Calcification of bioprosthetic heart valves. In Bodnar E, Frater R (eds): Replacement Cardiac Valves, Chapter 6. Elmsford, NY, Pergamon Press, 1991.
114. Schoen FJ, Levy RJ, Ratner BD, Lelah MD, Christie GW: Materials considerations for improved cardiac valve prostheses. In Bodnar E, Frater R (eds): Replacement Cardiac Valves, Chapter 15. Elmsford, NY, Pergamon Press, 1991.
115. Bortolotti U, Guerra F, Magni A, Milano A, Mazzucco A, Talenti E, Thien G, Gallucci V: Emergency reoperation for primary tissue failure of porcine bioprostheses. Am J Cardiol 1987;60:920–921.
116. Ionescu MI, Smith DR, Hasen SS, Chidambaram M, Tandon AP: Clinical durability of the pericardial xenograft valve: Ten years' experience with mitral replacement. Ann Thorac Surg 1982;34:265–276.
117. Gabbay S, Bortolotti U, Wasserman F, Tindel N, Factor SM, Frater RWM: Long-term follow-up of the Ionescu-Shiley mitral pericardial xenograft. J Thorac Cardiovasc Surg 1984;88:758–763.
118. Brais MP, Bedard JP, Goldstein W, Koshal A, Keon WJ: Ionescu-Shiley pericardial xenografts: Follow-up of up to 6 years. Ann Thorac Surg 1985, 39:105–111.
119. Reul GJ, Cooley DA, Duncan JM, Frazier OH, Hallman GL, Livesay JJ, Ott DA, Walker WE: Valve failure with the Ionescu-Shiley bovine pericardial bioprostheses: Analysis of 2680 patients. J Vasc Surg 1985;2:192–204.
120. Walley VM, Keon WJ: Patterns of failure in Ionescu-Shiley bovine pericardial bioprosthetic valves. J Thorac Cardiovasc Surg 1987;93:925–933.
121. Schoen FJ, Fernandez J, Gonzalez-Lavin L, Cernaianu A: Causes of failure and pathologic findings in surgically removed Ionescu-Shiley standard bovine pericardial heart valve bioprostheses: Emphasis on progressive structural deterioration. Circulation 1987;76:618–627.
122. Gallo I, Nistal F, Arbe E, Artinano E: Comparative study of primary tissue failure between porcine (Hancock and Carpentier-Edwards) and bovine pericardial (Ionescu-Shiley) bioprostheses in the aortic position at five- to nine-year follow-up. Am J Cardiol 1988;61:812–816.
123. Wheatley D, Fisher J, Reece IJ, Spyt T, Breeze P: Primary tissue failure in pericardial heart valves. J Thorac Cardiovasc Surg 1987;94:367–374.
124. Silver MD, Hudson REB, Trimble AS: Morphologic observations on heart valve prostheses made of fascia lata. J Thorac Cardiovasc Surg 1975;70:360–366.
125. Osinowo O, Monro JL, Ross JK: The use of glycerol-preserved homologous dura mater grafts in cardiac surgery: The Southampton experience. Ann Thorac Surg 1985;39:367–370.
126. Clarke DR, Karp RB: Transplantation techniques and use of cryopreserved allograft cardiac valves: A symposium. J Cardiac Surg 1987;2(suppl):1987.
127. Yankah AC, Hetzer R, Miller DC, Ross DN, Somerville J, Yacoub MH (eds): Cardiac Valve Allografts 1962–1987. New York, Springer-Verlag, 1988.
128. O'Brien MF, Stafford EG, Gardner MAH, McGiffin DC, Kirklin JW: A comparison of aortic valve replacement with viable cryopreserved and fresh allograft valves, with a note on chromosomal studies. J Thorac Cardiovasc Surg 1987;94:812–823.
129. Barratt-Boyes BG, Roche AHG, Subramanyan R, Pemberton JR, Whitlock RML: Long-term follow-up of patients with the antibiotic sterilized aortic homograft valve inserted freehand in the aortic position. Circulation 1987;75:768–777.
130. Matsuki O, Robles A, Gibbs S, Bodnar E, Ross DN: Long-term performance of 555 aortic homografts in the aortic position. Ann Thorac Surg 1988;46:187–191.
131. Rahimtoola SH: The problem of valve prosthesis-patient mismatch. Circulation 1978;58:20–24.
132. Steward S, Cianciotta D, Hicks GL, DeWeese JA: The Lillehei-Kaster aortic valve prosthesis. J Thorac Cardiovasc Surg 1988;95:1023–1030.
133. Schoen FJ, Schulman LJ, Cohn LH: Quantitative anatomic analysis of "stent creep" of explanted Hancock standard porcine bioprostheses used for cardiac valve replacement. Am J Cardiol 1985;56:110–114.
134. Roberts WC: Complications of cardiac valve replacement: Characteristic abnormalities of prostheses pertaining to any or specific site. Am Heart J 1982;103:113–122.
135. Williams DB, Pluth JR, Orszulak TA: Extrinsic obstruction of the Björk-Shiley valve in the mitral position. Ann Thorac Surg 1980, 32:58–62.
136. Solem JO, Kugelberg J, Stahl E: Acute immobilization of the disk in the Björk-Shiley aortic tilting disk valve prosthesis. Scand J Thorac Cardiovasc Surg 1983;17:217–219.
137. Ross EM, Roberts WC: A precaution when using the St. Jude Medical prosthesis in the aortic valve position. Am J Cardiol 1984;51:231–233.
138. Jarvinen A, Virtanen K, Peltola K, Maamies T, Ketonen P, Mannikko A: Postoperative disk entrapment following cardiac valve replacement. A report of ten cases. J Thorac Cardiovasc Surg 1984;32:152–156.
139. Moke CK, Cheung DLC, Chiu CSW, Aung-Khin M: An unusual lethal complication of preservation of chordae tendineae in mitral valve replacement. J Thorac Cardiovasc Surg 1988;95:534–536.

140. Jackson GM, Wolfe PL, Bloor CM: Malfunction of mitral Björk-Shiley prosthetic valve due to septal interference. Am Heart J 1982;104:158–159.
141. Murphy SK, Rogler WC, Fleming WH, McManus BM: Retraction of bioprosthetic heart valve cusps: A cause of wide-open regurgitation in the right-sided heart valves. Human Pathol 1988;19:140–147.
142. Ziemer G, Luhmer I, Oelert H, Borst HG: Malfunction of a St. Jude medical heart valve in mitral position. Ann Thorac Surg 1982;33:391–395.
143. Lester WM, Roberts WC: Fatal bioprosthetic regurgitation immediately after mitral and tricuspid valve replacements with Ionescu-Shiley bioprostheses. Am J Cardiol 1985;55:590–592.
144. Jones M, Rodriguez ER, Eidbo EE, Ferrans VJ: Cuspal perforations caused by long suture ends in implanted bioprosthetic valves. J Thorac Cardiovasc Surg 1985;90:557–563.
145. Ross EM, Roberts WC: A precaution when using the St. Jude Medical prosthesis in the aortic valve position. Am J Cardiol 1984;51:231–233.
146. Antunes MJ, Colsen PR, Kinsley RH: Intermittent aortic regurgitation following aortic valve replacement with the Hall-Kaster prosthesis. J Thorac Cardiovasc Surg 1982;84:751–754.
147. Jett GK, Jett MD, Bosco P, van Rijk-Swikker GL, Clark RE: Left ventricular outflow tract obstruction following mitral valve replacement: Effect of strut height and orientation. Ann Thorac Surg 1986;42:299–303.
148. Febres-Roman PR, Bourg WC, Crone RA, Davic RC, Williams TH: Chronic intravascular hemolysis after aortic valve replacement with Ionescu-Shiley xenograft: Comparative study with Björk-Shiley prostheses. Am J Cardiol 1980;46:735–738.
149. Harrison EC, Roschke EJ, Meyers HI, Edmiston WA, Chan LS, Tater D, Lau FYK: Cholelithiasis: A frequent complication of artificial heart valve replacement. Am Heart J 1978;95:483–488.
150. Clark RE, Grubbs FL, McKnight RC, Ferguson TB, Roper CL, Weldon CS: Late clinical problems with Beall model 103 and 104 mitral valve prostheses: Hemolysis and valve wear. Ann Thorac Surg 1976;21:475–482.
151. Wong PH, Nandi PL, Ho FCS, Chan TK: Acute intravascular hemolysis indicating thrombosis of Björk-Shiley aortic prosthesis. Arch Intern Med 1983;143:1471–1472.
152. Lader E, Kronzon I, Trehan N, Colvin S, Newman W, Roseff I: Severe hemolytic anemia in patients with a porcine aortic valve prosthesis. J Am Coll Cardiol 1983;1:1174–1176.
153. Goffin YA, Bartik MA, Hilbert SL: Porcine aortic vs. bovine pericardial valves: A morphologic study of the Xenomedica and Mitroflow bioprostheses. Z Kardiol 1986;75(suppl 2):213–222.
154. Ishihara T, Ferrans VJ, Jones M, Boyce SW, Roberts WC: Occurrence and significance of endothelial cells in implanted porcine bioprosthetic valves. Am J Cardiol 1981;48:443–454.
155. Ishihara T, Ferrans VJ, Barnhart GR, Jones M, McIntosh CL, Roberts WC: Intracuspal hematomas in implanted porcine valvular bioprostheses. J Thorac Cardiovasc Surg 1982;83:399–407.
156. Thiene G, Bortolotti U, Talenti E, Guerra F, Valente M, Milano A, Mazzucco A, Gallucci V: Dissecting cuspal hematomas. A rare form of porcine bioprosthetic valve dysfunction. Arch Pathol Lab Med 1987;111:964–967.
157. Goffin YA, Gruys E, Sorenson GD, Wellens F: Amyloid deposits in bioprosthetic cardiac valves after long-term implantation in man. A new localization of amyloidosis. Am J Pathol 1984;114:431–442.
158. Ratliff NB, McMahon JT, Nabb TJ, Cosgrove DM: Whipple's disease in the porcine leaflets of a Carpentier-Edwards prosthetic mitral valve. N Engl J Med 1984;311:902–904.
159. Schoen FJ, Hausner RJ, Howell JF, Beasley HL, Titus JL: Porcine heterograft valve replacement in carcinoid heart disease. J Thorac Cardiovasc Surg 1981, 81:100–105.

Bodnar, E. and Frater, R. W. M., editors
(1991) *Replacement Cardiac Valves,*
Pergamon Press, Inc. (New York), pp. 125–148
Printed in the United States of America

CHAPTER 6

CALCIFICATION OF BIOPROSTHETIC HEART VALVES

FREDERICK J. SCHOEN AND ROBERT J. LEVY

Sterile mechanical failure is the major cause of dysfunction of the most widely used heart valve bioprostheses (stent-mounted glutaraldehyde-preserved porcine aortic valve or bovine pericardium), providing the indication for approximately three-quarters of reoperations on patients with these valve replacement devices (1, 2). Structural dysfunction necessitates replacement of approximately 20 to 30% of porcine aortic valves within 10 years following implantation (1–4). Three processes account for the overwhelming majority of bioprosthetic valve failures: (1) cuspal mineralization, with or without secondary tearing (Fig. 6–1), (2) noncalcific mechanical failure (i.e., "fatigue") of the cuspal structure, and (3) design-related cuspal tears.

Calcification is causal or contributory to almost all degenerative failures of porcine valves (1–8). Of 90 porcine valves removed at reoperation at the Brigham and Women's Hospital during a 4½-year interval, 63 (70%) had primary tissue failure, 42 (67%) of these cases had calcification with secondary tearing leading to predominant regurgitation, 13 (21%) had calcific stenosis, and 8 (13%) had pure noncalcific defects with pure regurgitation (8). Noncalcific tears due to specific design and fabrication features of porcine valves are unusual. Although bioprostheses constructed of glutaraldehyde-treated bovine pericardium also fail as a result of calcification, design feature–related noncalcific tears occur frequently (9–11). The specific proportions of pericardial valve failures caused by the various mechanisms of dysfunction are not yet known. Deposition of calcium-containing apatite mineral also occurs widely in association with homografts (12–15) and other tissue valve replacements (16, 17), with other experimental and clinical cardiovascular and noncardiovascular medical devices and biomaterials (18, 19), including mechanical blood pumps (20–22), polymeric heart valves (23–26), and in cardiovascular disease in general (27–29).

This chapter describes the pathology and pathobiology of bioprosthetic valve calcification, its morphology, chemistry, determinants, and mechanisms. In addition, since bioprosthetic valve and other pathologic cardiovascular calcification share key pathologic features with physiologic (i.e., skeletal and dental) mineralization, a unified hypothesis for the key events in normal and abnormal mineralization is proposed. Research into the prevention of heart valve calcification is described in detail chapter 15 (30).

CALCIFICATION: TYPES AND CHARACTERIZATION

Physiologic Versus Pathologic Calcification

Calcification is a normal, or *physiologic,* event in the formation of bone, dentin, and tooth enamel. Long bone growth results from cellular proliferation and maturation of osteoblast precursors at the cartilaginous epiphyseal growth plate (31, 32). Physiologic

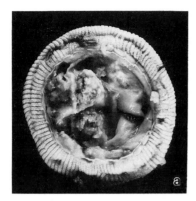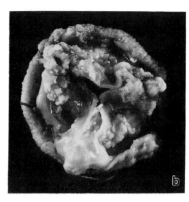

FIG. 6-1. Gross photographs showing mineralization of clinical porcine aortic valve and bovine pericardial bioprosthetic heart valves; gross photographs. (a) Marked calcification and calcification-related tear of porcine valve (inflow aspect); (b) massive calcific stenosis of pericardial bioprosthesis (outflow aspect). (a) Reproduced by permission of the American Heart Association, Inc., from Schoen FJ, et al: Chemically determined mineral content of explanted porcine aortic valve bioprostheses: Correlation with radiographic assessment of calcification and clinical data. Circulation 1987; 76:1061-1066. (b) is reproduced with permission from Schoen FJ: Cardiac valve prostheses: Pathological and bioengineering considerations. J Cardiac Surg 1987;2:65-108. Copyright, 1987, Futura Publishing Company, Inc.

mineralization is a directed, active, and energy-requiring process. The predominant crystalline mineral phase present in bone and other normally mineralized tissues is calcium hydroxyapatite $[Ca_{10}(PO_4)_6(OH)_2]$ (33).

Calcification occurring in functional soft tissues is abnormal, or *pathologic.* Two types of pathologic calcification occur: *metastatic,* in hypercalcemic hosts with otherwise normal tissues; and *dystrophic,* in necrotic or otherwise altered tissues in normocalcemic subjects (34). Dystrophic accumulation of crystalline calcium phosphate mineral in necrotic, injured, or altered soft tissues occurs frequently in cardiovascular diseases. In contrast to the orderly and regulated progression of physiologic mineralization, dystrophic calcification is haphazard. The term *calcific diseases* has been used to describe the dystrophic calcification that occurs in a variety of clinically important states such as atherosclerosis, aortic valve stenosis, crystal deposition arthritis, dental calculus, ischemic myocardial calcification, and the calcification associated with implanted medical devices (35).

Calcification can occur within natural cardiovascular tissues (e.g., homograft valves and associated tissue, stented autologous tissue valves, calcific aortic stenosis, atherosclerosis), with biological substrates rendered nonviable by chemical treatment (i.e., *bioprosthetic* materials), or in association with entirely synthetic materials (30, 36). The mineral phase in pathologic mineralization is apatitic, being structurally related to poorly crystalline calcium hydroxyapatite (37, 38). Mineral nucleation can be *intrinsic,* that is, within the boundaries of the tissue or biomaterial, involving its original constituents; or *extrinsic* to the substrate, that is, associated with elements or tissue not initially present or implanted, such as thrombus, endocarditic vegetations, or pseudointima (Fig. 6-2). The primary determinants of mineralization include factors related to both host metabolism and substrate structure and chemistry (30). Furthermore, pathologic mineralization is generally enhanced at the sites of the most intense dynamic mechanical defor-

LOCALIZATION OF CALCIFICATION

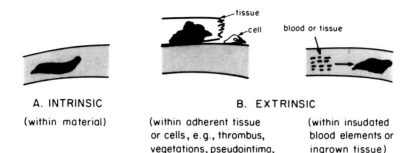

A. INTRINSIC

(within material)

B. EXTRINSIC

(within adherent tissue
or cells, e.g., thrombus,
vegetations, pseudointima,
neointima, cell debris)

(within insudated
blood elements or
ingrown tissue)

FIG. 6–2. Sites of localization of biomaterial-associated mineralization. Mineral nucleation and growth can be (A) within the boundaries of the biomaterial, involving its originally implanted constituents *(intrinsic)* or (B) associated with elements or tissue not initially implanted such as thrombus, vegetations, or pseudointima *(extrinsic)*. Reproduced with permission from Schoen FJ et al: Biomaterial-associated calcification. Pathology mechanisms and strategies for prevention. J Biomed Mater Res: Appl Biomater 1988;22(A1):11–36. Copyright 1988, John Wiley & Sons, Inc.

mations (20, 21, 39) and is potentiated when abnormal stress states exist, for example, in a bicuspid aortic valve (27).

Assessment of Extent and Location of Mineralization

Calcification of bioprosthetic valves is investigated by an integrated, multifaceted evaluation of specimens that includes gross examination, radiography, and light microscopy for routine cases, and atomic absorption spectroscopy, transmission electron microscopy (TEM), and scanning electron microscopy (SEM), with or without energy-dispersive x-ray analysis (EDXA), for investigative purposes (1, 6, 20, 26, 28, 40–42). Gross localization and intensity of mineral deposits are determined radiographically. Semiquantitative grading of the degree of calcification done on properly prepared specimen radiographs correlates well with chemically determined mineral (43, 44). Accurate comparisons among valves are facilitated by the use of carefully selected standards (Fig. 6–3). Quantification of calcium content is most reliably performed using atomic absorption spectroscopy (40–43). However, although extremely useful for comparative studies, bulk chemical analysis averages mineral over an entire specimen and thereby does not provide details of site localization. Morphology of calcific deposits is characterized by examination of histologic sections stained by von Kossa's method (for calcium phosphates) or by alizarin red (for calcium) (40–42, 45). SEM-EDXA permits the quantitative mapping of calcium, yielding both concentration and localizations of mineral. Conventional TEM is useful in investigating the ultrastructural morphology of calcific deposits and the relationship of mineral to structural features of the substrate tissue (40–42).

PATHOLOGY OF BIOPROSTHETIC VALVE CALCIFICATION

Calcific deposits in bioprosthetic valves are grossly nodular, often friable, yellow-white masses, which predominate at the cuspal commissures and basal attachments, the sites of greatest dynamic mechanical activity during valve function (1, 2, 6, 9, 39). Calcific

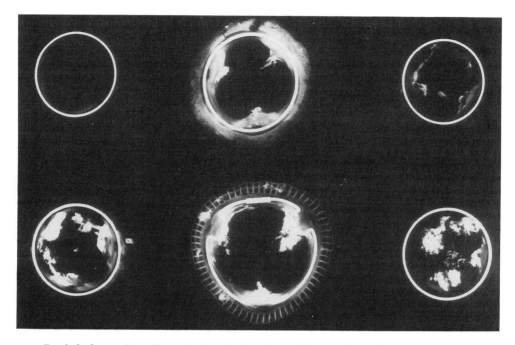

FIG. 6–3. Composite radiograph of calcified porcine aortic valve bioprostheses demonstrating various levels of mineralization, 1+ through 4+, and providing radiographic standards for examination. (Top) Uncalcified (0), 1+, and 2+; (bottom) 3+, 3+, and 4+. All specimens illustrated are Hancock porcine valves except for the middle one on the bottom row, which is a Carpentier-Edwards valve. Reproduced with permission of the American Heart Association, Inc., from Schoen FJ et al: Chemically determined mineral content of explanted porcine aortic valve bioprostheses: Correlation with radiographic assessment of calcification and clinical data. Circulation 1987;76:1061–1066.

deposits are initially intracuspal (i.e., intrinsic) but often ulcerate through the cuspal surface when extensive (1, 2, 6, 9) (Fig. 6–4). The earliest deposits in porcine aortic valves are usually confined to the valvular fibrosa, but later deposits clearly predominate in the spongiosa (6, 46); calcific deposits in pericardial valves are localized to the fibrosa (9). Intrinsic calcification causes clinical valve failure by cuspal stiffening, leading to stenosis, or by cuspal structural disruption, leading to valvular incompetence (1, 2, 6, 9). In calcified, torn valves, there is a correlation between the locations of calcific deposits and the sites of cuspal ruptures (4, 7). Ultrastructural studies of clinical valve tissue demonstrate that calcific deposits are related to cuspal connective tissue cells and their fragments, and collagen (46, 48).

Extrinsic calcific deposits form within thrombi, infected vegetations, or tissue overgrowth on bioprosthetic valves (1, 2, 46). Although intrinsic degenerative mineralization generally requires several years to develop to clinical significance, calcific deposits extrinsic to the cusps can form rapidly (within several days) in the necrotic inflammatory cells of superficial thrombotic accumulations, or in the vegetations of infective endocarditis (4, 9). Endocarditis-associated mineral deposits predominate within central areas of the valve, particularly along the free cuspal edges (1, 2). The extent to which there is extrinsic mineralization related to insudated plasma constituents *(sponge phenomenon)* (50) or frank cuspal hematomas (51, 52) is uncertain. Isolated extrinsic mineralization rarely causes failure of bioprosthetic valves.

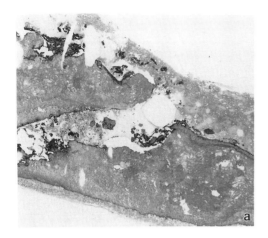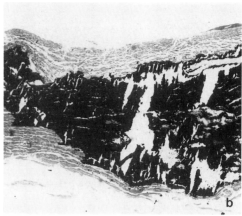

FIG. 6–4. Histology of clinical bioprosthetic valve calcification in leaflet cross sections. (a) Porcine bioprosthetic valve calcification, intrinsic, with ulceration through the valve surface (partially decalcified specimen). (b) Bovine pericardial bioprosthesis with calcification limited to the cuspal matrix. (a) Hematoxylin and eosin; (b) von Kossa stain (calcium phosphates—black); both × 150. (a) is reproduced with permission from Schoen FJ and Levy RJ: Bioprosthetic heart valve failure: Pathology and pathogenesis. Cardiol Clin 1984;2:717–739. Copyright, 1984, WB Saunders, Inc. (b) is reproduced with permission of the American Heart Association, Inc., from Schoen FJ: Causes of failure and pathologic findings in surgically removed Ionescu-Shiley standard bovine pericardial heart valve bioprostheses: Emphasis on progressive structural deterioration. Circulation 1987;76:618–627.

Bioprosthetic valve calcification is a progressive, time-dependent process. The extent of calcification in removed bioprosthetic valves varies widely (6, 43). In adults, intrinsic mineral accumulation is minimal in valves implanted for less than 3 years, but almost all porcine bioprostheses removed following function for longer duration have an increased mineral content. Some bioprostheses have minimal or no calcification after functioning for more than 10 years. In a recent study, valves with calcific deposits and degenerative failure were found to have a mean of 113 μg/mg calcium (range 3 to 239), following a mean of 87 months (range, 36–150) duration (43). Almost all valves removed for either calcific cuspal stiffening or tears secondary to mineralization had greater than 34 and 67 μg/mg calcium, in mitral and aortic valves, respectively. This suggests that bioprosthetic valve calcific failure usually requires a threshold mineral level and implies that although complete prevention of mineralization would be desirable, inhibition of mineralization to modest levels could make an important impact on patient prognosis. Mineralization is accelerated in younger patients (1, 2) (see below). No differences in either the propensity of pathology of mineralization have been noted between the two most widely used porcine bioprostheses (Hancock and Carpentier-Edwards).

PATHOBIOLOGY OF BIOPROSTHETIC VALVE CALCIFICATION

Animal Models

Experimental models used to investigate the pathophysiology (and prevention) of bioprosthetic tissue calcification include orthotopic tricuspid or mitral replacements or conduit-mounted valves in sheep (53–57) or calves (41, 58, 59) and heterotopic tissue sam-

TABLE 6–1. *Key Host and Tissue Determinants of Calcification of Subcutaneous Implants of Bioprosthetic Tissue (21 days)*

Experiment	Calcium content* (μg/mg)	References
Unimplanted PAV† cusp	3 ± 1	40,41
Unimplanted BP†	2 ± 1	42
3-week-old recipient rat		
Glutaraldehyde-treated PAV cusp	108 ± 16	40,41
Untreated (fresh) PAV cusp	6 ± 1	40
Glutaraldehyde-treated BP	114 ± 18	42
Millipore chamber–enclosed PAV cusp	92 ± 18	40
Purified glutaraldehyde cross-linked type I collagen	57 ± 6	88
6- to 8-month-old recipient rat	13 ± 4	40
3-week-old recipient mouse with PAV cusp		
Control mouse (BALB c)	102 ± 5	63
Nude (thymus-deficient)	96 ± 25	63

*Mean $\pm$ SEM.

†PAV = porcine aortic valve; BP = bovine pericardium.

ples implanted either in artificial hearts (60), in and around the heart in large animals (61, 62), or subcutaneously in mice (63), rabbits (64), or rats (40–42, 65). In all experimental models, either circulatory or heterotopic, including subcutaneous locations, bioprosthetic tissue calcifies progressively, with morphology similar to that observed in clinical specimens, but with markedly accelerated kinetics.

Tricuspid or mitral replacements in sheep or calves are the most widely used in vivo systems (41, 53–59). While tricuspid valves are generally easier to implant, the extent of calcific deposit accumulation is less than that of mitral valve replacements. Orthotopic valve replacements in sheep or calves calcify extensively and equivalently in 3 to 6 months, compared with the several years normally required for calcification of adult clinical bioprostheses (41, 53–59). Large-animal circulatory models closely mimic the clinical environment, but technical difficulties and expense limit their utility in elucidating the pathophysiology of calcification.

Subcutaneous implants of bioprosthetic tissue in small animals, primarily rats, provide a convenient, economical, and well-controlled model that simulates the essential metabolic requirements for mineralization. We have found that 3-week-old weanling rats yield the most reproducible and reliable data (40–42). This model yields specimens suitable for detailed biochemical, kinetic, and morphologic investigation and allows sufficient data replicates of specific experimental conditions for reliable quantitative comparisons of determinants of mineralization (Table 6–1).

Progression of Mineralization

Calcific deposits in either porcine valve or bovine pericardial tissue are evident morphologically and chemically within 48 h following subcutaneous implantation (41, 42). The progressive histologic and ultrastructural morphology, virtually identical in these two materials, is illustrated in Fig. 6–5. Initial deposits are localized to transplanted connective tissue cells and do not involve extracellular collagen fibers. Initial nucleation sites appear to be cell membranes, the nucleus, and intracellular organelles, such as mitochondria. With increasing duration of implantation, cell-associated deposits increase in

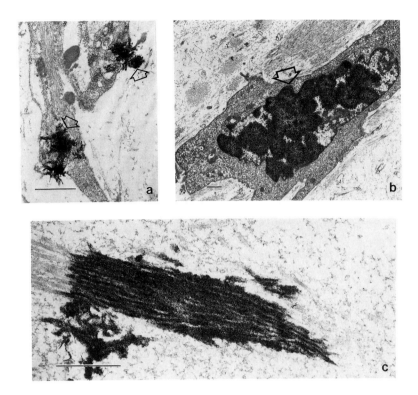

FIG. 6–5. Ultrastructure of porcine connective tissue cell- and collagen-associated calcific deposits in subcutaneous implants of bioprosthetic valve tissue in rats. (a) Focal deposits at cell surface and cytoplasm (arrows); (b) extensive intranuclear calcification (arrow); (c) collagen calcification. (a) 48 h, (b) 72 h, (c) 21 days. Bar = 1 μm. Sections stained with uranyl acetate and lead citrate. (a) is reproduced with permission from Schoen FJ, Kujovich JL, Levy RJ, St John Sutton M: Bioprosthetic valve failure. Cardiovasc Clin 1988;18(2):289–317. Copyright FA Davis, 1987. (b) and (c) are reproduced with permission from Schoen FJ, Levy RJ, Nelson AC, Bernhard WF, Nashef A, Hawley M: Onset and progression of experimental bioprosthetic heart valve calcification. Lab Invest 1985;52:523–532, © by US & Canadian Academy of Pathology (1985).

size and number, obliterating cells and dissecting among the collagen bundles. Direct collagen involvement subsequently occurs. As in clinical valves, the calcific deposits in porcine valves are predominantly in the spongiosa, and to a lesser extent in the fibrosa (calcium content in the spongiosa is 15 times that in the fibrosa at 28 days following implantation) (41).

Proliferation of nucleation sites and crystal growth result in progressive confluence of diffusely distributed microcrystals into macroscopic nodules, which focally obliterate implant architecture and ulcerate through the cuspal surface. These gross nodules are analogous to those responsible for clinical valve failures. Calcification is dramatically accelerated in subcutaneous implants of bioprosthetic tissue in young rats, with maximal accumulation of mineral within 8 weeks, to levels comparable to those of failed clinical explants (200 to 225 μg of calcium per milligram of tissue (41, 42). Half-maximal levels of mineralization are accumulated in approximately 3 weeks. The kinetics of mineralization are virtually identical for porcine aortic valve and bovine pericardium (66) (Fig. 6–6).

The similar morphologic progression of calcification in the different experimental

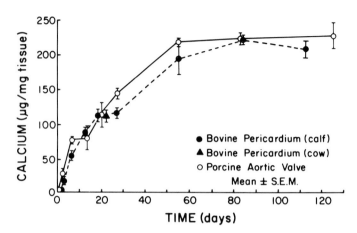

FIG. 6–6. Progression of calcification (as determined by atomic absorption spectroscopy) of glutaraldehyde-pretreated porcine aortic valve and bovine pericardium implanted subcutaneously in
rats. Reproduced with permission from Schoen FJ, Levy RJ: Pathophysiology of bioprosthetic
heart valve calcification in biologic and bioprosthetic valves. In Bodnar E and Yacoub M (eds):
Biologic and Bioprosthetic Valves, New York, Yorke Medical Books, 1986, p 418. Copyright now
held by Butterworth Publishers, Stoneham, MA.

models and in clinical bioprostheses, and in the different materials, suggests a common
pathophysiology, independent of implant site, which is summarized in Fig. 6–7 (41).
Calcification appears to depend only on exposure of a susceptible substrate to extracellular fluid in either a mechanically static or dynamic environment. Moreover, blood–
material interactions are clearly not required. This concept does not rule out possible
regulatory roles for circulating blood-borne substances, including inhibitors, and for
mechanical factors.

Effect of Mechanical Deformation

Extensive mechanical deformation during function accelerates calcification of bioprosthetic valves (1, 2, 39). Macroscopic calcification of functioning clinical and experimental bioprosthetic valves begins and is enhanced in areas of leaflet flexion where
deformations are maximal, especially the cuspal commissures and bases (recall Fig. 6–
3). Some data suggest that the degree of calcification on clinical porcine valves varies
according to the pressure differential across the valve during the closed phase of the car-

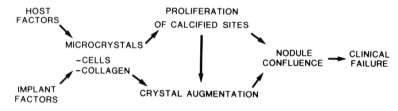

FIG. 6–7. Schematic model for critical events in bioprosthetic heart valve calcification. Reproduced with permission from Schoen FJ, Levy RJ, Nelson AC, Bernhard WF, Nashef A, Hawley
M: Onset and progression of experimental bioprosthetic heart valve calcification. Lab Invest
1985;52:523–532, © by US & Canadian Academy of Pathology (1985).

diac cycle (i.e., mitral > aortic > tricuspid), but although the left-versus-right-sided difference is well established, the aortic-versus-mitral difference has not been uniformly observed (67–69). Cuspal stiffening by calcific deposits induces new and substantial sites of stress concentration between the deposits and the surrounding tissue, potentiating leaflet rupture (70). Nevertheless, both the morphology and the extent of calcification in subcutaneous implants are analogous to those observed in clinical and experimental circulatory studies, despite the absence of dynamic mechanical activity characteristic of the circulatory environment (40–42).

The effects on calcification of mechanical deformation are complex (Fig. 6–8). In the subcutaneous model, enhanced calcification is noted in areas of tissue folds and bends, suggesting that static (as well as dynamic) mechanical deformation potentiates mineral-

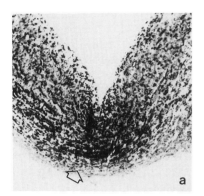
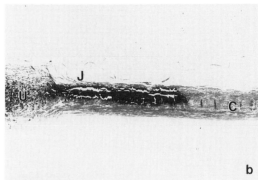

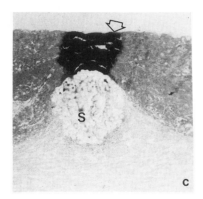

FIG. 6–8. Effects of static mechanical deformation on bioprosthetic tissue calcification. (a) Accentuation of calcific deposits in tissue folds of subcutaneously implanted specimen (arrow). (b) Inhibition of calcification in pericardium compressed prior to subcutaneous implantation, except at junction (J) of compressed area (C) with uncompressed tissue (U), where there is enhanced mineralization in disrupted tissue. (c) Focal mineralization (arrow) associated with anchoring sutures in pericardium covering stationary strut of unileaflet valve implanted as mitral replacement in sheep. von Kossa stain. (a) is reproduced by permission from Levy RJ, Schoen FJ, Levy JT, Nelson AC, Howard SL, Oshry LJ: Biologic determinants of dystrophic calcification and osteocalcin deposition in glutaraldehyde-preserved porcine aortic valve leaflets implanted subcutaneously in rats. Am J Pathol 1983;113:143–155. Copyright 1983, JB Lippincott Company. (c) is reproduced with permission from Shemin RJ, Schoen FJ, Hein R, Austin J, Cohn LH: Hemodynamic and pathologic evaluation of a unileaflet pericardial bioprosthetic valve. J Thorac Cardiovasc Surg 1988;95:912–919. Copyright 1988, CV Mosby Company.

ization (40). Moreover, nonmobile pericardial tissue covering the stationary frame of a new design unicuspid pericardial valve has exceedingly minimal calcification, except in areas where the tissue has been compressed by sutures (57). Compression perpendicular to the plane of the pericardium may mitigate calcification, while tissue disruption increases the degree of calcification (71, 72).

The above data suggest that circulatory dynamic stress promotes, but is not obligatory for, calcification of bioprosthetic tissue, and that the host metabolic environment and the inherent properties of the implant per se are responsible for the propensity of bioprosthetic tissue to calcify (1, 2). The mechanisms by which stress enhances calcification are unknown, but stress-generated crystal nucleation sites, structural disruption of the collagen architecture creating internal spaces that facilitate crystal growth, piezoelectric crystal augmentation, or increased fluid insudation deep into bioprosthetic valve cusps could be contributory factors (1, 2). The above results may explain the seemingly conflicting effects of deformation on bioprosthetic tissue calcification previously reported, in that tissue structure alteration by compressive deformation could either inhibit growth of calcific deposits by decreasing the spacing between collagen bundles and/or interfere with fluid and ion flow into the compressed region (72). In contrast, mechanical tissue disruption could allow increased fluid insudation, create new spaces into which calcific deposits could grow, or create new crystal nucleation sites (72).

Host Factors

The rate of clinical and experimental bioprosthetic tissue calcification is dependent on host metabolic factors (1, 2, 19, 40). Calcification in particular and valve failure in general are markedly accelerated in children, adolescents, and young adults (1, 2, 73, 74). In some studies, the age dependence of bioprosthetic valve failure continues to age 35 (75). The age dependence of calcification rate is simulated in the rat subcutaneous model, in which the amount of calcium accumulated in bioprosthetic tissue implanted for 21 days in 8-month-old rats is less than 15% of that accumulated in tissue implanted in 3-week-old rats (40). The basis for this differential rate of calcification is probably due to poorly understood age-related differences in calcium and phosphorus metabolism. Renal failure enhances mineralization (76). It has also been suggested that calcification is accelerated by increased dietary calcium (77). Although patient sex per se is not a determinant of calcification or valve failure, the physiologic conditions of pregnancy might potentiate mineralization (78).

Neither nonspecific inflammation nor specific immunologic responses appear to mediate bioprosthetic tissue calcification (1, 2, 40–42). Inflammation induces neither mineral deposition nor resorption. Morphologic examination of both circulatory and subcutaneous porcine valve implants reveals a classic foreign body reaction, composed primarily of nonlymphocytic mononuclear cells. Furthermore, inflammatory cell penetration into bioprosthetic tissue and host cell reaction to mineral deposits are minimal and inconsistent. In experiments in which enclosure of valve cusps in chambers prevents host cell contact with tissue but allows free diffusion of extracellular fluid, neither the extent nor the morphology of mineralization in rat subcutaneous implants is altered (40). Moreover, valve tissue implanted in congenitally athymic ("nude") mice, in whom T-cell function is grossly diminished, calcifies to the same extent as implants in immunologically competent hosts (63). Second bioprosthetic valve replacements fail no sooner than initial replacements. Previous clinical and experimental data detecting antibodies to valve tissue after implantation are probably a reflection of secondary response to valve damage and resultant exposure of new antigenic determinants, rather than a cause of failure (79, 80). Taken together, these studies strongly suggest that calcification is independent of both general inflammatory or specific immunologic processes.

Whether anticoagulation retards bioprosthetic valve and other pathologic calcification remains a controversial and unsettled issue. It has been hypothesized that warfarin therapy might limit calcification of bioprosthetic heart valves by inhibiting vitamin K–dependent synthesis of γ-carboxyglutamic acid–containing calcium-binding proteins, which are associated with normal and pathologic calcification (81, 82). Nevertheless, several studies from our laboratories have failed to demonstrate an effect of warfarin on calcification of porcine aortic valves implanted in the calf circulatory system or rat subcutaneous space, or on calcification of functioning cardiac assist device bladders (40, 58, 82). In contrast, an inhibitory effect of sodium warfarin on mineralization was suggested by a retrospective study of patients with clinical bioprosthetic valves (83) and by experimental investigations of elastomeric cardiac assist pump sacs (84, 85). However, since most calcification of smooth blood pumps is extrinsic, the latter results may be a reflection of decreased calcification due to decreased adherent thrombus.

Implant Factors

The propensity of bioprosthetic tissue to calcify is dependent on tissue preparation. Pretreatment of tissue with an aldehyde cross-linking agent is a prerequisite for calcification in the subcutaneous experimental environment; nonpreserved cusps implanted subcutaneously in rats do not mineralize (40, 86). More specifically, the amount of glutaraldehyde incorporated controls the extent of cross-links, which in turn probably determines the propensity toward calcification (Fig. 6–9) (86). However, a recent report suggests that prolonged incubation of bioprosthetic valve tissue in glutaraldehyde inhibits mineralization (87). Valves having formalin pretreatment also mineralize (88), and an

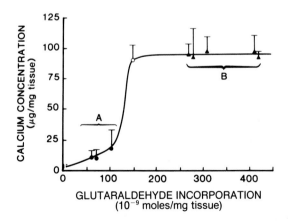

FIG. 6–9. Calcification of glutaraldehyde-treated bovine pericardial tissue after 21 days of a subdermal implant in rats as a function of glutaraldehyde incorporation. Specimens in group A had a low degree of both cross-linking and tissue stability, while specimens in group B had a high degree of cross-linking and stability. Reproduced with permission from Golumb G et al: The role of glutaraldehyde-induced cross-links in calcification of bovine pericardium used in cardiac valve bioprostheses. Am J Pathol 1987;127;122–133. Copyright 1987, JB Lippincott Company.

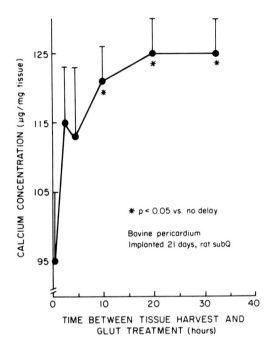

FIG. 6-10. Effect of fixation delay on the calcification of bovine pericardium. When delay between tissue harvest and fixation exceeds 10 h, calcification is significantly increased over levels associated with immediate glutaraldehyde treatment. Reproduced with permission from Maranto A, Schoen FJ: Effect of delay between tissue harvest and glutaraldehyde pretreatment on the calcification of bovine pericardium used in bioprosthetic heart valves. J Biomed Mater Res 1988;22:819–825.

experimental study suggests that formalin enhances mineralization (relative to glutaraldehyde) of implanted purified type I collagen sponges (89).

There has been concern that delayed glutaraldehyde treatment of bioprosthetic tissue during valve fabrication could potentiate calcification by autolytic generation of mineralization nucleation loci. We recently investigated the effects on mineralization of variable delays between harvest of bovine pericardium and initial glutaraldehyde pretreatments, using tissue implanted in rats (90). Susceptibility to mineralization increased only modestly with delays to 34 hours, suggesting that mineralization is not significantly altered by the usual temporal variation in tissue processing (Fig. 6–10). Considerable additional work will be necessary before the relative roles of specific tissue and preparation variables are understood.

Despite differences in composition and structure, glutaraldehyde-treated porcine aortic valve and bovine pericardium calcify comparably with respect to kinetics, extent, and morphology (8, 41, 42) (recall Figs. 6–1, 6–4, and 6–6). This suggests that the fundamental mechanisms of bioprosthetic tissue mineralization depend on specific biochemical modifications of implant microstructural components induced by aldehyde pretreatment, and common to both tissues. Moreover, the role of the critical effects of those processes on cells is emphasized by experiments that show that 24-hours incubation of glutaraldehyde-pretreated bioprosthetic tissue in 5% sodium dodecyl sulfate (SDS) solution both removes over 80% of endogenous phospholipids and reduces calcification by over 80% (91). While some studies have suggested that buffering of pretreatment solutions with phosphate buffers may be undesirable, others have found little effect of altering the buffer (62, 92). Surprisingly, there has been little meaningful work on pretreatment solutions alternative to aldehydes.

OTHER CARDIOVASCULAR AND PROSTHETIC CALCIFICATION

Calcification of Other Tissue Valve Replacements

Calcification occurs and can contribute to the ultimate failure of nonpreserved biological valves, including aortic and right ventricular outflow tract aortic valve homografts, and stented autologous fascia lata, autologous pericardial, and homologous dura mater valves (12–17, 93, 94). The only valve type in which calcification has not been observed is the nonstented pulmonary valve autograft to the aortic valve site. In one study, calcification was noted in 18% of 80 homograft failures, 19% of 27 fascia lata failures, and 5% of dura mater failures, but none of 14 pulmonary valve autograft failures (95).

As with bioprosthetic valves, calcification is more common and develops earlier and more severely in younger patients with aortic homografts (13, 15). Calcification of aortic homografts is less in "fresh" antibiotic-sterilized (and probably in cryopreserved) homografts than in chemically treated grafts (14). Calcification in homografts involves the cusps, or graft wall, or both (13–15). Mineralization limited to the graft wall is infrequently of hemodynamic significance (13–15).

The histologic appearances of homograft valve and aortic wall mineralization are not well described. We have studied homograft aortic wall calcification in clinical material and dog explants of right ventricular outflow tract reconstructions, and subcutaneous implants of homograft aortic walls in rats. In each case, a predominant site of mineralization was the laminar elastic tissue elements of the aortic wall (Fig. 6–11). In addition, in subcutaneous specimens, in which electron microscopy could be done, cell-associated and collagen-associated mineralization were also prominent (C. L. Webb, F. J. Schoen, and R. J. Levy, unpublished research).

Failure of fascia lata and other stented autologous and homologous tissue valves can be due to calcification. The morphology of such failures is similar to that of calcified pericardial bioprosthetic valves, with mineral occurring deep in the valve fibrosa (16, 17, 93) (Fig. 6–12).

Calcification of Vascular Connective Tissue

Native cardiovascular connective tissue is a common site of clinically important dystrophic calcification. Vascular calcification often begins in the young, progressively increases with age, and gives rise to a variety of clinical syndromes. Calcification is often prominent in atherosclerosis and contributes to the resultant clinical sequelae (28, 29). Calcification is the major pathologic process in degenerative aortic valve sclerosis/stenosis, the most common form of valvular heart disease (27). The mechanisms of vascular calcification have been studied through TEM of human vascular connective tissue and atheromatous plaques, and in vivo and in vitro experiments with rat aorta and fibroblasts cultured from canine heart valves (19, 28, 95, 96). Calcification of calcific aortic valves and atheromatous plaques is noted mainly in association with cellular degradation products (19, 20, 28, 35, 96, 97).

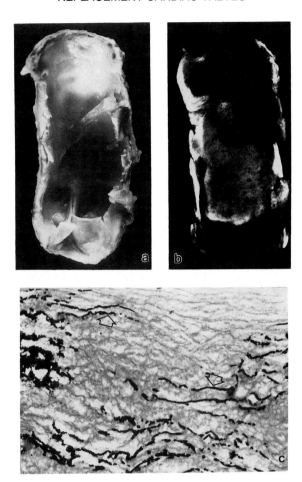

Fig. 6–11. Homograft aortic wall calcification. (a) gross photograph, (b) specimen radiograph, and (c) histologic cross-section of an aortic root homograft used as a right-sided valve conduit in a patient with congenital heart disease. The aortic wall but not the valve has calcified. (c) Shows the prominent mineralization of elastin (arrows) in homograft aortic wall. (c) von Kossa stain. Reproduced with permission from Schoen FJ: Interventional and Surgical Cardiovascular Pathology: Clinical Correlations and Basic Principles. WB Saunders, 1989. Copyright 1989, WB Saunders Company.

Large-sized vesicular structures, several microns in diameter, frequently occur in vascular connective tissue. Needle-shaped calcific crystals are frequently embedded in the thick wall of the vesicles. In view of their occurrence in the vicinity of disintegrated cells and the occasional observation of trilamellar membranes associated with larger vesicles, they presumably originate from the plasma membrane of the disintegrated cells (28). Red cell ghosts placed in Millipore chambers and implanted in the peritoneal cavities of inbred rats develop similar large, thick-walled vesicles that undergo calcification (28). This suggests that the vesicles originate from plasma membrane. The altered membrane may serve as the nidus of apatite nucleation.

The above experiments, taken in aggregate, suggest that a disturbance of calcium homeostasis, probably largely induced by and superimposed upon mechanical cell

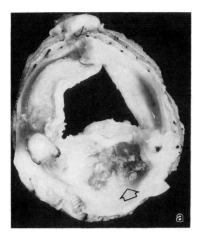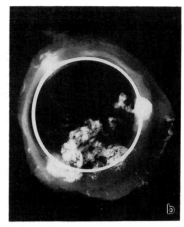

FIG. 6-12. Autologous fascia lata valve removed following 13 years and having one stiff, heavily calcified cusp (arrow). (a) Gross photograph; (b) specimen radiograph. Specimen courtesy of MI Ionescu, MD Reproduced with permission from Schoen FJ: Interventional and Surgical Cardiovascular Pathology: Clinical Correlations and Basic Principles. WB Saunders, 1989. Copyright 1989, WB Saunders Company.

injury, and that caused by aging, plays the central role in vascular calcification (19, 28). Failure of phagocytic cells to scavenge and digest cellular degradation products (thereby eliminating potential nucleation sites), alteration of membrane structure, and formation of apatite precursors are additional important features.

Calcification of Flexing Polymers

Deposition of calcific crystals on flexing surfaces can limit the functional longevity of polymeric leaflet heart valve prostheses and blood pumps (20, 21, 23, 26, 97, 98). The rigid mineral deposits can cause deterioration of valve or pump performance through loss of bladder pliability or through initiation of tears, or can become a site for thrombi and yield a source of emboli. Mechanical factors play an important promoting role (20–22, 99). Although most studies have been on specimens derived from experimental models, early calcific deposits were noted on two of the long-term clinical Jarvik artificial hearts (100).

Two types of calcified lesions are observed on trileaflet polymeric heart valves and smooth-surfaced blood pump bladders (22, 98). Most deposits are clearly extrinsic (Fig. 6–13). In these cases, dystrophic calcification occurs in the blood-derived pseudointimal surface deposits of leukocytes, erythrocytes, platelets and their fragments, and fibrin. Another type of calcified lesion, referred to as a *"plaque lesion,"* is a localized, slightly elevated area with an irregular but well-recognizable margin. This lesion is noted on cross-sectional examination to invade into the polymer bulk with fingerlike projections. The specific site of nucleation of the latter type of crystals is unknown, but it could be intrinsic. Calcific deposits are reported as being frequently associated with polymer surface defects, perhaps originating during fabrication or resulting from environmental stress cracking (22). Surface defects and subsurface voids may serve as preferred sites for calcific deposits in smooth polymer surfaces, perhaps through accumulating calcium-

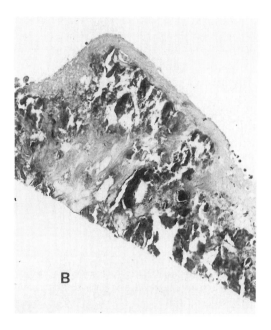

FIG. 6–13. Extrinsic calcification of smooth polyurethane pumping bladder (B) of an artificial heart following implantation and several months function in a calf. Hematoxylin and eosin. Specimen courtesy of DL Coleman, PhD, University of Utah. Reproduced with permission from Schoen FJ et al: Biomaterial-associated calcification. Pathology, mechanisms and strategies for prevention. J Biomed Mater Res: Appl Biomater 1988;22(A1):11–36. Copyright 1988, John Wiley & Sons, Inc.

binding proteins and lipids, but not necessarily secondary to thrombus formation. Although the soft segment portions of polyurethane (see Ref. 30) may have an affinity for calcium ions and calcium can be absorbed into the polymer (101), the mechanism by which calcium is crystallized at the polymer surface is not yet known.

The mechanism by which mechanical effects promote polymer calcification is unknown. Dynamic mechanical deformation may promote damage to adherent cells. It has been suggested that the stress concentrations raise local polymer temperature in dynamic regions, thereby altering the polymer domain structure, potentially facilitating intrinsic deposition of calcium phosphate and its transformation to apatite. Nevertheless, a direct mechanism by which crystallization of calcium phosphate occurs directly on or in a polyurethane or other elastomeric surface in the absence of dead and degraded cells or cellular components acting as nucleation sites remains to be demonstrated.

SIMILARITIES BETWEEN PHYSIOLOGIC AND PATHOLOGIC CALCIFICATION

Physiologic calcification in skeletal tissue and pathologic mineralization in calcific diseases share essential features (19, 35, 102). The mineral deposited initially in both normal and pathologic calcification is almost always a poorly crystalline form of hydroxyapatite, often substituted in carbonate. The typical molar ratio of Ca to P in calcified bioprosthetic tissue (approximately 1.6) and crystal structure determined by x-ray diffraction are analogous to those of hydroxyapatite, the predominant mineral phase in bone, and to those of the less well defined mineral phases that develop in most instances of pathologic calcification. A second feature common to virtually all forms of calcification is crystal formation associated with cell membranes, usually in the form of extracellular vesicles. Thus, in complicated atherosclerotic plaque, cardiac valvular degeneration, bioprosthetic heart valves, and blood pumps, calcification occurs in association with vesicular membrane fragments associated with aging or devitalized cells.

Current theories of crystal initiation in physiologic mineralization center on either cellular structures or extracellular matrix, especially collagen (31, 32, 101, 103). A leading theory considers that mineral initiation in developing bones, in the dentin of teeth, and in the growth plate cartilage of long bones results from the deposition of apatite crystals within and upon extracellular *matrix vesicles* (101). Rich in lipids, phospholipids, and calcium, matrix vesicles mineralize by concentrating calcium and phosphorus. Calcium may be attracted by its affinity for acidic phospholipids of the matrix vesicle membrane, and phosphate may be concentrated by the action of transmembrane phosphatases. Mechanisms for the direct participation of collagen in the nucleation of calcific deposits have been proposed (102).

MECHANISM OF BIOPROSTHETIC VALVE CALCIFICATION

Intrinsic and extrinsic biomaterial-associated mineralization, other dystrophic calcification, and physiologic mineralization may occur via a common mechanism (19, 28, 35). As in physiologic mineralization, dystrophic mineral is generally nucleated initially within cells and their organelles and membranous fragments and later in the extracellular connective tissue, particularly collagen. It is thus reasonable to hypothesize that dystrophic calcification in general, and mineralization of bioprosthetic valves in particular, occurs in situations in which cells are unable to compartmentalize their normally low calcium content relative to the extracellular environment (19).

The intracellular free-calcium concentration of intact living animal cells is approximately 10^{-7} M, while extracellular calcium is approximately 10^{-3} M (Fig. 6–14). This leads to a 10,000-fold gradient across the plasma membrane. Low cellular calcium levels are usually maintained by energy-requiring metabolic pumps that extrude Ca^{2+}, as well as by intracellular buffering mechanisms. Nevertheless, calcium and phosphorus levels may be relatively high in membrane-bound organelles, such as mitochondria, and phosphorus is prevalent both within the organellar and plasma membranes themselves, largely in phospholipids, and within the nucleus, in nucleic acids.

The hypothesized detailed mechanism and determinants of bioprosthetic valve mineralization are summarized in Fig. 6–15. In cells modified by aldehyde cross-linking or mechanical injury, cell membranes are disrupted (leading to increased permeability), the mechanisms for calcium extrusion are no longer fully functional, and the high-energy phosphates (particularly ATP) required to fuel these mechanisms are largely unavailable. Thus, calcium accumulation occurs unimpeded and extrusion is prevented. The net effect is a dramatic increase in intracellular calcium concentration. Crystal nucleation and growth occur and resultant clinical effect may follow. Modification of influential host or implant factors or interruption of the critical events summarized in Fig. 6–15 will likely reduce bioprosthetic valve mineralization (30).

The imbalance between influx and efflux induced by loss of cell vitality is analogous to the mitochondrial calcification that occurs when cardiac myocytes are irreversibly damaged by severe ischemia and exposed to plasma during reperfusion (104). The plasma membranes of necrotic myocytes, similar to connective tissue cells devitalized by

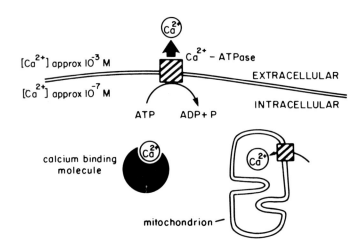

$[Ca^{2+}]$ approx 10^{-3} M

$[Ca^{2+}]$ approx 10^{-7} M

Ca^{2+} – ATPase

EXTRACELLULAR

INTRACELLULAR

ATP   ADP + P

calcium binding
molecule

mitochondrion

MAINTENANCE OF LOW INTRACELLULAR FREE CALCIUM

FIG. 6–14. Schematic representation of the physiologic gradient of free calcium across mammalian cell membranes. Maintenance of this gradient is energy-dependent. Binding of calcium ions occurs intracellularly in conjunction with calcium-binding molecules and organelles. Paralysis or saturation of these mechanisms can increase intracellular calcium concentrations. Reproduced with permission from Schoen FJ et al: Biomaterial-associated calcification. Pathology, mechanisms and strategies for prevention. J Biomed Mater Res: Appl Biomater 1988;22(A1):11–36. Copyright 1988, John Wiley & Sons, Inc.

glutaraldehyde, are incapable of excluding massive quantities of calcium ions, in the presence of transport systems that are no longer functional. The pathologic calcification that occurs in bioprosthetic valves, degenerative senile native aortic valve sclerosis, and nonfixed tissue valve implants (such as homografts and fascia lata valves) may be similar to the extent that, in each case, cell injury secondary to mechanically induced damage probably renders the tissue more susceptible to mineralization. Moreover, cell injury may be enhanced by local hypoxia in each of these poorly vascularlized tissues.

The initial phosphorus required for crystal nucleation is almost certainly readily available from the membranes (42). In this respect, using a newly available technique called electron energy loss spectroscopy (EELS), we have recently demonstrated focally high concentrations of phosphorus, associated with cell membranes and nuclei in unimplanted glutaraldehyde-preserved porcine valve and bovine pericardium, which probably provide initial nucleation sites for calcium phosphate. We hypothesize that the cells involved as nucleation sites could be cells of the implant itself, as in bioprosthetic valve mineralization, or in the adherent hematogenous cells, as in blood pump calcification. In contrast, in physiologic mineralization, matrix vesicles actively concentrate ions and thereby provide the means for crystal nucleation (102).

Future Directions

The key features of bioprosthetic valve calcification are summarized in Table 6–2. Future research objectives include (1) continued development of animal models, (2) determination of initial crystal nucleation events and sites, (3) elucidation of the relative

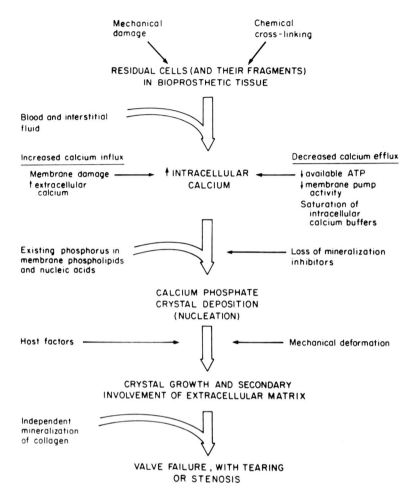

FIG. 6–15. Hypothetical model for the calcification of bioprosthetic tissue. This model takes into account host factors, implant factors, and mechanical damage and relates the initial nucleation sites to increased intracellular calcium levels, in residual cells and their fragments in the bioprosthetic tissue. The end result is valve failure, with tearing or stenosis. This model assumes that calcification is a product only of a susceptible substrate in a permissive environment. The key role of existing phosphorus in membrane phospholipids and nucleic acids in controlling the initial sites of crystal nucleation is emphasized, and a possible role for the independent mineralization of collagen is included. Mechanical deformation contributes to both nucleation and growth of calcific crystal.

TABLE 6–2. *Key Features of Bioprosthetic Heart Valve Calcification*

Substrate: glutaraldehyde-treated tissue
Sites/models: circulatory of subcutaneous
Mineral: poorly crystalline apatite
Mineral location: mostly intrinsic, occasionally extrinsic
Factors/determinants: host, implant, and mechanical
Nucleation sites: cells and collagen
Mechanism and early events: under investigation

roles of host, implant, and mechanical determinants, and (4) development of approaches for the inhibition of mineralization (19). The extent to which mechanisms of physiologic and pathologic calcification are analogous is yet unknown. For example, it should be determined whether alkaline phosphatase and/or related enzymes (important in skeletal mineralization) (102) play any role in pathologic calcification. Glutaraldehyde-fixed bovine pericardium retains biochemically measurable and histochemically stainable alkaline phosphatase activity (105), but whether this enzyme is contributory to mechanisms of bioprosthetic tissue mineralization, as it probably is to skeletal mineralization, is unknown.

It is presently unknown whether cell- and collagen-associated bioprosthetic valve calcification occur independently or cell-associated calcification somehow facilitates mineralization of the extracellular matrix. Purified preparations of type I collagen undergo intrinsic mineralization, independent of cells, when implanted subcutaneously in rats (88), and specific collagen-mineralization mechanisms likely exist in bone (103). Nevertheless, the role of collagen calcification in bioprosthetic valve tissue has not been elucidated. The biochemical rationale for the dependence of mineralization on cross-linking of cells and collagen is as yet uncertain. The specific metabolic causes of age-related potentiation of mineralization are also unknown. Finally, the mechanism for the mineralization-promoting effect of mechanical deformation has not been determined.

Acknowledgment—Supported in part by Grants HL38118 and HL36574 from the National Institutes of Health.

REFERENCES

1. Schoen FJ: Cardiac valve prostheses: Pathological and bioengineering consideration. J Cardiac Surg 1987;2:65–108.
2. Schoen FJ, Kujovich JL, Levy RJ, St. John Sutton M: Bioprosthetic valve failure. Cardiovasc Clin 1988;18/2:289–316.
3. Magilligan DJ, Lewis JW, Tilley B, Peterson E: The porcine bioprosthetic valve. Twelve years later. J Thorac Cardiovasc Surg 1985;89:499–507.
4. Gallo I, Nistal F, Blasquez R, Arbe E, Artinano E: Incidence of primary tissue valve failure in porcine bioprosthetic heart valves. Ann Thorac Surg 1988;45:66–70.
5. Milano A, Bortolotti U, Talenti E, Valfre C, Arbustini E, Valente M, Mazzucco A, Gallucci V, Thiene G: Calcific degeneration as the main cause of porcine bioprosthetic valve failure. Am J Cardiol 1984;53:1066–1070.
6. Schoen FJ, Hobson CE: Anatomic analysis of removed prosthetic heart valves: Causes of failure of 33 mechanical valves and 58 bioprostheses, 1980 to 1983. Human Pathol 1985;16:549–559.
7. Reul GJ, Cooley DA, Duncan JM, et al: Valve failure with the Ionescu-Shiley bovine pericardial bioprostheses: Analysis of 2680 patients. J Vasc Surg 1985;2:192–204.
8. Schoen FJ, Cohn LH: Explant analysis of porcine bioprosthetic heart valves: Modes of failure and stent creep. In Bodnar E, Yacoub M (eds): Biologic and Bioprosthetic Valves. New York, Yorke Medical Books, 1986; pp 356–365.
9. Schoen FJ, Fernandez J, Gonzales-Lavin L, Cernaianu A: Causes of failure and pathologic findings in surgically-removed Ionescu-Shiley standard bovine pericardial heart valve bioprostheses: Emphasis on progressive structural deterioration. Circulation 1987;76:618–627.
10. Gallo I, Nistal F, Arbe E, Artinano E: Comparative study of primary tissue failure between porcine (Hancock and Carpentier-Edwards) and bovine pericardial (Ionescu-Shiley) bioprostheses in the aortic position at five- to nine-year follow-up. Am J Cardiol 1988;61:812–816.
11. Walley VM, Keon WJ: Patterns of failure in Ionescu-Shiley bovine pericardial bioprosthetic valves. J Thorac Cardiovasc Surg 1987;93:925–933.
12. Wallace RB, Londe SP, Titus JL: Aortic valve replacement with preserved aortic valve homografts. J Thorac Cardiovasc Surg 1974;67:44–50.
13. Saravalli OA, Somerville J, Jefferson KE: Calcification of aortic homografts used for reconstruction of the right ventricular outflow tract. J Thorac Cardiovasc Surg 1980;80:909–920.

14. Ross DN: Evolution of the biological concept in cardiac surgery: A Pilgrim's progress. In Yankah AC, Hetzer R, Miller DC, Ross DN, Somerville J, Yacoub MH (eds): Cardiac Valve Allografts 1962–1987. New York, Springer-Verlag, 1988, pp 1–12.

15. Somerville J: Late results of homograft function used for right ventricular outflow obstruction. In Yankah AC, Hetzer R, Miller DC, Ross DN, Somerville J, Yacoub MH (eds): Cardiac Valve Allografts 1962–1987. New York, Springer-Verlag, 1988, pp 249–260.

16. McEnany MT, Ross DN, Yates AK: Valve failure in seventy-two frame-supported autologous fascia lata mitral valves. Two-year follow-up. J Thorac Vasc Surg 1972;63:199–214.

17. Silver MD, Hudson REB, Trimble AS: Morphologic observations on heart valve prostheses made of fascia lata. J Thorac Cardiovasc Surg 1975;70:360–366.

18. Schoen FJ: Biomaterial-associated infection, neoplasia, and calcification. Clinicopathologic features and pathophysiologic concepts. Trans Am Soc Artif Intern Organs 1987;33:8–18.

19. Schoen FJ, Harasaki H, Kim KM, Anderson HC, Levy RJ: Biomaterial-associated calcification: Pathology, mechanisms, and strategies for prevention. J Biomed Mater Res: Appl Biomater 1988;22,A1:11–36.

20. Whalen RL, Snow JL, Harasaki H, Nose Y: Mechanical strain and calcification in blood pumps. Trans Am Soc Artif Intern Organs 1980;26:487–491.

21. Coleman D: Mineralization of blood pump bladders. Trans Am Soc Artif Intern Organs 1981;27:708–713.

22. Cumming RD: Mechanical etiology of calcification. Presented at Devices and Technology Branch Contractors Meeting, NIH, December 16–18, 1985.

23. Braunwald NS, Morrow AG: A late evaluation of flexible Teflon prostheses utilized for total aortic valve replacements. J Thorac Cardiovasc Surg 1965;49:485–496.

24. Hennig E, Bucherl ES: Mineralization of circulatory devices made of polymers. In Planck H, Egbers G, Syre I (eds): Polyurethanes in Biomedical Engineering. Amsterdam, Elsevier, 1984, pp 109–134.

25. Wisman CB, Pierce WS, Donachy JH, Pae WE, Myers JL, Prophet GA: A polyurethane trileaflet cardiac valve prosthesis: In-vitro and in-vivo studies. Trans Am Soc Artif Intern Organs 1982;28:164–168.

26. Hilbert SL, Ferrans VJ, Tomita Y, Eidbo EE, Jones M: Evaluation of explanted polyurethane trileaflet cardiac valve prostheses. J Thorac Cardiovasc Surg 1987;94:419–429.

27. Schoen FJ, St. John Sutton M: Contemporary issues in the pathology of valvular heart disease. Human Pathol 1987;18:568–576.

28. Kim KM: Role of membranes in calcification. Surv Synth Pathol Res 1983;2:215–228.

29. Wissler RW: Principles of the pathogenesis of atherosclerosis. In Braunwald E (ed): Heart Disease. Philadelphia, WB Saunders, 1984, pp 1183–1204.

30. Schoen FJ, Levy RJ, Ratner BD, Lelah MD, Christie GW: Materials considerations for improved cardiac valve prostheses. In Bodnar E, Frater R (eds): Repalcement Cardiac Valves, Chapter 15. Elmsford NY, Pergamon Press, 1991.

31. Glimcher MJ: Composition, structure, and organization of bone and other mineralized tissues and the mechanism of calcification. In Greep RO, and Astwood ED (eds): Handbook of Physiology. Washington, DC, American Physiological Society, 1976, vol 2, pp 25–116.

32. Glimcher MJ: On the form and function of bone: From molecules to organs. Wolff's law revisited, 1981. In Weiss A (ed): The Chemistry and Biology of Mineralized Connective Tissues. Amsterdam, Elsevier/North-Holland, 1981, pp 617–673.

33. Posner AS: The mineral of bone. Clin Orthop 1985;200:87–99.

34. Robbins SL, Cotran RS, Kumar V (eds): Pathologic Basis of Disease. Philadelphia, WB Saunders, 1984, pp 35–36.

35. Anderson HC: Calcific diseases. Arch Pathol Lab Med 1983;107:341–348.

36. Woodward SC: Mineralization of connective tissue surrounding implanted devices. Trans Am Soc Artif Intern Organs 1981;27:697–702.

37. Tomazic BB, Etz ES, Brown WE: Nature and properties of cardiovascular deposits. Scan Microsc 1987;1:95–105.

38. Tomazic BB, Brown WE, Queral LA, Sadovnik M: Physiochemical characterization of cardiovascular calcified deposits: I. Isolation, purification and instrumental analysis. Atherosclerosis 1988;69:5–19.

39. Thubrikar MJ, Deck JD, Aouad J, Nolan SP: Role of mechanical stress in calcification of aortic bioprosthetic valves. J Thorac Cardiovasc Surg 1983;86:115–125.

40. Levy RJ, Schoen FJ, Levy JT, Nelson AC, Howard SL, Oshry LJ: Biologic determinants of dystrophic calcification and osteocalcin deposition in glutaraldehyde-preserved porcine aortic valve leaflets implanted subcutaneously in rats. Am J Pathol 1983;113:142–155.

41. Schoen FJ, Levy RJ, Nelson AC, Bernhard WF, Nashef A, Hawley M: Onset and progression of experimental bioprosthetic heart valve calcification. Lab Invest 1985;52:523–532.

42. Schoen FJ, Tsao JW, Levy RJ: Calcification of bovine pericardium used in cardiac valve bioprostheses. Implications for mechanisms of bioprosthetic tissue mineralization. Am J Pathol 1986;123:143–154.

43. Schoen FJ, Kujovich JL, Webb CL, Levy RJ: Chemically determined mineral content of explanted porcine aortic valve bioprostheses: Correlation with radiographic assessment of calcification and clinical data. Circulation 1987;76:1061–1066.

44. Cipriano PR, Billingham ME, Oyer PE, Kutsche LM, Stinson EB: Calcification of porcine prosthetic heart valves: A radiographic and light microscopic study. Circulation 1982;66:1100–1104.
45. Luna LG (ed): Manual of Histologic Staining Methods of the Armed Forces Institute of Pathology. New York, McGraw-Hill, 1968, vol 3, pp 175–177.
46. Ferrans VJ, Boyce SW, Billingham ME, Jones M, Ishihara T, Roberts WC: Calcific deposits in porcine bioprostheses: Structure and pathogenesis. Am J Cardiol 1980;46:721–734.
47. Stein PD, Kemp SR, Riddle JM, Lee MW, Lewis JW, Magilligan DJ: Relation of calcification to torn leaflets of spontaneously degenerated porcine bioprosthetic valves. Ann Thorac Surg 1985;40:175–180.
48. Valente M, Bortolotti U, Thiene G: Ultrastructural substrates of dystrophic calcification in porcine bioprosthetic valve failure. Am J Pathol 1985;119:12–21.
49. Ishihara T, Ferrans VJ, Jones M, Cabin HS, Roberts WC: Calcific deposits developing in a bovine pericardial bioprosthetic valve 3 days after implantation. Circulation 1981;63:718–723.
50. Goffin YA, Hilbert SL, Bartik MA, Salmon I: Cusp degeneration and calcification in explanted porcine aortic bioprostheses: Role of the sponge phenomenon. In Bodnar E, Yacoub M (eds): Biologic and Bioprosthetic Valves. New York, Yorke Medical Books, 1986, pp 405–417.
51. Ishihara T, Ferrans VJ, Barnhart GR, Jones M, McIntosh CL, Roberts WC: Intracuspal hematomas in implanted porcine valvular bioprostheses. J Thorac Cardiovasc Surg 1982;83:399–407.
52. Thiene G, Bortolotti U, Talenti E, Guerra F, Valente M, Milano A, Mazzucco A, Gallucci V: Dissecting cuspal hematomas. A rare form of porcine bioprosthetic valve dysfunction. Arch Pathol Lab Med 1987;111:964–967.
53. Barnhart GR, Jones M, Ishihara T, Chavez AM, Rose DM, Ferrans VJ: Bioprosthetic valvular failure. Clinical and pathological observations in an experimental animal model. J Thorac Cardiovasc Surg 1982;83:618–631.
54. Arbustini E, Jones M, Moses RD, Eidbo EE, Carroll RJ, Ferrans VJ: Modification by the Hancock T6 process of calcification of bioprosthetic cardiac valves implanted in sheep. Am J Cardiol 1984;53:1388–1396.
55. Jones M, Eidbo EE, Walters SM, Ferrans VJ, Clark RE: Effects of 2 types of preimplantation processes on calcification of bioprosthetic valves. In Bodnar E, Yacoub M (eds): Biologic & Bioprosthetic Valves. New York, Yorke Medical Books, 1986, pp 451–459.
56. Gallo I, Nistal F, Artinano E, Fernandex D, Cayon R, Carrion M, Garcia-Martinex V: The behavior of pericardial versus porcine valve xenografts in the growing sheep model. J Thorac Cardiovasc Surg 1987;93:281–290.
57. Shemin RJ, Schoen FJ, Hein R, Austin J, Cohn LH: Hemodynamic and pathological evaluation of a unileaflet pericardial bioprosthetic valve. J Thorac Cardiovasc Surg 1988;95:912–919.
58. Levy RJ, Zenker JA, Bernhard WF: Porcine bioprosthetic valve calcification in bovine left ventricle to aorta shunts: Studies of the deposition of vitamin K-dependent protein. Ann Thorac Surg 1982;62:313–318.
59. Dewanjee MK, Solis E, Mackey ST, Lenker J, Edwards WD, Didisheim P, Chesbro JH, Zollman PE, Kaye MP: Quantification of regional platelet and calcium deposition on pericardial tissue valve prostheses in calves and effect of hydroxyethylene diphosphonate. J Thorac Cardiovasc Surg 1986;92:337–348.
60. Harasaki H, Kiraly R, Nose Y: Three mechanisms of calcification in tissue valves. In Bodnar E, Yacoub M (eds): Biologic and Bioprosthetic Valves. New York, Yorke Medical Books, 1986.
61. Gabbay S, Bortolotti U, Factor S, Shore DF, Frater RWM: Calcification of implanted xenograft pericardium: Influence of site and function. J Thorac Cardiovasc Surg 1984;87:782–787.
62. Frasca P, Buchanan JW, Soriano RZ, Dunn JM, Marmon L, Melbin J, Buchanan SJ, Chang SH, Colub EE, Shapiro IM: Mineralization of short-term pericardial cardiac patch grafts. SEM/1984/II; 1984;973–977.
63. Levy RJ, Schoen FJ, Howard SL: Mechanism of calcification of porcine bioprosthetic aortic valve cusps: Role of T-lymphocytes. Am J Cardiol 1983;52:629–631.
64. Fishbein MC, Levy RJ, Ferrans VJ, Dearden LC, Nashef A, Goodman AP, Carpentier A: Calcification of cardiac valve bioprostheses: Biochemical histologic and ultrastructural observations in a subcutaneous implantation model system. J Thorac Cardiovasc Surg 1982;83:602–609.
65. Rossi MA, Braile DM, Teixeira MDR, Carillo SV: Calcific degeneration of pericardial valvular xenografts implanted subcutaneously in rats. Int J Cardiol 1986;12:331–339.
66. Schoen FJ, Levy RJ: Pathophysiology of bioprosthetic heart valve calcification. In Bodnar E, Yacoub M (eds): Biologic and Bioprosthetic Valves. New York, Yorke Medical Books, 1986, pp. 418–429.
67. Warnes CA, Scitt ML, Silver GM, Smith CW, Ferrans FJ, Roberts WC: Comparison of late degenerative changes in porcine bioprostheses in the mitral and aortic valve position in the same patient. Am J Cardiol 1983;51:965–968.
68. Cohen SR, Silver MA, McIntosh CL, Roberts WC: Comparison of late (62 to 140 months) degenerative changes in simultaneously implanted and explanted porcine (Hancock) bioprostheses in the tricuspid and mitral valve positions in six patients. Am J Cardiol 1984;53:1599–1602.

69. Cipriano PR, Billingham ME, Miller DC: Calcification of aortic versus mitral porcine bioprosthetic heart valves: A radiographic study comparing amounts of calcific deposits in valves explanted from the same patient. Am J Cardiol 1984;54:1030–1032.

70. Sabbah HN, Hamid MS, Stein PD: Estimation of mechanical stresses on closed cusps of porcine bioprosthetic valves: Effects of stiffening, focal calcium and focal thinning. Am J Cardiol 1985;55:1091–1096.

71. Buchanan JW, Buchanan SJ: Absence of mineralization in subcutaneous pericardial xenografts subjected to compressive trauma. Trans Soc Biomater 1986;9:78.

72. Tsao JW, Levy RJ, Schoen FJ: Compressive mechanical deformation inhibits calcification of bovine pericardium used in cardiac valve bioprostheses. Trans Soc Biomater 1987;10:180.

73. Kopf GS, Geha AS, Hellenbrand WE, Kleinman CS: Fate of left-sided cardiac bioprosthesis valves in children. Arch Surg 1986;121:488–490.

74. Sanders SP, Levy RJ, Freed MD, Norwood WI, Castaneda AR: Use of Hancock porcine xenografts in children and adolescents. Am J Cardiol 1980;46:429–438.

75. Magilligan DJ, Lewis JW, Heinzerling RH, et al: Fate of a second porcine bioprosthetic valve. J Thorac Cardiovasc Surg 1983;85:362–368.

76. Fishbein MC, Gissen SA, Collins JJ, Barsamian EM, Cohn LH: Pathologic findings after cardiac valve replacement with glutaraldehyde-fixed porcine valves. Am J Cardiol 1977;40:331–337.

77. Moront MG, Katz NM: Early degeneration of a porcine aortic valve bioprosthesis in the mitral valve position in an elderly woman and its association with long-term calcium carbonate therapy. Am J Cardiol 1987;59:1006–1007.

78. Bortolotti U, Milano A, Mazzucco A, Valfre C, Russo R, Valente M, Schivazappa L, Thiene G, Gallucci V: Pregnancy in patients with a porcine valve bioprosthesis. Am J Cardiol 1982;50:1051–1054.

79. Rocchini AP, Weesner KM, Heidelberger K, et al: Porcine xenograft valve failure in children: An immunologic response. Circulation 1981;64(Suppl II):II-162–II-171.

80. Bajpai PK, Salgaller ML: Immune responses to glutaraldehyde-treated xenografts. In Szycher M (ed): Biocompatible Polymers, Metals, and Composites. Westport, CT, Technomic Publishing, 1982, pp 373–394.

81. Gallop PM, Lian JB, Hauschka PV: Carboxylated calcium-binding proteins in vitamin K. N Engl J Med 1980;302:1460–1466.

82. Lian JB, Levy RJ, Bernhard W, Szycher M: LVAD mineralization of gamma-carboxyglutamic acid containing proteins in normal and pathologically mineralized tissue. Trans Am Soc Artif Intern Organs 1981;26:683–689.

83. Stein PD, Riddle JM, Kemp SR, et al: Effect of warfarin on calcification of spontaneously degenerated porcine bioprosthetic valves. J Thorac Cardiovasc Surg 1985;90:119–125.

84. Pierce WS, Donachy JH, Rosenberg G, et al: Calcification inside artifical hearts: Inhibition by warfarin sodium. Science 1980;208:601–603.

85. Hughes SD, Coleman DL, Dew PA, Burns GL, Olsen DB, Kolff WJ: Effects of Coumadin on thrombus and mineralization in total artificial hearts. Trans Am Soc Artif Intern Organs 1984;30:75–79.

86. Golomb G, Schoen FJ, Smith MS, Linden J, Dixon M, Levy RJ: The role of glutaraldehyde-induced cross-links in calcification of bovine pericardium used in cardiac valve bioprostheses. Am J Pathol 1987;127:122–130.

87. Schryer PJ, Tomasek ER, Starr JA, et al: Anticalcification effect of glutaraldehyde-preserved valve tissue stored for increasing time in glutaraldehyde. In Bodnar E, Yacoub M (eds): Biologic and Bioprosthetic Valves. New York, Yorke Medical Books, 1986, pp 471–477.

88. Bortolotti U, Talenti E, Milano A, Thiene G, Gallucci V: Formaldehyde- versus glutaraldehyde-processed porcine bioprostheses in the aortic valve position: Long-term follow-up. Am J Cardiol 1984;54:681–682.

89. Levy RJ, Schoen FJ, Sherman FS, Nichols J, Hawley MA, Lund SA: Calcification of subcutaneously implanted type I collagen sponges. Effects of formaldehyde and glutaraldehyde pretreatments. Am J Pathol 1986;122:71–82.

90. Maranto AR, Schoen FJ: Effect of delay between tissue harvest and glutaraldehyde pretreatment on the calcification of bovine pericardium used in bioprosthetic heart valves. J Biomed Mater Res 1988;22:819–825.

91. Levy RJ, Schoen FJ, Golomb G: Bioprosthetic heart valve calcification: Clinical features, pathobiology, and prospects for prevention. CRC Crit Rev Biocomp 1986;2:147–187.

92. Levy RJ, Schoen FJ, Howard SL, Levy JT, Oshry L, Hawley M: Calcification of cardiac valve bioprostheses. Host and implant factors. In Rubin RP, Weiss GB, Putney JW (eds): Calcium in Biological Systems. New York, Plenum Publishing, 1985, pp 661–668.

93. Yarbrough JW, Roberts WC, Reis RL: Structural alterations in tissue cardiac valves implanted in patients and in calves. J Thorac Cardiovasc Surg 1973;65:364–375.

94. Bodnar E, Rose D: Mode of failure in 170 explanted biological valves. Trans Soc Biomater 1982;5:128.

95. Tanimura A, McGregor DH, Anderson HC: Matrix vesicles in atherosclerotic calcification. Proc Soc Exp Biol Med 1983;172:173–177.

96. Kim KM, Valigorsky JM, Mergner WJ, Jones RT, Pendergrass RF, Trump BF: Aging changes in the human aortic valve in relation to dystrophic calcification. Human Pathol 1976;7:47–60.
97. Harasaki H, Kambic H, Whalen R, Murray J, Snow J, Murabayashi S, Hillegass D, Ozawa K, Kiraly R, Nose Y: Comparative study of flocked vs. biolized surface for long-term assist pumps. Trans Am Soc Artif Intern Organs 1980;26:470–474.
98. Bernhard WF, Gernes DG, Clay WC, Schoen FJ, Burgeson R, Valeri RC, Melaragno AJ, Poirier VL: Investigations with an implantable, electrically actuated ventricular assist device. J Thorac Cardiovasc Surg 1984;88:11–21.
99. Harasaki H, Moritz A, Uchida N, Chen JF, McMahon JT, Richards TM, Smith WA, Murabayashi S, Kambic HE, Kiraly RJ, Nose Y: Initiation and growth of calcification in polyurethane-coated blood pump. Trans Am Soc Artif Intern Organs 1987;33:643–649.
100. Taylor KD, Coldthorpe SH, Topaz SR, Jarvik RK: Analysis of blood diaphragms from three long term clinical Jarvik-7 total artificial heart implants. Trans Soc Biomater 1987;10:243.
101. Thoma RJ, Phillips RE: Calcification of poly (ether) urethanes. Trans Soc Biomater 1987; 10:245.
102. Anderson HC: Mineralization by matrix vesicles. Scan Elect Microsc 1984;2:953–964.
103. Glimcher MJ: The role of collagen and phosphoproteins in the calcification of bone and other collagenous tissues. In Rubin RP, Weiss GB, Putney JW, (eds): Calcium in Biological Systems. New York, Plenum Press, 1985, pp 607–616.
104. Hagler HK, Lopez LE, Murphy ME, et al: Quantitative x-ray microanalysis of mitrochondrial calcification in damaged myocardium. Lab Invest 1981;45:241–247.
105. Maranto AR, Schoen FJ: Alkaline phosphatase activity of glutaraldehyde-treated bovine pericardium used in bioprosthetic cardiac valves. Circ Res 1988;63:844–848.

Bodnar, E. and Frater, R. W. M., editors
(1991) *Replacement Cardiac Valves,*
Pergamon Press, Inc. (New York), pp. 149–186
Printed in the United States of America

CHAPTER 7

CAGED-BALL VALVES: THE STARR-EDWARDS AND SMELOFF-SUTTER PROSTHESES

JAMES I. FANN, CARLOS E. MORENO-CABRAL, AND D. CRAIG MILLER

HISTORICAL VIGNETTE

One of the most important achievements in the history of cardiac surgery is that associated with the conception, development, and clinical application of mechanical heart valve prostheses. Ideas in this area were coming to fruition at the same time that many other advances were occurring in this evolving field, including the advent of extracorporeal circulation.

In the early 1950s, the pioneering efforts of Charles Hufnagel and J. Moore Campbell, who independently designed a mechanical valve consisting of a lucite tube and a mobile spherical poppet, led to the first successful placement of a totally mechanical valvular prosthesis in a human (1, 2). Hufnagel accomplished this feat in September 1952 by implanting the device into the descending aorta of a patient with severe aortic regurgitation (1). The concept of a ball-and-cage one-way valve, interestingly, was originally patented in the United States as a bottle stopper in 1858 (3).

These efforts preceded the evolution of the most successful of the caged-ball valves, the Starr-Edwards (S-E) prosthesis. The development of this particular mechanical valve was initiated by an energetic man who wanted to create an artificial heart more than 30 years ago (3). M. Lowell Edwards, a retired engineer, presented himself in Albert Starr's office in Portland, Oregon, offering his services to accomplish such an ambitious objective. He was dissuaded of this idea, and the more logical concept of creating a valvular prosthesis matured. Two years later, in August 1960, the first S-E prosthesis was implanted in the *mitral* position by Starr (4). Earlier that year, Dwight Harken had successfully implanted a similar caged-ball prosthesis in the subcoronary position in patients with aortic regurgitation (5); this location was clearly physiologically advantageous compared with Hufnagel's prosthesis in the descending thoracic aorta. The first clinical S-E *aortic* valve implantation was performed in September 1961 (3). Experimentally, the caged-ball valve had been evaluated previously in the mitral position in dogs by F. Henry Ellis (6) and in the aortic position by W. Sterling Edwards (7), both in 1958.

The following decade was punctuated by an explosion in the use of these and many other mechanical prostheses. After early design improvements, the silastic ball, non-cloth-covered S-E mechanical valves became the standard against which all other valve substitutes were measured.

Shortly after the introduction of the caged-ball concept, a number of similar designs appeared in clinical use. These included the Servelle-Arbonville, Harken-Davol, Cooley-Cromie, Magovern-Cromie, Braunwald-Cutter, DeBakey-Surgitool, and Smeloff-Cutter [now Smeloff-Sutter (S-S)] prostheses (3). Because of high complication rates and problems with durability and structural design, all but the S-E, S-S, and Magovern-Cromie prostheses have been removed from the market. In this chapter we will review the two caged-ball valves currently widely available for clinical use: the S-E and the S-S prostheses.

STARR-EDWARDS PROSTHETIC VALVE

The basic construction of the early S-E valves consisted of a stainless steel four-strut cage housing a silastic ball. Subsequently, the cage was cast of Stellite 21, which is an alloy of cobalt (61–63.5%), chromium (25.5–29%), molybdenum (5–6%), and nickel (1.75–3.75%) (8).

The first S-E mitral valve implanted in humans was the model 6000, which contained a large area of exposed metal on its atrial surface. Due to an unacceptably high thromboembolic (TE) rate (freedom from TE of only 29% at 5 years (9)), a larger area of the inflow portion of the metal base was covered with cloth, leaving only the surface in contact with the ball uncovered. This modification, the addition of barium sulfate (2% by weight) to the poppet to make it radiopaque, and a decrease in the thickness of the metal struts resulted in the model 6120 (Fig. 7–1). The model 6120 valve has remained structurally unchanged since its clinical introduction in 1966 and is the only S-E mitral valve currently available. The modifications resulting in the model 6120 were thought to be associated with a substantial decrease in TE events. In an attempt to reduce this complication further, the struts and the entire base were covered with cloth (model 6300, released in 1967), inspired by experiments in dogs that showed complete neointimal covering of cloth-covered surfaces (10). The poppet was changed to a hollow metal (Stellite) ball. There was a documented decrease in TE rates, but two new problems appeared: cloth disruption from wear, and hemolytic anemia, which caused a sharp increase in reoperation rates (4 to 15% after 7 years) (9). Further modifications in design, aimed at reducing cloth wear, included placing small metal studs at the ball contact area on the orifice (models 6310 and 6320) and creating metal tracks to line the inner part of the struts, while leaving the outside portion covered with cloth (model 6400). All these

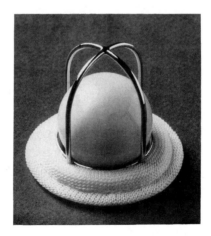

Fig. 7–1. The Starr-Edwards model 6120 mitral prosthesis. Courtesy of Baxter-Edwards Corporation.

changes, however, contributed no additional improvements, and these valves (models 6300, 6310, 6320, and 6400) were discontinued after 2 to 9 years of clinical use.

A similar parallel evolution of the S-E aortic valve prosthesis occurred. Although its original design was similar to that of the mitral prosthesis, the S-E aortic valve, first implanted in 1961, was subsequently changed to a three-strut cage, with three projecting feet on the inflow portion giving it a "double cage" effect, and a foam sewing ring for compressibility (model 1000, introduced in 1962). The problems encountered with this pioneering prosthesis were of different nature than those encountered with the mitral valve. The most serious defect, first reported in 1965 by Krosnick (11), was embolization of a silastic poppet from the cage of a model 1000 aortic prosthesis. This problem, later found to be due to *ball variance,* was felt to be secondary to abrasion damage and/or lipid infiltration of the silastic ball that resulted in (1) poppet embolization and acute aortic regurgitation, (2) hemolytic anemia, and (3) formation of thrombus on the ball surface, causing peripheral thromboemboli. From 1962 to 1964, 67% of recovered valves showed some degree of ball variance (9). This problem, however, has not been reported for valves implanted after 1965. The original model 1000 valve was subsequently modified by converting the ball seat from a spherical to a convex design and removing the projecting feet from the inflow surface of the valve. Simultaneously, the curing process of the silastic ball was changed, creating the model 1200 valve (introduced in 1965) (Fig. 7–2a). To reduce the amount of exposed metal further, the ring on the outflow aspect of the orifice was scalloped at the level of the struts, resulting in the introduction of the model 1260 in 1968 (Fig. 7–2b). The next generations of S-E aortic valves, that is, aortic models 2300, 2310, 2320, and 2400, followed a parallel course to their mitral counterparts and were ultimately also discontinued. The only currently available prostheses are the models 1200 (diameters 16 and 18 mm) and 1260 (diameters 21 to 31 mm). Recent evaluation of the S-E models 1200/1260 aortic and model 6120 mitral prostheses (mandated by the 1976 medical devices legislation) by the United States Food and Drug Administration (FDA) in 1988 has resulted in the approval of the models 1260 and 6120

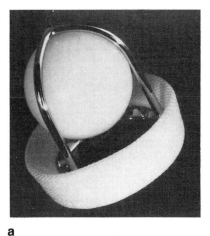   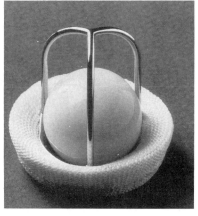

a   b

FIG. 7–2. The two currently available Starr-Edwards aortic prostheses. (a) Model 1200. (b) Model 1260. Courtesy of Baxter-Edwards Corporation.

(with the exception of sizes 20M and 22M); approval of the model 1200 and the smaller-sized mitral prostheses is pending at this time. The following discussion will focus on the two aortic models and the mitral model 6120.

Hydrodynamics and Hemodynamics

Areas of obstruction to forward flow in prosthetic valves with central occluders, such as the S-E and the S-S caged-ball valves, include (1) the valve ring (inflow or primary orifice), (2) the truncated cone (frustum) from the circumference of the valve ring to the occluder in the open position (outflow or secondary orifice), and (3) the place between the equator of the occluder and the surrounding ventricular or aortic wall (tertiary orifice) (12) (Fig. 7–3). Turbulent flow resulting from central obstruction may lead to intimal thickening and secondary endocardial fibroelastosis (13–15). The intimal thickening, composed mainly of fibrous tissue and devoid of foam cells, can occur in the aortic root, coronary ostia, and proximal coronary arteries and may lead to myocardial ischemia (13, 14). Endocardial fibroelastosis of various degrees has been reported in patients with mitral prostheses (13–15). The functional consequences of extensive, or focal, acquired left ventricular (LV) endocardial fibroelastosis is uncertain but may lead to myocardial failure (15).

The assessment of hemodynamic performance of a valvular prosthesis by measurement of transvalvular gradients alone is inadequate since a mildly stenotic prosthesis may produce significant gradients when the cardiac output is high or the transvalvular flow period is shortened. Reporting of valve areas, therefore, is essential since gradient, flow, and time are taken into consideration (16).

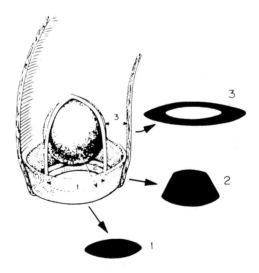

FIG. 7–3. Areas of obstruction to forward flow in the caged-ball valve: (1) the valve ring (inflow or primary orifice), (2) the truncated cone (frustum) from the circumference of the valve ring to the occluder (outflow or secondary orifice), and (3) the place between the equator of the occluder and the surrounding tissues (tertiary orifice). Reproduced with permission from Behrendt and Austen: Current status of prosthetics for heart valve replacement. Prog Cardiovasc Dis 1973;15:369–401.

Aortic Prosthesis

Inherent in the caged-ball design are some degree of transvalvular gradient and regurgitation. For example, in vitro studies of the smaller S-E aortic valves (e.g., size 9A, currently marketed as 23A with 23-mm annulus diameter; see Table 7–1) revealed a mean transvalvular gradient of 11.2 mmHg at a simulated cardiac output of 4.9 L/min with a calculated effective orifice area of approximately 1.5 cm² (Table 7–2) (17, 18). For sizes 24A to 27A aortic prostheses, the mean transvalvular gradient was 15.9 to 16.1 mmHg with a calculated valve area ranging from 1.61 to 1.86 cm² (18, 19). Components of backflow associated with prosthetic valves include closure backflow (required to close the valve) and leakage backflow (occurs after the valve is closed); prosthetic valves generally have a percentage backflow that varies directly with heart rate and inversely with cardiac output (20). The backflow was 3% with the size 23A S-E prosthesis at a simulated cardiac output of 4.9 L/min and heart rate of 70 beats/min (17). For the size 27A valve, backflow was 7.4% at a simulated cardiac output of 4.0 L/min and rate of 50 to 80 beats per minute (20). Comparative studies have shown that the percentage backflow with the S-E valve is lower than that associated with the St. Jude or Björk-Shiley valves because of absence of leakage backflow with the S-E valve and less closure backflow associated with the S-E than with the bileaflet valves (20).

In vivo hemodynamic evaluation of the models 1200/1260 aortic prostheses demonstrated, as would be expected, a higher peak systolic gradient with the smaller-sized prostheses; average peak systolic gradients ranged from 29 mmHg (calculated orifice area of 1.0 cm²) for size 21A valves to 13 mmHg (calculated valve area of 1.8 cm²) for the size

TABLE 7–1. *Specifications for Starr-Edwards Prostheses*

Size*	Annulus diameter (mm)	GOA† (cm²)
Model 1200		
16A (6A)	16	0.90
18A (7A)	18	1.19
Model 1260		
21A (8A)	21	1.41
23A (9A)	23	1.67
24A (10A)	24	1.79
26A (11A)	26	1.94
27A (12A)	27	2.16
29A (13A)	29	2.57
31A (14A)	31	2.89
Model 6120		
20M (00M)	20	1.27
22M (0M)	22	1.54
26M (1M)	26	2.14
28M (2M)	28	2.49
30M (3M)	30	2.86
32M (4M)	32	3.24
34M (5M)	34	3.66

*Old nomenclature in parentheses.

†Geometric orifice area, as reported by the manufacturer.

TABLE 7–2. *In Vitro Hydrodynamics of the Starr-Edwards Model 1260 Aortic Prosthesis*

Reference	Size	Mean transvalvular gradient (mmHg)	Simulated cardiac output (L/min)	Effective orifice area (cm²)	% backflow
18	21A	—	5.0	1.23	—
17	23A	11.2	4.9	—	3 (at 70 min⁻¹)
18	23A	—	5.0	1.46	—
19	24A	15.9	—	1.62	—
18	26A	—	5–7.2	1.86	—
19	27A	16.1	—	1.61	—
20	27A	—	4.0	—	7.4 (at 50–80 min⁻¹)

27A prostheses (16) (Table 7–3). More recently, Doppler echocardiography studies in patients with valves of various sizes showed an average peak systolic gradient of 29 mmHg; mild aortic regurgitation was seen in two of six patients studied (21).

Mitral Prosthesis

There is a direct relationship between mitral prosthetic size and hydrodynamic and hemodynamic performance. For the smaller-sized S-E mitral prostheses, for example, 26M, the mean diastolic gradient in vitro was 5.2 mmHg at a mean flow of 5 L/min, yielding an effective calculated orifice area of 1.43 cm²; the gradient increased to 16.5 mmHg at a mean flow of 9.0 L/min (22). For size 28M S-E prostheses, the mean diastolic gradient was 7.7 mmHg with a simulated cardiac output of 3.5 to 4.8 L/min (23). For a larger valve, for example, 30M, the gradient varied from 3.5 mmHg at a mean flow of 5.0 L/min to 11.3 mmHg at 9.0 L/min (22) (effective orifice area of 1.72 cm²) (Table 7–4).

In vivo hemodynamic studies have shown the mean diastolic gradient at rest for sizes 26M to 30M S-E mitral prostheses to be between 6 and 10 mmHg with an average effective orifice area of 1.4 to 2.39 cm² (16, 24–25) (Table 7–5). Glancy et al. noted that for the size 28M mitral prosthesis, the mean diastolic gradient was 6 mmHg at rest (effective orifice area of 2.39 cm²), which increased to 12.0 mmHg with exercise (effective orifice area of 2.15 cm²) (25). Similarly, for the larger sizes 30M and 32M valves, the mean initial gradient of 2.6 mmHg increased to 6.6 mmHg with exercise (25). Horskotte et al.

TABLE 7–3. *In Vivo Hemodynamics of the Starr-Edwards Model 1200 or 1260 Aortic Prosthesis*

Reference	Size	No. of patients	Peak pressure gradient (mmHg)	Effective orifice area (cm²)
At rest				
16	21A	5	29 (13–54)	1.0 (0.7–1.4)
16	23A	7	18 (1–32)	1.1 (0.8–1.5)
16	24A	7	13 (6–26)	1.3 (0.9–1.7)
16	26A	6	21 (16–26)	1.3 (1.1–1.5)
16	27A	1	13	1.8

TABLE 7-4. *In Vitro Hydrodynamics of the Starr-Edwards Model 6120 Mitral Prosthesis*

Reference	Size	Mean diastolic gradient (mmHg)	Mean flow (L/min)	Effective orifice area (cm²)
22	26M	5.2	5.0	1.43
22	26M	16.5	9.0	1.43
23	28M	7.7	3.5–4.8	—
22	30M	3.5	5.0	1.72
22	30M	11.3	9.0	1.72

reported the mean diastolic gradient for size 30M prostheses to be 6.3 mmHg at rest (effective orifice of 1.8 cm²), increasing to 11.9 mmHg (effective orifice area of 2.0 cm²) with exercise (26). For the largest valve evaluated, size 34M, the mean diastolic gradient was 5 mmHg with a calculated orifice area of 2.6 cm² (16). Late hemodynamic assessment showed a general reduction of mean pulmonary artery and left atrial pressure 1 year postoperatively in subjects who underwent mitral valve replacement (MVR) with a 30M mitral prosthesis; left atrial pressure, however, remained abnormally elevated (15 mmHg at rest, 26 mmHG with exercise) (26).

Clinical Performance with the Aortic Prosthesis

Survival

Hospital and late mortalities have not been linked directly to the particular prosthesis used, but are related to patient and disease-related factors and the era when the operation was performed. Therefore, mortalities per se cannot accurately reflect the advantages of

TABLE 7-5. *In Vivo Hemodynamics of the Starr-Edwards Model 6120 Mitral Prosthesis*

Reference	Size	No. of patients	Mean pressure gradient (mmHg)	Cardiac Index [L/(min · m²)]	Effective orifice area (cm²)
At rest					
16	26M	1	10	—	1.4
25	28M	9	6.0 (2–10)	2.6 (1.8–3.2)	2.39 (1.8–3.1)
16	28M	18	8 (4–13)	—	1.4 (0.8–1.8)
24	28M	17	7.5	—	—
16	30M	9	10 (3–15)	—	1.4 (0.8–2.7)
24	30M	18	7.6	—	—
26	30M	12	6.3	2.6	1.8
25	30 + 32M	12	2.6 (0–6)	2.72 (1.5–3.5)	—
16	32M	10	5 (3–9)	1.9 (1.2–2.7)	—
24	32M	2	5.5	—	—
16	34M	1	5	—	2.6
With exercise					
25	28M	9	12.0 (6–20)	3.59 (2.5–4.3)	2.15 (1.7–2.5)
26	30M	12	11.9	4.1	2.0
25	30 + 32M	12	6.6 (1–9)	3.82 (2.8–4.5)	—

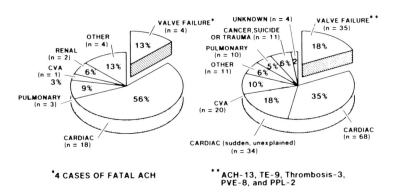

FIG. 7–4. Distribution of causes of hospital and late deaths after aortic valve replacement with the S-E model 1260 prosthesis in the Stanford experience. Valve failure was responsible for 13% of the early and 18% of the late deaths. CVA = cerebrovascular accident; ACH = anticoagulant-related hemorrhage; TE = thromboembolism; PVE = prosthetic valve endocarditis; PPL = periprosthetic leak. Reproduced with permission from Miller et al: Performance characteristics of the Starr-Edwards Model 1260 aortic valve prosthesis beyond ten years. J Thorac Cardiovasc Surg 1984;88:193–207.

one prosthesis over another; nevertheless, it is notable that one-eighth (4/32) of the hospital deaths in our series of patients undergoing aortic valve replacement (AVR) with S-E model 1260 prostheses at Stanford University were valve-related (27) (Fig. 7–4). The overall hospital mortality in this remote era (1968–1975) was 7%. Others have reported operative mortalities ranging from 6 to 14% (28–33) (Table 7–6). Wain et al. in London reported a higher hospital mortality (24.8%) in patients with relatively high preoperative risk factors (34).

Late survival and long-term morbidity, in addition to being strongly influenced by patient and disease-related risk factors, are also functions of the type of prosthesis used (35). The Stanford series included 449 patients who underwent AVR using the S-E model 1260 prosthesis; 417 were discharged from the hospital (27). The survival rates of those discharged were 72% ± 2% after 5 years and 52% ± 3% after 10 years (27), somewhat lower than that in other reports (28–34) (Table 7–6). Longer follow-up showed a survival rate of 41% after 14 years for patients discharged from the hospital (34). The hazard function for late death was highest during the first year and declined thereafter (27, 36). This characteristic nonconstant hazard over time makes reporting late deaths as a linearized rate somewhat misleading.

In the Stanford series, 18% of all late deaths after S-E AVR were related to valve failure (defined as any valve-related complication leading to reoperation or death) (see below); 18% were sudden deaths, 35% were cardiac-related deaths, and 10% were due to cerebrovascular accident (27) (Fig. 7–4). In a multivariate analysis studying risk factors affecting late survival in patients undergoing AVR with either a S-E or a Hancock porcine xenograft valve, we found that advanced NYHA functional class, the type of valve used (S-E > xenograft), aortic regurgitation (vs. stenosis), advanced age, diabetes, renal dysfunction, and atrial fibrillation portended decreased long-term life expectancy (35).

Table 7–6. *Clinical Results with the Starr-Edwards Model 1200 or 1260 Aortic Prosthesis*

Institution	Time of operation	Model	Hospital mortality	Late survival (discharged pts) (% at n years)		Mortality (% per pt-yr)
Stanford Univ. (27)	1968–75	1260	7.1	72	5	—
				52	10	
Univ. Oregon (31–33)	1965–79	1200/1260	12–14	84	3	—
				79–81	5	
				70	8	
				67	10–12	
(pre-1973)			14	81	5	3.6
				67	10	
(post-1973)				77	5	5.7
Mass. Gen. Hospital (29)	1973–77	1260	6	80	5	—
Mayo Clinic (28)	1963–72	—	6	—	—	—
		1200	—	80	5	
		1260	—	80	3	
Cardiothoracic Institute, London (34)	1964–80	—	24.8	—	—	
		1200/1260	—	41	14	
				52.8	10	
(1966–71)				68.9	5	—
(1975–80)				88.4	5	—
Royal Postgrad. Med. School, London (30)	1979–83	1260	—	89	5	4.26

Valve-related Morbidity with the Aortic Prosthesis

Valve Thrombosis

Because of its immediate life-threatening potential, valve thrombosis is a serious complication of valve replacement. Thrombus may occur without interfering with valve function, or—more importantly—may render the valve stenotic, incompetent, or both (14). Because the caged-ball valve has a high hydraulic safety margin (the area of the secondary orifice is equal to 120% of the primary orifice area), pannus and/or thrombus formation on the downstream side of the valve must encroach on a large portion of the secondary flow pathway before it becomes hemodynamically consequential (37). Since the buildup of pannus and clot is usually gradual in S-E valves, the resultant gradient across the prosthesis may develop slowly in some cases, thereby allowing early detection and reoperation (38).

The incidence of valve thrombosis in patients with S-E prostheses has been reported to be lower in recent years in both the mitral and aortic positions (39). The linearized rate of aortic valve thrombosis was 0.25% per patient year from 1965 to 1973 (27, 39), but no thrombosed valves were identified in the Oregon series between 1973 and 1984 (39, 40). This complication was associated with a high mortality; Metsdorff et al. reported one death in two patients with S-E aortic valve thrombosis (38), and there were no survivors in three cases in the Stanford series (27).

Thromboembolism

Another distinct disadvantage of any mechanical prosthesis is the tendency for clot formation on the thrombogenic surfaces with the potential for embolization. This risk of TE mandates indefinite anticoagulation therapy (warfarin sodium) despite its inherent

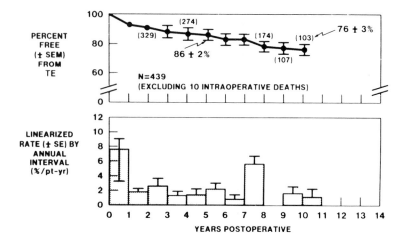

FIG. 7–5. Overall actuarial incidence of thromboembolism and instantaneous hazard of this complication by year after aortic valve replacement with the S-E model 1260 prosthesis in the Stanford experience. TE = thromboembolism; SEM = standard error of the mean; SE = standard error. Reproduced with permission from Miller et al: Performance characteristics of the Starr-Edwards model 1260 aortic valve prosthesis beyond ten years. J Thorac Cardiovasc Surg 1984;88:193–207.

complications. Even when strict anticoagulation is carried out, TE complications still unfortunately occur. In the Stanford experience, 14% ± 2% of patients after S-E AVR had sustained a TE event by 5 years, and 24% ± 3% by 10 years (linearized rate = 2.7% ± 0.3% per patient year) (27) (Fig. 7–5). As seen in Fig. 7–5, the risk was highest during the first year. Of these episodes, 94% were manifested by cerebral ischemia or infarction. Of the 72 patients with cerebral symptoms, 49% had only transient cerebral insults, 40% were left with a permanent neurologic deficit, and 11% died. Table 7–7 compares the incidence of morbid events from several institutions. The TE rates at these institutions were generally lower than that in the Stanford series, probably reflecting differences in definitions of complications, era of operation, and patient populations rather than true differences. In the Oregon series, the TE rate decreased after 1973 (39, 40), presumably the result of more intense and better control of anticoagulation, although this has been questioned by others (41); certainly, changes in patient characteristics over time may have been responsible. It is important to note, moreover, that once a TE event has occurred, these patients remain at much higher risk for subsequent TE events—approximately 7.7 to 8.4% per patient year (40).

In a multivariate analysis of all valve patients in our experience, the risk of TE was significantly increased if the patient had received a S-E prosthesis rather than a porcine xenograft, was older, and had had a prior TE or previous cardiac operation (35). Interestingly, neither atrial fibrillation nor endocarditis were identified as independent incremental risk factors for TE (35).

Anticoagulant-related Hemorrhage

After AVR with the S-E model 1260 valve, anticoagulant-related hemorrhage (ACH) of sufficient severity to warrant hospitalization, transfusion, or nontrivial outpatient care occurred in 18% ± 2% of the Stanford patients after 5 years and 26% ± 3% after 10

TABLE 7-7. Valve-related Morbidity with the Starr-Edwards Models 1200 or 1260 Aortic Prosthesis

Institution	TE*			ACH*			PVE*			Reoperation			Valve failure			Composite morbidity and mortality		
	% free	at n yrs	% per pt-yr	% free	at n yrs	% per pt-yr	% free	at n yrs	% per pt-yr	% free	at n yrs	% per pt-yr	% free	at n yrs	% per pt-yr	% free	at n yrs	% per pt-yr
Stanford Univ. (27)	86	5	2.7	82	5	3.1	95	5	0.9	95	5	1.1	87	5	2.2	66	5	6.0
	76	10	—	74	10	1.6	92	10	—	90	10	—	82	10	—	51	10	—
Univ. of Oregon (31–33, 39, 40, 54)	78–87	5	3.8–5.0	—	—	—	95	5	—	99	5	—	95	5	—	—	—	—
	71–77	10–12	—							92	11	—	94	7	—			
	66	15	—										88	10	—			
													82	15	—			
(pre-1973)	77–78	5	4.6–5.0	—	—	1.4				—	—	1.0	—	—	1.5			
	67	10	—															
(post-1973)	87–90	5	1.8–3.4	—	—	3.0				—	—	0.6	—	—	1.1			
Mass. Gen. Hospital (29)	90	5	—	88	5	—	94	5	—				95†	5	—			
Mayo (28, 41)	80	5	—															
	70	10	—															
(Model 1260)	>95	3	—															
(Model 1200)	80	5	—															
Cardiothoracic Inst., London (34)	75.8	13–14	—				85.5	13–14	—	63.1	13–14	—						
1966–71	92.9	5	—															
1975–80	84.6	5	—															
Royal Postgraduate, London (30)	93	5	3.13	—	—	0.85	—	—	1.14	—	—	3.69				84	5	6.25‡

*TE = thromboembolism; ACH = anticoagulant-related hemorrhage; PVE = prosthetic valve endocarditis.

†Valve failure includes infective endocarditis resulting in death or prosthetic replacement, or dysfunction of prosthesis resulting in regurgitation or stenosis with prosthetic replacement or death.

‡Total valve-related morbidity including TE, ACH, PVE hemolysis, paraprosthetic regurgitation, and mechanical failure.

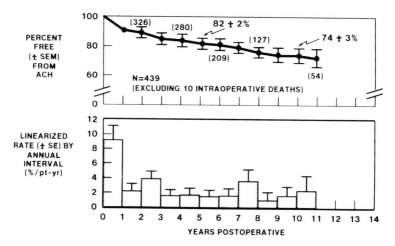

FIG. 7–6. Actuarial estimate of the occurrence of anticoagulant-related hemorrhage and the instantaneous hazard of this complication by year after aortic valve replacement with the S-E model 1260 prosthesis in the Stanford series. ACH = anticoagulant-related hemorrhage. SEM = standard error of the mean. Reproduced with permission from Miller et al: Performance characteristics of the Starr-Edwards model 1260 aortic valve prosthesis beyond ten years. J Thorac Cardiovasc Surg 1984;88:193–207.

years (the overall linearized rate was 3.1% ± 0.3% per patient year) (27) (Fig. 7–6). Similar to TE complications, the hazard of ACH was higher during the first year of operation. ACH rates from different centers are listed in Table 7–7. The higher incidence of ACH in the Oregon series (31) after 1973 appeared to parallel the decrease in TE rate, thereby probably conferring no net benefit to the patient. In our series, 89 patients out of 449 developed one or more ACH complications (27). Four of seven patients (57%) who developed ACH during the early postoperative period died of this complication, and 16% (13/82) of the late ACH complications were fatal; therefore, the overall ACH mortality was 19%. In actuarial terms, 94% ± 2% of patients were free of fatal ACH after 10 years (27). Factors found to correlate with increased risk of ACH in all Stanford AVR patients were S-E prosthesis (versus xenograft), increasing severity of congestive heart failure (NYHA class), gender (females > males), and advanced age (35). Interestingly, the likelihood of ACH was not higher for patients with hepatic dysfunction, renal insufficiency, or endocarditis (35).

Prosthetic Valve Endocarditis

Prosthetic valve endocarditis (PVE) following implantation of the S-E models 1200/1260 aortic prostheses occurred at a constant linearized rate of 0.9% ± 0.2% to 1.14% per patient year (27, 30) (Table 7–7). Actuarially, in the Stanford experience, 95% ± 1% of patients were free of PVE after 5 years and 92% ± 2% after 10 years (27); other investigators have reported similar results (29, 34) (Table 7–7). The risk continues into the second decade after valve replacement, as 86% of patients were estimated to be free of PVE after 13 to 14 years (34). The linearized rate of fatal PVE was 0.3% ± 0.1% per patient year (98% ± 1% were free of fatal PVE after 7 years) (27). With regard to treatment of PVE, 9 of 25 patients in our institution were treated medically with a 33% mortality; similarly, there were five deaths among the 16 patients (31%) who underwent surgical reintervention (27).

Hemolysis

Red blood cell survival is decreased in patients with native aortic valve disease and after prosthetic valve replacement (42). Mechanical ball valves may be associated with slightly more hemolysis than tilting disk and bioprosthetic valves (43). Additionally, in patients with malfunctioning mechanical valves, hemolysis is increased because of greater red cell trauma (14). A low haptoglobin and a high serum lactate dehydrogenase (LDH) level indicate ongoing hemolysis; the degree of elevation of LDH correlates inversely with ^{51}Cr-tagged red cell survival time (44). Isoenzymes of LDH may assist in differentiating between hemolysis and liver disease, and the presence of methemalbumin in the serum indicates more severe hemolysis (44).

The silastic ball non-cloth-covered S-E valves (models 1200/1260 and 6120), as opposed to the cloth-covered S-E prostheses, are rarely associated with clinically important hemolytic anemia in the absence of perivalvular leaks, infective endocarditis, or ball variance (all of which are associated with increased blood turbulence) (3, 30, 33, 40, 42). The majority of patients with S-E aortic prostheses have mildly elevated serum LDH levels, slightly shortened red cell survival, and a reticulocyte count of less than 5%, but are not clinically anemic (3). An unusual complication of chronic hemolysis following valve replacement is the appearance of biliary cholelithiasis, in particular pigment gallstones (45). The probability of freedom from clinically important hemolysis after AVR was 92% at 13 to 14 years (34).

Reoperation

Valve rereplacement in patients after AVR with the S-E model 1260 valve occurred at a constant linearized rate of $1.1 \pm 0.2\%$ per patient year in the Stanford series (27). After 5 years, $5\% \pm 1\%$ of patients had required reoperation, and after 10 years, $10\% \pm 2\%$. Indications for reoperation were TE (7 cases, no deaths), endocarditis (16 cases, 31% mortality), periprosthetic leak (PPL) (3 cases, no deaths), and miscellaneous (4 cases, 1 death), yielding an overall reoperative mortality of 19% (6/31) (27). A similar incidence of reoperation has been reported from the Oregon group; the incidence of reoperation was 1.0% per patient year before 1973 and 0.6% per patient year after 1973 (31–32) (Table 7–7). With longer follow-up, fully 37% of patients required reoperation after 13 to 14 years in a series from London (34). Independent predictors of reoperation among all valve patients in a multivariate study at Stanford included young age (particularly for patients with a bioprosthesis) and preoperative endocarditis. Neither valve type (S-E vs. xenograft) nor functional NYHA class were significant predictors of an increased risk of reoperation (35).

Valve Failure

As defined in our previous investigations of S-E prostheses, valve failure has been considered to be present if any of the following events require reoperation and/or cause death: (1) ACH, (2) prosthetic valve occlusion (thrombosis or tissue ingrowth), (3) TE, (4) PVE, (5) hemodynamic prosthetic dysfunction, including structural failure of prosthetic components (strut fracture, poppet escape, ball variance), (6) Reoperation for any other reason (e.g., hemolysis, noise, incidental), and (7) bland (PPL) (27, 46). This comprehensive definition serves a meaningful purpose in the choice of a particular type of valve for a specific individual and facilitates comparative analysis (46). For example, it is known that tissue valves have a higher incidence of structural valve failure while mechanical valves have a higher incidence of TE and ACH complications over the long term (>8–10 years). In order to compare adequately the overall performance of these two types of prostheses, a sensitive, precise, and standardized denominator, such as valve failure, should be employed.

In the Stanford series, 57% of valve failures in patients with S-E model 1260 aortic prostheses were due to TE, ACH, or valve thrombosis; 29% were caused by PVE (27). Almost half (31/65) of the patients who developed valve failure required reoperation (see above). The risk of valve failure was significantly higher during the first postoperative year (4.3% ± 1% per patient year vs. 1.9% ± 0.3% per patient year for years 2–14) (Fig. 7–7). The overall linearized rate of S-E aortic valve failure was 2.2% ± 0.3% per patient year (albeit of limited usefulness due to the changing hazard). In actuarial terms, 87% ± 2% of patients were free of valve failure after 5 years, and 82% ± 2% after 10 years (Fig. 7–7). For patients who developed valve failure, 62% (40/65) of cases were fatal ("valve-related death"). After 10 years, 88% of patients were free of fatal valve failure; the overall linearized rate was 1.3% ± 0.2% per patient year, but the hazard was nonconstant, being significantly higher during the first postoperative year (3.6% ± 1% per patient year) (27).

Using the Stanford definition of valve failure (except for the *exclusion* of deaths linked to preoperative endocarditis), Starr and colleagues noted valve failure rates of 1.5% per patient year and 1.2% per patient year before and after 1973, respectively (39).

Two other long-term reports focused on S-E aortic valve failure using similar definitions. Wain et al. diagnosed valve malfunction if mechanical failure, infection, TE, or

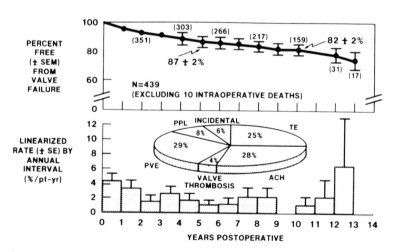

FIG. 7–7. Actuarial and annualized rates of valve failure after aortic valve replacement (S-E model 1260) using the Stanford definition (see text). TE = thromboembolism; ACH = anticoagulant-related hemorrhage; PVE = prosthetic valve endocarditis, PPL = periprosthetic leak; SEM = standard error of the mean. Reproduced with permission from Miller et al: Performance characteristics of the Starr-Edwards model 1260 aortic valve prosthesis beyond ten years. J Thorac Cardiovasc Surg 1984;88:193–207.

TABLE 7–8. *Clinical Results of Starr-Edwards Model 6120 Mitral Prosthesis*

Institution	Time of operation	Hospital mortality (%)	Late survival (discharged pts) (% at *n* years)		Mortality (% per pt-yr)
Stanford Univ. (46)	1965–76	10.6	90	1	7.3
			71	5	
			47	10	
Univ. Oregon (31–33, 49, 53)	1965–84	10–12	73–83	5	—
			54–61	10	
			50	12	
			36	15	
(pre-1973) (RR)		11	82	5	4.7
			62	10	
(post-1973)		13	77	5	6.3
			73	10	
Univ. Louvain, Brussels (24, 51–52)	1965–85	6.2–6.5	77–80	5	3.9
			61–72	10	
			70–73	12–13	
			48	19	
Mass. Gen. Hospital (29)	1973–77	10	77	5	—
Mayo Clinic (28)	1966–72	9	80	5	—

hemolysis/hemolytic anemia occurred (ACH was excluded in this definition); they reported the actuarial rate of freedom from valve-related death to be 74% after 13 to 15 years in patients with S-E model 1200/1260 valves (34). Using a definition of valve failure that included infective endocarditis resulting in death or prosthetic replacement, multiple TE events requiring prosthetic replacement, or dysfunction of the prosthesis resulting in regurgitation or stenosis with prosthetic replacement or death, Murphy et al. from the Massachusetts General Hospital reported that 95% of patients were free from valve failure after 5 years (29) (Table 7–8).

In our overall (S-E and bioprosthetic) multivariate study of risk factors following valve replacement, independent predictors of valve failure after AVR were younger age at operation, advanced degree of functional disability, and earlier operative year (35). Valve type (S-E vs. xenograft), however, was not a predictor of valve failure. The risk of fatal valve failure, on the other hand, was significantly influenced by valve type (S-E > xenograft), in addition to advanced NYHA functional class, hepatic dysfunction, and preoperative endocarditis (35).

Composite Valve-related Morbidity and Mortality

Combining the patients with TE, ACH, bland PPL, and PVE that did not result in reoperation or death with those who sustained valve failure generates a composite function or index that describes the incidence of all valve-related morbidity and mortality (46). This composite valve-related morbidity and mortality is the clinical "bottom line" of valve performance, since it goes beyond the question of simple prosthetic durability and considers the fact that some valve-related complications may simply offset each other (e.g., a lower incidence of TE at the expense of a higher rate of ACH) (27). This function, however, actually underestimates the true incidence of valve-related complications since an individual patient is entered into the actuarial analysis only once (even if more than one complication occurred in a single patient), and autopsies are not performed in all patients who die after operation.

In the Stanford series, a total of 174 out of 449 patients after AVR with the S-E model 1260 valve sustained one or more valve-related complications (27). These first events were ACH in 82 patients, TE in 63 patients, PVE in 22 patients, and miscellaneous complications in 7 patients. Actuarial analysis revealed that 66% ± 2% of patients were estimated to be free of a major valve-related complication after 5 years, and 51% ± 3% after 10 years (27). The overall linearized rate was 6.0% ± 0.5% per patient year, but these complications and/or deaths occurred at a nonconstant rate [the hazard being much higher during the first postoperative year (18.2% ± 2.2% per patient year) than thereafter (4.2% ± 0.4% per patient year)] (27) (Fig. 7–8). After the first year, there was no statistically significant change in the hazard function during the 2- to 5-year period compared with the 6- to ll-year interval (4.7% ± 0.6% per patient year versus 3.7% ± 0.6% per patient year), demonstrating no evidence that this overall risk declines even after many years have elapsed (Fig. 7–8). Hackett et al. from London recently documented that the valve-related morbidity rate (including TE, ACH, PVE, hemolysis, PPL, and mechanical failure) was equally high (6.25% per patient year) in patients with a S-E model 1260 prosthesis (30).

Using the concept of a composite valve-related morbidity and mortality function as an index with which to study newer mechanical and biological prostheses will permit assessment of whether or not these valves are truly superior in terms of overall clinical performance. At similar time intervals, lower complication rates must be demonstrated based on this criterion; furthermore, and perhaps most importantly, the long-term (10–20 years) function of the prosthesis must be equal or superior to these benchmark standards. Of course, it is implicitly understood that even this global reflection of clinical valve performance is likely to be related to factors other than the prosthesis per se, such that only multivariate analysis of retrospective results (which adjusts, in part, for differences in patient and disease-related factors) or—preferably—prospective, randomized clinical trials will actually be able to indicate if any particular valve substitute is substantially better or worse than another.

Structural and Mechanical Failure

Ball variance as seen with the original S-E prostheses has rarely been encountered with the S-E model 1200 aortic valves implanted after 1966 and model 1260 valves placed after 1968, both of which adopted a streamlined housing to reduce turbulence and a modified curing process of the silastic poppet (3, 36). In the Stanford series, no cases of ball variance, strut fracture, poppet escape, or any other structural fault was documented at autopsy or reoperation (27).

For the S-E model 1000 aortic valve, almost all cases of ball variance were discovered before 8 years; however, clinically occult ball variance can occur in patients with the model 1000 valves up to 20 years after implantation (47). There was a relationship between the year of valve implantation and the time (and severity) of ball variance in the past, but for the subgroup of patients currently alive and at risk, the sample sizes are too small to detect any difference if one still exists (47). Starr and his colleagues noted severe ball variance in only 3 of 12 patients in a subset of patients who received the model 1000 valve; at reoperation, simply changing the poppet was the procedure of choice.

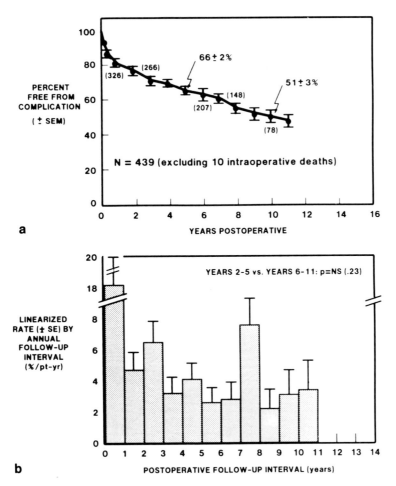

FIG. 7–8. (a) Actuarial curve illustrating the occurrence of all valve-related morbidity and mortality after aortic valve replacement with the S-E model 1260 prosthesis in the Stanford experience. Only 51% ± 3% of patients were free of a major valve-related complication at 10 years. SEM = standard error of the mean. (b) Instantaneous hazard by annual follow-up interval for all valve-related morbidity and mortality. This analysis takes into account only the first complications that occurred. Although the risk of a valve-related complication was highest for the first postoperative year, thereafter there was no statistically significant acceleration or decline in this risk. SE = standard error. Reproduced with permission from Miller et al: Performance characteristics of the Starr-Edwards model 1260 aortic valve prosthesis beyond ten years. J Thorac Cardiovasc Surg 1984;88:193–207.

Prophylactic reoperation is not indicated for patients with S-E model 1000 valves, but careful follow-up is recommended, and reoperation must be considered should symptoms develop (47). Clinical manifestations of ball variance are nonspecific and may include fatigue, dyspnea on exertion, palpitations, dizzy spells, angina, and syncopal episodes (48). The diagnosis is based on absence of the opening click, an abnormal phonocardiogram, recurrent embolic episodes, new onset of aortic regurgitation, and radiographic evidence of an abnormal appearance of the barium-impregnated poppet (48).

Clinical Performance with the Mitral Prosthesis

Survival

Although the hospital mortality was as high as 20% in the earliest years for patients receiving the S-E model 6000 mitral valve (49, 50), it has been reported to be between 6 and 13% with the present mitral prosthesis (model 6120), (24, 28, 29, 31–33, 46, 49, 51–52) (Table 7–8). This decrease in mortality is obviously secondary to generalized advances in cardiac surgery and postoperative care, rather than changes in the valve design per se (28, 53); it is also probably the result of changes in patient selection and timing of surgery. Valve design, nonetheless, might possibly be of some consequence, since 5.9 to 25% of hospital deaths have been due to valve failure (either valvular occlusion or TE) (24, 46, 53) (Fig. 7–9a).

The Stanford study of the S-E model 6120 valve included 509 patients undergoing MVR, 455 of whom were discharged from the hospital (46). The actuarial late survival rates of discharged patients were 71% ± 2% after 5 years, 47% ± 3% after 10 years, and 37% ± 3% after 14 years (Fig. 7–10). Similar survival rates have been reported from other institutions (Table 7–8). Linearized statistics show an overall attrition rate of 7.3% ± 0.5% per patient year for all late deaths, with 2.0% ± 0.3% per patient year for death due to valve failure (46). Causes of late death in this series included 27% related to valve

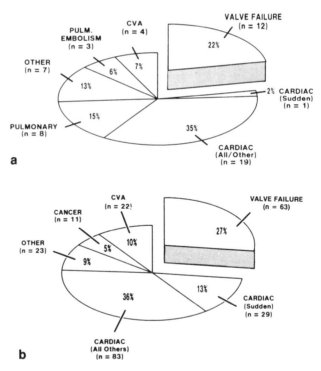

Fɪɢ. 7–9. (a) Causes of hospital deaths after mitral valve replacement with the S-E model 6120 prosthesis in the Stanford experience. Valve failure was responsible for 22% of these deaths. (b) Causes of late deaths. Note that 27% of these deaths were due to valve failure. CVA = cerebrovascular accident; Pulm = pulmonary. Reproduced with permission from Miller et al: Ten to fifteen year reassessment of the performance characteristics of the Starr-Edwards model 6120 mitral valve prosthesis. J Thorac Cardiovasc Surg 1983;85:1–20.

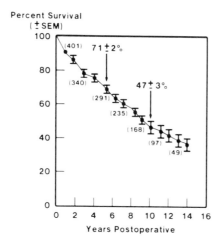

FIG. 7–10. Actuarial survival curve for 445 operative survivors after mitral valve replacement with the S-E model 6120 prosthesis in the Stanford experience. SEM = standard error of the mean. Reproduced with permission from Miller et al: Ten to fifteen year reassessment of the performance characteristics of the Starr-Edwards model 6120 mitral valve prosthesis. J Thorac Cardiovasc Surg 1983;85:1–20.

failure, 13% due to sudden cardiac events, and 36% associated with other cardiac causes (Fig. 7–9b).

Independent, statistically significant predictors of late death among patients receiving either S-E model 6120 or porcine xenograft valves at Stanford were older age, physiology (mitral regurgitation > stenosis), and valve type (S-E > xenograft) (35). Weaker associations included concomitant coronary artery bypass grafting, congestive heart failure, hypertension, and renal dysfunction. The presence of atrial fibrillation, diabetes mellitus, and ischemic origin of mitral valve disease were not significantly linked with a higher likelihood of late death (35).

Historically speaking, for MVR patients with a S-E model 6000 prosthesis, approximately 80% have died within 21 years of operation; the actuarial survival rates were 76, 58, and 22% after 5, 10, and 20 years, respectively (49, 50).

Valve-related Morbidity with the Mitral Prosthesis

Valve Thrombosis

Review of most investigations indicates that for any particular valve type, valve thrombosis is more common after MVR compared with AVR (27, 38–40, 46). In a report from the University of Oregon, the overall linearized rate of valve thrombosis in patients with the S-E model 6120 mitral valve was 0.4% per patient year (40); however, it was higher before 1973 (0.6% per patient year) than after (no reported episodes of thrombosis from 1973 to 1984) (39). Metsdorff et al. reported five patients with mitral valve thrombosis, all but one of whom were successfully managed by urgent or emergent valve rereplacement (20% reoperative mortality) (38). Miller et al. reported a total of 19 patients with mitral valve occlusion (thrombosis or tissue ingrowth) in the early and late postoperative periods associated with an overall mortality of 79%; reoperation for valve thrombosis per se carried a mortality risk of 43% (46).

Thromboembolism

The occurrence of TE complications is also more frequent after MVR than after AVR. In the Stanford series of MVR patients with the S-E model 6120 prosthesis, 35% ± 2% of patients had suffered a first TE event by 5 years, 45% ± 3% by 10 years, and 51% ± 3% by 14 years (46) (Fig. 7-11). The overall linearized rate for the first event was 5.7% ± 0.4% per patient year, but TE events occurred with a nonconstant hazard (higher incidence during the first postoperative year). If all TE events were taken into account (301 TE events in 179 patients), the overall linearized rate was 9.5% ± 0.5% per patient year (46). TE complications were manifested in the central nervous system (CNS) in 89% (160/179) of patients; this subgroup had a mortality of 16% (25/160), with 34% sustaining a permanent neurologic deficit and 50% having only transient symptoms. Figure 7-11 shows the actuarial rates of fatal TE; after 10 years, 92% ± 2% of patients were free from a fatal TE (46). Table 7-9 compares the rates of all morbid events after MVR with a S-E model 6120 valve from different institutions. Although the results were generally comparable to our results, some reports did show a lower incidence of TE complications (probably due to differences in definitions, year of operation, management of anticoagulation, and patient populations). Like the AVR data, the data from the Oregon group indicated a decreased incidence of TE after 1973 (from 6.6% per patient year to 0.8% per patient year) (31); the overall linearized rate was 1.4% per patient year after the first postoperative year (40). Those patients who suffered a TE complication, however, were at a much higher risk of a subsequent TE event (as high as 8.8% per patient year) (32, 40).

In a study assessing TE risk factors after MVR with various valve types, we found that the rate of this complication was significantly higher if a S-E valve (vs. xenograft) had been used and if preoperative endocarditis was present (35). Other significant, indepen-

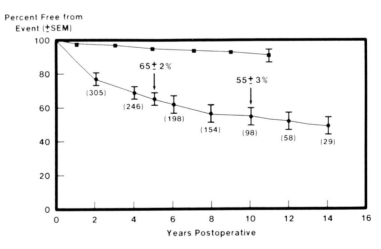

FIG. 7-11. Actuarial depiction of the incidence of thromboembolism and fatal thromboembolism after mitral valve replacement with the S-E model 6120 prosthesis in the Stanford experience. The instantaneous hazard of thromboembolism was high (17% ± 2% per patient year) for the first postoperative year but significantly lower (3.9% ± 0.4% per patient year) and constant thereafter. SEM = standard error of the mean. Reproduced with permission from Miller et al: Ten to fifteen year reassessment of the performance characteristics of the Starr-Edwards model 6120 mitral valve prosthesis. J Thorac Cardiovasc Surg 1983;85:1-20.

TABLE 7-9. Valve-related Morbidity with the Starr-Edwards Model 6120 Mitral Prosthesis

Institution	TE*			ACH*			PVE*			Reoperation			Valve failure			Composite morbidity and mortality		
	% free	at n yrs	% per pt-yr	% free	at n yrs	% per pt-yr	% free	at n yrs	% per pt-yr	% free	at n yrs	% per pt-yr	% free	at n yrs	% per pt-yr	% free	at n yrs	% per pt-yr
Stanford Univ. (46)	65	5	5.7	82	5	3.7	95	10	0.5	93	5	1.7	78	5	3.8	54	5	8.5
	55	10	—	67	10	—	—	—	—	84	10		71	10		38	10	
	49	14		52	14					80	14		62	14		25	14	
Univ. Oregon (31-33, 39-40, 49, 53-54)	72-83	5	5.1-6.1	94	6	1	94	6		88	10-12	0.6	91-92	5		—	—	—
	51-64	10		83	10		91	10	0.6				83	10		—	—	—
	56	15											76	15		—	—	—
(pre-1973)	68-70	5	6.0-6.6	—	—	1.4						0.9	—	—	1.9	—	—	—
	47-53	10																
(post-1973)	92-96	5	0.8-2.9	—	—	3.0						1.5	—	—	1.2	—	—	—
	84	9																
Univ. Louvain (24, 51-52)	80-81	5	3.1-4.7	95	5	1.08	97	5	0.26	—	—	—	92	5	1.4	70	5	4.9
Mass. Gen. Hospital (29)	77	10		90	10		95	10					85	10		59	10	
	67-74	13-15														55	13	
	83	5		93	5		95	5				0	95†	5				
Mayo (28)	75	5		—	—	—	—	—	—	—	—	—	—	—	—	—	—	—

*TE = thromboembolism; ACH = anticoagulant-related hemorrhage; PVE = prosthetic valve endocarditis.

†Valve failure as defined excludes ACH and incidental replacement.

dent predictors of TE complications were congestive heart failure, previous cardiac operation, and prior (preoperative) TE (35). Interestingly, atrial fibrillation was not linked
significantly to an increased risk of TE. In a study from the Mayo Clinic, variables predicting TE were the adequacy of anticoagulation, the presence of left atrial thrombus (at
the time of operation), and left atrial size (28). On the other hand, in our experience
(dichotomizing the patient population based on the presence or absence of left atrial
thrombus), the estimated proportions of patients free of TE after 10 years were similar
(55 vs. 56%) (46). This observation was confirmed in another study from Stanford using
multivariate analysis—left atrial thrombus was not predictive of TE complications (35).

With the older S-E model 6000 mitral prosthesis, only 31 and 21% of patients were
free of TE after 5 and 15 years, respectively (49).

Anticoagulant-related Hemorrhage

The risk of major hemorrhage after MVR with the S-E model 6120 valve was 3.7% ±
0.3% per patient year (constant hazard) in the Stanford series (46). In actuarial terms,
8% ± 2% of our patients had sustained a major ACH by 5 years, 33% ± 3% by 10 years,
and 48% ± 5% by 14 years (46) (Fig. 7–12). Central nervous system hemorrhage constituted 19% (22/116) of the ACH complications, 86% (19/22) of which were fatal; the
three surviving patients were left with a permanent neurologic deficit. The gastrointestinal tract was the most frequent site of ACH (31%), but only 4 of 36 cases (11%) were
fatal. Actuarial estimates of freedom from fatal ACH (Fig. 7–12) were 95% ± 1%, 94%
± 1%, and 92% ± 2% after 5, 10, and 14 years, respectively (46). Table 7–9 illustrates
the various ACH rates after MVR from a number of different institutions. Importantly,
the higher incidence of ACH complications after 1973 in the Oregon series (with a concomitant decrease in TE rates) probably reflects changing practices in anticoagulation
management.

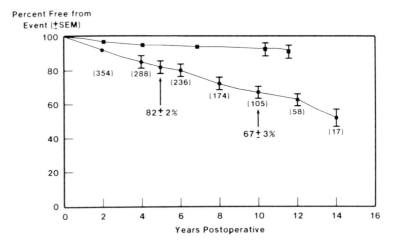

FIG. 7–12. Actuarial probability of anticoagulant-related hemorrhage and fatal bleeding complications after mitral valve replacement with the S-E model 6120 prosthesis in the Stanford experience. The risk was constant (3.7% ± 0.3% per patient year) throughout the postoperative follow-up period. SEM = standard error of the mean. Reproduced with permission from Miller et
al: Ten to fifteen year reassessment of the performance characteristics of the Starr-Edwards
model 6120 mitral valve prosthesis. J Thorac Cardiovasc Surg 1983;85:1–20.

Three variables were significant, independent predictors of ACH after MVR in our multivariate analysis: valve type (S-E > xenograft), advanced functional class, and (earlier) operative year (35).

Prosthetic Valve Endocarditis

In the Stanford series, endocarditis following MVR with the S-E model 6120 valve occurred at a constant rate of 0.5% ± 0.1% per patient year (46). After 5 years, 97% ± 1% were free of PVE, as were 95% ± 1% after 10 years. Unfortunately, the overall mortality of patients who developed PVE was high [53% (9/17)]; the linearized rate of fatal PVE was 0.3% ± 0.1% per patient year (46). Reoperation for PVE was carried out in 35% (6/17) of patients with a 33% mortality (see below). Other groups have reported similar results for PVE in patients with a S-E model 6120 mitral prosthesis (Table 7–9).

Hemolysis

The silastic ball non-cloth-covered mitral prosthesis, that is, S-E model 6120, is rarely associated with hemolytic anemia in the absence of PPL or infective endocarditis (3, 33, 49, 51). As noted with the S-E aortic valves, a significant fraction of patients have mildly elevated levels of LDH, slightly shortened red cell survival, and a reticulocyte count less than 5% (3), but clinically significant hemolytic anemia in the absence of PPL and PVE is not a problem with the present S-E model 6120 mitral prosthesis (49).

Reoperation

Valve reoperation after MVR with S-E model 6120 prosthesis was required by 7% ± 1% of patients after 5 years, 16% ± 2% after 10 years, and 20% ± 3% after 14 years in the Stanford experience, yielding a constant, linearized rate of 1.7% ± 0.2% per patient year (46). The indications for reoperation (and associated reoperative mortalities) are summarized in Table 7–10. The majority of reoperations were necessary for recurrent TE complications (64%) and were associated with a low mortality (5.9%). An inordinately high mortality, on the other hand, followed reoperation for valve thrombosis (43%) and endocarditis (33%) (46). At the University of Oregon, reoperation after MVR

TABLE 7–10. *Reoperative Mortalities According to the Reason for Valve Replacement*

	No.	%	Reoperative mortality
Multiple thromboemboli	34	64	2/34 = 5.9%
Valve thrombosis	7	13	3/7 = 43%
Prosthetic endocarditis	6	11	2/6 = 33%
Bland periprosthetic leak	2	4	0/2 = 0%
Anticoagulant-related hemorrhage	1	2	0/1 = 0%
Other*	3	6	0/3 = 0%
Totals	53	100	7/53 = 13%

*One case of possible ball variance in conjunction with partial valve thrombosis and two cases of incidental prosthesis replacement (due to thrombus on the cage and poppet at the time of subsequent aortic valve replacement). Reproduced with permission from Miller et al: Ten to fifteen year reassessment of the performance characteristics of the Starr-Edwards model 6120 mitral valve prosthesis. J Thorac Cardiovasc Surg 1983;85:1–20.

with a S-E mitral prosthesis was required by 12% of patients by 10 to 12 years (53) (Table 7–9).

In the multivariate analysis of risk factors portending morbid complications and late death following MVR at Stanford, only age at operation was found to be an independent determinant (increased risk in younger patients) of reoperation (35). Valve type (S-E vs. xenograft), endocarditis, and functional class had no significant influence on the likelihood of reoperation.

Valve Failure

Utilizing the previous definition of valve failure (see above), the following results were obtained in our study of the S-E model 6120 mitral prosthesis (46). The global linearized rate was 3.8% ± 0.3% per patient year, but the hazard function was nonconstant (higher during the first year). At 5, 10, and 14 years after the operation, 78% ± 2%, 71% ± 2%, and 65% ± 3% of patients were free of valve failure, respectively (Fig. 7–13); 62% of the patients who sustained valve failure died (46). The most lethal modes of valve failure at Stanford were ACH, valvular occlusion, and PVE (with associated mortalities of 96%, 79%, and 69%, respectively). The most frequent mode of valve failure was multiple TE events (48% of all cases); this was associated with a 45% mortality. Valve occlusion (associated with a fatality rate of 79%) comprised 16% of valve failures. The rate of fatal valve failure (valve-related deaths) occurred at a linearized rate of 2.4% ± 0.3% per patient year (46). Actuarial freedom from valve-related death was 87% ± 2% after 5 years, 80% ± 2% after 10 years, and 77% ± 3% after 14 years (46) (Fig. 7–13). Fully 22% of hospital deaths and 27% of late deaths were due to valve failure. These morbid and fatal events represent the overall biologic behavior (or "natural history") of a particular mechanical prosthetic valve (46).

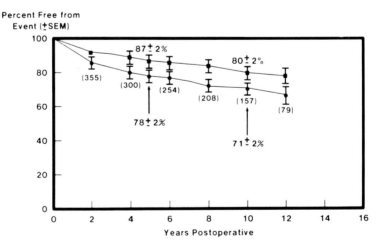

Fig. 7–13. Actuarial estimates of valve failure, using the Stanford definition, and fatal valve failure after mitral valve replacement with the S-E model 6120 prosthesis. Valve failure occurred at an overall linearized rate of 3.8% ± 0.3% per patient year, but the rate was nonconstant. The risk of valve failure was high (10% ± 1.5% per patient year) for the first postoperative year but was lower and constant between year 2 and year 13 (2.9% ± 3% per patient year). SEM = standard error of the mean. Reproduced with permission from Miller et al: Ten to fifteen year reassessment of the performance characteristics of the Starr-Edwards model 6120 mitral valve prosthesis. J Thorac Cardiovasc Surg 1983;85:1–20.

Using the Stanford definitions (excluding operative death from preexisting bacterial endocarditis), Starr and colleagues reported a valve failure rate after MVR with the S-E model 6120 prosthesis of 1.9% per patient year from 1965 to 1973 and 1.2% per patient year from 1973 to 1984 (39, 49, 54). Murphy et al. from the Massachusetts General Hospital noted that 95% of patients were free of valve failure 5 years after MVR with the model 6120 valve; however, ACH and incidental valve rereplacement were not included (29). Although limited by differences in patient populations, the rates of valve failure from various institutions are compared in Table 7–9. This scenario underscores the need for universal acceptance of standardized definitions of valve-related complications when reporting the performance of cardiac valve prostheses (55). A more recent study from the University of Louvain (using our definitions of valve failure) reported better results at 5 and 10 years of follow-up (24) (Table 7–9).

In a larger study from Stanford examining patients with all types of valves, earlier operative year, hypertension, and younger age were identified as being independent risk factors for valve failure after MVR (35). Neither valve type (S-E vs. xenograft) nor advanced disability (NYHA class) were significant predictors. For fatal valve failure, however, valve type was the single most important predictor (S-E > bioprosthesis), followed by older age (35).

Composite Valve-related Morbidity and Mortality

Analysis focused on all morbidity and mortality revealed that only 54% ± 2% of patients after MVR with S-E model 6120 prosthesis at Stanford University were free of all valve-related morbidity and mortality after 5 years, 38% ± 3% after 10 years, and 25% ± 4% after 14 years (46) (Fig. 7–14). In linearized terms, this rate was 8.5% ± 0.5% per patient year (considering each patient at risk for only one event), but this function

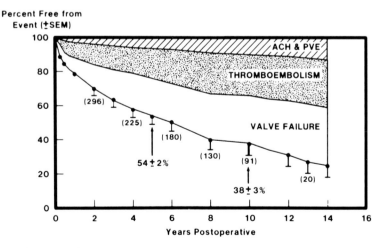

Fig. 7–14. Composite function incorporating all valve-related morbidity and mortality after mitral valve replacement with the S-E model 6120 prosthesis in the Stanford experience. The instantaneous hazard was nonconstant (23% ± 2% per patient year for the first postoperative year versus 6.2% ± 0.5% per patient year thereafter). ACH = anticoagulant-related hemorrhage; PVE = prosthetic valve endocarditis. SEM = standard error of the mean. Reproduced with permission from Miller et al: Ten to fifteen year reassessment of the performance characteristics of the Starr-Edwards model 6120 mitral valve prosthesis. J Thorac Cardiovasc Surg 1983;85:1–20.

occurred at a nonconstant hazard. Moreover, the linearized incidence of all morbid events (accounting for more than one event in any individual patient) exceeded 15% per patient year (46). A recent study from the University of Louvain using the same definitions for morbid events revealed somewhat better long-term statistics (Table 7–9); freedom from all valve-related morbidity and mortality was 70% ± 2%, 59% ± 3%, and 55% ± 3% after 5, 10, and 13 years, respectively (24).

In the multivariate regression analysis of patients receiving all types of valves at Stanford, valve type (S-E > xenograft) and previous cardiac operation were the significant independent predictors for all valve-related morbidity and mortality following MVR (35).

Structural and Mechanical Failure

Although ball variance occurred in patients with the S-E model 6000 mitral valves (48, 56, 57), it has been rare with the model 6120 valve (56). There was only one case of suspected ball variance in a partially thrombosed prosthesis in the Stanford experience; no case of poppet fracture, embolization, or strut fracture was evident among 3170 patient years of follow-up (46). In the University of Oregon MVR series, there was no case of intrinsic valve failure among 1369 patient years of follow-up (49).

SMELOFF-SUTTER PROSTHETIC VALVE

The original open-cage design of the present Smeloff-Sutter caged-ball prosthesis was introduced in 1962 by Cartwright and Palich (58). This valve was redesigned by Smeloff, Cartwright, Davey, and Kaufman in 1963 and became known as the SCDK prosthesis (59). Structural modifications in 1964 resulted in the Smeloff-Cutter prosthesis, which had a rounder annulus, larger sewing ring, and a silastic poppet that had been preswollen by heating at body temperature (60). Reports of ball variance prompted the reduction of the curing temperature of the silastic ball in 1966. After Sutter Biomedical, Inc. (San Diego) acquired the prosthetic valve division from Cutter Laboratories (Berkeley) in 1980, the valve became known as the Smeloff-Sutter (S-S) prosthesis.

The S-S prosthesis (Fig. 7–15), constructed from a single piece of medical-grade titanium, has an open-cage design that eliminates any structural material in this area of potential stasis. This design therefore has a theoretical advantage of fewer TE complications, in addition to less hemolysis and valve thrombosis. A potential hazard of open-cage valves in the mitral position, however, is the possible erosion of the LV myocardium by the struts of the prosthesis (61). The S-S valve uses the full-orifice principle, in which the equator of the ball returns to the level of the sewing ring or annulus when in the closed position by virtue of a double-cage architecture (59). These two features permit a smaller poppet, which clears the orifice by 0.003 to 0.005 in., and a lower cage profile downstream; thus, this type of valve may be advantageous in smaller hearts (60, 62). In the mitral position, the S-S valve encroaches less upon the ventricular septum and minimizes obstruction of the LV outflow tract during systole (62). In the aortic position, there may be less interference with coronary filling since the ball moves backward into the orifice during diastole (62). Additionally, the S-S is designed to permit regurgitation around the poppet to produce a self-washing effect, which potentially might reduce TE complications (63).

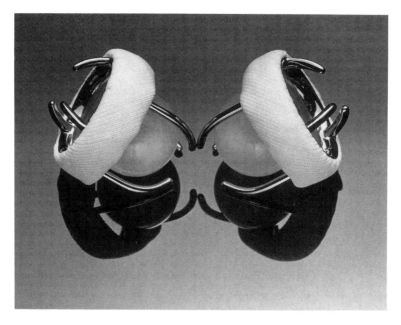

Fɪɢ. 7–15. The Smeloff-Sutter prosthetic valve. Courtesy of Sutter Biomedical, Inc.

Hydrodynamics and Hemodynamics

Current specifications, including old and new nomenclature, of the S-S valves are shown in Table 7–11. For the smaller valve sizes, the geometric orifice area of the S-S valve is similar to that of the S-E valve (see Tables 7–1 and 7–11); the larger sizes of the S-S prostheses have a comparatively larger cross-sectional area than do the S-E prostheses in both aortic and mitral positions (e.g., a 34-mm S-S mitral valve has an orifice area of 4.67 cm^2, while the same size S-E prosthesis has an orifice area of 3.66 cm^2).

Aortic Prostheses

In vitro evaluation of the S-S aortic valve revealed a peak transvalvular gradient of 55 mmHg for the size A-19 (19-mm external diameter) prosthesis at a mean flow rate of 4 L/min (peak flow rate of 13 L/min) and an effective orifice area of 1.19 cm^2 (64) (Table 7–12); this is compared with a peak transvalvular gradient of 47 mmHg for the Björk-Shiley tilting disk (60°) valve with a similar annulus diameter at equivalent flow rates. For the size A-24 S-S prosthesis, the peak systolic gradient was 18 mmHg (compared with 12 mmHg for the Björk-Shiley (size 25 mm) valve) at a mean flow rate of 4.5 L/min (peak flow rate of 17 L/min) and calculated effective orifice area of 2.05 cm^2 (64). The mean gradient for the size A-24 S-S valve was 3.8 mmHg compared with 2.5 mmHg for the 23-mm Björk-Shiley valve and 11.2 mmHg for the size 23A S-E valve (mean flow rate of 4.9 L/min and simulated "aortic" pressure of 125/75) (17). Regurgitant fraction was least in the smaller S-S valves (0.5% for size A-19) (64); in the moderate sizes (A-24), the regurgitant fraction varied from 3.2 to 7% (17, 64). For comparison, regurgitant fractions in the 23- to 25-mm Björk-Shiley and the size 23A S-E valves were 2.8 to 10 and 3%, respectively (17, 64).

TABLE 7–11. *Specifications for the Smeloff-Sutter Prostheses*

Size*	Annulus diameter (mm)	GOA† (cm^2)
Aortic		
A-19 (A-1)	19	1.20
A-21 (A-2)	21	1.56
A-23 (A-3)	23	1.82
A-24 (A-4)	24	2.10
A-26 (A-5)	26	2.36
A-29 (A-6)	29	2.90
A-31 (A-7)	31	3.56
A-33 (A-8)	33	4.14
A-34 (A-9)	34	4.67
A-38 (A-10)	38	4.67
Mitral		
M-22 (M-2)	22	1.56
M-23 (M-3)	23	1.82
M-24 (M-4)	24	2.10
M-26 (M-5)	26	2.36
M-29 (M-6)	29	2.90
M-31 (M-7)	31	3.56
M-33 (M-8)	33	4.14
M-34 (M-9)	34	4.67
M-38 (M-10)	38	4.67

*Old nomenclature in parentheses.

†Geometric orifice area, as reported by the manufacturer.

In vivo hemodynamic studies revealed the mean systolic gradient to be 13 mmHg across the size A-24 S-S aortic prosthesis with a calculated valve area of 2.05 cm^2 (65); for the slightly larger size A-26 prosthesis, the mean gradient was 8 mmHg with a calculated valve area of 2.31 cm^2 (65). Additional clinical comparisons of transvalvular gradients for the entire range of S-S aortic valve sizes have not been reported. Table 7–13 shows the available hemodynamic data.

Mitral Prosthesis

Experimental animal studies have shown small transvalvular gradients (less than 5 mmHg) with the S-S mitral prosthesis (66). In vitro evaluations revealed that a S-S mitral prosthesis (of unspecified size) was associated with a transvalvular gradient of 13 mmHg

TABLE 7–12. *In Vitro Hydrodynamics of the Smeloff-Sutter Aortic Prosthesis*

Reference	Size	Mean transvalvular gradient (mmHg)	Mean flow rate (L/min)	Peak flow rate (L/min)	Effective orifice area (cm^2)	% backflow
64	A-19	55 (peak)	4	13	1.19	0.5
64	A-24	18 (peak)	4.5	17	2.05	3.2
17	A-24	3.8	4.9	—	—	7
67	(not stated)	10	4.5	15	—	4

TABLE 7–13. *In Vivo Hemodynamics of the Smeloff-Sutter Aortic Prosthesis*

Reference	Size	No. of patients	Mean systolic gradient (mmHg)	Cardiac index [L/(min · m²)]	Valve area (cm²)
At rest					
65	A19	—	—	—	1.19
	A21	—	—	—	1.54
	A24	—	13	—	2.05
	A26	—	8	—	2.31
	(Various)	13	20	2.89	—
66	(Various)	7	19 (5–27)	—	1.54–3.12
69	(Various)	26	18.4	5.4*	—
With exercise					
66	(Various)	7	29 (8–38)	—	1.54–3.12
69	(Various)	26	28.4	7.8*	—
65	(Various)	13	26.1	4.39	—

*Cardiac output.

(peak flow of 15 L/min), compared with 12 mmHg and 7 mmHg for the comparable sized S-E and the Björk-Shiley valves, respectively; the mean regurgitant backflow was 5.6% for the S-S valve compared with 0.8 and 2% for the S-E and the Björk-Shiley valves, respectively (67). Evaluation of the size M-26 S-S mitral prosthesis revealed a mean diastolic gradient of 4.8 mmHg at a mean flow rate between 3.5 and 4.8 L/min (peak flow rate of 21 L/min); total regurgitation constituted 5% in this valve (23).

Clinically, Rouleau et al. noted the mean transvalvular gradient for the size M-29 to M-33 mitral prostheses to be unmeasurable at a cardiac index of 3.1 L/(min · m²) (68) (Table 7–14). In other reports, the mean gradient in valves of various sizes (specific sizes not given) ranged from 3.7 to 6 mmHg at rest (calculated valve areas 3.45 to 4.1 cm²) and increased to 3.9 to 15 mmHg with exercise (65–66, 69–70). The majority of the resting transvalvular differential occurred in the first ⅛ to ½ of diastole, regardless of the length of diastolic filling period (66). Transvalvular gradients persisted, possibly due to

TABLE 7–14. *In Vivo Hemodynamics of the Smeloff-Sutter Mitral Prosthesis*

Reference	Size	No. of patients	Mean pressure gradient (mmHg)	Cardiac index [L/(min · m²]	Valve area (cm²)
At rest					
68	M-29 to M-33	9	End-diastole 0	3.1	—
66	(Various)	8	6 (2–12)	1.5–2.9	3.45–4.1
69	(Various)	14	3.7	3.3*	—
65	(Various)	14	4.13	2.85	—
70	(Various)	7	6 (5–8)	2.6	—
With exercise					
66	(Various)	8	15 (4–20)	2.3–4.0	—
69	(Various)	14	3.9	4.8*	—
65	(Various)	14	7.7	3.13	—
70	(Various)	7	12 (11–13)	3.6	—

*Cardiac output.

the rigid metal ring in the annulus, increased ball mass, ball swelling, and decreased LV compliance (66).

Clinical Performance with the Aortic and Mitral Prostheses

The long-term performance of the S-S prosthetic valves has been analyzed less extensively than that of the S-E prostheses. Furthermore, the newer, more comprehensive definitions of valve failure (as used in the Stanford reports (27, 46) has yet to be applied to analysis of the S-S valve. Therefore, a precise comparative evaluation of this prosthesis and the S-E valve is not possible at this time.

Survival—Aortic Prosthesis

In an early study of the SCDK aortic prosthesis, the hospital mortality was 9% for isolated AVR (62). The hospital mortality with the S-S aortic valve in subsequent series was between 6.5 and 12.8% (65, 71–73) (Table 7–15). As noted, the operative mortality is more a function of the patient's preoperative status and era of operation and not necessarily a function of the type of valve used.

Long-term follow-up with the S-S aortic prosthesis has not been as comprehensive as that with the S-E aortic valves. The actuarial late survival rates of discharged patients ranged from 70 to 88% after 5 years, 61 to 80% after 8 years, and 57% after 10 years in the series from different institutions (63, 65, 71–73) (Table 7–15). The linearized mortality was between 2.7 and 4% per patient year (71, 72). These late survival rates with the S-S aortic prosthesis were comparable to those with the S-E prosthesis at 5 and 10 years follow-up; however, actuarial data for longer follow-up periods have not been reported.

TABLE 7–15. *Clinical Results and Valve-related Morbidity with the Smeloff-Sutter Aortic Prosthesis*

Institution	Time of operation	Hospital mortality (%)	Late survival (discharged pts) (% at n years)		Mortality (% per pt-yr)	TE % free	at n yrs	TE % per pt-yr	ACH % free	at n yrs	ACH % per pt-yr
Baylor College,	1969–77	8.5	80	5	4	(With coumadin)		2.6	—	—	2.9
Houston			71	8		(No anticoag.)		5.4	—	—	
(71)			57	10		(ASA/pers.)		2.9	—	—	
Sutter Hosp.,	1966–74	9	76.5	5	—	—	—	1.56	—	—	—
Sacramento	1970–82		48	7		—	—		—	—	
(63, 65)		7.4	66*	5	—	91	5	3.8	—	—	—
			49*	10	—	85	10		—	—	
						(With coumadin)		1.8			
Hôpital Charles	1972–80	6.5	88	5	2.73	96	5	1.2	—	—	1.81
Nicolle,			~ 80	8		93	8		—	—	
Rouen,											
France (72)											
Univ. Alberta	1966–72	12.8	~70	5	—	15.7% of total			—	—	—
			61	8		—	—		—	—	

*Including operative mortality.

TABLE 7–16. *Clinical Results and Valve-related Morbidity with the Smeloff-Sutter Mitral Prosthesis*

Institution	Time of operation	Hospital mortality	Late survival (discharged pts) (% at n years)		TE % free	at n yrs	% per pt-yr	ACH % free	at n yrs	% per pt-yr
Sutter Hosp. Sacramento (65)	1966–74	11	73.6 70	5 9	9.5% of total —	—		9.5% of total —	—	
UCSF (74)	1966–70	12	~60	5	—	—	6.5	24% of total		
Mayo Clinic (75)	1965–70 after 1966	6	~70	6	73 82	5 5	6.1	— —	— —	—
Univ. Alberta (76)	1966–71	16	~65	4	23% of total			—	—	—

Survival—Mitral Prosthesis

The hospital mortality with the early SCDK mitral prosthesis was 9% for isolated MVR (62). Subsequent series revealed an operative mortality associated with use of the S-S mitral prosthesis to be in the range of 6 to 16% for isolated MVR (65, 74–76) (Table 7–16).

The late survival rates of discharged patients after S-S MVR were between 60 and 74% after 4 to 5 years, and 70% after 6 to 8 years (Table 7–16) (65, 74–76). Oxman et al. at the Mayo Clinic reported no significant difference in survival rates in patients who underwent MVR with the S-S prosthesis and those with S-E mitral prostheses (models 6000 and 6120) over the same period of time (i.e., after 6 years) (75).

Valve-related Morbidity with the Aortic and Mitral Prostheses

Valve Thrombosis

A number of authors have reported no cases of S-S aortic valve thrombosis at variable lengths of follow-up (63, 71–72). Sarma et al. evaluated 21 aortic prostheses recovered at autopsy or reoperation and found only two valves to have "minimal evidence of thrombus" with the remainder thrombus-free (77). None of the deaths in this series were related to valve thrombosis, and the clinical relevance of "minimal thrombus formation" was not clear (77).

Although the incidence of mitral valve thrombosis as a result of ingrowth of fibrin or pannus or clot formation preventing proper excursion of the ball with the S-S prosthesis was low in the early studies (76, 78–79), Magilligan et al. noted that 13 of 107 discharged patients developed evidence of mitral valve thrombosis with incomplete poppet opening (80). This was diagnosed by auscultation, phonocardiography (delay in the valve opening sound), and echocardiography (delayed opening of ball as well as delayed cage motion) (78–80). Freedom from mitral valve thrombosis was 98% ± 2% and 84% ± 5% after 5 and 10 years, respectively (80). The mortality associated with this S-S mitral valve dysfunction was quite high (46%) (80), and was comparable to the mortality (79%) associated with S-E mitral valve thrombosis in the Stanford experience (46).

Thromboembolism

In early series, TE complications rarely occurred after AVR with the S-S prosthesis over relatively short follow-up periods (60, 65, 77). With more comprehensive definitions and stringent follow-up in subsequent studies, the linearized rate of TE in patients after S-S AVR was in the range of 1.2 to 3.8% per patient year (63, 71, 72) (Table 7–15). When only patients who received continuous anticoagulation therapy were considered, the risk of TE after AVR declined from 3.8 to 1.8% per patient year in a series from Sutter Hospital (Sacramento, California) (63); the linearized risk of major or lethal thromboembolic events was 0.7 to 1.9% per patient year (63, 71). For patients not receiving continuous anticoagulation for various reasons, there was a twofold increase in the risk of TE (5.4% per patient year versus 2.6% per patient year) (71). It is not surprising that inadequate and poor anticoagulation management contributed to this increased risk (60, 65, 71, 73); those receiving no medication had a higher incidence of minor embolic events, probably reflecting platelet emboli (71). Interestingly, after AVR with the S-S prosthesis, the linearized incidence of TE complications was 1.8% per patient year in a small group of selected patients who were switched to antiplatelet agents after being on continuous anticoagulation therapy for at least 1 year (63). Because this rate was comparable to that reported for patients who received continuous anticoagulation therapy indefinitely, Harlan et al. suggested that patients who had received at least 1 year of anticoagulation could be switched to antiplatelet agents if this was absolutely medically necessary; however, it was still their policy to recommend anticoagulation therapy in all patients if possible (63). After AVR with the S-S prosthesis, the actuarial TE-free rate was 91 to 96% after 5 years, 93% after 8 years, and 85% after 10 years (63, 72); these figures are similar to rates for the S-E and the Björk-Shiley aortic prostheses (63).

The linearized rate of TE complications with the S-S mitral prosthesis was 6.1 to 6.5% per patient year (74, 75) (Table 7–16). The risk of this complication was nonconstant and higher in the early postoperative period (5% risk within 30 days) and progressively declined thereafter (40% of all systemic emboli occurred in the first year, 72% in the first 2 years, and 91% in the first 3 years) (75). After MVR with the S-S prosthesis, the actuarial estimate of freedom from TE was 73% after 5 years, which was comparable to that associated with the non-cloth covered S-E mitral valve (75). Analysis of patients who underwent MVR with the S-S prosthesis after 1966 (vs. before 1966) revealed a slightly higher embolus-free rate of 82% after 5 years of follow-up (75) (Table 7–16).

Anticoagulant-related Hemorrhage

Anticoagulation appears to protect against major episodes of TE, but the associated morbidity (i.e., bleeding) among patients receiving warfarin is considerable. Following AVR with the S-S prosthesis, the linearized rate of ACH was 1.8 to 2.9% per patient year in two recent studies (71, 72) (Table 7–15); the linearized risk of major bleeding (defined as that resulting in death or permanent disability or requiring blood transfusion) was 2.1% per patient year (71). McHenry et al. reported an ACH morbidity rate of 9.3% and fatality rate of 3.3% in 217 patients after single AVR or MVR at an average follow-up of 37.7 months (65); no actuarial data were presented.

ACH appeared to be as frequent after mitral replacement with the S-S valve as after aortic replacement (65); however, there have been no comprehensive follow-up studies of patients after isolated S-S MVR. Bleeding problems (minor and major) occurred in 9.5 to 24% of the survivors after MVR with the S-S prosthesis at follow-up periods ranging from 14 to 37.7 month (65, 74) (Table 7–16). Unfortunately, no actuarial data have been reported.

Prosthetic Valve Endocarditis

In the reported series evaluating the clinical performance of the S-S aortic and mitral prostheses, PVE was rare. The incidence of this complication in patients with the S-S aortic prosthesis was approximately 1 to 3% during follow-up periods ranging from 6 months to 10 years (63, 72, 73). In a recent series of 365 survivors with a follow-up period of 13 years, Harlan et al. reported that only one AVR patient developed endocarditis and subsequently died of this complication (63). Sarma et al. noted a much higher incidence of aortic PVE (15%) at an average follow-up period of 4.9 years; however, their patient population was skewed, since 57% of the patients who developed this disease were intravenous drug users and continued such illicit drug abuse after the operation (77). Again, comparative evaluation with other series, particularly the long-term follow-up studies of patients with S-E aortic valves, is handicapped by the lack of actuarial analysis in most series of patients after AVR with S-S prostheses.

Follow-up is also incomplete for patients after MVR with the S-S mitral prosthesis; there have been reports of rare episodes of PVE in this population (74).

Hemolysis

Hemolytic complications do occur in patients with caged-ball prosthetic valves; however, they have not been as extensively evaluated or followed in patients who have undergone AVR or MVR with the S-S prostheses as in those with the S-E valves. As in patients after AVR or MVR with S-E prostheses, clinical evidence of hemolysis is rare in patients with the S-S prostheses except in cases of perivalvular leaks (71). In early reports of patients after AVR and MVR with the Cartwright-Palich, SCDK, and S-S prostheses, of those selected for hematologic evaluation, all had elevated levels of LDH, and 19% had decreased red cell survival; fewer than 50% of those patients, however, were clinically anemic at the time of evaluation (60). Of the patients evaluated by Soyer et al., significant hemolysis was evident in 7.5%, two-thirds of whom had valvular regurgitation requiring reoperation (72). Further follow-up studies revealed that about 33% of patients had evidence of hemolysis (72, 77); clinically important hemolytic anemia, however, was present in only 2.4% of the patients in the early series and rarely in subsequent series (71, 73).

Valve Failure

The combination of complications leading to reoperation or death (valve failure) has not been reported as such following AVR or MVR with the S-S prostheses. Similarly, the composite index of all valve-related morbidity and mortality as applied in the analysis of the clinical performance of the S-E valves have not been used in evaluating the long-term results of the S-S prosthesis.

Structural and Mechanical Failure

The occurrence of mechanical valve dysfunction has been rare in patients with the S-S aortic valve (63, 65, 71–75, 77). There have been occasional reports of ball variance (63, 65, 81), similar to that reported for the silastic ball S-E aortic valves.

In 1970, Lee et al. at the University of Alberta reported three cases of S-S mitral valve malfunction, the *sticky mitral ball syndrome,* as a result of impaction of the ball in the seating ring due to ball variance; this was detected by clinical and hemodynamic findings of intermittent mitral valve obstruction (82). Physical findings included a fluctuating pulse volume and arterial pressure coupled with varying intensity of the mitral closing sound, intermittent opening click, and a variable second sound opening click duration (82). One may also find an asynchronous sound of the prosthetic valve with simultaneous electrocardiographic evidence of sinus rhythm (83). The mechanical failure rate at the University of Alberta was 9% after placement of 32 S-S mitral valves (82).

McHenry et al. also reported two cases of mitral valve obstruction as a result of ball variance (81). Analysis of these poppets indicated that swelling and obstruction was principally due to infiltration of complex lipids and not the result of fissuring or cracking. The double-caged SCDK valve, the earlier version of the present S-S prosthesis, may be particularly vulnerable to lipid absorption and swelling of the silastic poppet, which may result in its sticking in the annulus, conversion to an orifice seating system, or its obstruction within the cage (81). Ball variance has not been detected with the newer, more recent prostheses, either because lipid absorption is a time-dependent phenomenon and not clinically apparent at the time of follow-up, or because the concentricity and cure standards in ball production have improved.

CONCLUSION

There is little question that the introduction of the S-E aortic and mitral non-cloth-covered prosthetic valves was a major advance in the treatment of patients with valvular heart disease. The place of S-E aortic and mitral prostheses in history remains undisturbed as they continue to serve as a benchmark against which newer generations of valve substitutes are evaluated. A somewhat turbulent evolution has resulted in the currently available S-E aortic and mitral models. The double-caged S-S valvular prostheses have also had a relatively long history (approaching 25 years), although they have not been as extensively used or as comprehensively evaluated as their S-E counterparts. It is clear that these seemingly indestructible mechanical prosthetic valves carry an array of associated complications, the majority of which are related to TE and the need for indefinite anticoagulation therapy. In this context, it may not be realistic to expect newer mechanical prostheses requiring warfarin anticoagulation therapy to have any substantial advantages. Taking this into account, important issues in the future center on eliminating the need for anticoagulation or minimizing the associated complications or the development of new, safer anticoagulant drugs. Although clear advantages—concerning TE and ACH—exist with both modern xenografts and allograft valves, tissue failure becomes an increasingly important consideration with these bioprostheses. The use of universally accepted definitions of prosthetic valve complications and valve failure (55), and the reporting of indices such as the composite valve-related morbidity and mortality index, will aid in defining the overall advantages, if any, of new introduced prostheses. A recent triinstitutional, retrospective study investigated the long-term performance of xenografts versus mechanical (S-E) prostheses (54). Evaluated according to structural failure, the mechanical valve is superior to the tissue valve at all time frames; using the Stanford definition of valve failure, the mechanical valve becomes superior after 5 to 10 years. This is not surprising since structural failure requiring reoperation (a component of valve failure) becomes an increasingly greater factor with bioprostheses at longer follow-up periods. Concerning fatal valve failure, however, we have previously shown that the risk is significantly and independently increased by the valve type (S-E > xenograft) (35), as complications with mechanical valves, in general, tend to be more catastrophic. Further studies will be necessary to confirm these findings, preferably in a prospective fashion.

In the Stanford experience, the type of valve used for AVR was the most significant determinant for TE, ACH, and fatal valve failure (S-E > xenograft) and the second most powerful predictor of decreased late survival (S-E > xenograft) (35). Similarly, for patients undergoing MVR, valve type was the most significant independent predictor of TE, ACH, fatal valve failure, and all valve-related morbidity and mortality (S-E > xenograft); it was also highly significant for predicting a decreased late survival (35). Reoperation, however, was related significantly to younger age (not necessarily with valve type), probably reflecting the early degeneration of tissue valves in this age group.

The position of the valvular prosthesis is important regarding complication rates, with the patients undergoing MVR being at an obvious disadvantage. The rates of combined valve-related morbidity and mortality found in our study of patients after MVR with the S-E prosthesis are very high (Fig. 7–14); fully 62% of these patients had a serious complication or died in a manner directly related to the valve by 10 years, and 75% by 14 years (46). Therefore, selecting the type of mitral valve prosthesis is an even more sensitive, challenging issue.

REFERENCES

1. Hufnagel CA, Harvey WP, Rabil PJ, McDermott TF: Surgical correction of aortic insufficiency. Surgery 1954;35:673–683.
2. Campbell JM: An artificial aortic valve. J Thorac Surg 1950;19:312–318.
3. Lefrak EA, Starr A (Eds): Caged ball valves. In Cardiac Valve Prostheses. New York, Appleton-Century-Crofts, 1979, pp. 67–166.
4. Starr A, Edwards ML: Mitral replacement: Clinical experience with a ball-valve prosthesis. Ann Surg 1961;154:726–740.
5. Harken DE, Soroff HS, Taylor WJ, Lefemine AA, Gupta SK, Lunzer S: Partial and complete prostheses in aortic insufficiency. J Thorac Cardiovasc Surg 1960;40:744–762.
6. Ellis FH, Bulbulian AH: Prosthetic replacement of the mitral valve: I. Preliminary experimental observations. Proc Mayo Clinic 1958;33:532–534a.
7. Edwards WS, Smith L: Aortic valve replacement with a subcoronary ball valve. Surg Forum 1958;9:309–313.
8. Staff A, Pierie WR, Raible DA, Edwards ML, Siposs GG, Hancock WD: Cardiac valve replacement: Experience with the durability of silicone rubber. Circulation 1966;38/39(suppl I):115–123.
9. Freimanis I, Starr A: The unnatural history of valvular heart disease: Late results with silastic ball valve prostheses. J Cardiovasc Surg 1984;25:191–198.
10. Braunwald NS, Bonchek LI: Prevention of thrombus formation on rigid prosthetic heart valves by the ingrowth of autogenous tissue. J Thorac Cardiovasc Surg 1967;54:630.
11. Krosnick A: Death due to migration of the ball from an aortic valve prosthesis. JAMA 1965;191:1083–1084.
12. Behrendt DM, Austen WG: Current status of prosthetics for heart valve replacement. Prog Cardiovasc Dis 1973;15:369–341.
13. Roberts WC, Morrow AG: Late postoperative pathologic findings after cardiac valve replacement. Circulation 1967;35/36(suppl I):48–62.
14. Roberts WC, Morrow AG: Topics in clinical medicine: Anatomic studies of hearts containing caged-ball prosthetic valves. Johns Hopkins Med J 1967;121:271–295.

15. Roberts WC, Morrow AG: Secondary left ventricular endocardial fibroelastosis following mitral valve replacement. Circulation 1968;38/39(suppl II):101–109.
16. Pyle RB, Mayer JE, Lindsay WG, Jorgensen CR, Wang Y, Nicoloff DM: Hemodynamic evaluation of Lillei-Kaster and Starr-Edwards Prostheses. Ann Thorac Surg 1978;26:336–343.
17. Björk VO, Olin C: A hydrodynamic comparison between the new tilting disc aortic valve prosthesis (Bjork-Shiley) and the corresponding prostheses of Starr-Edwards, Kay-Shiley, Smeloff-Cutter and Wada-Cutter in the pulse duplicator. Scand J Thorac Cardiovasc Surg 1979;4:31–36.
18. Yoganathan AP, Harrison EC, Corcoran WH: Prosthetic heart valves: Proceedings of a symposium of the 14th Annual Meeting of the Association for the Advancement of Medical Instrumentation. Pasadena, Cal Tech Press, 1980, p 181.
19. Yoganathan AP: Cardiovascular fluid mechanics: I. Fluid dynamics of prosthetic aortic valves. II. Use of the fast Fourier transform on the analysis of cardiovascular sounds. Doctoral thesis, California Institute of Technology, 1978.
20. Dellsperger KC, Wieting DW, Baehr DA, Bard RJ, Brugger J, Harrison EC: Regurgitation of prosthetic heart valves: Dependence on heart rate and cardiac output. Am J Cardiol 1983;51:321–328.
21. Williams GA, Labowitz AJ: Doppler hemodynamic evaluation of prosthetic (Starr-Edwards and Bjork-Shiley) and bioprosthetic (Hancock and Carpentier-Edwards) cardiac valves. Am J Cardiol 1985;56:325–332.
22. Gabbay S, McQueen DM, Yellin EL, Beecher RM, Frater RWM: In vitro hydrodynamic comparison of mitral valve prostheses at high flow rates. J Thorac Cardiovasc Surg 1978;76:771–787.
23. Bjork VO, Olin C: Hydrodynamic evaluation of the new tilting disc valve (Bjork-Shiley) for mitral valve replacement. Scand J Thorac Cardiovasc Surg 1970;4:37–43.
24. Schoevaerdts JC, Buche M, el Garvani A, Lichsteiner M, Jaumin P, Ponlot R: Twenty years' experience with the model 6120 Starr-Edwards valve in the mitral position. J Thorac Cardiovasc Surg 1987;94:375–382.
25. Glancy DL, O'Brien KP, Reis RL, Epstein SE, Morrow AG: Hemodynamic studies in patients with 2M and 3M Starr-Edwards prostheses: Evidence of obstruction of left atrial emptying. Circulation 1969;39/40(suppl I):113–118.
26. Horstkotte D, Haerten K, Seipel L, Korfer R, Budde T, Bircks W, Loogen F: Central hemodynamics at rest and during exercise after mitral valve replacement with different prostheses. Circulation 1983;68(suppl II):161–168.
27. Miller DC, Oyer PE, Mitchell RS, Stinson EB, Jamieson SW, Baldwin JC, Shumway NE: Performance characteristics of the Starr-Edwards model 1260 aortic valve prosthesis beyond ten years. J Thorac Cardiovasc Surg 1984;88:193–207.
28. Barnhorst DA, Oxman HA, Connolly DC, Pluth JR, Danielson GK, Wallace RB, McGoon DC: Long-term follow-up of isolated replacements of the aortic or mitral valve with the Starr-Edwards prosthesis. Am J Cardiol 1975;35:228–233.
29. Murphy DA, Levine FH, Buckley MJ, Swinski L, Daggett WM, Akins CW, Austen WG: Mechanical valves: A comparative analysis of the Starr-Edwards and Bjork-Shiley prostheses. J Thorac Cardiovasc Surg 1983;86:746–752.
30. Hackett D, Fessatidis I, Sapsford R, Oakley C: Ten year clinical evaluation of Starr-Edwards 2400 and 1260 aortic valve prostheses. Br Heart J 1987;57:356–363.
31. Macmanus Q, Grunkemeier GL, Lambert LE, Teply JF, Harlan BJ, Starr A: Year of operation as a risk factor in the late results of valve replacement. J Thorac Cardiovasc Surg 1980;80:834–841.
32. Macmanus Q, Grunkemeier GL, Lambert LE, Starr A: Non-cloth-covered caged-ball prostheses: The second decade. J Thorac Cardiovasc Surg 1978;76:788–794.
33. Bonchek LI, Starr A: Ball valve prostheses: Current appraisal of late results. Am J Cardiol 1975;35:843–854.
34. Wain WH, Drury PJ, Ross DN: Aortic valve replacement with Starr-Edwards valves over 14 years. Ann Thorac Surg 1981;33:562–569.
35. Mitchell RS, Miller DC, Stinson EB, Oyer PE, Jamieson SW, Baldwin JC, Shumway NE: Significant patient-related determinants of prosthetic valve performance. J Thorac Cardiovasc Surg 1986;91:807–817.
36. Best JF, Hassanein KM, Pugh DM, Dunn M: Starr-Edwards aortic prosthesis: A 20 year retrospective study. Am Heart J 1986;111:136–142.
37. Starr A, Grunkemeier GL: Selection of a prosthetic heart valve. JAMA 1984;251:1739–1742.
38. Metsdorff MT, Grunkemeier GL, Pinson CW, Starr A: Thrombosis of mechanical cardiac valves: A quantitative comparison of the silastic ball valve and the tilting disc valve. J Am Coll Cardiol 1984;4:50–53.
39. Starr A: The Starr-Edwards valve. J Am Coll Cardiol 1985;6:899–903.
40. Macmanus Q, Metsdorff MT, Grunkemeier GL, Starr A: Thrombotic and embolic complications with silastic ball prosthetic valves. Eur Heart J 1984;5:59–63.
41. Fuster V, Pumphrey CW, McGoon MD, Chesebro JH, Pluth JR, McGoon DC: Systemic thromboembolism in mitral and aortic Starr-Edwards prostheses: A 10–19 year follow-up. Circulation 1982;66(suppl I):157–161.

42. Brodeur MTH, Sutherland DW, Koler RD, Starr A, Kimsey JA, Griswold HE: Red blood cell survival in patients with aortic valvular disease and ball-valve prostheses. Circulation 1965;32:570–581.
43. Roberts D, Bake B, William-Olsson G: Improved red cell survival in patients with chronic subclinical hemolysis due to artificial heart valve. Scand J Thorac Cardiovasc Surg 1984;18:115–118.
44. Walsh JR, Starr A, Ritzmann LW: Intravascular hemolysis in patients with prosthetic valves and valvular heart disease. Circulation 1969;39/40(suppl I):135–140.
45. Merendino KA, Manhas DR: Man-made gallstones: A new entity following cardiac valve replacement. Ann Surg 1973;177:694–704.
46. Miller DC, Oyer PE, Stinson EB, Reitz BA, Jamieson SW, Baumgartner WA, Mitchell RS, Shumway NE: Ten to fifteen year reassessment of the performance characteristics of the Starr-Edwards model 6120 mitral valve prosthesis. J Thorac Cardiovasc Surg 1983;85:1–20.
47. Grunkemeier GL, Starr A: Late ball variance with the model 1000 Starr-Edwards aortic valve prosthesis. J Thorac Cardiovasc Surg 1986;91:918–923.
48. Hylen JC, Kloster FE, Starr A: Aortic ball variance: Diagnosis and treatment. Ann Int Med 1970;72:1–8.
49. Cobanaglu A, Grunkemeier GL, Aru GM, McKinley CL, Starr A: Mitral replacement: Clinical experience with a ball-valve prosthesis. Ann Surg 1985;202:376–383.
50. Levine FH, Copeland JG, Morrow AG: Prosthetic replacement of the mitral valve: Continuing assessments of the 100 patients operated upon during 1961–1965. Circulation 1973;47:518–526.
51. Sala A, Schoevaerdts J, Jaumin P, Ponlot R, Chalant C: Review of 387 isolated mitral valve replacements by the model 6120 Starr-Edwards prosthesis. J Thorac Cardiovasc Surg 1982;84:744–750.
52. Schoevaerdts JC, Jaumin P, Ponlot R, Chalant CH, Grunkemeier GL: Twelve year results with a caged-ball prosthesis. Thorac Cardiovasc Surg 1979;27:45–47.
53. Starr A, Grunkemeier G, Lambert L, Okies JE, Thomas D: Mitral valve replacement: A 10-year follow-up of non-cloth-covered vs. cloth-covered caged ball prostheses. Circulation 1976;54(suppl III):47–56.
54. Cobanoglu A, Jamieson WRE, Miller DC, McKinely C, Grunkemeier GL, Floten S, Miyagishima RT, Tyers GFO, Shumway NE, Starr A: A tri-institutional comparison of tissue and mechanical valves using a patient-oriented definition of "treatment failure." Ann Thorac Surg 1987;43:245–253.
55. Weisel RD, Miller DC: Guidelines for reporting the performance of cardiac valve prostheses. Cardiac Surg: State Art Rev 1987;1:159–170.
56. Joyce LD, Emery RW, Nicoloff DM: Ball variance and fracture of mitral valve prosthesis causing recurrent thromboemboli. J Thorac Cardiovasc Surg 1978;75:309–312.
57. Roberts WC, Levinson GE, Morrow AG: Lethal ball variance in the Starr-Edwards prosthetic mitral valve. Arch Intern Med 1970;126:517–521.
58. Cartwright RS, Palich WE, Ford WB, Ciacobine JW, Zubritzky SA, Ratan RS: Combined replacement of aortic and mitral valves: An original transatrial approach to the aortic valve. JAMA 1962;180:6–10.
59. Cartwright RS, Smeloff EA, Davey TB, Kaufman B: Development of a titanium double-caged full-orifice ball valve. Trans Am Soc Artif Int Organs 1964;10:231–236.
60. McHenry MM, Smeloff EA, Hattersley PG: Complications of heart valve replacement. Calif Med 1968;109:1–8.
61. Ibarra-Perez C, Rodriguez-Trujillo F, Perez-Redondo H: Engagement of ventricular myocardium by struts of mitral prosthesis. J Thorac Cardiovasc Surg 1971;61:401–404.
62. Cooley DA, Bloodwell RD, Beall AC, Gill SS, Hallman GL: Total cardiac valve replacement using SCDK-Cutter prosthesis: Experience with 250 consecutive patients. Ann Surg 1966;164:428–444.
63. Harlan BJ, Smeloff EA, Miller GE, Kelly PB, Junod FL, Ross KA, Shankar KG: Performance of the Smeloff aortic valve beyond ten years. J Thorac Cardiovasc Surg 1986;91:86–91.
64. Messmer BJ, Hallman GL, Liotta D, Martin C, Cooley DA: Aortic valve replacement: New techniques, hydrodynamics, and clinical results. Surgery 1970;68:1026–1037.
65. McHenry MM, Smeloff EA, Matlof HJ, Rice J, Miller GE: Long-term survival after single aortic or mitral valve replacement with the present model of Smeloff-Cutter valves. J Thorac Cardiovasc Surg 1978;75:709–715.
66. McHenry MM, Smeloff EA, Davey TB, Kaufman B, Fong WY: Hemodynamic results with full-flow orifice prosthetic valves. Circulation 1967;35/36(suppl I):24–33.
67. Liotta D, Messmer BJ, Hallman GL, Hall RJ, Martin G, Chafizadeh GN, Cooley DA: Prosthetic and fascia lata valves: Hydrodynamics and clinical results. Trans Am Soc Artif Int Organs 1970;16:244–254.
68. Rouleau CA, Frye RL, Ellis FH: Hemodynamic state after open mitral valve replacement and reconstruction. J Thorac Cardiovasc Surg 1969;58:870–878.
69. McHenry MM, Smeloff EA, Matlof HJ, Miller GE: Long-term follow-up of patients with present model Smeloff-Cutter valve. Circulation 1975;51/52(suppl II):215. Abstract.
70. Hawe A, Frye RL, Ellis FH: Late hemodynamic studies after mitral valve surgery. J Thorac Cardiovasc Surg 1973;65:351–358.
71. Starr DS, Lawrie GM, Howell JF, Morris GC: Clinical experience with the Smeloff-Cutter prosthesis: 1- to 12-year follow-up. Ann Thorac Surg 1980;30:448–454.
72. Soyer R, Brunet A, Redonnet M, Hubscher C, Letac B: Aortic valve replacement with Smeloff-Cutter prosthesis: 1 to 8 year follow-up. J Cardiovasc Surg 1983;24:138–143.

73. Lee SJK, Barr C, Callaghan JC, Rossall RE: Long-term survival after aortic valve replacement using Sme-loff-Cutter prosthesis. Circulation 1975;52:1132–1137.
74. Fishman NH, Edmunds LH, Hutchinson JC, Roe BB: Five-year experience with the Smeloff-Cutter mitral prosthesis. J Thorac Cardiovasc Surg 1971;62:345–356.
75. Oxman HA, Connolly DC, Ellis FH: Mitral valve replacement with the Smeloff-Cutter prosthesis. J Thorac Cardiovasc Surg 1975;69:247–254.
76. Lee SJK, Lees G, Callaghan JC, Couves CM, Sterns LP, Rossall RE: Early and late complications of single mitral valve replacement: A comparison of eight different prostheses. J Thorac Cardiovasc Surg 1974;67:920–925.
77. Sarma R, Roschke EJ, Harrison EC, Edmiston WA, Lau FYK: Clinical experience with the Smeloff-Cutter aortic valve prosthesis: An 8-year follow-up study. Am J Cardiol 1977;40:338–344.
78. Pfeifer J, Goldschlager N, Sweatman T, Gerbode F, Selzer A: Malfunction of mitral ball valve prosthesis due to thrombus: Report of 2 cases with notes on early clinical diagnosis. Am J Cardiol 1972;29:95–99.
79. Belenkie I, Carr M, Schlant RC, Nutter DO, Symbas PN: Malfunction of a Cutter-Smeloff mitral ball valve prosthesis: Diagnosis by phonocardiography and echocardiography. Am Heart J 1973;86:399–403.
80. Magilligan DJ, Oyama C, Alam M: Comparison of dysfunction with mechanical and porcine mitral valve prostheses. Circulation 1985;72(suppl II):129–134.
81. McHenry MM, Smeloff EA, Fong WY, Miller GE, Ryan PM: Critical obstruction of prosthetic heart valves due to lipid absorption by Silastic. J Thorac Cardiovasc Surg 1970;59:413–425.
82. Lee SJK, Zaragoza AJ, Callaghan JC, Couves CM, Sterns LP: Malfunction of the mitral valve prosthesis (Cutter-Smeloff): Clinical and hemodynamic observations in three cases. Circulation 1970;41:479–484.
83. Leatherman LL, Leachman RD, McConn RG, Hallman GL, Cooley DA: Malfunction of mitral ball-valve prostheses due to swollen poppet. J Thorac Cardiovasc Surg 1969;57:160–163.

Bodnar, E. and Frater, R. W. M., editors
(1991) *Replacement Cardiac Valves,*
Pergamon Press, Inc. (New York), pp. 187–200
Printed in the United States of America

CHAPTER 8

TILTING DISK VALVES

WILLIAM H. BAIN AND S. A. M. NASHEF

HISTORICAL PERSPECTIVE

The concept of the tilting disk valve arose out of the recognition that caged-ball valves were unnecessarily bulky and that their hemodynamic characteristics were less than ideal (Fig. 8–1). In an attempt to reduce the profile of such valves, a flat disk, instead of a ball, was used as an occluder in caged-disk valves. These were of a lower profile than caged-ball valves, but still suffered from the hemodynamic problem of having an occluder that remained relatively obstructive in the open position. Thus the concept of a disk that tilted within the valve ring, causing minimal obstruction to blood flow in the open position, was especially attractive.

The earliest examples of the tilting disk concept were *flap valves.* These had a ring with a straight segment along which a disk was hinged, much like the lid of a toilet seat. Blood flowed entirely along the inflow surface of the disk, and the stasis on the outflow side resulted in thrombus formation that obstructed disk movement (1, 2).

In 1964, Melrose and colleagues introduced a valve in which a free-floating polypropylene disk was equipped with integral hooks that retained it within the valve ring and limited its travel (3). In clinical application, however, severe wear of the polypropylene hooks occurred within 2 years of implantation, with subsequent valve malfunction (4).

In 1966, Juro Wada developed a tilting disk valve without a hinge. In this ingenious design a disk, which was Z-shaped in profile, would pivot around an eccentric waist restrained by guide lugs projecting from the ring (5). Unfortunately, the disk was made of Teflon and was susceptible to deformation where it impinged on the lugs. This resulted in an unacceptable incidence of thrombosis in early clinical trials, and the valve was withdrawn (6, 7).

A valve with an aerofoil-shaped disk that pivoted along an eccentric axis was developed by MacLeod in Edinburgh in the early 1970s (8). The mechanism, however, was susceptible to thrombosis and tissue ingrowth, and the valve did not find clinical application.

Currently available tilting disk valves are all based on hingeless designs that rely on struts or guide lugs to restrain the disk within the valve ring. There are three major designs to which most current and recent tilting disk valves are related: the Björk-Shiley, the Omniscience, and the Medtronic-Hall. A time scale of availability of various models is shown in Fig. 8–2.

The Björk-Shiley Valves

In 1969 Björk and Shiley collaborated to produce a valve in which the free-floating disk was restrained by two low-profile M-shaped struts. These allowed the disk to pivot to an opening angle of 60 degrees (9, 10). The disk was originally made of acetal resin

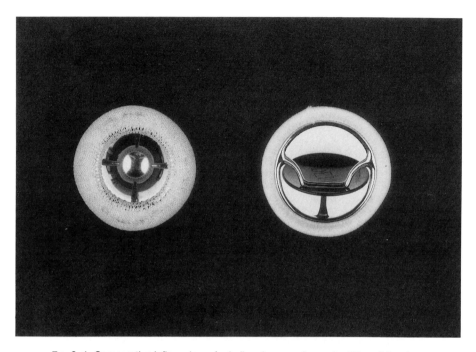

FIG. 8–1. Comparative inflow view of a ball-and-cage valve and a tilting disk valve.

(Delrin) and could absorb moisture when autoclaved; it was therefore replaced in 1971 with a pyrolytic carbon disk. In 1975 a tantalum radiopaque circular marker was incorporated into the disk so that its movement could be confirmed by radiologic screening. The valve can be rotated within its Teflon sewing ring and is often referred to as the *standard disk* or SD model of the Björk-Shiley valve.

In 1978 the struts were modified to allow the disk to move 2.5 mm downstream as it tilted, and the disk profile was changed from planoconvex to convexoconcave (11) (the

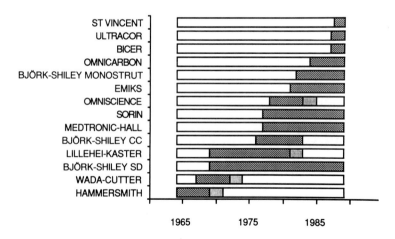

FIG. 8–2. Time scale of availability of tilting disk valves.

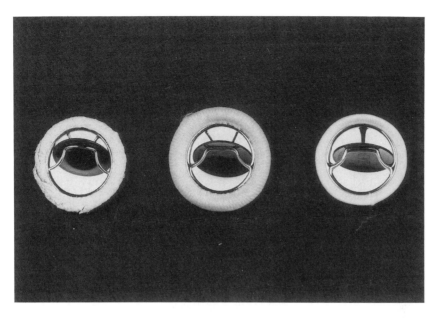

FIG. 8–3. Björk-Shiley valves. (Left to right) Standard disk valve, convexo-concave valve (60 degree), monostrut valve.

C-C model). This valve was available in two versions: the 60 degree and the 70 degree valve, depending on the disk opening angle. In 1981 the valve ring was altered to replace the outlet strut with a heavier single "hook" and the entire valve ring and struts were machined from one piece with no welds (the *monostrut* valve) (12). Versions of the Björk-Shiley valve are shown in Fig. 8–3.

The Lillehei-Kaster, Omniscience, and Omnicarbon Valves

A collaboration between C. W. Lillehei, a surgeon, and R. L. Kaster, an engineer, in the 1960s produced a number of experimental valves. In 1969 they introduced a tilting disk valve with a flat, pyrolytic carbon disk that tilted within a titanium valve ring with projecting hornlike struts (13–15). Subsequent clinical experience with the Lillehei-Kaster valve in the 1970s showed a high incidence of thrombotic obstruction (16–18).

The Omniscience valve was introduced clinically in 1978. Its thin convexoconcave pyrolytic carbon disk fits between four angled projections, or guide lugs, arising eccentrically from the valve ring (Fig. 8–4). The ring and guide lugs are machined from a single block of titanium. The valve can be rotated within its knitted polyester sewing ring.

The disk opens to 80 degrees but is inclined 12 degrees in the closed position. The disk does not move downstream on opening but is in permanent contact with part of the ring throughout the cardiac cycle. Its regurgitant flow in the closed position is significantly smaller than that of other tilting disk prostheses (19). In 1984 a new development of this prosthesis was introduced as the Omnicarbon valve. It has a similar design, but the entire valve mechanism is made of pyrolytic carbon, and early models also have a carbon-covered sewing ring.

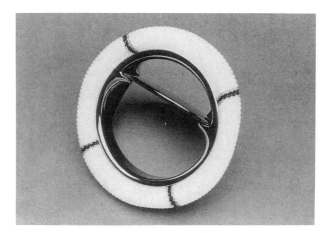

FIG. 8–4. The Omniscience valve.

The Medtronic-Hall Valve

This tilting disk valve was introduced into clinical practice in 1977. The valve was designed to offer an improved ratio of effective orifice to external diameter with the minor section of the orifice as large as possible (20). It has a thin and flat pyrolytic carbon disk that is guided by a sigmoid strut that passes through a hole in the center of the disk and is restrained by another strut and two guide lugs projecting from the ring (Fig. 8–5). The entire ring, with its struts and lugs, is machined from a single block of titanium. The opening angle is 75 degrees for aortic prostheses and 70 degrees for mitral prostheses.

The D16 modification of the Medtronic-Hall valve was introduced in 1979 in order to reduce subclinical hemolysis noted with the standard version. In this modification the flat surface of the minor strut was contoured to effect line contact with the disk in the closed position, and the two guide lugs were tilted slightly so that they too established

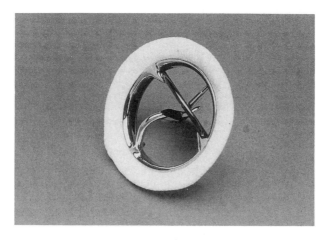

FIG. 8–5. The Medtronic-Hall valve.

only line contact with the disk. About one-third of Medtronic-Hall valves manufactured since 1977 are of the D16 configuration.

OPERATIVE CONSIDERATIONS

The surgical technique for the insertion of tilting disk prostheses is similar to that for other heart valve substitutes. Some aspects of technique, however, require special consideration.

Knots and Suture Ends

All tilting disk valves are constructed to exact and fine tolerances. The small space between the edge of the closed disk and the valve ring represents a design compromise that allows a "washing action" to prevent buildup of thrombus without permitting an unacceptable regurgitant volume. It is apparent, therefore, that an excessively long suture end may intrude between the ring and the disk and wedge the valve shut, with catastrophic consequences. Care should be taken to cut suture ends short and, where possible, to insert and ligate sutures a few millimeters away from the valve ring.

Tissue Interference

In common with other mechanical valves, it is important not to leave any tissue protruding within the range of excursion of the disk. In mitral valve replacement, chordae and papillary muscles must be divided clear of the edge of the opened disk. In aortic valve replacement, calcific protrusions below the annulus, particularly in relation to the lesser orifice, must be carefully removed.

Orientation

The primary objective governing the orientation of a tilting disk valve is to ensure that the full range of disk travel is not impeded by tissue above or below the valve. The secondary objective is to obtain the optimal flow pathway between the free edge of the open disk and the surrounding endocardium or aorta. Within these limitations, precise orientation is not critical. It is the authors' usual practice to implant tilting disk valves with the large orifice posteroinferiorly in the mitral position and toward the noncoronary/left coronary commissure in the aortic position. It is possible that a tilting disk valve with a large opening angle be implanted in such a way that the disk opens beyond the aortic flow axis. Theoretically, such a valve might not close in diastole (21). Valves that can be rotated within their sewing ring can be reoriented after implantation if necessary, taking great care to avoid damaging or weakening the valve mechanism. Forceps and other standard surgical instruments must never be used to rotate the valve: the appropriate valve holder is the only instrument suitable for this purpose.

CLINICAL RESULTS

The following data on the clinical performance of tilting disk valves are derived from major published series, including those from Glasgow, and expressed in linearized and actuarial terms with regard to the major valve-related complications: death, hemorrhage, embolism, periprosthetic leak, endocarditis, hemolysis, thrombotic obstruction, and structural failure. Unless otherwise specified, these events are defined in accordance with the system advocated by the authors (21).

Survival

The hospital mortality of valve replacement with well-established prostheses is related more to the preoperative status of the patients and the operative technique than to the choice of prosthesis. Reported medium-term survival (4–7 years) is 92 to 96% following aortic valve replacement and 82 to 87% following mitral valve replacement. Long-term survival (8–12 years) is 89 to 91% (aortic) and 78 to 82% (mitral). In view of the different patient characteristics in various institutions, crude survival figures cannot be relied upon to reflect valve performance. In a single-center comparison, Cortina et al. found no significant difference in late mortality after mitral valve replacement with three tilting disk prostheses (22).

Anticoagulation

Like all mechanical valves, tilting disk valves require lifelong anticoagulation therapy. Recently, some patients with the monostrut version of the Björk-Shiley valve were managed without anticoagulation therapy, but the incidence of embolism and valve thrombosis was relatively high (23). Thus one of the causes of morbidity following valve replacement with tilting disk valves remains anticoagulant-related hemorrhage. The reported incidence of serious hemorrhage varies between 0.3 and 1.1 per hundred patient years (%/py), and the varying incidence reflects differences in patient characteristics and compliance and the adequacy of the anticoagulant service in different institutions.

Systemic Embolism

Even with careful anticoagulation therapy, patients with tilting disk valves have a small but important incidence of systemic embolism, and a smaller but more serious risk of valve thrombosis (see below). The continuing occurrence of these complications has provided the impetus to develop tilting disk valves with a view to reducing the former and abolishing the latter. Unfortunately such developments, although successful in reducing the incidence of embolism and thrombosis, have introduced new problems (see the section on structural failure, below).

The incidence of systemic embolism after valve replacement with tilting disk valves compares favorably with that of alternative prostheses in compliant patient populations. Reported incidences of systemic embolism are detailed in Tables 8–1 and 8–2. The tables clearly indicate a wide variation in the reported incidence of emboli between different institutions assessing tilting disk valves. These differences are reduced, but not abolished, when different institutions report results for the same valve. This is due to several reasons:

1. Different institutions use different definitions of systemic embolism.
2. The interpretation of embolic symptoms is subjective.

TABLE 8–1. *Embolism Following Aortic Valve Replacement*

Valve assessed	Author and year	Number in series	Mean follow-up (years)	Linearized incidence (%/py)	Actuarial freedom	Comments
Björk-Shiley SD	Bain (41) (1985)	188	7.5	0.4	99% (5 years) 96% (15 years)	
	Sethia (29) 1986	184	4.8	0.4	98% (5 years) 91% (12 years)	
	Flemma (30) 1988	227	9	1.6	90% (5 years) 74% (15 years)	
Björk-Shiley C-C	Bain (41) 1985	136	4.3	0.2	99% (5 years) 99% (9 years)	
Björk-Shiley monostrut	Bain (42) 1988	180	1.8	0.5	98% (5 years)	
Medtronic-Hall	Beaudet (43) 1986	164	3.5	2.1	90% (5 years)	
	Butchart (44) 1987	233	3.1		92% (5 years)	
	Antunes (45) 1988	257	3.5	3.5	82% (5 years)	Third-world population
Lillehei-Kaster	Stewart (46) 1988	193	4.6	1.5	94% (5 years)	
Omniscience	Rabago (33) 1984	32	1.2	4.7	Not available	
	Carrier (27) 1987	33	???	3.8	88% (4 years)	Includes mitral valves and thrombosis

TABLE 8–2. *Embolism Following Mitral Valve Replacement*

Valve assessed	Author and year	Number in series	Mean follow-up (years)	Linearized incidence (%/py)	Actuarial freedom	Comments
Björk-Shiley SD	Bain (41) 1985	336	7.5	1.5	93% (5 years) 84% (15 years)	
	Sethia (23) 1986	323	4.8	1.5	93% (5 years) 86% (12 years)	
	Flemma (30) 1988	268	10	1.8	90% (5 years) 83% (15 years)	
Björk-Shiley C-C	Bain (41) 1985	232	4.3	2.0	90% (5 years) 89% (9 years)	
Björk-Shiley monostrut	Bain (42) 1988	274	1.7	3.0	92% (5 years)	
	Beaudet (43) 1986	163	3.5	2.3	90% (5 years)	
Medtronic-Hall	Butchart (44) 1987	414	3.1		84% (5 years)	
	Antunes (45) 1988	386	3.5	3.1	89% (5 years)	Third-world population
	Fananapazir (32) 1983	87	1.8	3.4	50% (3 years)	Includes thrombosis
Omniscience	Rabago (33) 1984	65	1.8	2.0	Not available	
	Cortina (22) 1986	63	3.3	4.5	65%	Includes thrombosis
	Carrier (27) 1987	72	2.2	3.8	88% (4 years)	Includes aortic valves and thrombosis

3. There is a higher incidence of embolism in the early years after implantation. Consequently short series, such as those of new valves, will show a higher linearized rate of embolism.

4. Some centers still persist in regarding systemic embolism and valve thrombosis as the same complication. We maintain that they are different and should be evaluated separately (21).

5. The adequacy of the anticoagulation services varies between centers.

Despite these discrepancies, we can conclude that the reported incidence of systemic embolism with tilting disk valves is generally low and that most centers report a lower incidence for aortic than for mitral valve replacement. Our experience in Glasgow indicates that when used with meticulous anticoagulation therapy, the Björk-Shiley valve is associated with an incidence of systemic embolism that is for aortic valve replacement lower than, and, for mitral valve replacement, equal to that of porcine bioprostheses (24). Early experience with the new Omnicarbon valve, with a mean follow-up of 22 months suggests a similarly low incidence of embolism, with 95.5% free of embolic events at 3 years (25).

Periprosthetic Leak and Prosthetic Endocarditis

These complications are more patient- and surgeon-related than valve-related. The reported incidence of periprosthetic leak varies between 0.7 and 2.0%/py. Prosthetic valve endocarditis occurred at a rate of approximately 0.8%/py for all three tilting disk valves (22).

Hemolysis

A degree of subclinical hemolysis can be detected in a majority of patients with tilting disk valves. Clinical hemolysis, resulting in anemia, has rarely been reported in the absence of a periprosthetic leak. Nevertheless, the detection of subclinical hemolysis with the Medtronic-Hall valve led to the D16 modification with subsequent disk fracture in a small subset of these valves (see below). One year after implantation, the first 100 patients to receive the Björk-Shiley monostrut valve in Glasgow had a mean hemoglobin level of 14.4 g/dL, a reticulocyte count of less than 2.5%, and a mean lactate dehydrogenase concentration of 550 μmol/L (normal range 230–525). Similarly low levels of subclinical hemolysis with this valve were reported in a multicenter evaluation by Thulin et al. (26). A more significant degree of hemolysis was reported by Carrier and associates for the Omniscience valve (27).

Thrombotic Obstruction

Limitation of disk movement by the accumulation of thrombus has been the commonest acute life-threatening complication of earlier tilting disk valves. The reported incidence of this complication with different tilting disk valves is detailed in Table 8–3. Reoperation for thrombotic obstruction was reviewed by Martinell and colleagues in 1986 (28).

The incidence of thrombotic obstruction of the Björk-Shiley standard disk valve in our experience was 0.6%/py, with most events occurring after mitral valve replacement (29). A similar experience has been reported recently by Flemma and associates (30).

TABLE 8–3. *Thrombotic Obstruction Following Mitral Valve Replacement*

Valve assessed	Author and year	Number in series	Mean follow-up (years)	Linearized incidence (%/py)	Actuarial freedom	Comments
Björk-Shiley SD	Bain (41) 1985	336	7.5	0.9	94% (5 years) 85% (15 years)	
	Sethia (29) 1986	323	4.8	1.1	96% (5 years) 92% (12 years)	
Björk-Shiley C-C	Bain (41) 1985	232	4.3	none	100% (9 years)	
Björk-Shiley monostrut	Bain (42) 1988	274	1.7	none	100% (5 years)	
Medtronic-Hall	Beaudet (43) 1986	163	3.5	none	100% (5 years)	
	Butchart (44) 1987	414	3.1	none	100% (5 years)	
	Antunes (45) 1988	386	3.5	1.1	96% (5 years)	Third-world population
	Fananapazir (32) 1983	87	1.5	9.4	Not available	
Omniscience	Rabago (33) 1984	65	1.5	2.6	Not available	
	Cortina (22) 1986	63	3.3	4.5	65%	Includes embolism

The introduction of the convexo-concave disk models has abolished this complication in Glasgow with no episodes of thrombotic obstruction in more than 1000 patients over an 8-year period. Current experience with the monostrut version of the Björk-Shiley valve from several centers has revealed no incidence of thrombotic obstruction in anti-coagulated patients (26).

In a single-center comparison of three tilting disk valves, Cortina and associates found that the incidence of thrombotic obstruction of the Omniscience valve was significantly higher than that of either the Medtronic-Hall or the Björk-Shiley 70 degree C-C valves (22). Other reports have also indicated high rates of thrombotic obstruction for the Omniscience valve in the mitral position (31–33). Longer follow-up of the new Omni-carbon version will be necessary to determine whether the pyrolytic carbon valve ring will prevent the problem of thrombotic obstruction that has been associated with this valve design.

Structural Failure

Two tilting disk valves are known to have suffered from structural failure, a rare but catastrophic complication: the Medtronic-Hall valve (in a small subset of its D16 config-uration) and, to a much greater extent, the Björk-Shiley (in its 60 degree and 70 degree C-C versions).

Three instances of disk fracture of the Medtronic-Hall valve have been reported to the manufacturers. All instances occurred in a subset of 317 valves with the D16 configu-ration that had an asymmetric pyrolytic coating. The suspect valves have been withdrawn.

Fracture of the outlet (minor) strut of the Björk-Shiley valve has been reported in both the 60 degree and the 70 degree C-C versions (34). Some 80,000 such valves have been implanted worldwide, and more than 300 such fractures have been reported to date. All C-C valves have now been withdrawn from the market. The linearized incidence of strut fracture for the C-C 60 degree valve is less than 0.5%/py and decreasing with time. The

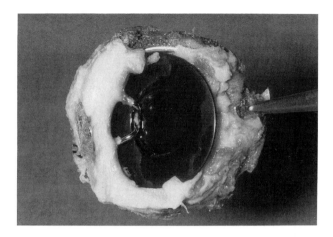

FIG. 8–6. Tissue ingrowth obstructing a Björk-Shiley standard disk valve in the tricuspid position.

incidence of this complication has been shown to be higher for mitral valve replacement with larger valves (29 to 33 mm). Recent statistical analysis appears to indicate that the risk of strut fracture in the C-C 60 degree valves, even in the higher-risk groups, is smaller than the risk of reoperation and that the hazard rate continues to decrease with time. There are therefore no current indications for elective valve rereplacement in asymptomatic patients with the C-C 60 degree valve (35). The incidence of strut fracture in the C-C 70 degree valves is higher. There may be an indication for elective rereplacement of these valves, in particular larger valves from the early manufacturing period. Statistical assessment of the comparative risks has been performed recently by Lindblom (47).

Tilting Disk Valves in the Tricuspid Position

On the rare occasions when tricuspid valve replacement is indicated, the best choice of prosthesis remains controversial. The authors have assessed 79 patients who had tricuspid valve replacement with the Björk-Shiley SD valve between 1971 and 1981. There was only one episode of thrombotic obstruction, which was successfully treated by reoperation. However, seven patients developed valve malfunction due to tissue ingrowth into the valve ring (Fig. 8–6), giving a linearized incidence of 1.4%/py. Fortunately this problem develops slowly and is readily recognized by echocardiography and Doppler ultrasound examination; reoperation is usually successful in our experience. It remains to be seen whether the newer tilting disk valves with their improved hemodynamic characteristics will be less liable to this complication.

OTHER TILTING DISK VALVES

The Sorin Valve

In 1977 Sorin Biomedical (Saluggia, Italy) produced a tilting disk valve that closely resembles the Björk-Shiley standard disk pyrolytic carbon disk valve. The disk is plano-convex and contains a radiopaque tantalum ring. It tilts within M-shaped struts that have a tapered cross-sectional contour to reduce turbulence on their downstream aspect. The sewing ring is of knitted Teflon fabric, and a carbon-coated version is available. The disk opening angle is 62 degrees.

Although this prosthesis has been available to centers in Europe and South America for 10 years, few detailed long-term reports have appeared in the literature. The prosthesis has been assessed by Pellegrini and associates (36) in Milan (mean follow-up 19.5 months), and a prospective randomized trial comparing the Sorin with the Björk-Shiley C-C valve was reported by Alfieri (37) at the Dutch Society of Thoracic Surgery in 1985. Overall performance was satisfactory, but both studies were too small for any meaningful conclusions.

A larger series of 504 single valve replacements with the Sorin valve was recently reported by Cotrufo and associates (38). In this series late mortality was remarkably low at 1.7%/py with 6-year actuarial survival of 91% for aortic valve replacement and 93% for mitral valve replacement. The incidence of systemic embolism for mitral valve replacement was 1.4%/py and compares favorably with reports on other tilting disk valves. Thrombotic obstruction, however, remains a problem and occurred in nine patients with mitral valve replacement, giving an incidence of 2.1%/py, somewhat similar to that of the SD Björk-Shiley valve used in the 1970s. The authors point out that thrombotic obstruction in their experience was associated with an overgrowth of fibrotic endothelial pannus.

The Emiks Valve

The Emiks valve appears to be very similar to the monostrut version of the Björk-Shiley valve and is manufactured and distributed in the Soviet Union. Follow-up of 148 patients yielded a survival rate of 94% for mitral and 78% for aortic valve replacement at 4 years. The incidence of systemic embolism was 2.0%/py for mitral replacement (39).

The Ultracor Valve

The Ultracor valve, designed by Kaster and reminiscent of the Lillehei-Kaster and Hall-Kaster prostheses, has a planoconvex, pyrolytic carbon disk equipped with a recess that engages an M-shaped retaining strut. The opening angle is 73 degrees in aortic valves and 68 degrees in mitral valves. The valve ring and strut are machined from one block of titanium without welds. There are as yet no substantial reports on the clinical performance of this valve.

The St. Vincent Valve

The St. Vincent valve became available in Europe in 1988 and is made in Singapore. It is reminiscent of the Björk-Shiley SD model but uses a Delrin flat disk. The valve ring and strut are machined from titanium, and the valve can be rotated within its Dacron sewing ring. The contact surfaces between the disk and struts are flat, a feature that was associated with hemolysis in other designs. The results of clinical trials with this valve have not yet appeared.

The Bicer Valve

The Bicer valve, developed in Buenos Aires and now manufactured in Canada, features a thin, biconvex lens-shaped disk that is retained by two short inflow lugs and a single outflow strut. The disk does not move downstream on opening and remains close to the ring in the region of the inflow guide lugs. The opening angle is 80 degrees and offers a relatively large effective orifice area. Clinical results are not yet available.

CURRENT PROBLEMS AND FUTURE PROSPECTS

In common with other mechanical heart valve substitutes, the use of tilting disk valves has been associated with a certain incidence of embolism, anticoagulant complications, periprosthetic leak, endocarditis, thrombosis, and structural failure. These complications may be patient-related, surgeon-related, or valve-related to varying degrees. For instance, not every embolus in a patient with a prosthetic valve is directly due to the valve: patients who have undergone closed or open mitral valvotomy have a linearized incidence of systemic embolism of 0.3 to 1.5%/py (40). The occurrence of a periprosthetic leak is related to the surgical technique and the quality of the host annulus. Anticoagulant-related hemorrhage is commonest in noncompliant patients who abuse alcohol. However, a review of the long-term performance of prosthetic valves indicates that some complications, such as thrombotic obstruction and structural failure, are clearly related to the prosthesis itself. The incidence of such complications may therefore be reduced or abolished by changes in the design of the valve or the materials used in its manufacture.

Tilting disk valves continue to occupy an important position in the range of prostheses available to today's valve surgeon. Their functional results are good, and, with careful anticoagulation, the overall incidence of systemic embolism is low. Structural failure has not been a problem with the Omniscience valve, but several reports have indicated that the incidence of thrombotic obstruction is significantly higher with this valve than with Björk-Shiley and Medtronic-Hall valves. The overall performance of the Medtronic-Hall valve has been good, and the incidence of thrombotic obstruction is low. The problem of disk fracture in a small subset of valves appears to be limited, and the valves at risk have been withdrawn. The problem of minor strut fracture in the C-C versions of the Björk-Shiley valves continues to be a source of concern in view of the large number of patients who have received these prostheses, now withdrawn. There is, however, evidence that for the 60 degree C-C valve the hazard rate is decreasing, and elective rereplacement is not advisable. The monostrut version of the Björk-Shiley valve has now been in clinical use for 8 years and has been free from both thrombotic obstruction and structural failure to date.

Prosthetic valves continue to improve, but as complication rates fall, more patients and longer follow-up are needed to detect subtle differences in clinical performance. This emphasizes the importance of continuous monitoring of patients with prosthetic heart valves in order to detect complications, recognize improvements, and thus bring the search for the perfect valve substitute closer to its successful fruition.

REFERENCES

1. Kernan MC, Newman MM, Levowitz BS, Stuckey JH: A prosthesis to replace the mitral valve. J Thorac Cardiovasc Surg 1957;33:698–706.
2. Pierce WS, Behrendt DM, Morrow AG: A hinged prosthetic cardiac valve fabricated of rigid components. J Thorac Cardiovasc Surg 1968;56:229–335.

3. Melrose DG, Bentall HH, McMillam IKR, Flege JB, Diaz FRA, Nahas RA, Fautley R, Carson J: The evolution of a mitral valve prosthesis. Lancet 1964;2:623.
4. Shaw TDR, Gunstensen J, Turner RWD: Sudden mechanical malfunction of Hammersmith mitral valve prostheses due to wear of polypropylene. J Thorac Cardiovasc Surg 1975;67:579–583.
5. Wada J: Knotless suture method and Wada hingeless valve. Jpn J Thorac Surg 1967;15:88.
6. Björk VO: Experiences with the Wada-Cutter valve prosthesis in the aortic area. One year follow-up. J Thorac Cardiovasc Surg 1970;60:26–33.
7. Cokkinos DV, Voridis E, Bakoulas G, Theodossiou A, Skalkeas GD: Thrombosis of two high-flow prosthetic valves. J Thorac Cardiovasc Surg 1971;62:947–949.
8. Knight CJ, McLeod N, Taylor DEM: Physical principles of the Edinburgh prosthetic heart valve. Med Biol Eng Comput 1977;14:264–272.
9. Bjork VO: A new tilting disc valve prosthesis. Scand J Thorac Cardiovasc Surg 1969;3:1–10.
10. Bjork VO: The central-flow tilting disc valve prosthesis (Bjork-Shiley) for mitral valve replacement. Scand J Thorac Cardiovasc Surg 1970;4:15–23.
11. Bjork VO: The improved Bjork-Shiley tilting disc valve prosthesis. Scand J Thorac Cardiovasc Surg 1978;12:81–89.
12. Vogel JHK: The monostrut Bjork-Shiley heart valve. J Am Coll Cardiol 1985;6:1142.
13. Kaster RL, Lillehei CW: A new cageless free-floating pivoting disc prosthetic heart valve: Design, development and evaluation. In Digest of the 7th International Conference of Medical and Biological Engineering, Stockholm 1967;387.
14. Kaster RL, Lillehei CW, Starek PJK: The Lillehei-Kaster pivoting disc aortic prosthesis and a comparative study of its pulsatile flow characteristics with four other prostheses. Trans Am Soc Artif Intern Organs 1970;16:233.
15. Lillehei CW, Kaster RL, Starek PJ, Bloch JH, Rees JR: A new central flow pivoting disc aortic and mitral prosthesis: Initial clinical experience. Am J Cardiol 1970;26:688. Abstract.
16. Chun PKC, Nelson WP: Common cardiac prosthetic valves. J Am Med Assoc 1977;238:401.
17. Costa IA, Faraco DL, Sallum FS: Disfuncaõ de protes de Lillehei-Kaster em posicaõ mitral. Rev Bras Med 1976;33:33.
18. Forman R, Beck W, Barnard CN: Results of valve replacement with the Lillehei-Kaster disc prosthesis. Am Heart J 1977;94:282.
19. Scotten LN, Racca RG, Nugent AH, Walker DR, Brownlea RT: New tilting disc cardiac valve prostheses. In vitro comparison of their hydrodynamic performance in the mitral position. J Thorac Cardiovasc Surg 1981;82:136–146.
20. Hall KV, Kaster RL, Woien A: An improved pivotal disc type prosthetic heart valve. J Oslo City Hosp 1979;29:3.
21. Nashef SAM, Bain WH: Valve-related events: A system of definitions. Thorac Cardiovasc Surg 1987;35:232–234.
22. Cortina J, Martinell J, Artiz V, Fraile J, Rabago G: Comparative clinical results with Omniscience (STM1), Medtronic-Hall and Bjork-Shiley convexo-concave (70 degrees) prostheses in mitral valve replacement. J Thorac Cardiovasc Surg 1986;91:174–183.
23. Lindblom D, Lindblom U, Henze A, Bjork VO, Semb BKH: Three-year clinical results with the monostrut Bjork-Shiley prosthesis. J Thorac Cardiovasc Surg 1987;94:34–43.
24. Nashef SAM, Sethia B, Turner MA, Davidson KG, Lewis S, Bain WH: Bjork-Shiley and Carpentier-Edwards valves: A comparative analysis. J Thorac Cardiovasc Surg 1987;93:394–404.
25. Thevenet A, Albat B, Thevenet E: Clinical experience with the Omnicarbon cardiac valve prosthesis. J Cardiovasc Surg 1988;29:22. Abstract.
26. Thulin LI, Bain WH, Huysmans HH, Van Ingen G, Prieto I, Basile F, Lindblom DA, Olin CL: Heart valve replacement with the Bjork-Shiley monostrut valve: Early results of a multicenter clinical investigation. Ann Thorac Surg 1988;45:164–170.
27. Carrier M, Martineau JP, Bonan R, Pelletier LC: Clinical and hemodynamic assessment of the Omniscience prosthetic heart valve. J Thorac Cardiovasc Surg 1987;93:300–307.
28. Martinell J, Fraile J, Artiz V, Cortina P, Fresneda P, Rabago G: Reoperations for left-sided low-profile mechanical prosthetic obstruction. Ann Thorac Surg 1987;43:172–175.
29. Sethia B, Turner MA, Lewis S, Rodger RA, Bain WH: Fourteen years' experience with the Bjork-Shiley tilting disc prosthesis. J Thorac Cardiovasc Surg 1986;91:350–362.
30. Flemma RJ, Muller DC, Kleinman LH, Werner PH, Andersen AJ, Weirauch E: Survival and event-free analysis of 785 patients with Bjork-Shiley spherical disc valves at 10 to 16 years. Ann Thorac Surg 1988;45:258–272.
31. Ohlmeier H, Mannebach H, Greitemeier A: Clinical follow-up of patients with Omniscience cardiac valves. Can this valve be recommended? Z Kardiol 1982;71:350–356.
32. Fananapazir L, Clarke DB, Dark JF, Lawson RAM, Moussalli H: Results of valve replacement with the Omniscience prosthesis. J Thorac Cardiovasc Surg 1983;86:621–625.
33. Rabago G, Martinell J, Fraile J, Andrade IG, Montenegro R: Results and complications with the Omniscience prosthesis. J Thorac Cardiovasc Surg 1984;87:136–140.

34. Lindblom D, Bjork VO, Semb BKH: Mechanical failure of the Bjork-Shiley valve. J Thorac Cardiovasc Surg 1986;92:894–907.
35. Hiratzka LF, Kouchoukos NT, Grunkemeier GL, Miller DC, Scully HE, Wechsler AS: Outlet strut fracture of the Bjork-Shiley 60 degree convexo-concave valve: Current information and recommendations for patient care. J Am Coll Cardiol 1988;11:1130–1137.
36. Pellegrini A, Peronace B, Marcazzan E, Rossi C, Colombo T: Results of valve replacement surgery with mechanical prostheses. Int J Artif Organs 1982;5:27–32.
37. Alfieri O, Van Swieten H, Pryczkowski J, Vermeulen F, Knaefen P, De Geest R, Defann J, De La Riviere AB, Van Riempst AS: In Proceedings of Congress of the Dutch Society of Thoracic Surgery, Rotterdam, 11 May, 1985.
38. Cotrufo M, Festa M, Renzulli A, de Luca L, Sante P, Giannolo B: Clinical results after cardiac valve replacement with the Sorin prosthesis. Eur J Cardio-thorac Surg 1988;2:355–359.
39. Iskrenko AV, Tarichko UV, Konstantinov BA: Five years experience with the Emiks and Liks prosthetic valve: Early and late results of 162 valve replacements. J Cardiovasc Surg 1988;29:22. Abstract.
40. Silverton NP, Tandon AP, Ionescu MI: Thrombosis, embolism and anticoagulant-related haemorrhage in patients with mitral valve disease. In Ionescu MI and Cohn LH (eds): Mitral Valve Disease. London, Butterworths, 1985, pp 337–347.
41. Bain WH, Sethia B, Turner MA, Rodger R: Fifteen years experience with the Bjork-Shiley tilting disc prosthesis. Cardiac Prostheses Symposium. Montreux: Shiley Inc, pp 271–281, 1985.
42. Ban WH, Pollock JCS Rodger RA: Five years experience of the Bjork-Shiley monostrut prosthesis: Valve-related events and haemodynamic performance. J Cardiovasc Surg 1988;29:5. Abstract.
43. Beaudet RL, Poirier NL, Doyle D, Nakhle G, Gauvin C: The Medtronic Hall cardiac valve: 7 years clinical experience. Ann Thorac Surg 1986;42:644–650.
44. Butchart EG, Lewis PA, Grunkemeier GL, Kulatilake N, Breckenenridge IM: Low risk of thrombosis and serious embolic events despite low intensity anticoagulation: Experience with 1004 Medtronic-Hall valves. Poster presentation at American Heart Association, Anaheim, 1987.
45. Antunes MJ, Wessels A, Sadowski RG, Schultz JG, Vanderdonck KM, Oliveira J, Fernandes LE: Medtronic Hall valve replacement in a third-world population group. J Thorac Cardiovasc Surg 1988;95:980–993.
46. Stewart S, Hicks GL, De Weese JA: The Lillehei-Kaster aortic valve prosthesis: Long term results in 273 patients with 1273 patient-years of follow-up. J Thorac Cardiovasc Surg 1988;95:1023–1030.
47. Lindblom D, Rodriguez L, Björk VO: Mechanical failure of the Bjork-Shiley valve: Updated follow-up and considerations on prophylactic replacement. J Thorac Cardiovasc Surg 1989;97:95–97.

Bodnar, E. and Frater, R. W. M., editors
(1991) *Replacement Cardiac Valves,*
Pergamon Press, Inc. (New York), pp. 201–228
Printed in the United States of America

CHAPTER 9

BILEAFLET VALVES

Dieter Horstkotte and Endre Bodnar

HISTORICAL PERSPECTIVES

The bileaflet principle, a hinge mechanism, and a low profile are basic to the design features of currently used bileaflet heart valve prostheses. Certain elements of this design were used earlier in the Gott-Daggett (1), Kalke-Lillehei (2), and Wada prostheses (3).

Clinical experiences with the hinge bileaflet prosthesis were first reported in 1964 when the Gott-Daggett valve was introduced (1). This valve had two semicircular leaflets retained within the ring by four hinges. The leaflets opened on the two sides without creating a third, central orifice, hence the name "butterfly valve." The consequent lack of proper washout on the outflow surface was probably the most important cause of the marked thrombogenicity of this valve. Follow-up experiences with 67 operative survivors ranged from two to five years and revealed an incidence of prosthetic valve thrombosis as high as 5.9% per patient year, and of embolic complications of 12.8% per patient year (4).

The thrombogenicity of this valve could not be reduced by (for the first time in heart surgery) application of a colloid graphite coating on the synthetic surfaces (5). The prosthesis was, therefore, withdrawn from clinical use (4).

The Gott-Daggett prosthesis remains, however, not only a significant forerunner of the bileaflet design, but a milestone in the development of thromboresistant materials, leading eventually to the introduction of pyrolitic carbon, in particular Pyrolite®, to heart valve manufacture.

The Kalke-Lillehei and Wada designs had, in those days, the perceived advantage of a lack of hinges. They had a central orifice, in addition to the two lateral ones, to improve hemodynamic function and to facilitate washout on either side of the leaflets (2, 3). Neither the Kalke-Lillehei, nor the Wada valve reached the clinical stage.

Although these 1960s prostheses failed due to mechanical malfunctions and high thrombogenicity, the most striking finding from the early studies of bileaflet prostheses was that their hemodynamic performances were superior to that of all other prostheses available at that time.

In 1976, the bileaflet design was modified and refined for manufacture entirely from pyrolitic carbon (6), which replaced the titanium of the valve ring, as well as the different materials used earlier for the leaflets. In vitro and later clinical experiences showed that using pyrolitic carbon, the hinged bileaflet design was not prone to disastrous mechanical failures, and that, in addition, Pyrolite was particularly biocompatible and thromboresistant material. Shortly after the first clinical implants in 1977, data were forthcoming to show a superior hemodynamic performance and a near normal flow profile (7), contributing to excellent clinical results (8).

CURRENTLY AVAILABLE BILEAFLET PROSTHESES

The clinical evidence showed that by using the appropriate material, the hinged bileaflet design was durable, had a low thrombogenicity, and superior hemodynamics. These results led to intensive research to improve this type of mechanical valve. However, no more than three bileaflet valves have reached the clinical stage so far. The St. Jude Medical valve was introduced in 1977 and received FDA approval in 1983. The Hemex-Duromedics valve was first implanted in 1982 (9); FDA approval was granted in 1986. Clinical use of the CarboMedics prosthesis was started in 1986 (10). The FDA approval process for this valve is under way. A comparison of basic design characteristics and other data for these three prostheses are given in Table 9–1.

St. Jude Medical Prosthesis

Since the first clinical implant in 1977, about 300,000 mitral (model M101) and aortic (model A101) prostheses have been implanted worldwide. The design and manufacture of the prostheses remained unchanged until 1989, when a metal ring was incorporated into the sewing ring for better X-ray imaging. Currently, St. Jude Medical has two sources of carbon components: Pyrolite® from Carbomedics Inc. (Austin, TX) and, since 1986, St. Jude Medical's own pyrolitic carbon.

Edwards-Duromedics Prosthesis

Since its introduction in March 1982, about 23,000 mitral (model 3160R) and aortic (model 9120R) Duromedics valves have been implanted worldwide. The prosthesis was originally introduced to the market as the Hemex valve (Hemex Scientific, Inc.). During the early years of marketing, the assembly was done in Scotland (Thackeray, Ltd.), and

TABLE 9–1. *Design Characteristics and Implant Data for the Three Commercially Available Prostheses*

	St. Jude Medical	Edwards-Duromedics	CarboMedics
First implantation	1977	1982	1986
Estimated number of implants*	290,000	24,000	18,000
One year results	Available	Available	No peer review
Five year results	Available	Available	N/A
Ten year results	Available	N/A	N/A
Leaflets			
Shape	Flat	Curved	Flat
Content of tungsten	4–5 10%	20%	20%
Opening angle (degrees)	85(M)/85(A)	73(M)/77(A)	78(M)/78(A)
Closing angle (degrees)	120(M)†/180(A)‡	180(M)/180(A)	130(M)/130(A)
Travel angle (degrees)	55(M)†/60(A)‡	73(M)/77(A)	53(M)/53(A)
Housing	Pyrolitic carbon over graphite	Solid Pyrolite	Solid Pyrolite
Stiffener ring	NO	YES	YES
Cuff	Dacron	Dacron/Teflon	Dacron

*Up to October 1990

†Sizes 25 mm or less

‡Sizes 27 mm or larger

§All three valves have pyrolitic carbon over tungsten-enriched substrate those valves were marketed as "Duromedics valves." After the takeover of Hemex, Inc. by the Edwards CVS Division of the Baxter Healthcare Corporation in 1985, the name was changed to "Edwards-Duromedics valve." The prosthesis, however, remained the same.

The marketing of this valve was suspended in 1986 after a series of prosthetic valve malfunctions (leaflet escape). Following minor modifications of the construction, and refinements in production (in order to eliminate leaflet escape to as high a degree as possible), the valve returned to the market in 1990. The major changes to the refined Edwards-Duromedics prosthesis are:

1. Design tolerance adjustments. The housing seating lip radius, which was an unspecified dimension with a reference value, was specified. The pivot slot location tolerance was tightened to allow for only unloaded pivots. The flat-to-flat matchup orifices were also tightened and the reference radius within the circumference of the pivot slot was specified. The housing safety stop was modified to blend into the new specification for the seating lip radius, to avoid any dimensional conflict between the safety stop and the seating lip.

2. Modification of the mitral sewing ring by replacmeent of a Teflon felt with a silicone rubber filler. Within the sewing ring, the titanium retainer ring, which fits over the housing stiffener, was slightly changed in geometry and, in addition, a silicone rubber O-ring was placed between the retainer and stiffener to act as a shock wave absorber.

3. Modification of the aortic sewing ring by replacement of the Teflon felt with a silicone rubber filler, together with the addition of a Mylar ring and washer. As in the mitral ring modification, the outside dimensions remain identical. Also, the dacron cloth is stitched together on the inner portion of the ring. The sewing technique prevents cloth tail pullout.

4. Additional quality control inspections have also been added to the manufacturing process: dye penetrant inspection for microporosity with a criterion of no penetration allowed, contact mapping to confirm seating lip contact, and dimensional inspection and matching to confirm that unloaded pivot balls are in the closed position.

CarboMedics Prosthesis

The valve was released for clinical use in December 1986 by Carbomedics, Inc. (Austin, TX) and about 17,000 mitral (model 700) and aortic (model 500) valves have been implanted so far.

TECHNICAL CONSIDERATIONS AT SURGERY

The potential for impeded leaflet movement due to interference with cardiac structures is slim, as the open leaflets are positioned in the middle of the bloodstream and enclosed within the ring in the closed position. Leaflets of Edwards-Duromedics valves are relatively exposed, as they protrude the most from the cage during valve opening. In theory, the St. Jude valve is the most protected as the leaflets hardly protrude from the valve ring, even during maximum opening. This feature makes the St. Jude valve particularly beneficial in complex outflow tract obstruction, septum hypertrophy, and small aortic annulus.

For surgical technical considerations, the orientation of bileaflet valves within the heart seems to be of minor importance. However, for postoperative hemodynamics and consequent thromboembolic complications, as well as for noninvasive imaging, orientation may be important. With in vitro flow studies in pulse duplicators, it has not so far been demonstrated that orientation does affect the flow performance (11, 12). In clinical practice, the preferential orientations appear to contradict each other. For aortic replacement, it is recommended to place one pivot guard (or the axis of the leaflets if there is no pivot guard, as in the CarboMedics prosthesis) at the commissure between the right and noncoronary cusp and the other at the center of the left coronary cusp (13). In contrast, a 120 degree rotation has also been suggested, placing one pivot guard at the commissure between the left and the noncoronary cusp and the other at the middle of the right coronary cusp (14). These differences in recommended orientations relate to the perception of the potential influence of the intraventricular septum, especially in cases with asymmetrical septal hypertrophy on flow conditions across the prosthesis. There is, however, no evidence from the literature as to which of the placement methods lessens the potential for compromise of the anterior flow.

In the mitral position, anatomical positioning of the prosthesis by placing the two pivot guards at the natural commissures (13) is recommended, as well as rotating the prosthesis by 90 degrees and inserting the two pivot guards into the middle of the anterior and the posterior mitral leaflets (14). The rationale for the latter is to avoid the vicinity of the posterior ventricular wall, which might interfere with the full opening and closing of the adjacent leaflet of the prosthesis. This would carry the potential for an asynchronous leaflet movement and consequent thrombosis (15).

It has to be noted, however, that such interference is highly unlikely with the St. Jude Medical valve, where the leaflets are well protected within the housing. Valve related complications, including valve thrombosis, embolism, sudden death, perivalvular leaks, and hemolysis, were found to be identical whether the St. Jude valves in the mitral position were anatomically or anti-anatomically orientated (16). Another in vivo study, however, concludes that the anatomical orientation creates a smoother washout in the left ventricle (17).

CLINICAL INVESTIGATIONS WITH BILEAFLET PROSTHESES

Comparability of Published Results

A comparative review of the three bileaflet valves is hardly possible. The first difficulty arises from the fact that the length of time for the available follow-up information, as well as the numbers implanted, are widely different. In addition to this, discrepancies exist in the number of relevant publications; a computer search for the purpose of this chapter using DIMDI and MEDLINE databases and the three valves generated a total of 1040 references in peer review journals for the St. Jude Medical, 98 references for the Edwards-Duromedics and only two publications, not clinically oriented, for the CarboMedics valves. There is no publication available on the new generation Edwards-Duromedics valve. Not more than seven publications report on comparative assessment of the different bileaflet valves. There are neither level one (randomized trials with low false-positive and false-negative errors) nor level two studies (random errors) available for comparing the performances of the different bileaflet valves. The picture is further obscured by differences in the patient population, the presence of incremental risk factors, the late effects of myocardial protection during surgery, and several other factors (18, 19).

The potential bias introduced by these factors cannot be eliminated unless a truly randomised study is conducted (20). Such a study, however, is yet to be completed to compare the bileaflet valves. These are the reasons why a scientifically sound comparison is so difficult to make.

Those operative studies comparing the St. Jude Medical and the Edwards-Duromedics prostheses in a nonrandomised fashion could not reveal any difference in terms of clinical improvement, intrinsic dysfunction, or actuarial survival in a 48 months postoperative period (21).

It is very unfortunate that even in the case of a randomised study valid comparisons cannot necessarily be made, and scientific interpretation of the data may remain impossible, due to the way in which the data are presented. This is the case with a randomised comparison of the Björk-Shiley, St. Jude Medical, and Starr-Edwards valves, where the Björk-Shiley and Starr-Edwards subpopulations were grouped together, making it impossible to decide whether the complications were caused by one or the other of the two prostheses in the same group (22). It is stressed again that results from a randomised prospective trial involving different bileaflet prostheses are not available in the literature.

Subjective and Clinical Improvement

The subjective improvement after heart valve replacement depends on the postoperative status of the pulmonary circulation, and the function of the left ventricle.

If the preoperative diagnosis was mitral stenosis or mixed mitral valve disease, the pulmonary artery pressure will have a decisive role. In case of pure mitral incompetence or aortic valve disease indicating valve replacement, the postoperative left ventricular function will determine the degree of subjective as well as clinical improvement. However, significant differences may exist between subjective and clinical improvement in individual cases (23), which may be due to nothing more than the patient's unrealistic expectations prior to surgery. An important factor in this respect is the preoperative functional status which will serve as the point of reference for the patient.

As a consequence, the comparison of subjective and clinical improvement is impossible unless it is done as stage I of a randomized trial. However, this has not yet been attempted with the bileaflet prostheses.

Nevertheless, functional and clinical results for periods of up to 10 years have been reported with the St. Jude valve in a number of publications. It appears that on average, a NYHA class 1.5 improvement can be expected after isolated aortic valve replacement with this prosthesis (24, 25).

It is suggested that the correct timing of surgery (that is, before irreversible myocardiac damage can occur) will result in a marked improvement in the postoperative status.

Prosthetic Valve Noise

The sound generated by the opening and closing of mechanical valves can be found disturbing by some patients. The prostheses clicks are transmitted by the tissue layers and airways within the chest. Those with a high tone sound sensitivity may find the high tone clicks exceeding 8 kHz especially unpleasant, and cannot become accustomed to them. Sleeplessness and a desire to have the culprit valve replaced by another, less noisy model may result. The noise level of the bileaflet prostheses is less than that of the caged-ball valves. The noise level of the St. Jude valve is 40 ± 7 dB(A) and that of the Edwards-Duromedics valve is 47 ± 7 dB(A) at a 10 cm distance from the chest, and it is 24 ± 4 dB(A) and 39 ± 6 dB(A) respectively (p < 0.001) at a 1 m distance (26).

The 15 dB(A) difference between these two noise levels corresponds to a nine-fold increase in sound pressure on the logarithmic dB(A) scale. This is the explanation as to why patients with the Edwards-Duromedics valve suffer sleeplessness three times as often as those with the St. Jude prosthesis, and 11% of them feel disturbed during day time activities (26). This important difference is thought to be caused by pertinent design characteristics.

There is no published information on the noise generated by the CarboMedics valve. The sound pressure generated by a mitral prosthesis is higher than that of an aortic. This is due to the larger valve size and the consequent larger mass and closing impact of the leaflets. There is a positive correlation between measurable sound pressure and patient complaints. At present, however, it is not known whether a larger body surface area could dampen the sound pressures of a prosthesis (26).

Postoperative Functional Capacity

After mitral valve replacement, an increase in the functional capacity as assessed by exercise tests has been reported to be 40–100% (27). Differences in the increase of functional capacity may depend on hemodynamic properties of the implanted valve type and on the pulmonary vascular resistance which may remain elevated postoperatively.

Functional capacity was measured by having patients climb stairs until dypsnea appeared, and using this test, differences have been found between prostheses; for instance, the increase of functional capacity was 74% in patients with Ionescu-Shiley, 180% with St. Jude, 171% with Björk-Shiley, and 128% with Starr-Edwards prostheses. Although conclusions drawn from these findings may be restricted due to the fact that the comparison was not randomised, the greater increase of functional capacity after implantation of a bileaflet mechanical prosthesis compared with a pericardial tissue valve or a caged-ball prosthesis, and the correlation between functional capacity and simultaneously measured pulmonary artery pressures are obvious (28, 29).

In another study, the pulmonary artery pressure at rest and during bicycle exercise (in the supine position) was compared in four groups of patients, each having different prosthetic valves but matching preoperative clinical and hemodynamic parameters, as well as left ventricular function.

In the St. Jude Medical group of this study, the pulmonary artery pressure increased from 9.7 ± 9.1 mmHg at rest, to 26.1 ± 9.9 mmHg at 30 Watts bicycle exercise, and 37.4 ± 13.9 mmHg at 150 Watts. Twelve percent of patients with St. Jude Medical prostheses had to stop exercise at the 30 Watts level, while 51% could tolerate 150 Watts or more. In contrast, in the Ionescu-Shiley group the pulmonary artery pressure increased from 24.7 ± 4.9 mmHg at rest to 37.3 ± 7.5 mmHg at 30 Watts bicycle exercise, and to 58.1 ± 14.0 mmHg at 150 Watts bicycle exercise. Twenty-five percent of these patients had to stop at the 30 Watts level and only 22% tolerated 90 Watts, none reaching the 150 Watts level (Fig. 9–1). Results with the Starr-Edwards and Björk-Shiley prostheses have been found to be between those described for the St. Jude and the Ionescu-Shiley valves (25).

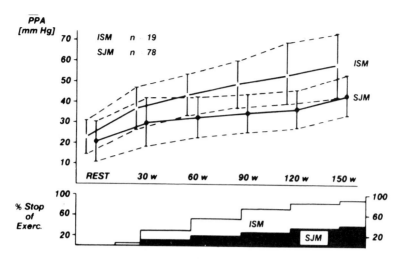

FIG. 9–1. Mean pulmonary pressure (PPA) during rest and exercise (measured in watts) after mitral valve replacement with St. Jude Medical (SJM) and Ionescu-Shiley (ISM) valves. % Stop of Exercise = percentage of patients who stopped at that level of exercise.

PROGNOSIS AFTER BILEAFLET VALVE REPLACEMENT

As none of the existing replacement valves are a perfect substitute for the natural valve, complications caused by these prostheses remain a subsequent source of mortality after valve replacement.

The cumulative survival rates and rates of freedom from complications which are commonly used to assess long term valve performances would have to be compared ideally to similar survival functions of an age- and sex-matched group of the general population and to the survival of those patients who received medical rather than surgical treatment. Unfortunately, the former is not always readily available and the latter could not be done in a randomised fashion for ethical reasons. However, a medically treated group of patients in whom heart valve replacement is indicated but not performed for different reasons can be used for comparisons. In such cases, patients have been used who either refused the recommended operation, or in whom the operation has not been performed because of a lack of operative capacity in the early 1970s (30, 31).

Comparing consecutive patients operated on between 1978 and 1980 who had received Björk-Shiley, St. Jude Medical, and Ionescu-Shiley pericardial valves for mitral valve replacement, revealed only slight differences in survival after 10 years of follow-up (Fig. 9–2). Survival was significantly more favorable than the prognosis of patients without operation (natural history group).

Cumulative survival of consecutive patients operated on for aortic valve replacement during the same time frame is shown in Fig. 9–3. All prostheses, irrespective of type or size, provided statistically significantly better survival compared with the natural history of patients with aortic valve disease. Another, comparative analysis of medically and surgically treated patients with aortic valve disease revealed higher differences between these two groups if the diagnosis was stenosis (p < 0.000001) than if it was insufficiency (p < 0.0001).

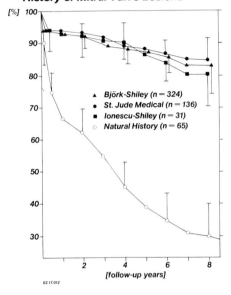

Cumulative Survival after Mitral Valve Replacement Compared to the Natural History of Mitral Valve Lesions

▲ Björk-Shiley (n = 324)
● St. Jude Medical (n = 136)
■ Ionescu-Shiley (n = 31)
○ Natural History (n = 65)

[follow-up years]

02.17.012

FIG. 9–2. Cumulative survival after mitral valve replacement compared to the natural history of mitral valve disease.

IN VIVO HEMODYNAMIC FINDINGS

The large effective orifice area of the bileaflet valves, especially that of the St. Jude valve with its theroretical 85 degree opening angle contributes to creating a flat, near normal flow profile with far less obstruction and turbulence, as compared with earlier generations of replacement valves (12, 32–37). It follows that there is development of only minor laminar shear forces as measured on the St. Jude valve.

In vitro studies of both the Edwards-Duromedics and the CarboMedics valves found a somewhat higher transvalvular pressure gradient but a lower closing reflux compared with the St. Jude valve (38).

In native mitral valves, clinical signs and symptoms of mitral stenosis are present if the orifice area is reduced to less than 1.5 cm^2 in adults (39). The most commonly used outer diameter of a prosthetic heart valve used in adult patients is 29 mm, where the in vivo measured valve orifice area varies between 1.7 and 3.2 cm^2, depending on the type of the prosthesis (24, 27, 28). Therefore, the design characteristics may determine whether a given prosthesis will produce signs and symptoms of mitral stenosis or not.

Taking into account the reported effective valve orifice areas of different mechanical and tissue valves, it can be demonstrated that all prostheses cause mild to moderate obstruction. For 29 mm mitral prostheses, the effective orifice area has been reported to be 2.2–2.5 cm^2 for Björk-Shiley, 1.9–3.2 cm^2 for Medtronic-Hall, 1.9–2.0 cm^2 for the Ionescu-Shiley pericardial tissue valve, 1.3–2.7 cm^2 for the Hancock prosthesis, and 2.2–3.0 cm^2 for the Carpentier-Edwards porcine valve. In comparison, the St. Jude valve has a calculated orifice area of 2.8–3.4 cm^2.

The flow/pressure relationship of five mechanical valves and the Ionescu-Shiley peri-

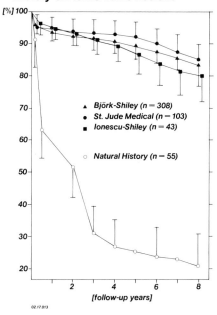

Cumulative Survival after Aortic Valve
Replacement Compared to the Natural
History of Aortic Valve Lesions

▲ Björk-Shiley (n = 308)
● St. Jude Medical (n = 103)
■ Ionescu-Shiley (n = 43)

○ Natural History (n = 55)

[follow-up years]

02.17.013

FIG. 9–3. Cumulative survival after aortic valve replacement compared to the natural history of aortic valve disease.

cardial valve, all of which are mitral valves with a tissue annulus diameter of 29 mm (or the nearest possible size when 29 mm size prostheses were not available) was compared under identical conditions at rest and during exercise. The results with Starr-Edwards, St. Jude medical, and Ionescu-Shiley mitral prostheses of equal size are given in Figs. 9–4 and 9–5, and they suggest that, with regard to the flow-pressure relationship, the bileaflet design seems to be superior to all other valve designs.

The flow/pressure relationship is similar after aortic and mitral valve replacements. The residual transaortic pressure gradient is of only minor importance with the usual valve sizes, with normal prosthetic function, and when left ventricular function is not severely impaired (40). However, in the case of a small aortic annulus, which only allows the implantation of valves less than 21 mm in outer diameter, high residual transaortic gradients may undermine the postoperative results (41, 42). To create an adequate effective orifice area, additional surgical procedures are recommended. Due to the favorable flow/pressure relationship, bileaflet prostheses may have significant advantages if only small aortic valves can be used.

We did not find a significant difference between effective and geometric orifice area with the 25 mm St. Jude Medical bileaflet aortic prosthesis. This is in contrast to a number of results with other replacement valves, especially with bioprostheses. A low pressure gradient was also measured across CarboMedics valves in the mitral position. Published data on comparative hemodynamic assessment of the St. Jude and Edwards-Duromedics prostheses are summarized in Table 9–2 for the mitral, and in Table 9–3 for the aortic positions (35, 43).

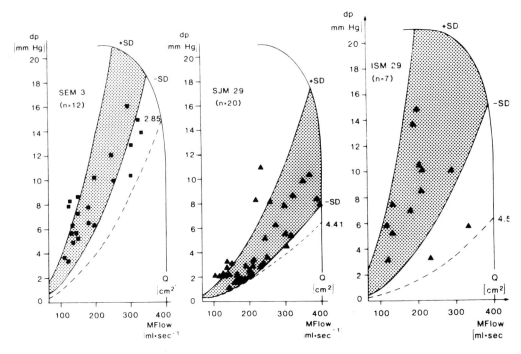

Fig. 9–4. Flow/pressure relationship of Starr-Edwards (SEM), St. Jude Medical (SJM), and Ionescu-Shiley (ISM) valves in the mitral position.

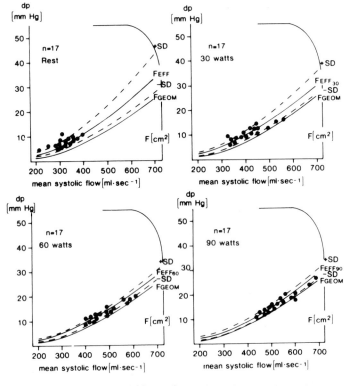

Fig. 9–5. Flow/pressure relationship of 29 mm St. Jude Medical mitral prostheses at rest and during exercise.

210

TABLE 9–2. *In Vivo Hemodynamic Findings for the St. Jude Mechanical (SJM) and the Edwards-Duromedics (ED)* Mitral Prostheses with an Outer Diameter of 29 mm*

	SJM 29 rest	SJM 29 30 watts	ED 29 rest
Total valve area (cm2)	6.61	6.61	6.61
Primary orifice area (cm^2)	4.52	4.52	4.25
Mitral FB-flow (mL/sec)	167 ± 42	291 ± 73	131 ± 16
dP† (mmHg)	2.3 ± 0.6	6.4 ± 3.0	4.1 ± 2.7
Effective orifice area (cm^2)	3.1 ± 0.8	3.4 ± 0.7	2.4 ± 1.8
Effective/primary orifice areas	0.69	0.73	0.56
PI†	0.47	0.51	0.36

*Calculated from the original published in JP Pomar et al. (1986)

†dP = mean diastolic pressure loss; PI = performance index (effective to total valve area ratio).

THERAPY AFTER VALVE REPLACEMENT

General Considerations

Long term medical therapy after valve replacement in general includes oral anticoagulation, endocarditis prophylaxis, and, in certain cases, the restoration of sinus rhythm. This is also true with bileaflet prostheses.

Special Considerations after Bileaflet Valve Replacement

The excellent biocompatibility and thromboresistance of Pyrolite®, combined with good hemodynamic characteristics gave rise to the assumption that patients with a St. Jude valve in the aortic position may not have to receive anticoagulant treatment. In reality, however, the contrary has been proved. Follow-up information on the St. Jude valve emerged, and data on the rate of thromboembolism, with and without anticoagu-

TABLE 9–3. *In Vivo Hemodynamic Findings for the St. Jude Medical (SJM) and the Edwards-Duromedics (ED)* Aortic Prostheses with Outer Diameters of 23 or 25 mm*

	SJM 23 rest	SJM 23 30 watts	ED 23 rest	SJM 25 rest	SJM 25 30 watts
Total valve area (cm^2)	4.15	4.15	4.15	4.91	4.91
Primary orifice area (cm^2)	2.55	2.55	2.36	3.09	3.09
Aortic flow (mL/sec)	299 ± 52	433 ± 64	229 ± 26	317 ± 50	433 ± 75
dP† (mmHg)	9.6 ± 3.1	15.7 ± 3.2	18.0 ± 7.1	7.7 ± 2.2	11.7 ± 2.2
Effective orifice area (cm^2)	2.2 ± 0.3	2.5 ± 0.3	1.3 ± 0.4	2.6 ± 0.4	2.9 ± 0.3
Effective/primary orifice areas ratio	0.86	0.96	0.55	0.84	0.93
PI†	0.53	0.59	0.31	0.53	0.58

*Calculated from the original data published in JP Pomar et al. (1980)

†dP = mean systolic pressure loss; PI = Performance index (effective to total valve area ratio).

lation, have made it clear that this valve is not exempt from the pitfalls of mechanical prostheses in general; lifelong anticoagulation is necessary, just as with any other mechanical valve (44). Platelet inhibitors alone proved to be inefficient.

Nonetheless, the relatively low thrombogenicity of the bileaflet valve is considered by Nair et al. to be such as to justify only a moderate level of anticoagulation, keeping the International Normalized Ratio (INR) between 1.5 and 2.5 (45). In the experience of the Düsseldorf Medical University, an INR of 2–2.5 and 2.5–3.5 is necessary with aortic and mitral St. Jude valve replacements, respectively.

The cumulative rate of thrombosis, embolism, and bleeding was assessed in 165 patients having at least one St. Jude valve, by Nair et al. (45). After nine years at risk, the cumulative rate for those who did not receive any treatment was 30%, for those on an aspirin/dipyrodamol regime 50%, for the warfarin group 11%, and for those who had dipyrodamol in addition to warfarin, 8%. Other studies confirm that prophylaxis with platelet inhibitors alone increases the risk of thromboembolism 3.4–4.3 times. Without any antithrombotic therapy, the risk increases by 19.8 times (46).

NONINVASIVE ASSESSMENT OF VALVE FUNCTION

Notwithstanding the progress that has been made in valve design, materials, and medical science, all replacement valves currently in clinical use carry a certain risk of valve related or valve induced complications (47, 48). Valve related complications include thrombosis, embolism, prosthetic valve endocarditis, mechanical dysfunction, and hemolysis; valve induced complications include occasional scar tissue ingrowth. The side effects of the long term medical therapy, that is, anticoagulant bleeding, are foremost among the variety of possible complications (49, 50).

The instantaneous rate of hazard for any complication is by far the highest during the first six months postoperatively. After that period some complications, like thrombosis and embolism, have a fairly constant hazard rate during the years of follow up, while others, like paravalvular leak or primary tissue failure of bioprostheses, appear to have a decreasing or increasing rate with time, respectively (18).

It cannot be stressed strongly enough that, although the hazard rates may increase or decrease during given periods of the follow up, the respective rates never reach zero for any of the above mentioned complications (19). This makes the regular control of patients after heart valve replacement mandatory. The bileaflet valves are not exempt from this rule.

Medical checkups after valve replacement cannot be limited to the diagnosis and/or treatment of complications. A thorough investigation has to be completed at regular intervals, partly to document the normal functioning of the prosthesis and partly to establish a base line of parameters for comparison if any complication is suspected.

Such lifelong series of investigations must not cause any discomfort to the patient, nor may they carry any risk. Furthermore, the cost/benefit ratio has to be acceptable for the health organizations of the individual countries. The noninvasive methods eminently qualify for this role. In a large series of patients with prosthetic valve malfunction, clinical examination, auscultation, and phonomechanocardiography led to correct diagnoses in 63% of all cases (51).

Auscultation and Phonomechanocardiography

Auscultation remains a basic method of clinical assessment after heart valve replacement, and it demands the knowledge of all those opening and closing clicks, and systolic and/or diastolic murmurs which are characteristic of the individual prosthesis types and are present without any malfunction of the prosthesis.

Grade 1/6 or 2/6 systolic murmur is present in about 25% of patients with a bileaflet valve in the aortic position. This is thought to be due to turbulent flow (51). Diastolic murmur is exceptional with these valves in the aortic position, in spite of the reflux across the closed valve, a feature inherent in the design. This backflow does not exceed 4%–8% of the forward flow; therefore, in the vast majority of cases it does not generate an audible murmur.

A mid-diastolic rumble can be present, though not frequently, with bileaflet valves in the mitral position. It most probably represents the asynchronous closing of the two leaflets, first reported in 1981 (53, 54). This asynchronous closing is a possibility, and has been confirmed clinically, with all bileaflet prostheses (Fig. 9–6). The time interval between the closing of the two leaflets is 5.5 ± 1.8 msec (range 1.0–16 msec) for mitral, and 4.4 ± 2.1 msec (range 1–7.5 msec) for aortic models of the St. Jude valve. It is 4.0 ± 2.4 msec (range 1.0–7.8 msec) for the aortic Edwards-Duromedics valve (55).

A closing click is audible in more than 90% of mitral, and nearly 100% of aortic bileaflet valves currently in clinical use, irrespective of the design and/or make (51).

A new regurgitant murmur or a regurgitant murmur of abnormal intensity was recorded in 100% of cases with paraprosthetic leak and in 73% with prosthetic valve thrombosis in the Düsseldorf experience. About 70% of prosthetic valve endocarditis cases present with a new regurgitant murmur due to the developing paravalvular leak. A new stenotic murmur was heard in 80% of patients with tissue ingrowth, in 85% with valve thrombosis, and in 23% with thrombendocarditis.

In patients followed up in Düsseldorf a weakening or loss of prosthetic clicks was present in 100% of patients with prosthetic valve thrombosis and in about 10% with thrombendocarditis. However, tissue ingrowth never created a regurgitant murmur, nor did it cause disappearance or even weakening of any of the prosthetic clicks. Although it is

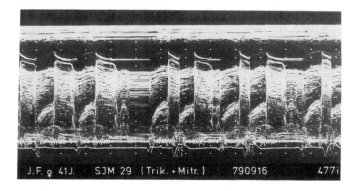

Fig. 9–6. Echocardiogram showing asynchronous closure of a St. Jude Medical prosthesis in the aortic position.

conceivable that the buildup of pseudoendothelium on valvular surfaces might weaken the clicks, this clinical sign should always be considered as alarming, since it is usually the consequence of the occluder hitting against the soft mass of a thrombus.

Chronic Intravascular Hemolysis

Red blood cell damage in patients with replacement valves is the consequence of shear stresses in turbulent and rapid blood flow. It can be diagnosed and accurately quantified by the assessment of the serum levels of lactate dehydrogenase (LDH) and haptoglobin (54).

Chronic intravascular hemolysis is of no clinical importance in the vast majority of patients with properly functioning bileaflet valves (56). Occasional cases of severe hemolysis in the absence of any valve malfunction or paravalvular leak have been reported with the St. Jude valve in the mitral position (56–58). Asynchronous closure has been suggested as one causative factor (55, 57, 59, 60).

It is interesting to note that the somewhat hemolytic values of LDH are at variance with other hemodynamic parameters of the St. Jude valve and differ from experiences with other mechanical prostheses where hemolysis is usually a secondary consequence of a hemodynamic problem. Another difference between the St. Jude Medical and other prosthetic valves is that the former produces more hemolysis in the mitral than in the aortic position (56).

In general, however, it has to be stressed that red blood cell damage is more pronounced with malfunctioning than with properly working valves ($p < 0.0005$). Therefore, the hemolytic behavior of a given prosthesis type is a good indicator of its functional integrity ($p < 0.05$) (Fig. 9–7). Nonetheless, the degree of hemolysis does not correlate with the hemodynamic severity of paravalvular or transvalvular regurgitation, nor with

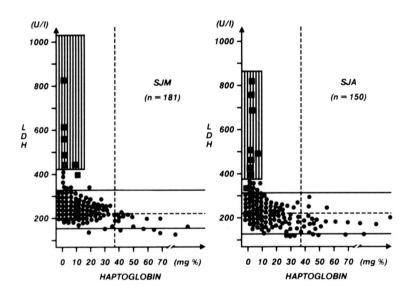

FIG. 9–7. Haptoglobin and LDH values after mitral (SJM) and aortic (SJA) valve replacement with St. Jude Medical prosthesis.

TABLE 9–4. *Continuous-Wave Doppler Echocardiographic Findings for St. Jude Medical (SJM)* and Edwards-Duromedics (ED)† Mitral Prostheses*

Prosthesis/OD‡	n	PHT‡	dP‡	MOA‡
SJM—27	17	85 ± 11	2.5 ± 0.6	2.6 ± 0.3
SJM—29	56	78 ± 16	2.3 ± 1.1	2.8 ± 0.5
SJM—31	34	74 ± 9	2.1 ± 0.5	3.0 ± 0.3
ED—27	5	67 ± 3	2.0 ± 0.4	3.3 ± 0.2
ED—29	10	75 ± 5	2.0 ± 0.1	3.0 ± 0.2
ED—31	8	68 ± 10	1.9 ± 0.4	3.2 ± 0.4

*University of Düsseldorf

†W Dimitri et al. (1986)

‡OD = Sewing ring diameter (mm); PHT = Pressure half time (msec); dP = calculated mean transprosthetic gradient (mmHg); MOA = calculated mitral opening area

a valve obstruction of any origin (55, 61, 62). The usual range of LDH for properly working St. Jude Medical and Edwards-Duromedics valves is given in Table 9–4. Relevant data are not available for the CarboMedics prosthesis.

Fluoroscopy

Fluoroscopy, especially with an amplifier is, together with auscultation, the method of choice for diagnosing an acute valve failure (63). An experienced investigator with an exact knowledge of the normal radiological appearance of the given prosthesis can easily recognize the abnormal movement of the prosthetic ring, inadequate opening or closing of the poppet, or the absence of a part of the valve, normally the (or a) disk, which has escaped.

To achieve good imaging of valve opening and closing, the fluoroscopy should be done parallel to the cross section of the prosthetic ring and parallel to the long axis of the leaflet(s). With systematic rotation even a poorly radiopaque valve, like the St. Jude, can easily be found. The asynchronous movement of the two leaflets is not an infrequent finding, and it is perfectly compatible with the proper function of the prosthesis (see above).

There are some major differences in the X-ray image of the three bileaflet valves. Both the CarboMedics and the Edwards-Duromedics valves have a radiopaque stiffener ring around the prosthetic annulus and have a high enough tungsten concentration within the leaflets to be clearly shown on standard X-ray equipment in almost all orientations.

The St. Jude Medical valve does not have any radiopaque material in or around the valve housing and has only a relatively low tungsten concentration within the leaflets. Therefore, imaging by fluoroscopy needs a somewhat more sophisticated approach, as well as the use of an amplifier. Nevertheless, in experienced hands both housing and leaflets can readily be imaged if two, sometimes three axis X-ray beams are used (Fig. 9–8). The selection of the appropriate plane is rather important, because the open leaflets hardly protrude from the valve housing. In spite of these obstacles the time needed for

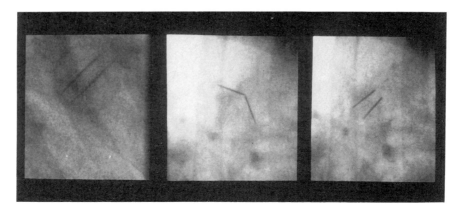

FIG. 9–8. X-ray appearance of the St. Jude valve in open and closed positions.

identifying the valve and for confirming, or otherwise, the proper excursion of the two leaflets is surprisingly short. In 640 consecutive fluoroscopy studies of St. Jude valves in Düsseldorf, the average time under radiation was 14 ± 5 sec (6–34 sec).

An abnormally wide tilting movement of the valvular ring is the sign of paravalvular dehiscence; restricted opening and/or closing of the leaflet(s) is the consequence of thrombus, whether sterile or infected, infringement of underlying cardiac structure, or a long suture end. The importance of fluoroscopy was well demonstrated in cases of leaflet escape of the Edwards-Duromedics valve when an instant differential diagnosis between escape and gross thrombosis had to be made (64).

It should be kept in mind when deciding for or against leaflet movement restriction that both the theoretical maximum opening angle and the travel angle are different in the three bileaflet valves. The former is 85 degrees for the St. Jude Medical, 77 degrees for the aortic and 73 degrees for the mitral Edwards-Duromedics valve, and 78 degrees for the CarboMedics prosthesis. The travel angle of the St. Jude valve is 55 degrees for valve sizes of 25 mm or less and 60 degrees for sizes 27 mm or larger, the closing angle being 120 degrees and 130 degrees, respectively. The Edwards-Duromedics leaflets meet the valve housing in the horizontal plane. The travel angle of the CarboMedics prosthesis is 53 degrees and the closing angle 130 degrees. These angles for any given valve undergoing fluoroscopy should always be assessed and the actual findings recorded for future reference.

Echocardiography

The M-mode echocardiographic appearance of bileaflet valves is the same as that of tilting disk prostheses, and depends on the orientation of the valve (52). In the aortic position, both leaflets can be imaged in only 26% of the cases, while in the mitral position both leaflets are shown in 95% of the cases. It is a frequent observation in these patients that the closure of the two leaflets is asynchronous due to the early closure during diastole of the one lying posteriorly (Fig. 9–7).

As stated previously (see above) the asynchronous closing is perfectly compatible with the proper function of the prosthesis. It is especially frequent when atrial fibrillation is present or when the cardiac index is low (56, 65). Left ventricular flow pattern and the effect of gravitation among others have been suggested as causative factors (66). This fairly usual finding should, however, be differentiated from the irregular closing and/or opening of a leaflet which occurs in case of thrombus apposition (52).

Doppler Echocardiography

Use of M-mode and 2D echocardiography provides only indirect information on the functional integrity of a prosthesis. Doppler echocardiography gives direct evidence of regurgitation and/or obstruction (67, 68, 69, 70). The sensitivity of the method is such that the pressure loss and regurgitant flow can be measured even in the case of normally functioning valves. Furthermore, Doppler echocardiography is an important tool in the assessment of intracardiac flow patterns, flow profiles, and regurgitant jets.

The reliability of the data derived from Doppler echocardiography is best confirmed by simultaneous catheter and echo studies. It is important to note that Doppler echo-cardiography can substantially overestimate bileaflet valve gradients when compared to catheter-obtained gradients. Base values for the acceptable, "normal" range of pressure gradient and reflux can thus be obtained and put in the perspective of past experience with invasive studies (Table 9–4). Pressure half-time is an important parameter in the assessment of transprosthetic gradient. The upper limit of tolerance for the St. Jude Medical prosthesis with a 29 mm outside diameter is 104 msec. It has been proved that day-to-day and inter-observer variation of the method is low. Prosthetic valve malfunction due to a significant obstruction can be detected with near 100% sensitivity and specificity.

The color-Doppler study is especially useful in the analysis of turbulent flow, and therefore in the imaging of regurgitation (71–75). The normally functioning St. Jude valve has two typical kinds of regurgitation (71, 75) which can be reliably differentiated from pathological trans- or periprosthetic regurgitation.

In sequence, the first of these two regurgitations occurs during valve closure with a 50–150 msec duration across prostheses in the mitral position, and up to 125 msec duration across those in the aortic. The regurgitant jet is broad and it does not extend much into the left atrium (mitral), or left ventricular outflow tract (aortic), due to the low pressure difference between the respective upstream and downstream cardiac chambers during the closing period.

The second regurgitation is holosystolic in the mitral and holodiastolic in the aortic position. It is located at the hinge area, the center of the valve, and, especially with the St. Jude valve, in the vicinity of the entire valve housing. This reflux is inherent in the design and it is nothing else than the washout necessary to prevent thrombus buildup. The backflow through the pivot area may be extremely turbulent and it may be imaged as minute jets penetrating deep (40 mm) into the left atrium through mitral prostheses, or into the left ventricular outflow tract through aortic prostheses. The depth of the jet depends on the pressure gradient across the closed valve (72).

It is interesting to note that bileaflet valves which have the lowest profile among the mechanical prostheses have probably the highest closing reflux. The total amount of reflux across the St. Jude valve varies between 4% and 15% of the forward flow, depending on valve size, pressure gradient across the closed valve, cardiac rhythm, stroke volume, heart rate, and the method used for assessment (24, 76).

It could well be suggested that the hemolysis associated with bileaflet valves is another consequence of these regurgitations.

The special value of transoesophageal echo- and Doppler echocardiography for bileaflet valves as well as for other designs (74) has been well established and documented. Especially in the mitral position where valve shadowing "masks" the region behind the prosthesis, transoesophageal echocardiography is the method of choice to demonstrate leakage, valve thrombosis, prosthetic endocarditis, and other kinds of valve malfunction.

MORBIDITY AFTER BILEAFLET VALVE IMPLANTATION

Many years' confusion regarding valve related and treatment related (anticoagulation) complications came to an end recently, when a comprehensive and standard set of definitions was proposed and became generally accepted in the relevant publications (18, 77). According to current guidelines, morbidity after valve replacmeent may be due to structural deterioration, nonstructural dysfunction, valve thrombosis, embolism, anticoagulant related hemorrhage, and prosthetic valve endocarditis. Structural deterioration denotes any change in the prosthetic valve's functional integrity arising from an intrinsic abnormality which causes higher pressure gradient or volume loss than given in the design specification of the prosthesis in question. Earlier these complications have often been referred to as "mechanical dysfunction."

Nonstructural dysfunction includes any abnormality which causes stenosis or regurgitation but is not an intrinsic fault of the valve itself. In the majority of cases it is due to paravalvular leak—less often to suture entrapment, pannus formation, or inappropriate sizing of the valve (77). Chronic intravascular hemolysis of clinical importance is also classified as a nonstructural dysfunction, but evidence has recently been emerging that in some cases it may be present without any apparent morphological reason, and therefore this should be reported separately as dysfunction inherent in the given design. Similar consideration should be given to hemolysis if it is caused by or accompanied by surface deterioration of the prosthesis.

For thrombosis, embolism, anticoagulant-related bleeding, and prosthetic endocarditis there are well-known and widely accepted definitions available.

Structural Deterioration (Mechanical Dysfunction)

The dysfunction of a mechanical prosthesis can be the consequence of wear and tear or other fault of any of the materials it incorporates, similarly to problems which might arise with any engineered product. The durability of the current generation of mechanical prostheses is acceptable, with the rare exception of certain models or limited production series. No more than 10 instances of structural deterioration with consecutive leaflet escape following fracture of the leaflet or the hinge mechanism of the St. Jude Medical prosthesis are known to the manufacturer. During the same period they have received implant information on more than 300,000 valves (78). Aortic prostheses were involved three times, mitral prostheses seven times.

According to information provided by the manufacturer, in six of these 10 cases the valves, during or immediately after insertion, were submitted to mishandling, such as attempting to rotate the valve which is not rotatable, or using sharp or traumatizing instruments when handling the Pyrolite®. It is conceivable that the damage caused during the operation remained undetected by the surgeon and the actual fracture was triggered later by a mechanical stress, like a high cardiac output. An instance where this was assumed to have happened is in the case of a 10-year-old boy who suffered leaflet escape during long-distance running (79).

In the early series of the St. Jude valve, leaflet escape and jamming were attributed to housing/leaflet mismatch. The potential for this mode of failure was eliminated in 1982 by the introduction of a computer driven automatic gauging machine.

Four leaflet escapes without fracture of any valve component have also been reported in the literature. Three of these occurred 10–23 months after mitral valve replacement and all were successfully reoperated (79–81). One fatal leaflet escape happened 25 days after an aortic valve replacement. In addition, an intermittent disturbance of leaflet motion leading to reoperation was described (82). A laboratory examination of the removed prosthesis revealed a small disproportion between leaflet and housing which caused intermittent dysfunction.

Seventeen mechanical failures of the Edwards-Duromedics valve have been reported to the manufacturer so far (83). The estimated incidence is higher than that of fracture with the St. Jude Medical valve, but it is much lower than the incidence of mechanical failure reported for other series of mechanical valves (84). The Duromedics valve was withdrawn by Baxter-Edwards Laboratories in May 1988. With some substantial improvements in valve design and manufacturing, the Edwards-Duromedics valve has been back on the market since June 1990.

The reason for the withdrawal of the valve was that in the failed valves returned to the manufacturer a certain microporosity was found on the surface of the pyrolitic carbon housing. With the closing motion of disk and bileaflet valve occluders, there is a Venturi effect causing formidable changes in pressure and creating cavitation bubbles. If there is a microporous surface close to the cavitation bubbles, cavitation erosion is most likely to occur. Microporosity, therefore, may predispose pyrolitic carbon valves to mechanical failure.

In the early 1980s, when the first large series of pyrolitic valves entered the market there were no appropriate quality control techniques available to demonstrate the presence of microporosity. Dye penetration, scanning electronmicroscopy, and other methods introduced since, now enable the manufacturers to detect microporosity in almost all cases.

Of the 17 cases reported, 15 had fractures occurring in mitral and only two in aortic Edwards-Duromedics prostheses. The mode of failure was not uniform. Leaflet fractures were present centrally or in the pivot ball area (85, 86), while housing fractures involved the hinge mechanism (87). The clinical picture and the management of leaflet escape with the Edwards-Duromedics valve have been the subject of several publications (85–88). There are no direct test data (wear test or animal experiments) available to compare the predicted durability of the redesigned Edwards-Duromedics valve.

There are no publications available to assess the mechanical reliability of the CarboMedics prosthesis. There has been no reported case of postoperative leaflet escape or fracture according to the manufacturer.

Nonstructural Dysfunction

Periprosthetic Dehiscence

Annular calcification and/or infection and/or degenerative lesion are the predisposing factors for perivalvular dehiscence with all mechanical valves. There is no evidence to show that bileaflet valves are different in any way from other valves in this respect (Fig. 9–9).

Excessively high hemolysis due to a paravalvular leak of no hemodynamic importance

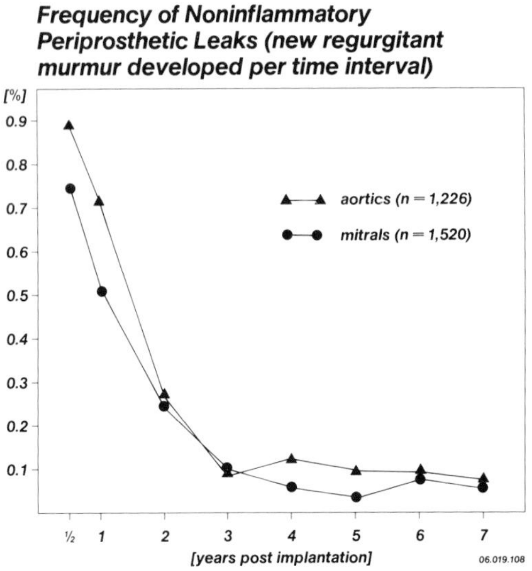

**Frequency of Noninflammatory
Periprosthetic Leaks (new regurgitant
murmur developed per time interval)**

FIG. 9–9. Time-related incidence of periprosthetic leaks.

has been reported with bileaflet, especially with St. Jude Medical, valves (89–91). However, a causative relationship between design and the extent of hemolysis due to para-valvular leak has not so far been established. Similar problems can occur with other mechanical, or even with bioprosthetic valves (92, 93).

Prosthetic Valve Obstruction

Sterile or infected thrombus, pannus formation, and, to a lesser extent, interference of cardiac or noncardiac (suture) structures with the occluder movement can lead to prosthesis obstruction.

Based on a review of the literature which includes 26 publications reporting 51,886 patient years total follow-up information, the rate of valve thrombosis for the St. Jude Medical valve was calculated to be 0.28%/py for valves in the aortic, and 0.21%/py for valves in the mitral position (24, 94–102).

Like any other mechanical valve, bileaflet valves, too, are prone to a relatively higher incidence of thrombosis in the tricuspid position (103). Nonetheless, bileaflet valves are preferred by many surgeons for tricuspid replacement because of the perceived low thrombogenicity of this design (104).

In case of valve thrombosis, lysis therapy can be completed with streptokinase, uro-kinase, and recombinant tissue-type plasminogen activator (rt-PA) (105–117). With prostheses in the mitral or aortic position, the rate of primary success is about 65%. Severe complications like bleeding and/or embolism have been reported in more than 25% of the cases (24). These facts should be given serious consideration before such an indication is made. The experiences with lysis therapy of thrombosed prostheses in the tricuspid position is entirely different. Due to the very low rate of complications, throm-bolytic therapy offers itself as a true alternative to reoperation in these cases (24, 116).

Jamming of the occluder of a bileaflet valve by suture entrapment is a rare clinical finding, although it has been reproduced experimentally (118). Such jamming may result in very high transprosthetic pressure gradients, and the risk of it is higher for the Edwards-Duromedics than for the St. Jude Medical valve (118). In any case, long suture ends should not be left around a bileaflet prosthesis.

Prosthetic Valve Induced Chronic Intravascular Hemolysis

Results from clinical studies involving consecutive series of patients show no difference in the LDH level between those having a bileaflet valve or a mechanical valve of any other design (56), whereas the plasma free hemoglobin is higher with bileaflet prostheses (58). Also, a marked hemolysis accompanies minute, hemodynamically insignificant paravalvular leaks with these valves.

Excessive late hemolysis may follow bileaflet valve implantation even in the absence of paravalvular leak or any other malfunction, according to reports on the St. Jude valve (119, 120). Microthrombi on the leaflets, or surface irregularities as assessed by electron microscopy, are thought to be the causative factors (119).

The potential role of cavitation associated with the leaflet closing cannot be dismissed. It may contribute to creating hemolysis, especially in the mitral position, as well as to promoting surface microporosity (Edwards-Durmedics valve); it is the subject of current intensive research.

Clinically manifest, severe hemolysis may follow double, mitral, and aortic valve replacement as a consequence of the regurgitant jet through the aortic valve striking the anterograde atrioventricular flow during systole (121). The acceleration of the leakage flow creates intensive turbulence, especially in the hinge area of the St. Jude Medical valve, and this too may have a potential role in hemolysis. On the other hand, the same turbulent flow around the hinges may be a key factor in the low thrombogenicity of the St. Jude valve.

A further possible cause of the high hemolysis with bileaflet valves is early, mid-diastolic closure of the posteriorly lying leaflet of a mitral or tricuspid prosthesis (Fig. 9–6) with atrial fibrillation causing a long diastole. This early closure is independent of posture and its mechanism awaits further clarification (56, 59, 60), but it appears as the major single reason why hemolysis with the St. Jude Medical valve, unlike any other mechanical valve, is higher in the case of atrial fibrillation than it is in sinus rhythm (56).

Prosthetic Valve Endocarditis

There is nothing specific to bileaflet valves in this respect, the incidence of late (>60 days after surgery) endocarditis is 0.1%–0.5%/py, the same as with any other mechanical prosthesis (24, 98, 101, 122–129). Higher rates are usually due to inadequate prophylaxis, and to invasive diagnostic or therapeutic procedures in high-risk patients.

Systemic Embolism and Bleeding

Embolism after heart valve replacement can be caused by the thrombogenicity of the implanted device (130). However, it can be caused by underlying cardiac anomalies, especially enlarged left atrium, weak or absent atrial contractions, compromised left ventricular function, and atrial fibrillation (131–134), and this makes it impossible to define which embolism was "valve related" and which was "non-valve related" (135). As a consequence, all postoperative embolism is denoted by definition as valve related. Only well-designed, prospective, randomised trials with identical incremental risk factors and

TABLE 9–5. *Reported Linearized Rate of Prosthetic Valve Thrombosis in Bileaflet Prostheses**

Author/year	Mitral n	Mitral %/py	Aortic n	Aortic %/py	Mitral plus aortic n	Mitral plus aortic %/py
St. Jude Medical						
Arom (1989)	464	0.2	698	0.0	1,162	0.18
Burckhardt (1988)	200	0.2	456	0.2	656	0.20
Czer (1987)	232	0.0	232	0.7	464	0.35
Horstkotte (1990)	577	0.2	413	0.1	990	0.12
Kinsley (1986)	330	0.8	335	0.1	665	0.45
Weighted mean	1,803	0.28	2,134	0.17	3,937	0.22
Edwards-Duromedics						
Dimitri (1987)	—	—	—	—	129	0.0
Jamieson (1987)	—	—	—	—	119	0.6
Klepetko (1987)	—	—	—	—	432	0.3
Weighted mean	—	—	—	—	680	0.30

*No data from peer review journals available for the CarboMedics prosthesis.

anticoagulant treatment within the patient population could reveal differences between prostheses with statistical certainty. Such data are not available for bileaflet valves (136, 137). Data obtained from reviewing the relevant literature are summarized in Tables 9–5 and 9–6 (10, 50, 78, 123–126, 133, 138–142).

The incidence of anticoagulant-related bleeding can be relatively high, reaching unacceptable levels in some cases. This should be taken into consideration when "exceptionally" low thrombosis and embolism rates are reported. Under ideal circumstances, the incidence of thromboembolic complications and that of bleeding should be identical or

TABLE 9–6. *Reported Linearized Rate for Systematic Embolism (TE) and Hemorrhage due to Anticoagulation Therapy (ACH) following St. Jude Medical Mitral (M) and Aortic (A) Valve Replacement*

Author/year	Implant period/position	n	TE (%/py)	ACH (%/py)	TE + ACH (%/py)
Arom (1985)	1977–1983 (M)	334	2.2	2.2	4.4
	1977–1983 (A)	349	0.7	4.6	5.3
Czer (1987)	1977–1984 (M)	139	2.0	2.6	4.6
	1977–1984 (A)	177	2.1	2.1	4.2
Duncan (1986)	1978–1983 (M)	188	0.4	0.0	0.4
	1978–1983 (A)	478	1.0	1.1	2.1
Horstkotte (1990)	1978–1989 (M)	577	1.6	2.4	4.0
	1978–1989 (A)	413	1.1	2.3	3.4
Le Clerc (1983)	1978–1982 (M)	320	3.9	1.7	5.6
	1978–1982 (A)	355	0.6	0.7	1.3
Weighted mean	(M)	1,558	2.09	1.94	4.03
	(A)	1,772	0.99	2.09	3.08

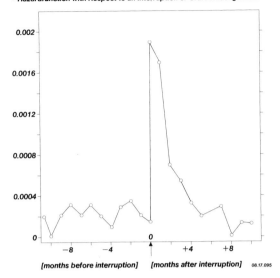

Monthly Incidence of Thrombembolic Complications
– Hazardfunction with Respect to an Interruption of Oral Anticoagulation –

[months before interruption]   [months after interruption]   08.17.095

FIG. 9–10. Instantaneous hazard of thromboembolism before and after interruption of oral anti-coagulant treatment.

at least stay within the same range. With bileaflet, as with any other mechanical prostheses, incorrect anticoagulation or the interruption of the anticoagulation therapy results in a significant and unacceptable increase of the instantaneous rate of hazard of thromboembolism (Fig. 9–10).

CURRENT PROBLEMS AND FUTURE PERSPECTIVES

Many features of the bileaflet design should be considered as an advance compared with those of the caged-ball and tilting disk prostheses. The majority of the available data demonstrates that clinical and hemodynamic results are at least as good as those obtained with tilting "mono"-disk valves. An overall superiority of the bileaflet valves, however, has not been established yet.

There is no scientifically sound evidence in terms of controlled studies to decide if there is any difference in clinical performance on hemodynamic function among the three bileaflet valves. It should be noted, however, that clinical studies comparing the St. Jude Medical and Edwards-Duromedics valves in a relatively large patient population over a relatively long time period, could not show a statistically significant difference in performance.

The scientific information in peer review journals on the CarboMedics prosthesis, five years after its introduction, is unusually scant. This makes futile any attempt to discuss it in comparative terms. As this book goes to press it remains to be demonstrated whether, and how, it lives up to expectations in terms of clinical performance, particularly in comparison with the other two bileaflet valves. Similarly, the durability of the new Edwards-Duromedics valve is yet to be proven.

The oldest and most broadly used member of the bileaflet family, the St. Jude Medical valve provided gratifying results in terms of survival and freedom from thrombosis and embolism during its first 13 years in clinical practice. The excellent hemodynamic characteristics, especially in small sizes, make it an ideal choice in children receiving a mechanical prosthesis and in case of a small aortic or mitral annulus.

REFERENCES

1. Gott VL, Daggett RL, Whiffen JD, et al: A hinged leaflet valve for total replacement of the human aortic valve. J Thorac Cardiovasc Surg 1964;48:713.
2. Kalke BR, Mantini EL, Kaster RL, et al: Hemodynamic features of a double-leaflet prosthetic heart valve of new design. Trans Am Soc Artif Intern Organs 1967;13:105.
3. Wada J, Komatsu S, Ikeda K, et al: A new hingeless valve. In: Brewer LA (ed): Prosthetic Heart Valves. Springfield IL, Charles C Thomas, 1969, pp 304–314.
4. Young WP, Daggett RL, Gott VL: Long-term follow up of patients with a hinged leaflet prosthetic heart valve. In: Brewer LA (ed): Prosthetic Heart Valves. Springfield IL, Charles C Thomas, 1969, p 622.
5. Gott VL, Koepke DE, Daggett RL: The coating of intravascular plastic prostheses with colloidal graphite. Surgery 1961;50:382.
6. Emery RW, Palmquist WE, Mettler E, et al: A new cardiac valve prosthesis: in vitro results. Trans Am Artif Intern Organs 1978;24:550.
7. Horstkotte D, Haerten K, Herzer JA, et al: Preliminary results in mitral valve replacement with the St. Jude Medical prosthesis: comparison with the Björk-Shiley valve. Circulation 1981;64(suppl 2):II-203.
8. Lillehei CW: The St. Jude Medical Prosthetic Heart Valve: results from a five-year multicentre experience. In: Horstkotte D, Loogen F (eds): Update in Heart Valve Replacement. New York, Springer, 1986.
9. Hemex Scientific Inc. Clinical data report 3, July 1984.
10. Neveux JY, Logeais Y: Eighteen months experience with Carbomedics valves. Proc First Internat Symp Carbomedics Prosth Heart Valve, Bordeaux, France, Silent Partners, 1988, p 3.
11. Scotten LN, Racca RG, Nugent AH, et al: New tilting disc cardiac valve prostheses. J Thorac Cardiovasc Surg 1981;82:136.
12. Bruss KH, Reul H, van Gilse J, et al: Pressure drops and velocity fields at four mechanical heart valve prostheses: Björk-Shiley standard, Björk-Shiley concave-convex, Hall-Kaster and St. Jude Medical. Life Support Syst 1983;1:3.
13. Nicoloff DM, Arom KV, Lindsay WG, et al: Techniques for implantation of the St. Jude valve in the aortic and mitral positions. In: DeBakey ME (ed): Advances in Cardiac Valves: Clinical Perspectives. New York, Yorke, 1983, p 191.
14. Baudet EM, Oca CC, Roques XF, et al: A 5½ year experience with the St. Jude Medical cardiac valve prosthesis: early and late results of 737 valve replacements in 671 patients. J Thorac Cardiovasc Surg 1985;90:137.
15. Aoyagi S, Tanaka K, Nishi Y, et al: Valve thrombosis of St. Jude Medical prosthesis: report of three cases. Nippon Kyobu Geka Gukkai Zasshi 1990;43:129.
16. Duveau D, Michaud JL, Desions P, et al: Mitral valve replacement with the St. Jude Medical prosthesis: 242 cases with clinical results and an evaluation of prosthesis positioning. In: DeBakey ME (ed): Advances in Cardiac Valves: Clinical Perspectives. New York, Yorke, 1983, p 183.
17. Chandran KB, Schoephoerster R, Dellsperger KC: Effect of prosthetic mitral valve geometry and orientation on flow dynamics in a model human left ventricle. J Biomechanics 1989;22:51–65.
18. Horstkotte D, Trampisch HJ: Long-term follow-up after heart valve replacement. Z Kardiol 1986;75:641.
19. Blackstone EH, Kirklin JW: Death and other time-related events after valve replacement. Circulation 1983;72:753.
20. Feinstein AR: Current problems and future challenges in randomised clinical trials. Circulation 1984;70:767.
21. Demertzis ST, Frank G, Lowes D, et al: Clinical results after prosthetic heart valve replacement with the St. Jude Medical and Duromedics prostheses. In: Bodnar E (ed): Surgery for Heart Valve Disease. London, ICR Publishers, 1990, p 560.
22. Mikaeloff P, Jegaden O, Ferrini M, et al: Prospective randomised study of St. Jude Medical versus Björk-Shiley or Starr-Edwards 6120 valve prostheses in the mitral position. Three hundred and fifty seven patients operated on from January 1979 to December 1983. J Cardiovasc Surg (Torino) 1989;30:966.
23. Horstkotte D, Loogen F, Bircks W: Is the later outcome of heart valve replacement influenced by the hemodynamics of the heart valve substitute? In: Horstkotte D, Loogen F (eds): Update in Heart Valve Replacement. Darmstadt, Steinkopff, 1986, pp 55.
24. Horstkotte D, Loogen F: Erworbene Herzklappenfehler. Munich, Urban and Schwarzenberg, 1987.
25. Horstkotte D: Improvement of prognosis and quality of life by mitral and aortic valve replacement. Comparative long-term follow-up study after implantation of different prostheses. In: D'Alessandro LC (ed): Heart Surgery 1987. Rome, Casa Editrice Scientifica Internazionale, 1987, pp 11–42.

26. Moritz A, Kobinia G, Steinseifer U, et al: Subjective noise perception and sound pressure levels after valve replacement with St. Jude Medical and Duromedics-Edwards bileaflet heart valve prostheses. Z Kardiol 1989;78:784.
27. Horstkotte D, Haerten K, Schulte HD, et al. Hemodynamic findings at rest and during exercise after implantation of different mitral valve prostheses with equal tissue annulus diameter. Z Kardiol 1983;72:385.
28. Horstkotte D, Friedrichs W, Schulte HD, Loogen F: Hamodynamik und Leistungsfahigkeit von Patienten nach prothetischem Herzklappenersatz. In: Loskot F (ed): Herzerkrankungen. Darmstadt, Steinkopff, 1986, p 387.
29. Horstkotte D: Prosthetic valves or tissue valves—a vote for mechanical prostheses. Z Kardiol 1985;74(suppl 6):19.
30. Horstkotte D, Loogen F, Kleikamp G, et al: The influence of heart valve replacement on the natural history of isolated mitral, aortic and multivalvular disease. Z Kardiol 1983;72:494.
31. Horstkotte D, Loogen F: The natural history of aortic valve stenosis. Eur Heart J 1988;9(suppl E):57–64.
32. Yoganathan AP, Chaux A, Gray RJ: Bileaflet tilting disc and porcine aortic valve prostheses: in vitro hydrodynamic characteristics. J Am Coll Cardiol 1984;3:313.
33. Schramm D, Baldauf W, Meisner H: Flow patterns and velocity fields distal to human aortic and artificial heart valves as measured simultaneously by ultramicroscope manometry in cylindrical glass tubes. Thorac Cardiovasc Surgeon 1980;28:133.
34. Stein PD, Sahhab HN: Measured turbulence and its effect on thrombus formation. Circ Res 1974;35:608.
35. Horstkotte D, Haerten K, Seipel L, et al: Central hemodynamics at rest and during exercise after mitral valve replacement with different prostheses. Circulation 1983;68(suppl 2):161–168.
36. Hasenkam JM, Giersiepen M, Reul H: Three-dimensional visualization of velocity fields downstream of six mechanical aortic valves in a pulsatile flow model. J Biomechanics 1988;21:647–661.
37. Heiliger R, Lambertz H, Gelles J, Mittermayer CH: Comparative study of mechanical cardiac valve prostheses for implantation in the mitral position. Herz 1987;12:405–412.
38. Chandran KM, Schoephoerster R, Fatemi R, Dove EL: An in vitro experimental comparison of Edwards-Duromedics and St. Jude bileaflet heart valve prostheses. Clin Phys Physiol Meas 1988;9:233–241.
39. Horstkotte D, Loogen F: Histoire naturelle des cardiopathies valvulaires acquises. In: Acar J (ed): Cardiopathies Valvulaires Acquises. Paris, Flammarion, 1985, p 225.
40. Horstkotte D, Haerten K, Korfer R, et al: Hemodynamic findings at rest and during exercise after implantation of different aortic valve prostheses. Z Kardiol 1983;72:429.
41. Wortham DC, Tri TB, Bowen TE: Hemodynamic evaluation of the St. Jude Medical valve prosthesis in the small aortic annulus. J Thorac Cardiovasc Surg 1981;81:615.
42. Teoh KH, Fulop JC, Weisel J, et al: Aortic valve replacement with a small prosthesis. Circulation 1987;76(suppl 3):123–131.
43. Pomar JL, Barriusco C, Cardone M, et al: Short-term clinical, echo and hemodynamic results with the new Duromedics bileaflet heart valve. J Cardiovasc Surg 1985;26:125.
44. Ribeiro PA, Zaibag AL, Idris M, et al: Antiplatelet drugs and the incidence of thrombembolic complications of the St. Jude Medical aortic prosthesis in patients with rheumatic heart disease. J Thorac Cardiovasc Surg 1986;91:92–98.
45. Nair CK, Mohiuddin SM, Hilleman DE, et al: Ten year results with the St. Jude Medical prosthesis. Am J Cardiol 1990;65:217–225.
46. Chaux A, Czer LKC, Matloff MJ, et al: The St. Jude Medical bileaflet valve prosthesis. J Cardiovasc Surg 1984;88:706–717.
47. Horstkotte D, Loogen F: Prosthetic valve-related or valve-induced complications. In: Horstkotte D, Loogen F (eds): Update in Heart Valve Replacement. Darmstadt, Steinkopff, 1986, p 79.
48. Schoen FF: Pathology of cardiac valve replacement. In: Morse D, Steiner RM, Fernandez J (eds): Guide to Prosthetic Cardiac Valves. New York, Springer, 1985, p 209.
49. Forfar JC: A seven-year analysis of hemorrhage in patients on long-term anticoagulant treatment. Br Heart J 1979;42:128.
50. Horstkotte D, Korfer R, Seipel L, et al: Late complications in patients with Björk-Shiley and St. Jude Medical heart valve replacement. Circulation 1983;68(suppl 2):175.
51. Horstkotte D, Curtius JM, Bircks W, Loogen F: Noninvasive evaluation of prosthetic heart valves. In: Rabago G, Cooley DA (eds): Heart Valve Replacement and Future Trends in Cardiac Surgery. New York, Futura Publishing, 1987, p 349.
52. DePace N, Lichtenberg R, Kotler MN, et al: Echocardiographic and phonocardiographic assessment of the St. Jude cardiac valve prosthesis. Chest 1981;80:272.
53. Horstkotte D, Korfer R: St. Jude Medical valve prosthesis for mitral valve replacement—preliminary results. Proceedings of the Second Int Symp on the St. Jude Valve, San Diego CA, 1981, p 113.
54. Horstkotte D, Haerten K, Leuner C, et al: Chronic intravascular hemolysis following mitral valve replacement with Björk-Shiley, Lillehei-Kaster and Starr-Edwards prosthesis. Z Kardiol 1978;67:629.
55. Donnerstein RC, Allen HD: Asynchronous leaflet closure in the normally functioning bileaflet mechanical valve. Am Heart J 1990;119:694–697.

56. Horstkotte D, Aul C, Seipel L, et al: Influence of valve type and valve function on chronic intravascular hemolysis following mitral and aortic valve replacement using alloprosthesis. Z Kardiol 183;72:119.
57. Yanai T, Aoyagi S, Isomura T, et al: Observation of two leaflets motion of the St. Jude Medical valve prosthesis in the mitral position and study on the possible causes of hemolysis in the postoperative periods. Jap J Artif Organs 1985;14:1343.
58. Ferrjere M, Saussine M, Delpech S, et al: Hemolyse chez les malades porteurs de prosthese valvulaire cardiaque. Comparison entre les valves de Björk-Shiley et Saint Jude Medical. Arch Mal Coeur 1985;78:RY3.
59. Yuda T, Morishita Y, Arikawa K, et al: Intravascular hemolysis after prosthetic valve replacement. Nippon Kyobu Gillia Gukkai Zasshi 1990;38:270.
60. Jansen W, Neihues B, Hombach V, et al: Echokardiographische Kriterien der St. Jude-Medical-Prothese in Mitralposition. Herz/Kreislauf 1980;12:309.
61. Horstkotte D, Pippert H, Korfer R, et al: Hemolytic anemia resulting from insignificant perivalvular deshiscence of St. Jude Medical aortic valve replacement. Z Kardiol 1986;75:502.
62. Sallam IA, Show A, Bain WH: Experimental evaluation of mechanical hemolysis with Starr-Edwards, Kay-Shiley and Björk-Shiley valves. Scand J Thorac Cardiovasc Surg 1976;10:117.
63. Sands MJ, Lachmann AS, O'Reilly DJ: Diagnostic value of cinefluoroscopy in the evaluation of prosthetic heart valve dsyfunction. Am Heart J 1982;104:622.
64. Denvaert FE, Dumont N, Primo GC: Fluoroscopic differentiation between leaflet escape and valve thrombosis of the Edwards-Duromedics mitral valve. Acta Cardiologica 1989;44:221–228.
65. Amann FW, Burckhardt D, Hasse J, Grodel E: Echocardiographic features of the correctly functioning St. Jude Medical valve prosthesis. Am Heart J 1981;101:45.
66. Feldman HJ, Gory RJ, Chaux A: Noninvasive in vivo and in vitro study of the St. Jude mitral valve prosthesis. Evaluation using two-dimensional and M-mode echocardiography, phonocardiography and cinefluoroscopy. Am J Cardiol 1982;49:1101.
67. Veyrat C, Cholot N, Abithol G, Kalmanson D: Noninvasive diagnosis and assessment of severity of aortic valve disease and evaluation of aortic prosthesis function using echo pulsed Doppler velocimetry. Br Heart J 1980;43:393.
68. Hoffman A, Amann FW, Gradel E, Burckhardt D: Nicht-invasive Bestimmung von Druckgradienten an Herzklappenprothesen mit Doppler-Ultraschall. Schwiez med Wschr 1982;112:1600.
69. Weistein IR, Marbarger JP, Perez JE: Ultrasonic assessment of the St. Jude prosthetic valve: M-mode, two-dimensional and Doppler echocardiography. Circulation 1983;68:897.
70. Simpson IA, Rodger JC, Tweddel AC, et al: Can Doppler echocardiography provide a hemodynamic assessment of mitral prosthetic function? Z Kardiol 1986;75(suppl 2):50.
71. Gioia, G, Rutsch W: Normal Echo-Doppler values in Duromedics valvular prosthesis. Giorn Ital Cardiol 1988;18:213–217.
72. Gibbs JC, Wharton GA, Williams GJ: Doppler ultrasound of normally functioning mechanical mitral and aortic valve prostheses. Int J Cardiol 1988;181:391–398.
73. Minardi G, DiSegni M, Boccardi L, et al: Doppler echocardiography in assessing mechanical and biological heart valve prostheses. G Ital Cardiol 1988;18:121–134.
74. Desideri A, Dreysse S, Schartl M: The Duromedics mitral valve mechanical prostheses: evaluation by means of transesophageal echocardiography. G Ital Cardiol 1989;19:680–685.
75. Alam M, Rosman HS, McBroom D, et al: Color flow Doppler evaluation of St. Jude Medical prosthetic valves. Am J Cardiol 1989;64:1387.
76. Kohler J, Schroder W: Closing volume and leaking volume of new prosthetic heart valves. Life Support Syst, Proceedings Ninth Annual Meeting ESAO. London, Saunders, 1982, p 115.
77. Edmunds LH, Clark RE, Cohn LH, et al: Guidelines for reporting morbidity and mortality after cardiac valvular operations. Ann Thorac Surg 1988;46:257–259.
78. von der Emde J, Eberlein V, Rein V: Bileaflet Prostheses. In: Horstkotte D, Bodnar E (ed): State of the Art in Valve Replacement. London, ICR Publishers, 1990.
79. Hasse J: Escaped leaflet in a St. Jude Medical mitral prosthesis. In: DeBakey ME (ed): Advances in Cardiac Valves: Clinical Perspectives. New York, Yorke, 1983, pp 115–123.
80. Hjelms E: Escape of a leaflet from a St. Jude Medical prosthesis in the mitral position. Thorac Cardiovasc Surgeon 1983;31:310–312.
81. Odell JA, Durandt J, Shama DM, Vythilingum S: Spontaneous embolization of a St. Jude prosthetic mitral valve leaflet. Ann Thorac Surg 1985;39:569–572.
82. Zeimer G, Luhmer I, Oelert H, Borst HG: Malfunction of a St. Jude Medical heart valve in mitral position. Ann Thorac Surg 1982;33:391–395.
83. Edwards CVS Division, Baxter Healthcare Corporation. Written communication, October 1990.
84. Ostermeyer J, Horstkotte D, Bennett J, et al: The Björk-Shiley 70° convexo-concave prosthesis strut fracture problem. Thorac Cardiovasc Surgeon 1987;35:71–77.
85. Klepetko W, Moritz A, Mlczoch J, et al: Leaflet fracture in Edwards-Duromedics bileaflet valves. J Thorac Cardiovasc Surg 1989;97:90–94.

86. Alvarez J, Deal CW: Leaflet escape from a Duromedics valve. J Thorac Cardiovasc Surg 1990;99:372.
87. Dimitri WR, Williams BT: Fracture of the Duromedics mitral valve housing with leaflet escape. J Cardiovasc Surg 1990;31:41–46.
88. Deuvaert FG, Deoriendt J, Massant J, et al: Leaflet escape of a mitral Duromedics prosthesis. Acta Chir Belg 1989;89:15–18.
89. Feld H, Roth J: Severe hemolytic anaemia after replacement of the mitral valve by a St. Jude Medical prosthesis. Br Heart J 1989;62:475.
90. Horstkotte D, Pippert H, Korfer R, et al: Hamolytische Anamie als Folge einer hamodynamisch unbedeutenden paravalvularen Dehiszenz nach St. Jude Medical Aortenklappenersatz. Z Kardiol 1986;75:502–504.
91. Okita Y, Miki S, Kusuhara K, et al: Intractable hemolysis caused by perivalvular leakage following mitral valve replacement with St. Jude Medical prosthesis. Ann Thorac Surg 1988;46:89–92.
92. Hockett RD, Krewson L, Weiss A, Chaplin H: Severe paravalvular mechanical hemolysis with a normal blood smear. Am J Clin Pathol 1989;92:513–515.
93. Mezger J, Weinhold CH, Kreuzer E, Erdmann E: Kunstliche Herzklappen und intravasale Hamolyse. Internist 1988;29:781–783.
94. Soubank DW, Yoganathan AP, Harrison EC, Corcoran WH: A quantitive method for the in vitro study of sounds produced by prosthetic heart valves, II: An experimental comparative study for the sounds produced by a normal and simulated Starr-Edwards series 2400 aortic prosthesis. Med Biol Eng Comput 1984;22:40.
95. Dunan JM, Cooley DA, Reul GJ: Experience with the St. Jude Medical valve and the Ionescu-Shiley bovine pericardial valve at the Texas Heart Institute. In: Matloff JM (ed): Cardiac Valve Replacement. Boston, Martinus Nijhoff, 1985, p 233.
96. Dupon H, Michaud JL, Duveau D: Mitral valve replacement with St. Jude Medical prostheses: a 60-month study of 350 cases at Centre Hospitalier Universitaire. In: Matloff JM (ed): Cardiac Valve Replacement. Boston, Martinus Nijhoff, 1985, p 179.
97. Horstkotte D, Korfer R, Budde TH: Spatkomplikationen nach Björk-Shiley-und St. Jude-Medical-Herzklappenersatz. Z Kardiol 1983;72:251.
98. Kingsley RH, Antunes MJ, Colsen PR: St. Jude Medical valve replacement. An evaluation of performance. J Thorac Cardiovasc Surg 1986;92:349–360.
99. Le Clerc JL, Wellens F, Deuvaert FE, Primo G: Long-term results with the St. Jude Medical valve. In: DeBakey ME (ed): Advances in Cardiac Valves. Scottsdale AZ, Yorke, 1983, p 33.
100. Lillehei CW: Worldwide experiences with the St. Jude Medical valve prosthesis: clinical and hemodynamic results. Contemp Surg 1980;20:11.
101. Nakano K, Imamura E, Hashimoto A, et al: Six-year experience with the St. Jude Medical prosthesis: early and late results of 540 valves in 462 patients. Jap Circ J 1987;51:275–283.
102. Nicoloff DM: Three years experience with the St. Jude Medical valve prosthesis: clinical and hemodynamic results. Proceedings of the Second Int Symp on the St. Jude valve. San Diego CA, 1981, p 171.
103. Minami K, Horstkotte D, Schulte HD, Bircks W: Thrombosis of two St. Jude Medical prostheses in one patient after triple valve replacement. Case report and review of the literature. Eur J Cardiothorac Surg 1988;2:48.
104. Aoyagi S, Tanaka K, Nishi Y, et al: Operative results of tricuspid valve replacement with St. Jude Medical prosthesis. Nippin Kyobu Gukkai Geka Zasshi 1989;37:2463.
105. Baille Y, Choffel J, Sicard P: Traitement thrombolytique des thromboses des prothese valvulaire. Nouv Presse Med 1974;3:1233.
106. Besse P, Ledain L, Roudant M, Ohayon J: Fibrinolytic treatment of valvular prostheses thrombotic obstruction. Eur Heart J 1985;6(suppl 1):75.
107. Czer LC, Weiss M, Bateman TM: Fibrinolytic therapy of St. Jude valve thrombosis under guidance of digital cinefluoroscopy. J Am Coll Cardiol 1985;5:1244.
108. Drour RA: Successful streptokinase therapy of prosthetic aortic valve thrombosis. Am Heart J 1984;108:605.
109. Gagnon RM, Beaudet R, Lemire J: Streptokinase thrombolysis of a chronically thrombosed mitral valve prosthetic valve. Cath Cardiovasc Diagn 1984;10:10.
110. Inberg MV, Havia T, Arstila M: Thrombolytic treatment for thrombotic complication of valve prosthesis after tricuspid valve replacement. Scand J Thorac Cardiovasc Surg 1977;11:195.
111. Joyce LD, Boucek M, McGought EC: Urokinase therapy for thrombosis complication of valve prosthesis after tricuspid valve replacement. Scand J Thorac Cardiovasc Surg 1977;11:195.
112. Ledain L, Lorient-Roudan MF, Gateau P: Fibrinolytic treatment of thrombosis of prosthetic heart valves. Eur Heart J 1982;3:371.
113. Laluaga IT, Carrera D, d'Oliviera J: Successful thrombolytic therapy after acute tricuspid valve obstruction. Lancet 1971;1:1067.
114. Neimann JL, Massin N, Westpaall JC: Guerison par les thrombolytiques des thromboses aigues de protheses valvulaires. Ann Med Nancy 1977;16:1171.

115. Page A, Gateau P, Roudaut R: Traitement thrombolytique dans les thromboses de protheses valvulaires. Nouv Presse Med 1980;9:3186.
116. Prieto-Palmomino MA, Ruiz-de-Elvira JJ, Ruiz-de-Elvira JM, et al: Successful thrombolysis on a mechanical tricuspid prosthesis. Eur Heart J 1989;10:1115.
117. Witchitz S, Veyrat C, Moisson P: Fibrinolytic treatment of thrombosis on prosthetic heart valves. Br Heart J 1980;44:545.
118. van Son JA, Steinseifer U, Reul H, et al: Jamming of prosthetic heart valves by suture trapping: experimental findings. Thorac Cardiovasc Surgeon 1989;37:288.
119. Morishita Y, Arikawa K, Yamashita M, et al: Fatal hemolysis due to unidentified causes following mitral valve replacement with bileaflet tilting disc valve prosthesis. Heart Vessels 1987;3:100–103.
120. Watanabe S, Nakano U, Misumi H, et al: St. Jude Medical valve replacement: clinical experience in 1,039 patients. Nippon-Geka, Gukkai-Zasshi 1989;90:1513.
121. Taggart DP, Spyt TJ, Wheatley DJ, Fisher J: Severe hemolysis with the St. Jude Medical prosthesis. Eur J Cardiothorac Surg 1988;2:137.
122. Lund O, Knudsen MA, Pilegaard HK, et al: Long-term performance of Starr-Edwards silastic ball valves and St. Jude Medical bi-leaflet valves. A comparative analysis of implantations during 1980–1986 for aortic stenosis. Eur Heart J 1990;11:108–119.
123. Arom UV, Nicoloff DM, Kersten TE, et al: Ten-year follow-up study of patients who had double valve replacement with the St. Jude Medical prosthesis. J Thorac Cardiovasc Surg 1989;98:1008.
124. Antunes MJ: Valve replacement in the elderly. Is the mechanical valve a good alternative? J Thorac Cardiovasc Surg 1989;98:485.
125. Klepetko W, Moritz A, Khunl-Brady G, et al: Implantation of the Duromedics cardiac valves prosthesis in 400 patients. Ann Thorac Surg 1987;44:303–309.
126. Arom KV, Nicoloff DM, Kersten TE, et al: Ten years' experience with the St. Jude Medical valve prosthesis. Ann Thorac Surg 1989;47:831–837.
127. Burckhardt D, Striebel D, Vogt S, et al: Heart valve replacement with St. Jude Medical valve prosthesis. Long-term experience in 743 patients in Switzerland. Circulation 1988;78(suppl 1):18–24.
128. Jamieson MPG, Bain WH, Wheatley OJ, Faichney A: The Duromedics bileaflet valve: clinical experience over four years. J Cardiovasc Surg 1987;28:16.
129. Dimitri WR, Williams BT: Intermediate term follow-up of Duromedics prolytic carbon valve. J Cardiovasc Surg 1987;28:15.
130. Dale J, Myhre E: Platelet function in patients with aortic ball valves. Am Heart J 1977;94:359.
131. Fuster V, Gersch BJ, Giuliani ER: The natural history of idiopathic dilated cardiomyopathy. Am J Cardiol 1981;47:525.
132. Hetzer R, Gerbode F, Kerth WJ: Thrombotic complications after valve replacement with porcine heterografts. World J Surg 1979;3:505.
133. Hinton RC, Kistler JP, Fallon JT: Influence of etiology of atrial fibrillation on incidence of systemic embolism. Am J Cardiol 1977;40:509.
134. Wright JO, Hiratzka LF, Brandt B, Doly DB: Thrombosis of the Björk-Shiley prosthesis: illustrative cases and review of literature. J Thorac Cardiovasc Surg 1982;84:138.
135. Horstkotte D, Schulte HD, Bircks W, Loogen F: The hazard of thrombembolia with chronic mitral lesions before and after valve replacement. Eur Heart J 1987;8(suppl 1):116.
136. Czer LSC, Matloff JM, Chaux A, et al: The St. Jude valve: analysis of thromboembolism, warfarin-related hemorrhage, and survival. Am Heart J 1987;114:389–397.
137. Kuntze CEE, Ebels T, Eijgelaar A, Homan van der Heide JN: Rates of thromboembolism with three different mechanical heart valve prostheses: randomised study. Lancet 1989;1:514–517.
138. Di Sesa VJ, Collins JJ, Cohn LH: Hematological complications with the St. Jude valve and reduced-dose coumadin. Ann Thorac Surg 1989;48:280–283.
139. Moritz A, Klepetko W, Khunl-Brady G, et al: Four year follow-up of the Duromedics-Edwards bileaflet valve prostheses. J Cardiovasc Surg (Torino) 1990;31:274–282.
140. Kinsley RH, Antunes MJ, Colsen RP: St. Jude Medical valve replacement. J Thorac Cardiovasc Surg 1986;92:349–360.
141. Fontan F, Roques X, Baudet E, et al: Is the Edwards-Duromedics bileaflet prosthesis the least thrombogenic mechanical cardiac valve? In: 1987 Mini-Symposium Series on the Edwards-Duromedics bileaflet valve. Austin TX, Silent Partners, Inc., 1987, pp 9–18.
142. Keen G, Bhatnager NK, Dhasmana JP, et al: Initial experience with 158 Carbomedics valves. In: Proceedings of the First International Clinical Symposium on the Carbomedics Prosthetic Heart Valve. Austin TX, Silent Partners, Inc., 1989, pp 11–20.

Bodnar, E. and Frater, R. W. M., editors
(1991) *Replacement Cardiac Valves,*
Pergamon Press, Inc. (New York), pp. 229–275
Printed in the United States of America

CHAPTER 10

PORCINE VALVES

W. R. E. Jamieson, V. Gallucci, G. Thiene, A. N. Gerein, U. Bortolotti, M. T. Janusz, A. Milano,
and R. T. Miyagishima

Glutaraldehyde-preserved porcine bioprostheses have been used as cardiac valve substitutes since 1971. The introduction of glutaraldehyde for the fixation of biological tissue by Carpentier and colleagues (1) in 1969 facilitated the use of bioprostheses, both porcine and bovine pericardium, as a satisfactory alternative to mechanical valves. The porcine bioprostheses have given patients an excellent quality of life with a low rate of serious thromboembolism, essential lack of thrombosis, and freedom from anticoagulant-related hemorrhage (2–19, 19a). The primary concern with bioprostheses is limited durability, which has been documented since the early 1980s (8–10, 20–29). The University of Padova has the most extensive experience with the Hancock standard porcine bioprosthesis; the prosthesis was introduced in 1971 (8, 20, 21, 30–37). The University of British Columbia has documented extensive experience with both the Carpentier-Edwards standard and supraannular porcine bioprostheses, introduced in 1975 and 1981, respectively (9, 38–54).

The porcine bioprostheses available for implantation as cardiac valve substitutes are both previous and new-generation porcine valves. The previous-generation prostheses, the Hancock standard and the Carpentier-Edwards standard, are high-pressure glutaraldehyde-fixed prostheses. These prostheses are presently used only in the United States. The new-generation bioprostheses are essentially treated with low-pressure glutaraldehyde fixation. The most extensive experience has been with the Carpentier-Edwards supraannular porcine valve, introduced in 1981, and the Hancock II porcine valve, introduced in 1982. The Medtronic-Intact pressure-free glutaraldehyde-fixed porcine bioprosthesis has been available since 1985. Porcine bioprostheses have been compared with other prosthesis types (4, 5, 55–62).

The clinical experience with replacement porcine valves will be documented from the worldwide literature, as well as the current experience from the University of British Columbia and the University of Padova. The clinical performance assessment will consider patient survival, hemodynamics, thromboembolism, anticoagulant-related hemorrhage, prosthetic valve endocarditis, structural valve deterioration (primary tissue failure), reoperation, and mortality (valve-related).

The following descriptive features of the various prostheses are presented to facilitate comparative evaluation.

The Hancock standard porcine valve has been in continuous use since 1981. The Hancock standard valve is high-pressure glutaraldehyde tissue fixed and is mounted into a Dacron-covered polypropylene stent. There are various sewing ring configurations to facilitate interrupted or continuous suturing techniques.

The Carpentier-Edwards bioprosthetic porcine valve is mounted on a totally flexible Elgiloy (cobalt-nickel alloy) stent, which is radiopaque. The porcine tissue is fixed in a 0.625% buffered glutaraldehyde solution at pressures of 40 to 60 mmHg. The sewing ring material is tubular knitted porous Teflon, which surrounds a silicone rubber insert.

The Hancock modified orifice porcine valve is a standard valve of a composite nature. The right coronary leaflet containing the muscle shelf has been replaced by a leaflet that does not contain the muscle bar from another porcine valve. This high-pressure-fixed valve is mounted into a Dacron-covered polypropylene stent.

The Carpentier-Edwards supraannular bioprosthesis is a second-generation porcine bioprosthetic valve that is mounted on a totally flexible Elgiloy (cobalt and nickel) stent, which is radiopaque. The valve design allows for supraannular placement of the prosthesis in the aortic position, maximizing the effective orifice of the prosthesis. The porcine tissue is fixed in a 0.625% buffered glutaraldehyde solution at low pressure (less than 4 mmHg). The valve design contains an inner Mylar support that is flared between the commissures to accommodate the much wider opening characteristic of low-pressure fixed leaflets, thus minimizing the risk of abrasion of the leaflets against the stent.

The Xenomedica valve is a porcine xenograft fixed with glutaraldehyde under low pressure (less than 4 mmHg). The construction is of a composite nature; the right coronary leaflet containing the muscle shelf has been excised and replaced with a leaflet that does not contain the muscle bar. This leaflet is obtained from another porcine valve.

The Hancock II porcine bioprosthesis is a second-generation bioprosthetic valve. The porcine tissue is initially fixed in glutaraldehyde at 1.5 mmHg and then at high pressure. The fixation methods are designed to ensure good tissue geometry. The tissue is mounted into a Dacron-covered Delrin stent to offer optimal hemodynamic performance. The prosthesis has a reduced valve profile and radiopaque markers. The prosthesis has T6 (surfactant notation) anticalcification treatment.

The Medtronic-Intact porcine bioprosthesis features stress-free glutaraldehyde fixation to preserve the normal anatomy and retain the mechanical functions inherent in natural valve tissue. The Delrin stent is Dacron-covered and features low stent rails and widened sinuses to facilitate leaflet excursion without abrasion. It is treated with toluidine blue for calcium retardation.

The St. Jude Bioimplant porcine bioprosthesis is a second-generation bioprosthetic valve. The prosthesis is low-pressure (4 mmHg) glutaraldehyde-fixed for maintenance of natural shape, low profile, and collagen crimp. The commissures and high rails support the tissue annulus and leaflet coaptation.

The Wessex porcine bioprosthesis has been implanted clinically since 1982. The Wessex valve features 0.2% glutaraldehyde fixation at a high pressure of 50 mmHg. The edges of the supporting frame are covered with a strip of glutaraldehyde-treated porcine pericardium with exposure of the parietal surface.

METHODS

The methods for assessing the clinical performance of cardiac valvular prostheses used at both the University of Padova and the University of British Columbia are essentially identical, facilitating comparison, and have been previously reported (8, 21, 34, 39, 41, 49, 63).

The valve-related complications under consideration are thromboembolism, anticoagulant-related hemorrhage, prosthetic valve endocarditis, and primary tissue failure

TABLE 10–1. *Summary of Freedom from Valve-Related Complications and Composites, Aortic Valve Replacement (Carpentier-Edwards vs. Hancock)*

Complications/ composites	CE	H	
	10 years (%)	10 years (%)	15 years (%)
Thromboembolism	85.1 ± 2.9	90.8 ± 3.5	90.8 ± 3.5
Primary tissue failure	83.1 ± 3.7	57.4 ± 5.5	37.0 ± 10.0
Reoperation	76.4 ± 4.3	51.7 ± 5.2	33.1 ± 8.9
Mortality	89.9 ± 2.3	88.3 ± 3.2	70.6 ± 16.0
Complications (Total)	62.3 ± 3.9	40.4 ± 5.0	23.2 ± 7.5

(structural valve deterioration). The composites of valve-related complications evaluated are valve-related reoperation and mortality. The clinical performance evaluation will also consider patient survival and in vivo hemodynamics.

Valve-related mortality includes all deaths (proved or suspected) from valve-related complications (thromboembolism, hemorrhage related to antithromboembolic therapy, prosthetic valve endocarditis, periprosthetic leak, structural valve deterioration, and clinical valve dysfunction). Sudden, unexplained deaths were not considered valve-related by the authors, for it is known that biological valves do not generally fail in a catastrophic manner.

PATIENTS

The University of Padova implanted the Hancock standard (H-S) porcine bioprosthesis between 1971 and 1978 in 796 patients [aortic valve replacement (AVR), 196; mitral valve replacement (MVR), 502; multiple replacements* (MAVR), 71]. The University of British Columbia used the Carpentier-Edwards standard (CE-S) porcine bioprosthesis between 1975 and 1986 (majority prior to 1982) in 1183 patients [AVR, 572; MVR, 509; multiple replacements* (MR), 211]. The experience from the University of British Columbia used for comparison will be the first 1000 operations performed between 1975 and 1981 (42). The mean age of the patient population at Padova was 47.5 years (range, 8–71 years), considerably younger than the mean age at the University of British Columbia of 56.8 years (8–85 years). The cumulative follow-up for the Hancock series was 5099 years (mean AVR, 7 years; MVR, 8 years; MAVR, 6 years) and for the Carpentier-Edwards series was 5937 years (mean AVR, 6.3 years; MVR, 5.7 years; MR, 5.3 years).

The clinical performance of the Hancock porcine bioprosthesis is available to 15 years and the Carpentier-Edwards porcine valve to 10 years (Tables 10–1 to 10–4).

AORTIC VALVE REPLACEMENT

The freedom from thromboembolism is similar with both prostheses, at 10 years 85% for CE-S and 91% for H-S (Figs. 10–1 and 10–2). The younger patient population in the H-S series may explain the better performance in this series. The major difference in the

---

*Multiple replacements are known as MAVR at the University of Padova and MR at the University of British Columbia.

TABLE 10-2. *Summary of Freedom from Valve-Related Complications and Composites, Mitral Valve Replacement (Carpentier-Edwards vs. Hancock)*

Complications/ composites	CE 10 years (%)	H 10 years (%)	H 15 years (%)
Thromboembolism	77.8 ± 5.2	83.5 ± 2.1	79.0 ± 3.4
Primary tissue failure	71.8 ± 4.9	78.8 ± 2.6	41.0 ± 5.5
Reoperation	67.6 ± 4.6	75.7 ± 2.7	39.8 ± 5.4
Mortality	82.2 ± 4.3	90.1 ± 1.6	84.6 ± 4.1
Complications (Total)	44.8 ± 5.0	56.0 ± 2.9	20.2 ± 4.1

TABLE 10-3. *Summary of Freedom from Valve-Related Complications and Composites, Multiple Valve Replacements (Carpentier-Edwards vs. Hancock)*

Complications/ composites	CE 10 years (%)	H 10 years (%)	H 12 years (%)
Thromboembolism	96.3 ± 2.1	87.2 ± 5.0	87.2 ± 5.0
Primary tissue failure	65.8 ± 7.9	59.5 ± 10.9	49.0 ± 13.0
Reoperation (VR)	55.3 ± 10.4	49.7 ± 10.2	40.7 ± 11.7
Mortality (VR)	87.8 ± 6.5	74.3 ± 6.7	74.3 ± 6.7
Complications (Total)	55.9 ± 7.2	26.5 ± 7.8	18.9 ± 8.5

TABLE 10-4. *Valve-Related Complications and Survival Summary (% per Patient Year)*

	AVR CE	AVR H	MVR CE	MVR H	Multiple CE	Multiple H
Late mortality	3.4	3.5	4.1	3.8	3.7	7.0
Thromboembolism	1.2	0.7	1.7	1.7	0.6	1.7
fatal	0.3	0.4	0.5	0.4	0.2	0.6
Primary tissue failure	1.0	3.9	1.9	2.6	3.3	4.1
Reoperation	1.6	4.9	2.7	3.0	3.8	6.1
Complications (Total)	3.3	6.3	5.6	5.5	6.5	12.0

two series is in primary tissue failure or structural valve deterioration. The freedom from primary tissue failure at 10 years with the CE-S valve is 83% and with the H-S valve is 57% (Figs. 10-3 and 10-4). The age discrepancy between the two groups, 47.5 years for H-S and 56.8 years for CE-S, may be the major factor in the occurrence of primary tissue failure. The characteristics of the prostheses must also be given consideration; the mechanical stress factors on the porcine tissue may be a factor.

The freedom from reoperation at 10 years for the CE-S prosthesis is 76% and for the H-S prosthesis is 52% (Figs. 10-5 and 10-6). This 24% discrepancy can be explained by the incidence of primary tissue failure. Prosthetic valve endocarditis and periprosthetic leak do not influence the performance of the prosthesis with regard to the discrepancy of the reoperative rates. The freedom from valve-related mortality at 10 years is identical for the two prostheses (Figs. 10-7 and 10-8). The freedom from all complications,

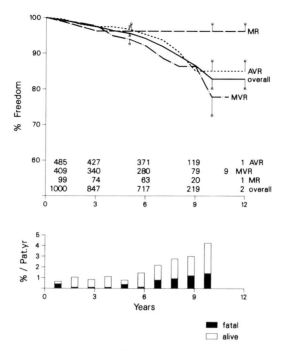

FIG. 10–1. Freedom from thromboembolism (University of British Columbia, Carpentier-Edwards standard).

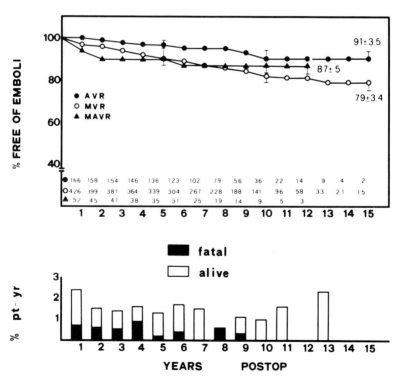

FIG. 10–2. Freedom from thromboembolism (University of Padova, Hancock standard).

233

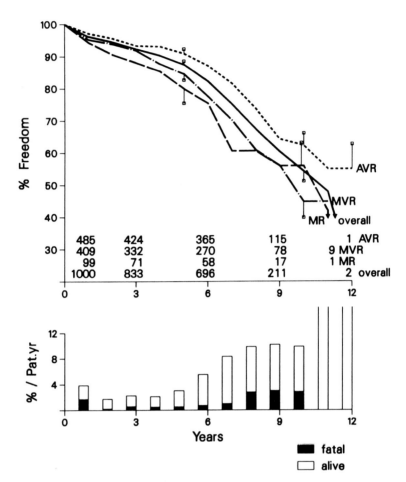

Fɪɢ. 10–3. Freedom from primary tissue failure (overall) (University of British Columbia, Carpentier-Edwards standard).

including thromboembolism, hemorrhage, primary tissue failure, prosthetic valve endocarditis, and periprosthetic leak is 62% for CE-S and 40% for H-S (Figs. 10–9 and 10–10). This difference is also explained by the incidence of primary tissue failure.

The freedom from primary tissue failure at 15 years is 37% with the H-S valve. This progressive deterioration of the prosthesis over time is also reflected in the freedom from reoperation and mortality due to valve-related causes. In the long-term, the CE-S prosthesis is considered to be related to progressive deterioration, but the superior performance at 10 years is encouraging even considering the older population base.

MITRAL VALVE REPLACEMENT

The performance of the two prostheses at 10 years does not show the same differences in the mitral as in the aortic position. The freedom from thromboembolism is 78% at 10 years for CE-S and 84% for H-S (Figs. 10–1 and 10–2). This difference may be explained

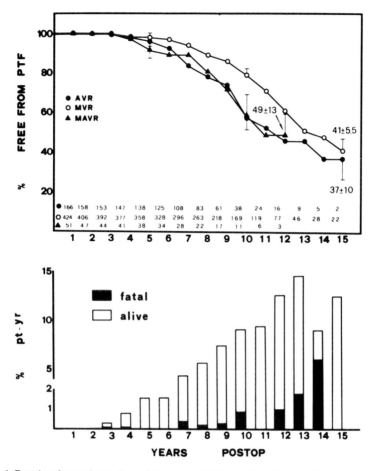

FIG. 10–4. Freedom from primary tissue failure (overall) (University of Padova, Hancock standard).

by differences in the anticoagulant management. The freedom from hemorrhage related to anticoagulants in the H-S group is 85% for mitral prostheses (91% for aortic prostheses) at 10 years. The CE-S experience shows a freedom from anticoagulant hemorrhage overall of 96% at 10 years (AVR 98%, MVR 93%).

The CE-S prosthesis performed less favorably than the H-S prosthesis in the mitral position with regard to primary tissue failure, 72% for CE-S and 79% for H-S at 10 years (Figs. 10–3 and 10–4). The freedom from primary tissue failure at 15 years for the H-S valve is 41%, illustrating a very progressive deterioration between 10 and 15 years. The valve-related reoperation and mortality experience with the CE-S valve is less favorable than that with the H-S valve and reflects the incidence of primary tissue failure (Figs. 10–5 to 10–8). The freedom from overall complications also reflects the performance with regard to primary tissue failure (Figs. 10–9 and 10–10).

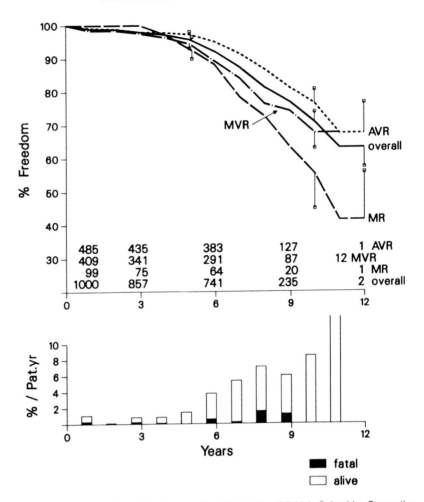

FIG. 10–5. Freedom from valve-related reoperation (University of British Columbia, Carpentier-Edwards standard).

MULTIPLE VALVE REPLACEMENTS

The performance of the two prostheses in multiple replacements shows less difference. The freedom from thromboembolism for CE-S was 96% and for H-S 87% at 10 years (Figs. 10–1 and 10–2). Anticoagulant management, between the series, would not explain this reverse of findings from mitral valve replacement. Earlier operation in the disease process could reduce persistent atrial fibrillation and reduce a risk factor for thromboembolism. The freedom from hemorrhage related to anticoagulant management was 76% for the H-S valve at 10 years for multiple replacements. The freedom from hemorrhage was 94.6% overall for the CE-S population (42).

There is no major difference in the freedom from primary tissue failure between the two prostheses, 66% for CE-S and 60% for H-S at 10 years (Figs. 10–3 and 10–4). This difference is reflected in the freedom from valve-related reoperation; 55% for CE-S and 50% for H-S (Figs. 10–5 and 10–6). The discrepancy is wider for freedom from valve-related mortality, 88% for CE-S and 74% for H-S (Figs. 10–7 and 10–8). This difference

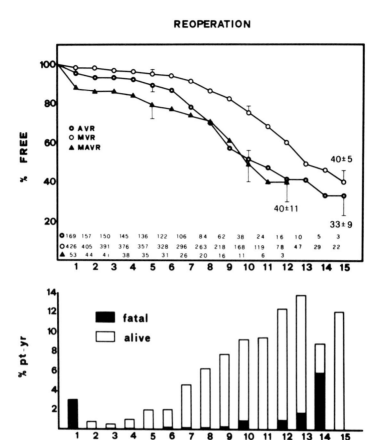

REOPERATION

FIG. 10-6. Freedom from valve-related reoperation (University of Padova, Hancock standard).

in performance reflects primary tissue failure and other complications, namely prosthetic valve endocarditis, periprosthetic leak, and hemorrhage. The linearized occurrence rate for prosthetic valve endocarditis following multiple replacements was 2.6% per patient year for the H-S group compared with 0.5% per patient year for the CE-S group. The related fatalities can explain the difference between the mortality of the prostheses. The prostheses per se will not explain the discrepancy in incidence of prosthetic valve endocarditis between them.

The performance with regard to overall complications shows a wide discrepancy, 56% freedom for CE-S and 27% for H-S (Figs. 10–9 and 10–10). The major determinant factor has been hemorrhagic complications (20%). Thromboembolism and prosthetic valve endocarditis are also influential factors.

PRIMARY TISSUE FAILURE

The clinical performance of the H-S and the CE-S prostheses with regard to primary tissue failure is illustrated in Figs. 10–11 to 10–16. The prostheses have been evaluated by valve position and by age groups, namely less than 25 years, 26 to 50 years, and 51

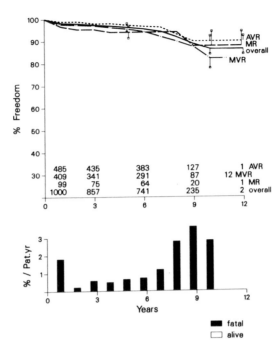

FIG. 10–7. Freedom from valve-related mortality (University of British Columbia, Carpentier-Edwards standard).

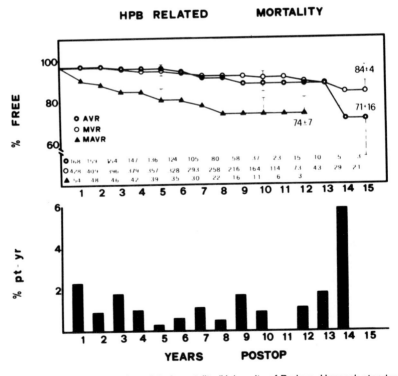

FIG. 10–8. Freedom from valve-related mortality (University of Padova, Hancock standard).

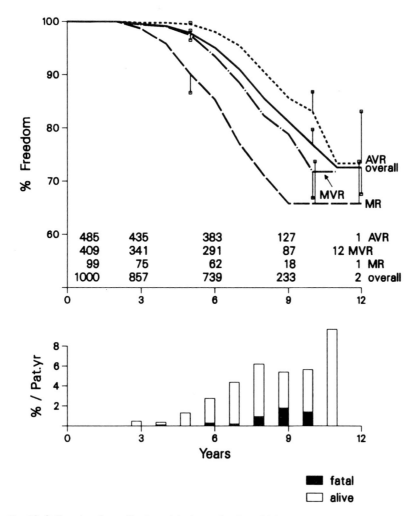

Fɪɢ. 10–9. Freedom from all valve-related complications (University of British Columbia, Carpentier-Edwards standard).

years and greater. The freedom from primary tissue failure of the CE-S for AVR is 83%, MVR 72%, and MR 65.5% at 10 years, while that of the H-S for AVR is 37% at 15 years, for MVR 41% at 15 years, and for MR 49% at 12 years. Comparison of the two prostheses at 10 years reveals better performance for CE-S in the aortic and multiple replacements and similar performance for both prostheses in mitral replacements.

The comparison of the prostheses by age groups for *each position* has revealed interesting observations. For AVR, the freedom from primary tissue failure for the H-S valve was 26% at 12 years for the less-than-25-years group, 34% at 15 years for the 26-to-50-years group, and 60% at 14 years for the 51-and-over group (Fig. 10–13). For AVR for the CE-S valve the freedom from primary tissue failure was 60% at 8 years for the less-than-25-years group, 63% at 10 years for the 26-to-50-years group, and 75% at 10 years

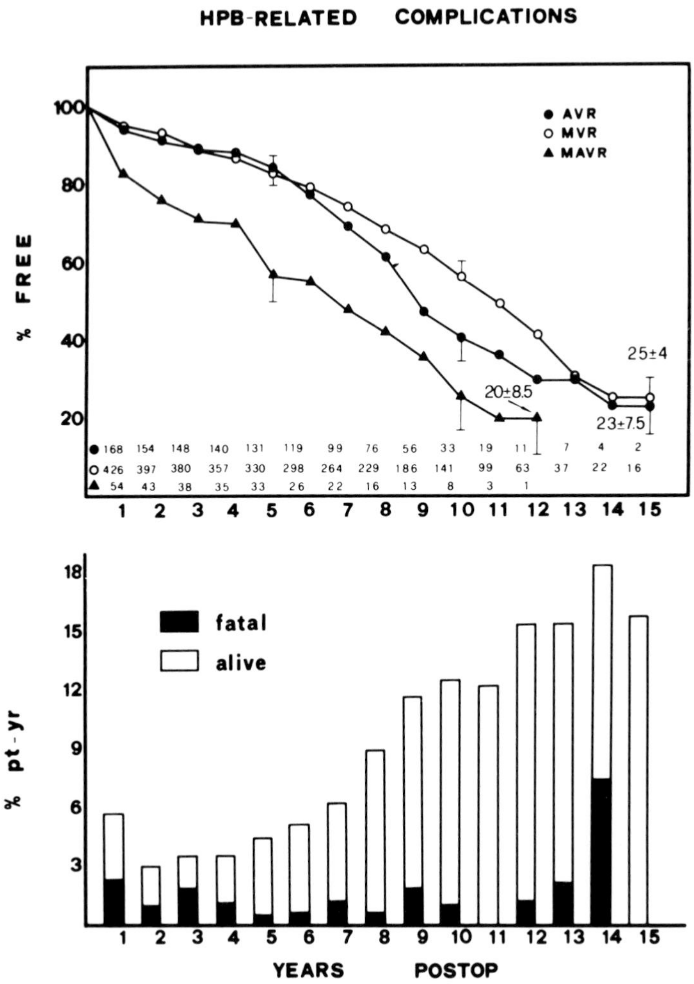

HPB-RELATED COMPLICATIONS

FIG. 10–10. Freedom from all valve-related complications (University of Padova, Hancock standard).

for the 51-and-over group (Fig. 10–12). Comparing the two valves, for AVR the CE-S valve performed better in the groups less than 50 years of age, but over 50 years the performances of both the CE-S and the H-S were similar. For MVR the freedom from primary tissue failure for the H-S valve was 22% at 15 years for the less-than-25-years group, 36% at 15 years for the 26-to-50-years group, and 77% at 15 years for the 51-and-over age group (Fig. 10–15). For MVR for the CE-S valve, the freedom was 29% at 8 years for the less-than-25-years group, 69% at 10 years for the 26-to-50-years group, and 83% at 8 years for the 51-and-over age group (Fig. 10–14). Comparing the two valves, for MVR the H-S valve performed better in the groups less than 50 years of age, but over 50 years the performances of both the CE-S and the H-S were similar.

The CE-S prosthesis was further extensively evaluated, and *overall* population was compared by specific age groups (Fig. 10–11). The freedom from primary tissue failure for the group less than 25 years of age was 46% at 8 years and for the groups 26 to 50 years and 51 years and over at 10 years was 65 and 66%, respectively. At 8 years there was a difference in the latter two groups, 72 and 86%, respectively. At the 8-year interval the differences were significant between the three groups. For the valve positions documented above, for AVR the difference was significant only for the age groups 26 to 50 years and 51 years and over, while for MVR the difference in primary tissue failure between the less-than-25-year group was significantly greater than that of either of the older groups, 26 to 50 years and 51 years and over.

Previously the CE-S group was evaluated by a different analysis of age groups (Fig. 10–16) (49). At 10 years there was a significant difference between all three groups, the freedom from primary tissue failure for overall patients less than 30 years was 27%, for those 30 to 59 years was 77%, and for those 60 and over years was 83%. When the total patient population was evaluated by decades of age at implantation, the long-term freedom from primary tissue failure was greater with each advancing decade of age.

The documented world experience for structural valve deterioration (primary tissue failure) with both previous and new-generation porcine bioprostheses is detailed in Table 10–5 (8, 9, 22, 33, 37, 39, 41, 42, 48–50, 53, 58, 64–80). The previous-generation porcine valves are the standard porcine prostheses, H-S and CE-S. The experience of the authors is the most extensive reported to date. The early experience with the new-generation prostheses, the Bioimplant and the Carpentier-Edwards supraannular, shows failure rates similar in the early stage of evaluation to those of the previous-generation prostheses at similar time frames. There is no available documentation on several prostheses, namely Hancock II, Wessex, Xenomedica, and Medtronic-Intact. The majority of these prostheses are formulated with low-pressure glutaraldehyde-fixed tissue. The Medtronic-Intact prosthesis is made with stress-free (pressure-free) glutaraldehyde fixation.

The new-generation prostheses have been in use since 1982 (81–84). Carpentier and colleagues (81) introduced the Carpentier-Edwards supraannular porcine bioprosthesis to reduce fatigue lesions and improve hemodynamics. This prosthesis was designed for implementation in the supraannular position, rather than within the annulus, to provide an orifice diameter of the same dimensions as the patient's annulus diameter. The valve was designed to optimize the stress–strain relationships by using the flexible Elgiloy wireform and low-pressure glutaraldehyde preservation. The stent height of the aortic supraannular prosthesis is lower than that of the standard valve, but the tissue height is not appreciably changed because of the lower mounting of the valvular tissue. The stent height of the mitral supraannular prosthesis is considerably lower than that of the mitral standard prosthesis. The Hancock II porcine bioprosthesis was introduced in 1982 by Wright and colleagues (84). The Hancock II incorporates low-pressure glutaraldehyde preservation in the preparation of the porcine tissue. The Hancock II porcine bioprosthesis is also designed for supraannular implantation in the aortic position. The Medtronic-Intact porcine bioprosthesis, an intraannular prosthesis, the latest of the new generation of biological valves, is formulated with pressure-free glutaraldehyde preservation. The stress-free or pressure-free fixation process is designed to preserve the normal collagen architecture of the porcine tissue, in an attempt to reduce fatigue injuries and increase durability.

The manufacturers, in formulating the new-generation porcine bioprostheses, attempted to retain the collagen crimp of valvular cusps by minimal pressurized fixation as recommended by Broom (85) in 1978, Broom and Thompson (86) in 1979, and Broom and Christie (87) in 1982. These authors have placed emphasis on maintaining the radial compliance of the cusp with maintenance of the collagen crimp to facilitate

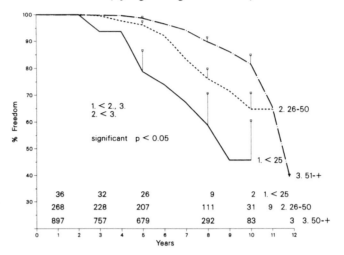

FIG. 10–11. Freedom from primary tissue failure (overall—age groups) (University of British Columbia, Carpentier-Edwards standard).

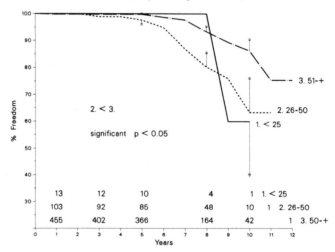

FIG. 10–12. Freedom from primary tissue failure (aortic valve replacement—age groups) (University of British Columbia, Carpentier-Edwards standard).

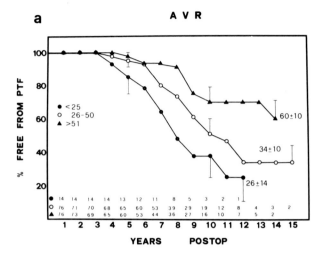

FIG. 10–13. Freedom from primary tissue failure (aortic valve replacement—age groups) (University of Padova, Hancock standard).

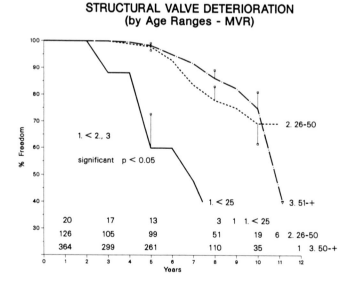

FIG. 10–14. Freedom from primary tissue failure (mitral valve replacement—age groups) (University of British Columbia, Carpentier-Edwards standard).

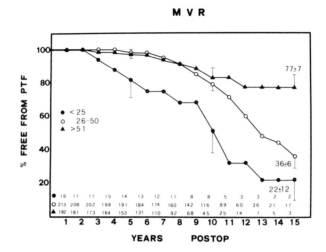

FIG. 10–15. Freedom from primary tissue failure (mitral valve replacement—age groups) (University of Padova, Hancock standard).

loading conditions. The Hancock II and the Carpentier-Edwards supraannular porcine bioprostheses incorporate fixation in glutaraldehyde at a pressure of less than 4 mmHg. The long-term influence on durability will be determined over time, but a mode of failure has been identified with the Carpentier-Edwards supraannular prosthesis (48). One aortic prosthesis and seven mitral prostheses have been explanted for commissural tears causing significant regurgitation. Two mitral prostheses explanted for regurgitation had the

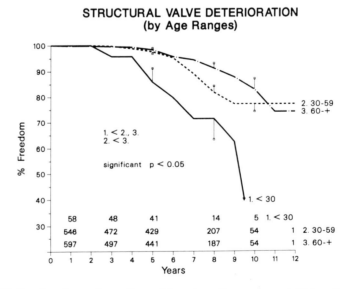

FIG. 10–16. Freedom from primary tissue failure (overall—age groups) (University of British Columbia, Carpentier-Edwards standard).

aortic wall detached from one stent post by tissue tear. The incidence of structural valve deterioration with the Carpentier-Edwards supraannular prosthesis is identical at the 5-year interval to that of the Carpentier-Edwards standard prosthesis, 98.9 and 97.9%, respectively. The experience with the Hancock II prosthesis is somewhat limited, with a shorter duration of exposure compared with the Carpentier-Edwards supraannular valve, and early durability has yet to be documented (88). The Medtronic-Intact also has limited exposure since introduction in 1985; there are two known failures due to perforations and tear, resulting in valvular incompetence.

The calcification of biological prostheses, particularly common in adolescent and preadolescent populations, has also received considerable attention. Carpentier and colleagues reported in 1982 that the rate of calcification could be reduced by decreasing the phosphate content in the tissue or blocking calcium-binding sites with magnesium and surfactant (83). In 1982, Carpentier used the surfactant Tween 80 (83). In 1984, Carpentier again reported on calcium-mitigation therapy, documenting that the surfactant *N*-lauroylsarcosine and Triton X-100 provided better calcification mitigation than Tween 80 and sodium dodecyl sulfate (82). The Hancock II prosthesis is pretreated with surfactant using sodium dodecyl sulfate in the T6 process (89, 90). Jones and colleagues evaluated calcium-mitigation therapies in an in vivo in situ sheep model and found that only polysorbate 80 and sodium dodecyl sulfate were effective, but only with porcine tissue (91). Toluidine blue, which is used for pretreatment of the Medtronic-Intact valve, was found to provide no substantial effect.

THROMBOEMBOLISM

The documented experience of thromboembolism for previous- and new-generation porcine bioprostheses is detailed in Table 10–6 (8, 9, 41, 42, 48–50, 53, 58, 65, 66, 68–71, 73, 76, 80, 91–96). For comparative use the data are shown as occurrence rates and percentage freedom from thromboembolic events with mean age at implantation. The occurrence rates are influenced by valve position and the mean age of the patient population. The incidence is higher for the mitral position than for the aortic position and increases with the mean age of the patient population. The increase in the incidence of thromboembolism with age is probably indicative of other unrecognized causes of thromboembolism such as extracranial cerebrovascular disease. The higher incidence of thromboembolism with MVR is at least partially related to preexisting atrial dysfunction and chronic atrial fibrillation. The freedom from thromboembolism for AVR is approximately 95% and for MVR 90% at 5 years. There appears to be no appreciable difference in the performance of previous- and new-generation porcine bioprostheses with regard to thromboembolism.

HEMORRHAGE RELATED TO ANTICOAGULANT THERAPY

The experience with hemorrhage related to anticoagulant therapy is shown in Table 10–7 (8, 9, 33, 41, 42, 48–50, 53, 65–67, 69–72, 76, 96). The lack of long-term need for anticoagulant therapy reduces hemorrhage as a significant complication. The incidence with mitral replacement is higher than that with aortic replacement because anticoagulants are used primarily in the presence of chronic atrial fibrillation, which is present in a significant proportion of patients with mitral valve disease. The freedom from hemorrhagic complications is over 95% at 5 to 10 years of observation.

Table 10–5. Structural Valve Deterioration (Primary Tissue Failure)

Prosthesis and author	Mean age (years)	Mean follow-up (years)	Occurrence (%/pt yr)*			Freedom (%) and length of follow-up*		
			AVR	MVR	Overall	AVR	MVR	Overall
Hancock Standard								
Bolooki et al. (64)	49 (range, 15–71)	6	—	1.5	1.3	NA	NA	NA
Brais et al. (65)	53	5.4		NA	2.7	—	NA	NA
Gallo et al. (67)	NA	7.1	—	—	—	97 at 5 yr, —69 at 10 yr	95 at 5 yr, 70 at 10 yr	65 at 7 yr
Gallo et al. (68)	42.5	AVR 5.8 MVR 6.2	1.11	1.93	NA	85 at 8 yr	85 at 8 yr	—
Gallucci et al. (33)	53	5.2	—	1.7	1.7	—	98 at 5 yr, 58 at 13 yr	
Miller et al. (72)	AVR 59 MVR 56	AVR 4.1 MVR 4.3	0.4	1.1	NA	89 at 8 yr	77 at 10 yr	NA
Nistal et al. (74)	48	59	NA	—	0.61	NA	—	93 at 6.9 yr
Schoen et al. (75)	57	—	NA	NA	NA	96 at 5 yr	98 at 5 yr	NA
Gallucci et al. (8)	47.5	AVR 7 MVR 8	3.9	2.6	NA	37 at 15 yr	41 at 15 yr	NA
Milano et al. (37)	48 (range, 17–70)	AVR 6.6	3.5			34.3 at 14 yr	75 at 10 yr	
Cohn et al. (66)	60					82 at 10 yr 59 at 15 yr	35 at 15 yr	
Carpentier-Edwards Standard								
Jamieson et al. (50)	NA	3.8	0	0.7	NA	NA	NA	NA
Jamieson et al. (53)	57 (range, 15–82)	4.3	1.16	1.0	NA	NA	NA	NA

Louagie et al. (70)	65 (range, 25–84)	2.43	NA	NA	0.77	NA	NA	NA
Soots et al. (76)	AVR 49 / MVR 48	AVR 2.85 / MVR 2.95	0.24	0.32	NA	NA	NA	NA
Jamieson et al. (42)	57	5.9 / AVR 6.3 / MVR 5.7	1.0	1.9	1.6	83.1 at 10 yr	71.8 at 10 yr	97.9 at 5 yr, 76.9 at 10 yr
Jamieson et al. (39)	NA	5.6	0.9	1.8	1.5	83.1 at 10 yr	72.1 at 10 yr	77.0 at 10 yr
Jamieson et al. (9)	57 (range, 8–85)		0.9	1.8	1.5	83 at 10 yr	72 at 10 yr	77 at 10 yr / 72.7 at 12 yr
Carpentier-Edwards and Hancock Standard								
Cohn et al. (58)	60.5 (range, 16–95)	4.6	0.79	—	0.79	90.7 at 9 yr	—	—
Hartz et al. (69)	59 (range, 19–88)	3.25	0.3	0.5	H 0.4 / CE 0.62	100 at 5 yr	96 at 5 yr	99 at 5 yr
Magilligan et al. (71)	NA	NA	NA	NA	NA	97 at 5 yr / 71 at 10 yr	96 at 5 yr / 71 at 10 yr	97 at 5 yr / 71 at 10 yr
Carpentier-Edwards Supraannular								
Jamieson et al. (41)	NA	AVR 1.2 / MVR 1.1	0	0	0	100 at 2.5 yr	100 at 2.5 yr	100 at 2.5 yr
Wahlers et al. (80)	55	1.65	1.2	—	NA	NA	—	NA
Jamieson et al. (48)	62 (range, 13–87)	2.8	0.05	0.3	0.2	99.4 at 5 yr	98.8 at 5 yr	100 at 3 yrs, 98.9 at 5 yr
Jamieson et al. (49)	61 (range, 13–85)	1.95	0	0.1	0.1	100 at 4 yr	98.6 at 4 yr	98.8 at 4 yr
Bioimplant								
Navia et al. (73)	54 (range, 17–76)	NA	NA	NA	NA	93.7 at 6 yr (735 yr) / 96.2 at 6 yr (35 yr)	100 at 6 yr	NA
Villemot et al. (79)	NA	NA	0.28	0.5	0.39	94 at 6 yr	90 at 6 yr	98 at 5 yr, 91 at 6 yr
Pavie et al. (19a)	52 (range, 9–76)	NA	—	—	1.5	94 at 5 yr	89 at 5 yr	92 at 5 yr

TABLE 10–6. *Thromboembolism*

Prosthesis and Author	Mean age (years)	Occurrence (%/pt yr)			Actuarial freedom (%) and length of follow-up		
		AVR	MVR	Overall	AVR	MVR	Overall
Hancock Standard							
Brais et al. (65)	53		5.8			86 at 3 yr, 73 at 6 yr	
Gallo et al. (68)	42.5 (range, 6–68)	0.97	1.93	NA	95 at 5 yr, 94 at 8 yr	91 at 5 yr, 88 at 8 yr	
Gallucci et al. (8)		0.70	1.7		91 at 15 yr	79 at 15 yr	
Magilligan et al. (71)	48 (range, 17–70)	0.70			89.4 at 14 yr	80 at 10 yr	
Cohn et al. (66)					84 at 10 yr, 78 at 15 yr	60 at 15 yr	
Carpentier-Edwards Standard							
Gallo et al. (94)	48.4 (range, 13–71)	0.5	2.3	NA	NA	NA	NA
Jamieson et al. (50)	NA	1.0	1.7	NA	NA	NA	NA
Jamieson et al. (53)	57 (range, 15–82)	1.1	1.7	1.5	NA	NA	NA
Louagie et al. (70)	65 (range, 25–84)	3.8	NA	3.1	86 at 3.5 yr	98 at 3 yr, 97 at 5 yr	
Soots et al. (76)	AVR 49 MVR 48	0.48	0.9	NA	98 at 3.5 yr		
Jamieson et al. (42)	57	1.2	1.7	1.3	85 at 10 yr	78 at 10 yr	83 at 10–12 yr
Jamieson et al. (9)	57 (range, 8–85)	1.3	1.8	1.5	84 at 10 yr	77 at 10 yr	82 at 10, 12 yr

	Age						
Carpentier-Edwards and Hancock Standard							
Cohn et al. (58)	60.5 (range, 16–95)	1.9		NA	85 at 9 yr	92.6 at 5 yr	97 at 5 yr
Hartz et al. (69)	59 (range, 19–88)	0.28	1.35	0.73	99.4 at 5 yr	89 at 3, 5 yr	
Magilligan et al. (71)	NA	NA	NA	NA	93 at 5 yr 88 at 10 yr	84 at 10 yr	
Spencer et al. (96)	NA	NA	NA	NA	87 at 5 yr	85 at 5 yr	85.4 at 5 yr
Carpentier-Edwards Supraannular							
Jamieson et al. (41)	NA	1.8	3.2	2.7	NA	NA	91 at 2 yr
Wahlers et al. (80)	55	0.3	—	0.3	NA	—	NA
Jamieson et al. (49)	61 (range, 13–85)	2.8	2.4	2.6	93 at 4 yr	92 at 4 yr	92 at 4 yr
Jamieson et al. (48)	62 (range, 13–87)	2.2	2.9	2.4	93 at 5 yr	87 at 5 yr	90.6 at 5 yr
Bioimplant							
Navia et al. (73)	54 (range, 17–76)	NA	NA	NA	97.5 at 6 yr	94 at 6 yr	97 at 5 yr
Pavie et al. (19a)	52 (range, 9–76)			0.7	98 at 5 yr	98 at 5 yr	

PROSTHETIC VALVE ENDOCARDITIS

The overall experience with previous- and new-generation porcine bioprostheses with regard to prosthetic valve endocarditis is shown in Table 10–8 (9, 33, 37, 38, 41, 42, 49, 54, 58, 65, 66, 69, 71–73, 76, 80, 96, 97). The clinical performance is documented as occurrence rates and percentage freedom from endocarditis. Prosthetic valve endocarditis is not a common problem with either previous- or new-generation porcine bioprostheses. There is no overall predilection for valve position. The freedom from prosthetic valve endocarditis for all porcine bioprostheses is over 95% with 5 to 10 years of observation.

REOPERATION (VALVE-RELATED)

The clinical performance of porcine bioprostheses with regard to valve-related reoperation is detailed in Table 10–9 (8, 9, 33, 41, 42, 48–50, 53, 65, 66, 68, 72, 76). Reoperation for bioprostheses failure is due to either prosthetic valve endocarditis, periprosthetic leak, or structural valve deterioration in the majority of cases. The freedom from reoperation decreases with younger age as structural valve deterioration becomes more evident. Both the occurrence rates and percentage freedom from reoperation are related to mean follow-up; the observation is particularly evident by observation of the experience of Gallucci et al (8) and Jamieson et al (42). The overall freedom from reoperation is approximately 95% at 5 years, 70% at 10 years, and 45% at 15 years. The early experience for the new-generation porcine valves is similar to that of the previous-generation prostheses at the respective times.

MORTALITY (VALVE-RELATED)

The documentation of valve-related mortality is limited and has been reported mainly by Jamieson and colleagues (Table 10–10) (9, 42, 48, 49, 66, 71). Valve-related mortality included deaths from thromboembolism, anticoagulant hemorrhage, prosthetic valve endocarditis, periprosthetic leak, and structural valve deterioration (primary tissue failure). The mortality from the last three complications is related primarily to reoperative mortality. The freedom from valve-related mortality is approximately 96% at 5 years and 86% between 10 and 15 years. The risk of reoperative surgery for structural valve deterioration is the major influence on valve-related mortality. The experience of Jamieson and colleagues, representing experience with reoperative surgery, has shown reduced risk between previous- and new-generation porcine bioprostheses.

HEMODYNAMICS

The in vivo hemodynamics of porcine bioprostheses have received extensive investigation, especially for the small aortic sizes of the standard previous-generation prostheses. Table 10–11 details the literature by valve position and prosthesis with regard to valve size, investigative cardiac output, effective orifice area, and mean transvalvular gradient (40, 81, 98–118). The data for rest and exercise conditions are provided as detailed by the various investigators. In the aortic position the small sizes of the standard pros-

Table 10–7. Hemorrhage Related to Antithromboembolic Therapy

Prosthesis and author	Mean follow-up (years)	Occurrence (%/pt yr)			Actuarial freedom (%) and length of follow-up		
		AVR	MVR	Overall	AVR	MVR	Overall
Hancock Standard							
Brais et al. (65)	5.4	—	NA	1.1	NA	NA	NA
Gallo et al. (67)	AVR 5.8 (range, 5.2–7.8) MVR 6.1 (range, 5.1–8.0)	NA	NA	0.5	NA	NA	NA
Gallucci et al. (33)	5.2 (range, 1.6–13.2)	—	0.4	0.4	—	NA	NA
Miller et al. (72)	AVR 4.1 MVR 4.3	0.8	1.2	NA	NA	NA	NA
Gallucci et al. (8)	—	0.3	0.6	NA	NA	NA	NA
Magilligan et al. (71)		0.1			97% at 10 yr 97% at 15 yr		96% at 10 yr 94% at 15 yr
Cohn et al. (66)	AVR 6.6						
Carpentier-Edwards Standard							
Jamieson et al. (50)	3.8	0	0.24	NA	100 at 7 yr	NA	NA
Jamieson et al. (53)	4.3	0	0.17	0.07	100 at 7 yr	NA	NA
Lougie at al. (70)	2.4	NA	NA	1.16	NA	NA	NA
Soots et al. (76)	AVR 2.9 MVR 3.0	1.2	1.1	NA	NA	NA	NA
Jamieson et al. (42)	5.9	0.3	0.6	0.5	NA	NA	NA
Jamieson et al. (9)		0.3	0.7	0.5	97.8 at 10 yr	93.4 at 10 yr	95.7 at 10–12 yr
Carpentier-Edwards and Hancock Standard							
Hartz et al. (69)	3.2	1.5	1.3	NA	NA	NA	NA
Spencer et al. (96)	3.5	NA	NA	NA	NA	NA	94 at 5 yr
Carpentier-Edwards Supraannular							
Jamieson et al. (41)	AVR 1.2 MVR 1.1	0	2.1	1.2	100 at 2½ yr	NA	NA
Jamieson et al. (48)	2.8	0.2	0.7	0.5	NA	NA	NA
Jamieson et al. (49)	1.95	0.3	1.2	0.7	99.5% at 4 yr	95.7% at 4 yr	97.7% at 4 yr

TABLE 10–8. *Prosthetic Valve Endocarditis*

Prosthesis and author	Occurrence (%/pt yr)			Actuarial Freedom (%) and length of follow-up		
	AVR	MVR	Overall	AVR	MVR	Overall
Hancock Standard						
Brais et al. (65)	—	1.3	1.3	—	98% at 3 yr, 92% at 6 yr	98% at 3 yr, 92% at 6 yr
Gallucci et al. (33)	—	0.2	0.2	—	NA	NA
Magilligan et al. (71)	NA	NA	NA	NA	NA	94 at 5 yr
Miller et al. (72)	0.9	0.5	NA	95 at 6 yr	96 at 6 yr	NA
Milano et al. (37)	0.6					
Cohn et al. (66)				94 at 10 yr 93 at 15 yr	94 at 10 yr 93 at 15 yr	
Carpentier-Edwards Standard						
Janusz et al. (54)	0.94	0.24	NA	NA	NA	NA
Jamieson et al. (38)	0.5	0.5	NA	NA	NA	NA
Soots et al. (76)	1.4	0.5	NA	NA	NA	NA
Jamieson et al. (42)	0.5	0.6	0.5	NA	NA	NA
Jamieson et al. (9)	0.5	0.6	0.6	93.6 at 10 yr	94.6 at 10 yr	94 at 10 yr 89 at 12 yr
Carpentier-Edwards and Hancock Standard						
Cohn et al. (58)	0.55	—	NA	95.5 at 9 yr	—	NA
Spencer et al. (96)	NA	NA	NA	NA	NA	95.7 at 5 yr
Hartz et al. (69)	0.65	1.18	NA	97% at 5 yr	95 at 5 yr	NA
Carpentier-Edwards Supraannular						
Jamieson et al. (41)	0.3	0.7	0.8	NA	NA	NA
Wahlers et al. (80)	NA	—	0.3	NA	—	NA
Jamieson et al. (49)	0.2	0.5	0.4	99.3 at 4 yr	98.9 at 4 yr	99 at 4 yr
Bioimplant						
Navia et al. (73)	NA	NA	NA	97 at 6 yr	96 at 6 yr	NA
Pavie et al. (19a)	NA	NA	NA	98 at 5 yr	97 at 5 yr	97 at 5 yr

thesis have been found to be relatively stenotic. The standard Hancock prosthesis is more stenotic than the standard Carpentier-Edwards. The modified-orifice Hancock valve has afforded improved hemodynamic performance over the standard prosthesis. The new-generation Carpentier-Edwards supraannular and Bioimplant prostheses provide improved hemodynamic performance over the standard Hancock and Carpentier-Edwards prosthesis in the smaller sizes, especially 19 to 23 mm. With the large aortic 25- to 31-mm prostheses, the hemodynamic performance of standard previous- and new-generation porcine bioprostheses is less striking. The standard prostheses and the new-generation Medtronic-Intact prostheses are intraannular and consequently have increased obstructive properties. The new-generation Hancock II, Carpentier-Edwards supraannular, and Bioimplant have been constructed for supraannular implantation and improved hemodynamics. In these prostheses the orifice can be of the same diameter as the patient's valve annulus if the supraaortic space can accommodate the prosthesis.

The hemodynamic performance of porcine prostheses in the mitral position have been generally satisfactory under both rest and exercise conditions. The new-generation porcine prostheses have not provided a significant change in hemodynamic performance over the standard ones (Table 10–11).

There is limited documentation of porcine biological valves by noninvasive Doppler techniques (119, 120). Simpson and colleagues (119) evaluated the Wessex porcine bio-

Table 10–9. *Valve-Related Reoperation*

Prosthesis and author	Mean age (years)	Patients			Mean follow-up (years)	Occurrence (%/pt yr)			Actuarial freedom (%) and length of follow-up		
		AVR	MVR	Overall		AVR	MVR	Overall	AVR	MVR	Overall
Hancock Standard											
Brais et al. (65)		—	111	111	5.4	—	3.3	3.3	NA	NA	NA
Gallo et al. (68)		131	202	403	AVR 5.8 MVR 6.1	1.7	3.0	2.4	NA	NA	NA
Gallucci et al. (33)		—	476	476	5.2	—	2.2	2.2	NA	NA	NA
Miller et al. (72)		857	794	1651	AVR 4.1 MVR 4.3	1.2	1.4	NA	NA	NA	NA
Gallucci et al. (8)		196	502	769	AVR 7.0 MVR 8.0	4.9	3.0	NA	NA	NA	NA
Cohn et al. (66)	60 (range, 17–95)								81 at 10 yr 59 at 15 yr	74 at 10 yr 29 at 15 yr	
Carpentier-Edwards Standard											
Jamieson et al. (50)		106	107	235	3.8	0.2	1.2	1.0	NA	NA	NA
Jamieson et al. (53)		155	154	355	4.25	0.5	1.3	1.0	NA	NA	NA
Soots et al. (76)		291	522	813	AVR 2.85 MVR 2.95	0.7	0.5	0.6	NA	NA	NA
Jamieson et al. (42)	57 (range, 8–85)	483	401	988	5.9 AVR 6.3 MVR 5.7	1.6	2.7	2.2	76.4 at 10 yr	67.6 at 10 yr	95.8 at 5 yr 70.8 at 10 yr 63.2 at 12 yr
Jamieson et al. (9)		569	500	1183		1.5	2.5	2.1	76.5 at 10 yr	68 at 10 yr 63 at 12 yr	71 at 10 yr
Carpentier-Edwards Supraannular											
Jamieson et al. (41)		286	259	592	AVR 1.2 MVR 1.1	0	1.1	0.5			
Jamieson et al. (49)	61 (range, 13–85)	546	525	1167	1.95	0.5	1.0	0.8	98.3 at 4 yr	93.1 at 4 yr	95.8 at 4 yr
Jamieson et al. (48)		733	678	1536	2.8 AVR 2.8, MVR 2.7	0.6	0.9	0.8	96.5 at 5 yr	95.8 at 5 yr	98.2 at 3 yr 95.9 at 5 yr

TABLE 10–10. *Valve-Related Mortality*

Prosthesis and author	Mean age (years)	Mean follow-up (years)	Occurrence (%/pt yr)			Actuarial freedom (%) and length of follow-up		
			AVR	MVR	Overall	AVR	MVR	Overall
Hancock Standard								
Magilligan et al. (71)	48 (range, 17–70)	AVR 6.6	3.8			66.3 at 14 yr		
Cohn et al. (66)	60 (range, 17–95)					60 at 10 yr 40 at 15 yr	58 at 10 yr 43 at 15 yr	
Carpentier-Edwards Standard								
Jamieson et al. (42)	57 (range, 8–85)	5.9 AVR 6.3 MVR 5.7	NA	NA	NA	89.9 at 10 yr	82.2 at 10 yr	96.3 at 5 yr 86.4 at 10, 12 yr
Jamieson et al. (9)	57 (range, 8–85)		NA	NA	NA	89.4 at 10 yr	82.3 at 10 yr	86.2 at 10, 12 yr
Carpentier-Edwards Supraannular								
Jamieson et al. (49)	61 (range, 13–85)	1.95	NA	NA	NA	98.7 at 4 yr	98.0 at 4 yr	98.4 at 4 yr
Jamieson et al. (48)	62 (range, 13–87)	2.8 AVR 2.8 MVR 2.7	NA	NA	NA	98.8 at 5 yr	94.5 at 5 yr	98.2 at 3 yr, 96.8 at 5 yr
Bioimplant								
Pavie et al. (19a)	52 (range, 9–76)		NA	NA	NA	90 at 5 yr	85 at 5 yr	88 at 5 yr

prosthesis and determined transvalvular gradients to be comparable to in vivo hemo-dynamic means of other porcine valves. The transvalvular gradient for the 23-mm aortic prosthesis was 21 mmHg and for the 29- and 31-mm mitral prosthesis, 3.7 and 3.3 mmHg, respectively. Williams et al. (120), evaluating a series of standard Hancock and Carpentier-Edwards aortic prostheses, found the mean gradient to be 23 mmHg and the mean effective orifice area to be 2.1 cm.

In vitro hemodynamics have been reported by Yoganathan et al. (121) and Walker et al. (122, 123). Yoganathan showed that the new-generation Hancock II valve had supe-rior pressure drop characteristics and better use of stent orifice area than the Hancock I (121). In 1980, Walker observed that the Carpentier-Edwards standard valve had supe-rior transvalvular pressure differences and energy loss characteristics than the Hancock standard valve (122). As further reported in 1984, the Carpentier-Edwards supraannular prosthesis had higher transvalvular pressure during forward flow than new-generation pericardial valves but less energy loss than most (122).

PATIENT SURVIVAL

The overall patient survival with the various porcine biological valves is detailed in Table 10–12 and Figures 10–17 and 10–18 (7–9, 33, 41, 42, 48–50, 53, 64, 65, 69–73, 76, 80, 96, 124). The patient survival information is documented by prosthesis, valve position, and mean age, and presented as early death (%), late death (% per patient year), and overall survival. In consideration of the survival data, the mean age of the patient population at implantation must always be considered. The survival data of the authors differ considerably because the mean age of the Gallucci series is 47.5 years and that of the Jamieson series is 57 years. The two series are also difficult to compare because the Jamieson data include operative (30-day) mortality while the Gallucci data were calcu-lated from operative survivors.

PORCINE VALVES IN CHILDREN AND ADOLESCENTS

The introduction of biological valves was considered a major advance for the man-agement of valvular disease in children and adolescents. Between 1978 and 1984 numer-ous reports expressed the concern of premature calcification of porcine bioprostheses (31, 125–146). In 1978 Kutsche and coauthors (135) presented one of the initial reports of premature calcification in children. Thandroyen and colleagues (143) in 1980 identified severe short-term calcification of porcine valves in children and postulated that dystro-phic calcification resulted from primary collagen degeneration. Silver and colleagues (142) identified calcification usually commencing near the commissures. These investi-gators felt that the positive calcium balance with a more labile calcium homeostasis was the contributing factor to premature calcification. Bortolotti and colleagues (31) reported the increasing frequency of calcification and fatigue-induced lesions in the left atrioven-tricular position and postulated that the cause was related to greater mechanical stress in the high-pressure ventricle.

The magnitude of the calcification problem has been detailed by several reports from South Africa (125, 140, 143, 147). Antunes and Santos (124) reported a primary failure rate of 21% per patient year for the population of 135 patients less than 20 years old; the freedom from degeneration was 20% at 6 years. In the same year, 1984, Antunes again

TABLE 10–11. Hemodynamics

Author	Prosthesis*	Valve size (mm)	Cardiac output (L/min)		Effective orifice area (cm²)		Mean transvalvular gradient (mmHg)	
			Rest	Exercise	Rest	Exercise	Rest	Exercise
Aortic Position								
Bove et al. (99)	CE-S	19			1.1	1.56	9.8	20.4
Foster et al. (105)	CE-S	19	5.8 ± 0.3		1.11 ± 0.23		33 ± 5	
Jones et al. (106)	H-S	19	3.9		0.98		2.5	
Craver et al. (103)	H-MO	19	2.53	3.96	0.89		32	70
Zusman et al. (117)	H-MO	19	4.9 ± 0.2		—	—	12.5 ± 3.5	
Bove et al. (99)	CE-S	21			1.35	1.57 ± 0.17	9.8 ± 18.3	25.5 ± 23.8
Rothkopf et al. (116)	CE-S	21			1.3		18.0	
Lee et al. (108)	CE-S	21			1.03		15.0	
Jones et al. (106)	H-S	21	5.1		1.61		18.0	
Craver et al. (103)	H-MO	21	3.9	6.21	1.59 ± 0.46	1.28	9.7	17.5
Zusman et al. (117)	H-MO	21	4.5 ± 0.9				10.0 ± 6.5	
Carpentier et al. (81)	CE-SA	21	4.9				13.6	
Foster et al. (105)	H-S	21			1.27		10.0	
Chaitman et al. (100)	CE-S	21-23	5.4	9.9	1.2 ± 0.1	1.3 ± 0.1	21 ± 3	28 ± 2
Jamieson et al. (40)	CE-SA	21-25			1.98		9.0	21.0
Pelletier et al. (112)	CE-S	21-23			1.14 ± 0.09	1.28 ± 0.09		
Pelletier et al. (113)	CE-S	21-23			1.4 ± 0.1		13.4 ± 2.2	
Lee et al. (108)	CE-S	23			1.60		17.3	
Rothkopf et al. (116)	CE-S	23			1.1		30.0	
Levine et al. (110)	CE-S	23	4.7 ± 0.9		1.2 ± 0.4		7.6 ± 6.2	
Cohen-Solal et al. (101)	CE-S	23			1.46		19.0 ± 8.0	
Borkon et al. (98)	H-S	23			1.29		7.0	
Jones et al. (106)	H-S	23	5.5		1.46		16.0	
Craver et al. (103)	H-MO	23	4.87			1.34	18.1	28.0
Zusman et al. (117)	H-MO	23	4.7 ± 1.5	1.84 ± 0.69		10.8 ± 5.9	10.5	
Carpentier et al. (81)	CE-SA	23	4.8		1.4 ± 0.5		18.6 ± 7.1	
Cosgrove et al. (102)	CE-SA	23						
Navia et al. (111)	Bioimplant	23/24	5.7 ± 1.3	7.3 ± 1.4			16.8 ± 9.3	23.7 ± 8.5
Navia et al. (111)	Bioimplant	22-28	5.9 ± 1.1	7.6 ± 1.5			16.0 ± 10.3	23.2 ± 16.7
Levine et al. (110)	H-MO	23	4.7 ± 1.5				10.8 ± 5.9	
Rossiter et al. (115)	H-S	21-25			1.9		21.0 ± 8.0	
Rossiter et al. (115)	H-MO	19-25			2.5		16.0 ± 2.0	
Cohen-Solal et al. (101)	CE-S	25			1.7 ± 0.4		15.0 ± 6.0	
Cosgrove et al. (102)	CE-S	25			1.6 ± 0.5		31.6 ± 7.3	
Rothkopf et al. (116)	CE-S	25			1.5		19.0	
Lee et al. (108)	CE-S	25	5.6		1.63		14.0	
Jones et al. (106)	H-S	25			1.44		17.0	
Borkon et al. (98)	H-S	25			1.72		7.0	
Cosgrove et al. (102)	CE-S	25			1.6 ± 0.52		31.6 ± 7.3	
Zusman et al. (117)	H-MO	25	5.2 ± 0.8				9.8 ± 5.8	
Levine et al. (110)	H-MO	25	4.6 ± 0.8		1.95 ± 0.47		11.9 ± 5.5	

Levine et al. (110)	CE-S	25					8.3 ± 5.9	
Craver et al. (103)	H-MO	25	4.6 ± 0.5				2.0	
Pelletier et al. (113)	CE-S	25/27	2.51		1.37 ± 0.07	1.57 ± 0.11	11.3 ± 1.5	
Cosgrove et al. (102)	CE-SA	25			2.1 ± 0.9		16.3 ± 10.1	
Pelletier et al. (112)	CE-S	25/27			1.37 ± 0.07		NA	
Chaitman et al. (100)	CE-S	25/27	5.5	9.9	1.2 ± 0.1	1.3 ± 0.1	21.0 ± 3.0	28.0 ± 2.0
Jones et al. (106)	H-S	27	4.4		1.61		9.0	
Cosgrove et al. (102)	CE-S	27			2.4 ± 0.7		15.7 ± 7.0	
Cohen-Salal et al. (101)	CE-S	27			2.0 ± 0.5		16.0 ± 5.0	
Cosgrove et al. (102)	CE-SA	27			2.4 ± 0.7		15.7 ± 7.0	
Borkon et al. (98)	H-S	27			1.97		5.5	
Pelletier et al. (113)	CE-S	27			2.1 ± 1.0		15.5 ± 11.1	
Levine et al. (110)	H-MO	27/29			5.3 ± 1.0		11.0 ± 6.0	
Levine et al. (110)	CE-S	27/29			5.5 ± 1.3		6.6 ± 5.0	
Rothkopf et al. (116)	CE-S	27			2.7		11.0	
Lee et al. (108)	CE-S	27			1.71		14.5	
Lee et al. (108)	CE-S	29			2.7		14.5	
Cosgrove et al. (102)	CE-S	29			2.9 ± 0.6		12.5 ± 4.6	
Levine et al. (110)	CE-S	29			4.7 ± 1.2		2.8 ± 1.1	
Cohen-Solal et al. (101)	CE-S	29-31	6.7	12.4	2.5 ± 0.4	2.4 ± 0.3	6.0 ± 2.0	
Chaitman et al. (100)	CE-S	29-31			1.9 ± 0.3		17.0 ± 2.7	18.0 ± 2.7
Levine et al. (110)	H-MO	29	5.0 ± 1.4		1.93 ± 0.25	2.43 ± 0.34	3.7 ± 1.2	
Pelletier et al. (112)	CE-S	29-31			1.4 ± 0.1			
Pelletier et al. (113)	CE-S	21-31			1.93 ± 0.25		11.4 ± 1.1	
Pelletier et al. (112)	CE-S	29-31					7.5 ± 2.2	
Mitral Position								
Pelletier et al. (112)	CE-S	27/29			2.33 ± 0.14		7.1 ± 0.6	
Chaitman et al. (100)	CE-S	27-29	4.5	6.9	2.1 ± 0.2		7.0 ± 0.8	
Rasmusson et al. (114)	CE-S	27-33	4.67 ± 1.47	10.1 ± 3.4	1.98 ± 0.86	2.4 ± 0.2	7.1 ± 2.6	17.0 ± 3.5
Pelletier et al. (113)	CE-S	27-33			2.5 ± 0.1		6.4 ± 0.4	
Pelletier et al. (112)	CE-S	31-33			2.68 ± 0.16		5.1 ± 0.3	
Chaitman et al. (100)	CE-S	31-33	4.6	6.8	2.9 ± 0.4	3.2 ± 0.6	5.0 ± 0.6	11.0 ± 1.8
Rasmusson et al. (114)	H-S	29-33	4.96 ± 1.15		1.94 ± 0.5	2.32 ± 0.54	3.6 ± 1.8	7.1 ± 2.3
Kagawa et al. (107)	H-S	29-31				7.96 ± 5.36	19.32 ± 8.49	
Navia et al. (111)	Bioimplant	28-30	5.1 ± 1.1	7.1 ± 1.4			2.0 ± 1.7	4.8 ± 2.8
Navia et al. (111)	Bioimplant	28-30	5.1 ± 1.3	6.7 ± 1.9			2.1 ± 1.8	3.7 ± 2.6
Levine et al. (110)	H-MO	31	4.4 ± 0.8				3.5 ± 1.0	
Levine et al. (110)	CE-S	31	4.8 ± 1.1				2.6 ± 0.7	
Pelletier et al. (112)	CE-S	27/29			2.33 ± 0.14		7.1 ± 0.6	
Carpenter et al. (81)	CE-SA	31	4.7				2.5	
Pelletier et al. (112)	CE-S	31-33			2.68 ± 0.16	2.8 ± 0.22	6.4 ± 0.4	
Pelletier et al. (113)	CE-S	27-33			2.5 ± 0.1	3.14 ± 0.24	7.0	
Jamieson et al. (40)	CE-SA	27-31			1.72		—	
Levine et al. (110)	H-MO	33-35	4.6 ± 1.4				3.2 ± 1.9	
Levine et al. (110)	CE-S	33-35	4.7 ± 0.7				2.1 ± 1.1	

*CE-S = Carpentier-Edwards Standard; H-S = Hancock Standard; H-MO = Hancock modified orifice; CE-SA = Carpentier-Edwards supraannular.

TABLE 10–12. *Patient Survival*

Prosthesis and author	Patients			Mean age (years)	Early death (%)	Late death (%/pt yr)	Survival (% + S.E.)	
	AVR	MVR	Overall				AVR	MVR
Hancock Standard								
Bolooki et al. (64)	20	63	177	49 (range, 15–71)	Overall 8.6	Overall 2.6	95 at 5 yr	87 at 5 yr
Brais et al. (65)	—	111	111	53	MVR 11.7	MVR 4.8		78 at 3 yr 70 at 6 yr
Gallo et al. (68)	131	202	403	42.5 (range, 6–68)	AVR 4.5 MVR 10.8	AVR 1.95 MVR 1.47	92 at 5 yr 85 at 8 yr	95 at 5 yr 86 at 8 yr
Gallucci et al. (33)	—	476	476	53 (range, 9–63)	MVR 13	MVR 3.1		87 at 5 yr 74 at 13 yr
Miller et al. (72)	857	794	1651	AVR 59 MVR 56		AVR 0.5 MVR 0.8		
Gallucci et al. (8)	196	502	769	47.5 (range, 8–71)		AVR 3.5 MVR 3.8	37 at 15 yr	52 at 15 yr
Magilligan et al. (71)	196			48 (range, 17–70)		AVR 3.8	51 at 14 yr	
Carpentier-Edwards Standard								
Jamieson et al. (50)	106	107	235	NA	AVR 2.8 MVR 8.4	Overall 3.9	82.5 at 6 yr	76.4 at 6 yr
Jamieson et al. (53)	155	154	355	57 (range, 15–82)	AVR 4.5 MVR 9.0	AVR 3.4 MVR 3.6	84 at 5 yr 8.14 at 6 yr	72 at 7 yr 70 at 6 yr
Lougie et al. (70)	88	38	122	65 (range, 25–84)	AVR 10.5 MVR 12.5	Overall 5.0	76 at 5 yr	60 at 5 yr
Soots et al. (76)	291	522	813	AVR 49.1 MVR 48.2	AVR 5.5 MVR 4.6	AVR 1.2 MVR 1.1	88 at 5 yr	91 at 5 yr

258

Study			Age				
Jamieson et al. (42)	483	401	57 (range, 8–85)	AVR 5.2 / MVR 9.5	AVR 3.4 / MVR 4.1	66 at 10 yr	55 at 10 yr
Jamieson et al. (9)	569	500	57 (range, 8–85)	AVR 5.1 / MVR 8.8	AVR 3.6 / MVR 4.2	65 at 10 yr	54 at 10 yr
Carpentier-Edwards and Hancock Standard							
Hartz et al. (69)	208	209	59 (range, 19–88)	AVR 6.2 / MVR 14.3	AVR 3.1 / MVR 4.4	79 at 5 yr	68 at 5 yr
Spencer et al. (96)	786	1492	NA	Overall 7.8	NA	89 at 5 yr	84 at 5 yr
Magilligan et al. (71)	NA	817	NA	AVR 6.3 / MVR 8.3	NA	79 at 5 yr / 57 at 10 yr	80 at 5 yr / 69 at 10 yr
Zussa et al. (124)	287	506	49 (range, 14–71)	AVR 4.5 / MVR 5.9	Overall 4.4	83 at 6 yr	77 at 7 yr
Carpentier-Edwards Supraannular							
Jamieson et al. (41)	286	259	NA	AVR 5.2 / MVR 10.0	Overall 6.2	87 at 2 yr	82 at 2 yr
Wahlers et al. (80)	222	234	55	AVR 5.8	Overall 2.6	94 at 2.5 yr	78 at 4 yr
Jamieson et al. (49)	546	1167	61 (range, 13–85)	AVR 5.3 / MVR 9.3	AVR 4.0 / MVR 4.8	81 at 4 yr	
Jamieson et al. (48)	733	1536	62 (range, 13–87)	AVR 5.3 / MVR 8.9	AVR 3.2 / MVR 4.8	82 at 5 yr	71 at 5 yr
Bioimplant							
Navia et al. (73)	132	279	54 (range, 17–76)	NA	NA	79 at 6 yr	86 at 6 yr
Pavie et al. (19a)	63	14	52 (range, 9–76)	AVR 1.6 / MVR 8.9 / MR 7.1 / Overall 6.0		87 at 5 yr	87 at 5 yr

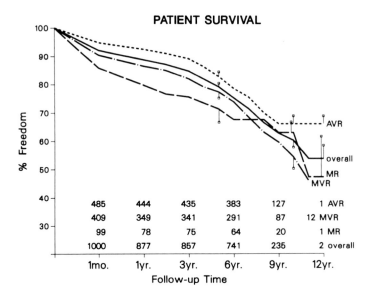

FIG. 10–17. Patient survival (University of British Columbia, Carpentier-Edwards standard).

reported a prohibitive failure rate in children, 22.5% per patient year (148). It was recommended that porcine valves not be implanted in children and that degenerating valves be replaced early rather than late. In 1982, Human et al. (133) indicated that valvular degeneration contributed to only 10% survival beyond 10 years. Williams et al. (145) reported the Mayo Clinic experience in 1982 with a 59% freedom from failure at 5 years and said that mechanical prostheses are preferable for children.

Miller and colleagues (138) reported the Stanford University experience in 1982 of isolated porcine valves and conduit-containing porcine valves. They found that porcine valves develop fibrocalcific degeneration with or without leaflet retraction or perforation,

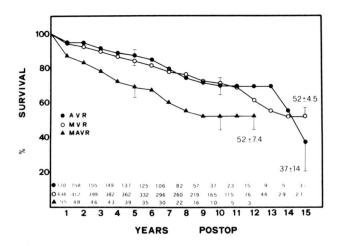

FIG. 10–18. Patient survival (University of Padova, Hancock standard).

whereas conduits fail because of pseudointimal proliferation of the proximal conduit. The incidence of valve failure requiring reoperation was 10.1% per patient year for free-standing valves, whereas the rate was 4.1% per patient year for conduits. The primary tissue failure rate was 8.1% per patient year, and the freedom from reoperation due to primary tissue failure at 5 years was 59%. Additional experience with porcine valve-containing conduits has been reported by Edwards and colleagues (128). Jamieson and colleagues (51) reported that the incidence of primary tissue failure in free-standing valves under the age of 20 years is 7.6% per patient year and the freedom from primary tissue failure at 5 years is 70% and at 10 years 43%. Milano and colleagues (36) in 1986 summarized the use of prosthetic valves in children, recommending mechanical valves in the aortic position and recommending that efforts be made to preserve the natural valve of the child because both porcine and mechanical valves are unsatisfactory in the systemic atrioventricular position.

The choice of prosthesis for women nearing childbearing age is extremely important (31, 47, 139). The porcine bioprosthesis is recommended because of the opportunity of management without anticoagulation (47). The warfarin anticoagulants are contraindicated during pregnancy because of fetal wastage, fatal hemorrhage, and malformations caused by the teratogenic effect of warfarin. The use of porcine prostheses avoids the necessity for anticoagulant management to prevent thromboembolism and the subsequent complications and management problems during pregnancy.

PATHOLOGY OF PORCINE VALVE DEGENERATION

The degeneration of porcine valves is related to leaflet rupture and leaflet calcification (12, 149–154). The high incidence of leaflet calcification in children is detailed in the previous section. It is felt that mechanical stress plays an important role and the calcification starts at the commissures and extends toward the center of the leaflet. Goffin and Bartik (151) have detailed the three characteristic features of calcification: (1) early intrinsic calcification that spreads along the fibrous cords from the commissures, (2) intrinsic calcification of the fibrous annulus of the three cusps and muscular shelf of the right coronary cusp, and (3) gross calcific nodules of extrinsic nature originating from the enlarged spongiosa in the central area of the cusp. Fiddler and colleagues (129) described this third type of calcification as the soaked sponge phenomenon, with massive insudation in the spongiosa of cellular elements and calcification-enhancing factors such as γ-carboxyglutamic acid and lipids. The first and third types of calcification result in Ishihara type I tears or gross calcific stenosis. Leaflet rupture is related to mechanical stress factors with or without calcification of the fibrous cords. The commonest forms of rupture are the Ishihara type I juxtacommissural radial rupture or Ishihara type IV pinpoint perforations due to collagen degeneration. In 1982, Ishihara (152) described four types of anatomic degeneration of biological valves, namely, type I, tears involving the free edges of the cusps; type II, linear perforations extending along the basal regions of the cusps forming an arc parallel to the sewing ring; type III, large, round or oval perforations that occupy the central regions of the cusps; and type IV, small, pinhole-like perforations, usually multiple and localized in central regions of the cusps, often in association with multiple calcific deposits. Goffin and Bartil (151) summarized degeneration of porcine valves as leaflet calcifications that are stress-induced and commence at commissures, and cusp rupture, which is predominantly radical or commissural and in most cases is associated with stress-induced calcification of the fibrous cords.

The initial reports on structural changes in glutaraldehyde-preserved porcine valves were presented by Spray and Roberts (155, 156), and Ferrans (157) in 1978. The long-term changes consisted of progressive disruption of collagen, erosion of valve surfaces, formation of aggregates of platelets, and accumulation of lipids. The progressive break-down of collagen and the sponge phenomenon of the spongiosa have been the main pathologic degenerative changes. Ferrans and colleagues (157) also described changes of thrombosis with short-term insudation of plasma proteins, penetration of erythrocytes into surface crevices, formation of a thin surface layer of fibrin, and deposition of mac-rophages, giant cells, and few platelets. The insudation of plasma proteins and lipids accompanies spongiosa loosening, collagen bundle separation, and extraction of proteoglycans.

The spectrum of pathologic changes contributing to late failure of the Hancock por-cine bioprosthesis has been documented by the University of Padova (21, 30, 32, 35, 158–164). The pathologic changes include dystrophic calcification, thrombosis, fibrous tissue overgrowth, primary tears, cuspal hematomas, and stent creep. Left ven-tricular wall rupture has also been a complication of porcine bioprostheses (35, 165–168).

Calcification

Calcification is the main factor influencing long-term durability (Figs. 10–19 to 10–21). In the experience with the standard Hancock porcine bioprosthesis at the University of Padova, 68% of the explant cases failed because of calcification. The calcification was progressive, a time-related phenomenon involving all bioprostheses in place for more than 6 years. Commissures are the first structures affected by calcium deposits, and their selective involvement may suffice to cause cuspal tears and severe incompetence, even if the remaining cuspal tissue is intact (160, 163) (Fig. 10–20). Cusp tearing may be abrupt, necessitating emergency reoperation (30). When the body of the cusp is infiltrated by calcific deposits, tissue stiffness impairs cusp pliability and causes valve stenosis. How-ever, mineralized leaflets disintegrate readily like an eggshell, leading to valve incompe-tence by tears, frayings, and loss of substance. Washout of fragments of calcific cusp tissue may be responsible for embolic events (159). The Padova experience indicates that no different propensity for calcification exists between mitral or aortic porcine bio-prostheses (21). Electron microscopic studies showed that calcific precipitation occurs on both collagen fibrils and cellular debris (164) (Fig. 10–21). Early nuclei of calcification consist of round or oval bodies with an electron-light or dense core, surrounded by one or more layers formed by radically arranged microneedle-shaped crystals, and occasion-ally by a few concentric layers of cytoplasmic membrane-like structures. X-ray diffrac-tion and energy-dispersion microanalysis identified the calcium deposits as crystals of hydroxyapatite (164).

Thrombus Formation

Thrombus formation related to Hancock porcine valves, in the Padova experience, is not rare and may be primary or secondary (160) (Fig. 10–22). Primary thrombosis occurs even in the absence of tissue failure; the thrombus fills the valve sinuses and impairs cusp movements. If thrombus organization does not intervene, systemic embolization may occur. Secondary thrombosis occurs in the setting of prosthetic mitral or tricuspid ste-

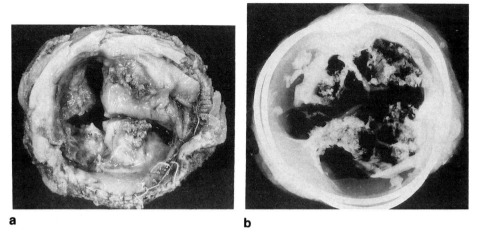

FIG. 10–19. (a) Pathology. (b) Calcification, general. (Hancock standard).

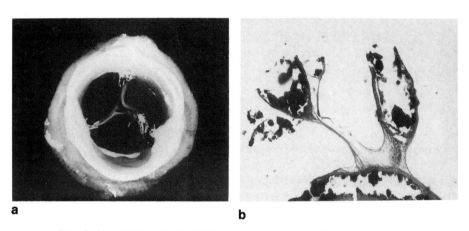

FIG. 10–20. (a) Pathology. (b) Calcification, commissures. (Hancock standard).

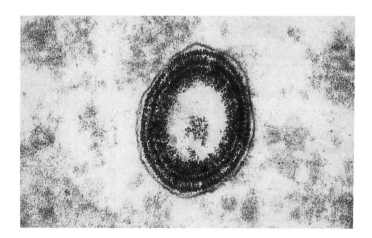

FIG. 10–21. Pathology and calcification (electron micrograph) (Hancock standard).

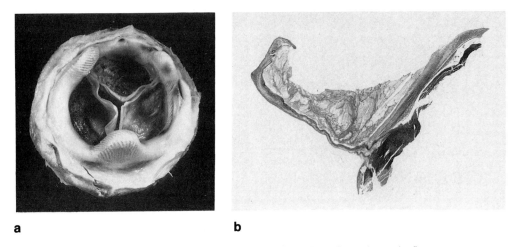

a   **b**

Fig. 10–22. (a) Pathology. (b) Thrombus formation. (Hancock standard).

nosis due to calcific cusp stiffness (32). The thrombus may be located on the valve itself, in the body, or in the auricle of the left atrium, in a fashion quite similar to that observed in rheumatic mitral valve stenosis.

Endocarditis

Endocarditis presents either as vegetations or polypoid masses obstructing the prosthetic orifice, or as cusp ulcerations causing prosthetic regurgitation (169) (Fig. 10–23). Paravalvular abscesses creating prosthetic dehiscence are rare, since unlike mechanical devices, the leaflets themselves are the site of microbial implantation and growth. Indeed, clusters of bacteria and leukocyte infiltrates are observed deep within the cusp tissue and are responsible for necrosis with tears or perforations (Fig. 10–23). A large spectrum of offending organisms are involved, including fungi. Secondary calcification is a regular finding in healed endocarditis. Sepsis and thromboembolic events with systemic dissemination of the septic, friable vegetations are a frequent finding and account for the poor patient outcome and extremely high mortality at reoperation (161).

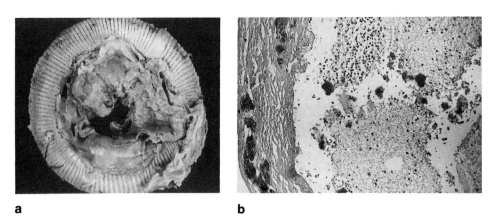

a   **b**

Fig. 10–23. (a) Pathology. (b) Endocarditis. (Hancock standard).

Fibrous Tissue Overgrowth

Fibrous tissue overgrowth appears as a thick host pannus covering mostly the atrial side of prosthetic valves implanted in an atrioventricular position (158) (Fig. 10–24). The reduction in the valve orifice may be so pronounced as to cause prosthetic valve stenosis, even in the presence of intact pliable leaflets. However, the host fibrous tissue itself may be the site of calcium deposition (160).

Cuspal Rupture

Tears causing prosthetic valve incompetence are usually calcium-related (35). In a few cases, however, cusp tissue may be disrupted even in the absence of mineralization (so called primary tears) (Fig. 10–25). Laceration may occur in correspondence to the muscular shelf of the right coronary cusp, as a possible consequence of immunoreaction against the porcine myocytes (162). Cusp disruption by massive lipid infiltration is another rare, isolated cause of leaflet tears and prosthetic valve incompetence (170) (Fig. 10–26).

Cuspal Hematomas

Cuspal hematomas are a potential but infrequent determinant of valve dysfunction, and only six cases were observed in 193 Hancock standard bioprosthetic explants (171) (Fig. 10–27). In most cases the cuspal hematomas contributed to valve failure; only in

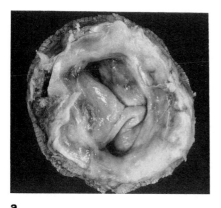
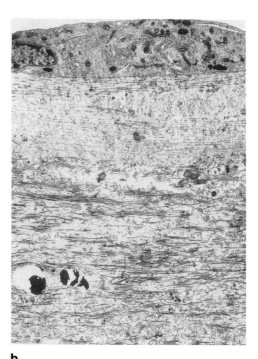

a   **b**

Fɪɢ. 10–24. (a) Pathology, fibrous tissue overgrowth. (b) Pathology, fibrous tissue overgrowth with calcification. (Hancock standard.)

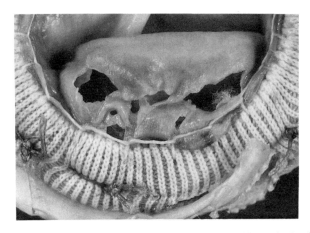

FIG. 10–25. Pathology, primary tear without calcification (Hancock standard).

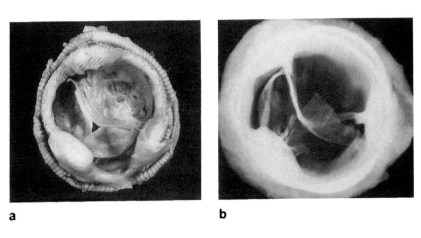

a

b

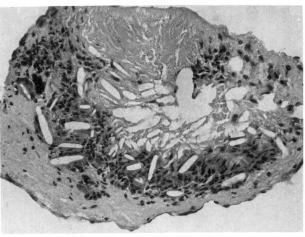

c

FIG. 10–26. (a, b, c) Pathology, lipid infiltration (Hancock standard).

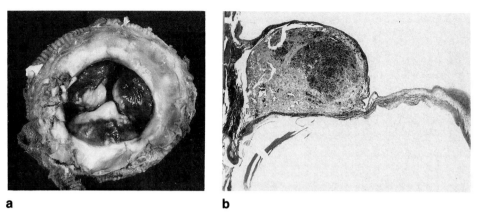

a   b

Fig. 10–27. (a) Pathology. (b) Cuspal hematoma. (Hancock standard).

one instance was it the sole factor determining stenosis by cusp thickening, requiring reoperation. Cuspal hematomas may involve bioprostheses implanted in both the mitral and aortic positions, and might reflect a complication of anticoagulant therapy (171).

Stent Creep

The initial Hancock bioprosthesis had a rigid stent, which was soon replaced by a new polypropylene flexible frame in order to reduce commissurial stresses; however, polypropylene frequently undergoes permanent deformation, with inward post bending due to the so-called creep (172, 173), which has a definite structure substrate, consisting of 0.7- to 1.0-μm large cracks, which are visible on the polypropylene surface by scanning electron microscopy (Fig. 10–28). In the Padova experience, post bending of the Hancock bioprosthesis was never an isolated cause of bioprosthetic dysfunction.

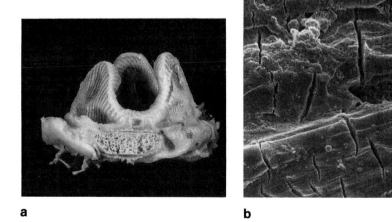

a   b

Fig. 10–28. (a) Stent creep. (b) Stent creep polypropylene surface.

CONCLUSIONS

Porcine bioprostheses have given patients an excellent quality of life with a low rate of serious thromboembolism, essential lack of thrombosis, and freedom from anticoagulant-related hemorrhage. The primary concern is that limited durability has compromised use in young populations and long-term performance in intermediate-age populations. Extended evaluation of new tissue preparation techniques will determine effect on long-term clinical performance.

The future of porcine bioprostheses will, in all likelihood, be favorably influenced by advanced chemical treatments of biological tissue and engineering advance in stent design and tissue configuration. The influence of these advances on clinical performance will require another 20 years of observation.

REFERENCES

1. Carpentier A, Lemaigre G, Ladislas R, Dubost C: Biological factors affecting long-term results of valvular heterografts. J Thorac Cardiovasc Surg 1969;58:467.
2. Acinapura AJ, Cunningham JN Jr, Jacobwitz IJ, Kramer MD, Rose DM, Zisbrod Z: A 7-year experience with 1,275 Carpentier-Edwards porcine prostheses. In Bodnar E, Yacoub M (eds): Biologic and Bioprosthetic Valves: Proceedings of the Third International Symposium. New York, York Medical Books, 1986, pp 98–104.
3. Angell WW, Angell JD, Kosek JC: Twelve-year experience with glutaraldehyde-preserved porcine xenografts. J Thorac Cardiovasc Surg 1982;83:493–502.
4. Bolooki H, Kaiser GA, Mallon SM, Palatianos GM: Comparison of long-term results of Carpentier-Edwards and Hancock bioprosthetic valves. Ann Thorac Surg 1986;42(5):494–499.
5. Cobanoglu A, Jamieson WRE, Miller DC, McKinley C, Grunkemeier GL, Floton HS, Miyagishima RT, Tyers GFO, Shumway NE, Starr A: A tri-institutional comparison of tissue and mechanical valves using a patient-oriented definition of treatment failure. Ann Thorac Surg 1987;43:245–253.
6. Di Sesa VJ, Allfred EN, Kowalker W, Shemin RJ, Collins JJ Jr, Cohn LH: Performance of a fabricated trileaflet porcine bioprosthesis. Midterm follow-up of the Hancock modified-orifice valve. J Thorac Cardiovasc Surg 1987;94(2):220–224.
7. Gallo I, Ruiz B, Duran CG: Isolated mitral valve replacement with the Hancock porcine bioprosthesis in rheumatic heart disease: Analysis of 213 operative survivors followed up to 4.5 to 8.5 years. Am J Cardiol 1984;53(1):178–181.
8. Gallucci V: The standard Hancock porcine bioprosthesis: Overall experience at the University of Padova. Proceedings of the Fourth International Symposium—Cardiac Bioprostheses. J Cardiac Surg 1988;3(3)Suppl:337–345.
9. Jamieson WRE, Allen P, Miyagishima RT, Gerein AN, Munro AI, Burr LH, Janusz MT, Ling H, Tutassaura H, Tyers GFO: The Carpentier-Edwards standard porcine bioprosthesis—A first generation tissue valve with excellent long-term clinical performance. J Thorac Cardiovasc Surg 1990;99:543–561.
10. Oyer PE, Stinson EB, Miller DC, Jamieson SW, Reitz BA, Baumgartner W, Shumway NE: Clinical analysis of the Hancock porcine bioprosthesis. In Cohn LH, Gallucci V (eds): Cardiac Bioprostheses: Proceedings of the Second International Symposium. New York: Yorke Medical Books, 1982, pp 539–551.
11. Oyer PE, Stinson EB, Miller DC, Jamieson SW, Mitchell RS, Shumway NE: Thromboembolic risk and durability of the Hancock bioprosthetic cardiac valve. Eur Heart J 1984;5(suppl D):81–85.
12. Paphitis CA, Lennox SC: Early experience with the Xenomedica bioprosthetic valve. In Bodnar E, Jacoub M (eds): Biologic and Bioprosthetic Valves: Proceedings of the Third International Symposium. New York, Yorke Medical Books, 1986, pp 652–658.
13. Pavie A, Gandjbakhch I, Baud R, Bors V, Fontanel M, Mattei MF, Cabrol C, Cabrol A: The low profile Liotta valve. Mid-term results. Arch Mal Coeur 1987;80:1395–1404.
14. Reece IJ, Anderson JD, Wain WH, Carr K, Toner PE, Tindale W, Black MM, Wheatley DJ: A new porcine bioprosthesis: In vitro and in vivo evaluation. Life Supp Syst 1985;3:207–227.
15. Reece IJ, Wheatley DJ, Munro JL, Wisheart JC, Keen G, Ross JK, Shore DF, Pollock JCS, Davidson KG: Early results with the Wessex porcine bioprosthesis in 245 patients. In Bodnar E, Jacoub M (eds): Biologic and Bioprosthetic Valves: Proceedings of the Third International Symposium. New York: Yorke Medical Books, 1986, pp 760–767.
16. Romano M, Sigal R, Lorente P, Piwnica A: Low profile bioprostheses for mitral valve replacement. Z Kardiol 1986;75(suppl 2):305–307.
17. Vrandecic MP, Gontijo B, Rabelo S: Clinical experience with a new generation porcine bioprostheses. In

Bodnar E, Jacoub M (eds): Biologic and Bioprosthetic Valves: Proceedings of the Third International Symposium. New York: Yorke Medical Books, 1986, pp 659–665.

18. Williams MA: The Intact bioprosthesis—Early results. Proceedings of the Fourth International Symposium—Cardiac Bioprostheses. J Cardiac Surg 1988;3(3)Suppl 347–351.

19. Hatcher CR Jr, Craver JM, Jones EL, Bone DK, Guyton RA: The porcine bioprosthesis. A review of 1,000 consecutive patients undergoing cardiac valve replacement. Am Surg 1983;49:6–10.

19a. Pavie A, Bors V, Piazza C, Desruennes M, Fontanel M, Jault F, Gandjbakheh I, Cabrol C: Mid-term results of the Liotta-Bioimplant Low Profile Bioprostheses. J Card Surg 1988;3:353–358.

20. Bortolotti U, Milano A, Mazzucco A, Valfre C, Talenti E, Guerra F, Thiene G, Gallucci V: Results of reoperation for primary tissue failure of porcine bioprostheses. J Thorac Cardiovasc Surg 1985;90:564–569.

21. Bortolotti U, Milano A, Thiene G, Guerra F, Mazzucco A, Talenti E, Gallucci V: Long-term durability of the Hancock porcine bioprosthesis following combined mitral and aortic valve replacement: An 11 year experience. Ann Thorac Surg 1987;44(2):139–144.

22. Cohen SR, Silver MA, McIntosh CL, Roberts WC: Comparison of late (62 to 140 months) degenerative changes in simultaneously implanted and explanted porcine (Hancock) bioprostheses and the tricuspid and mitral valve positions in six patients. Am J Cardiol 1984;53:1599–1602.

23. Foster AH, Greenberg GJ, Underhill DJ, McIntosh CL, Clark RE: Intrinsic failure of Hancock mitral bioprostheses: 10 to 15 year experience. Ann Thorac Surg 1987;44(6):568–577.

24. Gallo I, Nistal F, Ruiz B, Duran G: Incidence of primary tissue valve failure with the Hancock I cardiac bioprosthesis: A 6- to 10-year review. In Bodnar E, Yacoub M (eds): Biologic and Bioprosthetic Valves: Proceedings of the Third International Symposium. New York, Yorke Medical Books, 1986, pp 116–127.

25. Isomura T, Yanai T, Akagawa H, Aoyagi S, Kosuga K, Ohishi K, Koga M: Late pathological changes of Carpentier-Edwards porcine bioprostheses in the mitral position. J Cardiovasc Surg (Torino) 1986;27(3):307–315.

26. Klovekorn WP, Struck E, Holper K, Meisner H, Sebening F: Causes of valve failure and indications for reoperation after bioprosthetic cardiac valve replacement. In Cohn LH, Gallucci V (eds): Cardiac Bioprostheses: Proceedings of the Second International Symposium. (eds): New York, Yorke Medical Books, 1982, pp 530–538.

27. Magillian DJ Jr, Kemp SR, Stein PD, Peterson E: Asynchronous primary valve failure in patients with porcine bioprosthetic aortic and mitral valves. Circulation 1987;76(3 pt 2):141–145.

28. Pomar JL, Bosch X, Chaitman BR, Pelletier C, Grondin CM: Late tears in leaflets of porcine bioprostheses in adults. Ann Thorac Surg 1984;37(1):78–83.

29. Magilligan DJ Jr, Lewis JW Jr, Heinzerling RH, Smith D: Fate of a second porcine bioprosthetic valve. J Thorac Cardiovasc Surg 1983;85:362–370.

30. Bortolotti U, Guerra F, Magni A, Milano A, Mazzucco A, Talenti E, Thiene G, Gallucci V: Emergency reoperation for primary failure of porcine bioprostheses. Am J Cardiol 1987;60:920–921.

31. Bortolotti U, Milano A, Mazzucco A, Valfre C, Russo R, Valente M, Schivazappa L, Thiene G, Gallucci V: Pregnancy in patients with a porcine valve bioprosthesis. Am J Cardiol 1982;50:1051–1054.

32. Bortolotti U, Thiene G: Calcification of porcine heterografts implanted in children. Chest 1981;80:117–118.

33. Gallucci V, Bortolotti U, Milano A, Valfre C, Mazzucco A, Thiene G: Isolated mitral valve replacement with the Hancock bioprosthesis: A 13-year appraisal, Ann Thorac Surg 1984;38(6):571–578.

34. Gallucci V, Bortolotti U, Minalo A, Mazzucco A, Valfre C, Guerra F, Faggian G, Thiene G: The Hancock porcine valve 15 years later: An analysis of 575 patients. In Bodnar E, Yacoub M (eds): Biologic and Bioprosthetic Valves: Proceedings of the Third International Symposium; New York, Yorke Medical Books, 1986, pp 91–97.

35. Milano A, Bortolotti U, Talenti E, Valfre C, Arbustini E, Valente M, Mazzucco A, Gallucci V, Thiene G: Calcific degeneration as the main cause of porcine bioprosthetic valve failure. Am J Cardiol 1984;53:1066–1070.

36. Milano AD, Vouhe PR, Baillot-Vernant F, Donzeau-Gouge P, Trinquet F, Roux P-M, Leca F, Neveux J-Y: Late results after left-sided cardiac valve replacement in children. J Thorac Cardiovasc Surg 1986;92:218–225.

37. Milano AD, Bortolotti U, Mazzucco A, Guerra F, Stellin G, Talenti E, Thiene G, Gallucci V: Performance of the Hancock porcine bioprosthesis following aortic valve replacement: Considerations based on a 15-year experience. Ann Thorac Surg 1988;46:216–222.

38. Jamieson WRE, Allen P, Janusz MT, Germann E, Chan F, MacNab J, Munro AI, Miyagishima RT, Gerein AN, Burr LH, Tyers GFO: First-generation porcine bioprosthesis: Valve-related complications in the intermediate term. In Bodnar E, Yacoub M (eds): Biologic and Bioprosthetic Valves: Proceedings of the Third International Symposium. New York, Yorke Medical Books, 1986, pp 105–115.

39. Jamieson WRE, Allen P, Ling H, Miyagishima RT, Burr LH, Janusz MT, Gerein AN: Carpentier-Edwards porcine bioprostheses (previous and new generation)—Assessment of clinical performance. Can J Cardiol 1988;4(6):314–321.

40. Jamieson WRE, Gerein AN, Ricci DR, Janusz MT, Tyers GFO, Munro AI, Burr LH, Allen P, Ling H,

Hayden RI, Tutassaura H: Carpentier-Edwards supra-annular porcine bioprosthesis: A new generation tissue valve (clinical and hemodynamic assessment). In Bodnar E, Jacoub M (eds): Biologic and Bioprosthetic Valves: Proceedings of the Third International Symposium. New York, Yorke Medical Books, 1986, pp 141–151.

41. Jamieson WRE, Gerein AN, Tyers GFO, Janusz MT, Munro AI, Jyrala AJ, Miyagishima RT, Allen P: Carpentier-Edwards supra-annular porcine bioprosthesis: Clinical experience and implantation characteristics. J Thorac Cardiovasc Surg 1986;91:555–565.

42. Jamieson WRE, Janusz MT, Miyagishima RT, Munro AI, Gerein AN, Allen P, Burr LH, MacNab J, Chan F, Tyers GFO: The Carpentier-Edwards standard porcine bioprosthesis—Long-term evaluation of the high pressure glutaraldehyde fixed prostheses. Proceedings of the Fourth International Symposium—Cardiac Bioprosthesis. J Card Surg 1988;3(suppl I):321–336.

43. Jamieson WRE, Burr LH, Munro AI, Miyagishima RT, Gerein AN: Cardiac valve replacement in the elderly—Clinical performance of biological prostheses. Ann Thorac Surg 1989;48:173–185.

44. Jamieson WRE, Janusz MT, Miyagishima RT, Munro AI, Tutassaura H, Gerein AN, Burr LH, Allen P: Embolic complications of porcine heterograft cardiac valves. J Thorac Cardiovasc Surg 1981;81(4):626–631.

45. Jamieson WRE, Janusz MT, Munro AI, Allen P, Miyagishima RT, Gerein AN, Burr LH, Tyers GFO, MacNab J, Chan F: Carpentier-Edwards standard porcine bioprosthesis—Reliable performance at seven years. Thai J Surg 1986.

46. Jamieson WRE, Janusz MT, Tyers GFO, Allen P, Munro AI, Burr LH, Gerein AN, Ling H, Miyagishima RT, Tutassaura H: Early durability of the Carpentier-Edwards porcine bioprosthesis. In Kaplitt MJ and Borman JB (eds): Concepts and Controversies in Cardiovascular Surgery. Norwalk, Appleton-Century-Crofts, 1983, pp 111–133.

47. Jamieson WRE, Munro AI, MacNab J, Patterson MWH: Porcine bioprostheses in patients 20 years and younger: Is there a role for this prosthesis? In Bodnar E, Yacoub M (eds): Biologic and Bioprosthetic Valves: Proceedings of the Third International Symposium. New York: Yorke Medical Books, 1986, pp 290–298.

48. Jamieson WRE, Munro AI, Miyagishima RT, Allen P, Janusz MT, Gerein AN, Burr LH, Ling H, Hayden RI, Tutassaura H, MacNab J, Chan F, Tyers GFO: The Carpentier-Edwards supra-annular porcine bioprosthesis—New generation low pressure glutaraldehyde fixed prosthesis. Proceedings of the Fourth International Symposium—Cardiac Bioprostheses. J Card Surg 1988;3:507–521.

49. Jamieson WRE, Munro AI, Miyagishima RT, Burr LH, Gerein AN, Janusz MT, Tyers GFO, Allen P: The Carpentier-Edwards supra-annular porcine bioprosthesis—A new generation tissue valve with excellent intermediate clinical performance. J Thorac Cardiovasc Surg 1988;96:652–666.

50. Jamieson WRE, Pelletier LC, Janusz MT, Chaitman BR, Tyers GFO, Miyagishima RT: Five-year evaluation of the Carpentier-Edwards porcine bioprosthesis. J Thorac Cardiovasc Surg 1984;88(3):324–333.

51. Jamieson WRE, Rosado LJ, Munro AI, Gerein AN, Burr LH, Miyagishima RT, Janusz MT, Tyers GFO: Carpentier-Edwards porcine bioprosthesis—Primary tissue failure (structural valve deterioration) by age groups. Ann Thorac Surg 1988;46:155–162.

52. Jamieson WRE: Bioprostheses are superior to mechanical prostheses. Z Kardiol 1986;75(2):258–271.

53. Jamieson WRE: Tissue valves for cardiac valve replacement. Can J Surg 1985;28(6):499–505.

54. Janusz MT, Jamieson WRE, Allen P, Munro AI, Miyagishima RT, Tutassaura H, Burr LH, Gerein AN, Tyers GFO: Experience of the Carpentier-Edwards porcine valve prosthesis in 700 patients. Ann Thorac Surg 1982;34(6):625–633.

55. Bloomfield P, Kitchen AH, Wheatley DJ, Walbaum PR, Lutz W, Miller HC: A prospective evaluation of the Bjork-Shiley, Hancock and Carpentier-Edwards heart valve prostheses. Circulation 1986;73(6):1213–1222.

56. Borkon AM, Soule LM, Baughman KL, Aoun H, Baumgartner WA, Gardner TJ, Watkins L Jr, Gott VL, Reitz BA: Comparative analysis of mechanical and bioprosthetic valves after aortic valve replacement. J Thorac Cardiovasc Surg 1987;94(1):20–33.

57. Cohn LH, Allred EN, Cohn LA, Austin JC, Sabik J, DiDesa VJ, Shemin RJ, Collins JJ Jr: Early and late risk of mitral valve replacement: A 12 year concomitant comparison of the porcine bioprosthetic and prosthetic disc mitral valves. J Thorac Cardiovasc Surg 1985;90:872–882.

58. Cohn LH, Allred EN, DiSesa VJ, Sawtelle K, Shemin RJ, Collins JJ Jr: Early and late risk of aortic valve replacement. A 12 year concomitant comparison of the porcine bioprosthetic and tilting disc prosthetic aortic valves. J Thorac Cardiovasc Surg 1984;88:695–705.

59. Craver JM, Jones EL, McKeown P, Bone DK, Hatcher Jr CR, Dandrach M: Porcine cardiac xenograft valves: Analysis of survival, valve failure, and explanation. Ann Thorac Surg 1982;34(1):16–21.

60. Goffin YA, Bartik MA, Hilbert SL: Porcine aortic vs bovine pericardial valves: A morphologic study of the Xenomedica and Mitroflow bioprostheses. Z Kardiol 1986;74(suppl 2):213–222.

61. Hammond GL, Geha AS, Kopf GS, Hashim SW: Biological versus mechanical valves. Analysis of 1116 valves inserted in 1012 adult patients with a 4818 patient-year and a 5327 valve-year follow-up. J Thorac Cardiovasc 1987;93(2):182–198.

62. Nistal F, Artinano E, Gallo I: Primary tissue valve degeneration in glutaraldehyde-preserved porcine bioprostheses: Hancock I versus Carpentier-Edwards at four and seven year's follow-up. Ann Thorac Surg 1986;42:568–572.

63. Bodnar E, Wain WH, Haberman S: Assessment and comparison of the performance of cardiac valves. Ann Thorac Surg 1982;34:146–156.

64. Bolooki H, Mallon S, Kaiser GA, Thurer RJ, Kieval J: Failure of Hancock xenograft valve: Importance of valve position (4- to 9-year follow-up). Ann Thorac Surg 1983;36(3):246–252.

65. Brais MP, Bedard JP, Goldstein W, Koshal A, Keon WJ: Mitral valve replacement with Hancock porcine bioprostheses: Up to 7 year follow-up. Can J Surg 1985;28(2):119–123.

66. Cohn LH (personal communication): Fifteen year experience with Hancock porcine bioprosthetic valve replacements.

67. Gallo I, Nistal F, Artinano E: Six- to ten-year follow-up of patients with the Hancock cardiac bioprosthesis. J Thorac Cardiovasc Surg 1986;92:14–20.

68. Gallo I, Ruiz B, Nistal F, Duran CMG: Degeneration in porcine bioprosthetic cardiac valves: Incidence of primary tissue failure among 938 bioprostheses at risk. Am J Cardiol 1984;53:1061–1065.

69. Hartz RS, Fisher EB, Finkelmeier B, DeBoer A, Sanders JH Jr, Moran JM, Michaelis LL: An eight-year experience with porcine bioprosthetic cardiac valves. J Thorac Cardiovasc Surg 1986;91:910–917.

70. Louagie Y, Muteba P, Marchandise B, Kremer R, Schoevaredts JC, Chalant CH: Experience with the selective use of the Carpentier-Edwards bioprostheses. Thorac Cardiovasc Surg 1986;34(2):77–81.

71. Magilligan DJ Jr, Lewis JW Jr, Tilley B, Peterson E: The porcine bioprosthetic valve: Twelve years later. J Thorac Cardiovasc Surg 1985;89:499–507.

72. Miller DC, Oyer PE, Stinson EG, Shumway NE: Ten year durability and performance of porcine bioprostheses. Z Kardiol 1985;74(6):15–18.

73. Navia JA, Belzzitti J, Meletti J, Liotta D: Late follow-up of the flexible stent, low profile Liotta bioprosthesis. Z Kardiol 1986;75(suppl 2):254–257.

74. Nistal F, Garcia-Satue, E, Artinano E, Fernandez D, Riancho GG, Cayon R, Carrion F, Duran CG, Gallo I: Primary tissue failure in bioprosthetic glutaraldehyde-preserved heart valves: Bovine pericardial versus porcine tissue in the mid-term. In Bodnar E, Yacoub M (eds): Biologic and Bioprosthetic Valves: Proceedings of the Third International Symposium. New York: Yorke Medical Books, 1986, pp 233–244.

75. Schoen FJ, Schulman LJ, Cohn LH: Quantitative anatomic analysis of "stent creep" of explanted Hancock standard porcine bioprostheses used for cardiac valve replacement. Am J Cardiol 1985;56(1):110–114.

76. Soots G, Pieronne A, Roux JP, Stankowiak C, Warembourg H Jr, Watel A, Prat A, Segbeya A, Maatouk M, Crepin F: Experience with 813 aortic or mitral valve replacements with the Carpentier-Edwards bioprosthesis: Five year results. Eur Heart J 1984;5(suppl D):87–94.

77. Stein PD, Kemp SR, Riddle JM, Lee MW, Lewis JW Jr, Magilligan DJ Jr: Relation of calcification to torn leaflets of spontaneously degenerated porcine bioprosthetic valves. Ann Thorac Surg 1985;40(2):175–180.

78. Thubrikar MJ, Deck JD, Aonad J, Nolan SP: Role of mechanical stress in calcification of aortic bioprosthetic valve. J Thorac Cardiovasc Surg 1983;86:115–125.

79. Villemot JP: Liotta bioprosthesis. Seven years experience. Proceedings of the Fourth International Symposium—Cardiac Bioprostheses.

80. Wahlers T, Oclert H, Borst HG: The Carpentier-Edwards supra-annular bioprosthesis for aortic valve replacement. Clinical experience in 234 patients. J Cardiovasc Surg 1986;27(4):488–93.

81. Carpentier A, Dubost C, Lane E, Nashef A, Carpentier S, Relland J, Deloche A, Fabiani J-N, Chauvaud S, Perier P, Maxwell S: Continuing improvement in valvular prostheses. J Thorac Cardiovasc Surg 1982;83:27–42.

82. Carpentier A, Nashef A, Carpentier S, Ahmed A, Goussef N: Techniques for prevention of calcification of valvular bioprostheses. Circulation 1984;70(suppl I):I-165–I-168.

83. Carpentier A, Nashref A, Carpentier S, Goussef N, Relland J, Levy RJ, Fishbein MC, El Asmar B, Benomar M, El Sayed S, Donzeau-Gouge PG: Prevention of tissue valve calcification by chemical techniques. In Cohn LH, Gallucci L (eds): Cardiac Bioprostheses: Proceedings of the Second International Symposium. New York: Yorke Medical Books, 1982, pp 320–330.

84. Wright JTM, Eberhardt CE, Gibbs ML, Saul T, Gilpin CB: Hancock II—An improved bioprosthesis. In Cohn LH, Gallucci V (eds): Cardiac Bioprostheses: Proceedings of the Second International Symposium. New York, Yorke Medical Books, 1982, pp 425–444.

85. Broom ND: Fatigue induced damage in glutaraldehyde-preserved heart valve tissue. J Cardiovasc Thorac Surg 1978;76(2):202–211.

86. Broom ND, Thompson FJ: Influence of fixation conditions on the performance of glutaraldehyde treated porcine aortic valves: Towards a more scientific basis. Thorax 1979;34:166.

87. Broom ND, Christie CW: The structure–function relationship of fresh and glutaraldehyde-fixed aortic valve leaflets. In Cohn LH, Gallucci V (eds): Cardiac Bioprostheses: Proceedings of the Second International Symposium. New York, Yorke Medical Books, 1982, pp 476–494.

88. David TE, Uden DE: Hancock II Bioprosthesis: Clinical experience and hemodynamic assessment. In Bodnar E, Yacoub M (eds): Biologic and Bioprosthetic Valves: Proceedings of the Third International Symposium. New York, Yorke Medical Books, 1986, pp 152–158.

89. Arbustini E, Jones M, Moses RD, Eidbo EE, Carroll RJ, Ferrans VJ: Modification by the Hancock T6 process of calcification of bioprosthetic cardiac valves implanted in sheep. Am J Cardiol 1984;53:1388–1396.

90. Gallo I, Nistal F, Fernandez D, Factor SM, Frater RW: Comparative study of calcification in the T6 treated and standard Hancock I porcine xenografts: Experimental study in weanling sheep. Thorac Cardiovasc Surg 1986;34(5):310–315.

91. Jones M, Ferrans VJ: Comparative study of calcification in the T-6-treated and standard Hancock-I porcine xenografts: Experimental study in weanling sheep. Thorac Cardiovasc Surg 1987;35(3):189–190.

92. Croft CH, Buja LM, Floresca MZ, Nicod P, Estrera A: Late thrombotic obstruction of aortic porcine bioprostheses. Am J Cardiol 1986;57(4):355–356.

93. Edmunds LH Jr. Thromboembolic complications of current cardiac valvular prostheses. Ann Thorac Surg 1981;34(1):96–106.

94. Gallo I, Artinano E, Nistal F: Four to seven-year follow-up of patients undergoing Carpentier-Edwards porcine heart valve replacement. Thorac Cardiovasc Surg 1985;33:347–351.

95. Navia JA, Gimenez C, Meletti I, Liotta D: Thromboembolism with low profile bioprosthesis. Eur Heart J 1984;5(suppl D):95–100.

96. Spencer FC, Bauman FG, Grossi EA, Culliford AT, Galloway AC: Experiences with 1643 porcine prosthetic valves in 1492 patients. Ann Surg 1986;203(6):691–700.

97. Baumgartner WA, Miller DC, Reitz BA, Oyer PE, Jamieson SW, Stinson EB, Shumway NE: Surgical treatment of prosthetic valve endocarditis. Ann Thorac Surg 1980;30(3):747–758.

98. Borkon AM, McIntosh CL, Jones M, Lipson LC, Kent KM, Morrow AG: Hemodynamic function of the Hancock standard orifice aortic valve bioprosthesis. J Thorac Cardiovasc Surg 1981;82(4):604–607.

99. Bove EL, Marvasti MA, Potts JL, Reger MJ, Zamora JL, Eich RH, Parker FB Jr: Rest and exercise hemodynamics following aortic valve replacement. A comparison between 19 and 21 mm Ionescu-Shiley pericardial and Carpentier-Edwards porcine valves. J Thorac Cardiovasc Surg 1985;90:750–756.

100. Chaitman BR, Bonan R, Lepage G, Tubau JF, David PR, Dyrda I, Grondin CM: Hemodynamic evaluation of the Carpentier-Edwards porcine xenograft. Circulation 1979;60:(5):1170–1182.

101. Cohen-Solal A, Leroy G, Hittinger L, Fernandez F, Gay J, Gourgon R: Hemodynamic evaluation of the Carpentier-Edwards porcine bioprosthesis and the Hancock pericardial bioprosthesis in aortic position. Arch Mal Coeur 1986;79(3):346–354.

102. Cosgrove DM, Lytle BW, Gill CC, Golding LAR, Stewart RW, Loop FD, Williams GW: In vivo hemodynamic comparison of porcine and pericardial valves. J Thorac Cardiovasc Surg 1985;89(3):358–368.

103. Craver JM, King SB III, Douglas JS, French RH, Jones EL, Morris DC, Kopchak J, Hatcher CR Jr: Late hemodynamic evaluation of Hancock modified orifice aortic bioprosthesis. Circulation 1979;60(2), Pt 2):93–97.

104. Czer LS, Gray RJ, Bateman TM, De Robertis MA, Resser K, Chaux A, Matloff JM: Hemodynamic differentiation of pathologic and physiologic stenosis in mitral porcine bioprostheses. J Am Coll Cardiol 1986;7(2):284–294.

105. Foster AH, Tracy CM, Greenberg GJ, McIntosh CL, Clark RE: Valve replacement in narrow aortic roots: Serial hemodynamics and long-term clinical outcome. Ann Thorac Surg 1986;42(5):506–516.

106. Jones EL, Craver JM, Morris DC, King SB III, Douglas JS Jr, Franch RH, Hatcher CR Jr, Morgan EA: Hemodynamic and clinical evaluation of the Hancock xenograft bioprosthesis for aortic valve replacement (with emphasis on management of the small aortic root). J Thorac Cardiovasc Surg 1978;75(2):300–308.

107. Kagawa Y, Tabayashi K, Suzuki Y, Ito T, Sato N, Horiuchi T: Intermediate term results of isolated mitral valve replacement with glutaraldehyde-preserved porcine xenograft valve: Clinical and hemodynamic comparison between Hancock valve and Angell-Shiley valve. Tohoku J Exp Med 1986;150:37–50.

108. Lee G, Grehl TM, Joyce JA, Kaku RF, Harter W, DeMaria AN, Mason DT: Hemodynamic assessment of the new aortic Carpentier-Edwards bioprosthesis. Cathet Cardiovasc Diagn 1978;4:373–381.

109. Leroy G, Lelguen C, Juillard A, d'Auzac, Fernandez F, Gerbaux A: Hemodynamic evaluation of mitral and aortic bioprosthesis. Apropos of 27 Carpentier-Edwards and 7 Hancock (standard model prostheses). Arch Mal Coeur 1982;75(4):459–466.

110. Levine FH, Carter JE, Buckley MJ, Daggett WM, Akins CW, Austen WG: Hemodynamic evaluation of Hancock and Carpentier-Edwards bioprostheses. Circulation 1981;64(suppl II):192–195.

111. Navia JA, Tamashiro A, Gimenez C, Zambrana-Vidal D, Liotta D: Hemodynamic evaluation in valvular patients carrying low profile bioprostheses. In Cohn LH, Gallucci V (eds): Cardiac Bioprostheses: Proceedings of the Second International Symposium. New York, Yorke Medical Books, 1982, pp 104–112.

112. Pelletier C, Chaitman BR, Baillot R, Val PG, Bonan R, Dyrda I: Clinical and hemodynamic results with Carpentier-Edwards porcine bioprosthesis. Ann Thorac Surg 1982;34(6):612–624.

113. Pelletier C, Chaitman BR, Bonan R, Dryda I: Hemodynamic evaluation of Carpentier-Edwards standard

and improved annulus bioprostheses. In Cohn LH, Gallucci V (eds): Cardiac Bioprostheses: Proceedings of the Second International Symposium. New York, Yorke Medical Books, 1982, 91–103.

114. Rasmussen K, Vesterlund T, Vejlsted H: A hemodynamic study of the Carpentier-Edwards and Hancock porcine xenografts in the mitral position. Scand J Thorac Cardiovasc Surg 1984;18(1):37–40.

115. Rossiter SJ, Miller DC, Stinson EB, Oyer PE, Reitz BA, Moreno-Cabral RJ, Mace JG, Robert EW, Tsagaris TJ, Sutton RB, Alderman EL, Shumway NE: Hemodynamic and clinical comparison of the Hancock modified orifice and standard orifice bioprostheses in the aortic position. J Thorac Cardiovasc Surg 1980;80(1):54–60.

116. Rothkopf M, Davidson T, Lipscomb K, Narahara K, Hillis LD, Willerson JT, Estrera A, Platt M, Mills L: Hemodynamic evaluation of the Carpentier-Edwards bioprosthesis in the aortic position. Am J Cardiol 1979;44:209–214.

117. Zusman DR, Levine FH, Carter JE, Buckley MJ: Hemodynamic and clinical evaluation of the Hancock modified-orifice aortic bioprostheses. Circulation 1981;64(2 pt 2):189–191.

118. Sade RM, Ballenger JF, Hohn AR, Arrants JE, Riopel DA, Taylor AB: Cardiac valve replacement in children. Comparison of tissue with mechanical prosthesis. J Thorac Cardiovasc Surg 1979;76(1):123–127.

119. Simpson IA, Reece IJ, Houston AB, Hutton I, Wheatley DJ, Cobbe SM: Noninvasive assessment by Doppler ultrasound of 155 patients with bioprosthetic valves: A comparison of the Wessex porcine, low profile Ionescu-Shiley, and Hancock pericardial bioprostheses. Br Heart J 1986;56(1):83–88.

120. Williams GA, Labovitz AJ: Doppler hemodynamic evaluation of prosthetic (Starr-Edwards and Bjork-Shiley) and bioprosthetic (Hancock and Carpentier-Edwards) cardiac valves. Am J Cardiol 1985;56(4):325–332.

121. Yoganathan AP, Woo YR, Sung HW, Williams FP, Franch RH, Jones M: In vitro hemodynamic characteristics of tissue bioprostheses in the aortic position. J Thorac Cardiovasc Surg 1986;92(2):198–209.

122. Walker DK, Scotten LN, Brownlee RT: New generation tissue valves. Their in vitro function in the mitral position. J Thorac Cardiovasc Surg 1984;88:573–582.

123. Walker DK, Scotten LN, Modi VJ, Brownlee RT: In vitro assessment of mitral valve prostheses. J Thorac Cardiovasc Surg 1980;79:680–688.

124. Zussa C, Ottino G, di Summa M, Poletti GA, Zattera GF, Pansini S, Morea M: Porcine cardiac bioprostheses: Evaluation of long-term results in 990 patients. Ann Thorac Surg 1985;39(3):243–250.

125. Antunes MJ, Santos LP: Performance of glutaraldehyde-preserved porcine bioprosthesis as a mitral valve substitute in a young population group. Ann Thorac Surg 1984;37(5):387–392.

126. Curcio CA, Commerford PJ, Rose AG, Stevens JE, Barnard MS: Calcification of glutaraldehyde-preserved porcine xenografts in young patients. J Thorac Cardiovasc Surg 1981;81:621–625.

127. Deviri E, Yechezkel M, Levinsky L, Vidne BA, Levy MJ: Calcification of a porcine valve xenograft during pregnancy—a case report and review of the literature. Thorac Cardiovasc Surg 1984;32:266–268.

128. Edwards WD, Agarwal KC, Feldt RH, Danielson GK, Puga FJ: Surgical pathology of obstructed, right-sided, porcine-valved extracardiac conduits. Arch Pathol Lab Med 1983;107(8):400–405.

129. Fiddler GI, Gerlis LM, Walker DR, Scott O, Williams GJ: Calcification of glutaraldehyde-preserved porcine and bovine xenograft valves in young children. Ann Thorac Surg 1983;25(3):257–261.

130. Gardner TJ, Roland J-MA, Neill CA, Donahoo JS: Valve replacement in children. A fifteen-year perspective. J Thorac Cardiovasc Surg 1982;83:178–185.

131. Geha AS, Laks H, Stansel HC Jr, Cornhill JF, Kilman JW, Buckley MJ, Roberts WC: Late failure of porcine valve heterografts in children. J Thorac Cardiovasc Surg 1979;78:351–364.

132. Hellberg K, Ruschewski W, de Vevie ER: Early stenosis and calcification of glutaraldehyde-preserved porcine xenografts in children. Thorac Cardiovasc Surg 1981;29(6):369–374.

133. Human DG, Joffe HS, Fraser CB, Barnard CN: Mitral valve replacement in children. J Thorac Cardiovasc Surg 1982;83:873–877.

134. Kopf GS, Geha AS, Hellenbrand WE, Kleinman CS: Fate of left-sided cardiac bioprosthesis valves in children. Arch Surg 1986;121(4):488–490.

135. Kutsche LM, Oyer P, Shumway N, Baum D: An important complication of Hancock mitral valve replacement in children. Circulation 1979;60(2 pt 2):98–103.

136. Mathews RA, Park SC, Neches WH, Lenox CC, Zuberbuhler JR, Fricker FJ, Siewers RD, Hardesty RL, Lerberg DB, Bahnson HT: Valve replacement in children and adolescents. J Thorac Cardiovasc Surg 1977;73(6):872–876.

137. McGoon DC, Danielson GK, Puga FJ, Ritter DG, Mair DD, Ilstrup DM: Late results after extracardiac conduit repair for congenital cardiac defects. Am J Cardiol 1982;49(7):1741–1749.

138. Miller DC, Stinson EB, Oyer PE, Billingham ME, Pitlick PT, Reitz BA, Jamieson SW, Baumgartner WA, Shumway NE: Durability of porcine xenograft valves and conduits in children. Circulation 1982;66(suppl I)I-172–I-185.

139. Nunez L, Larrea JL, Aguado MG, Reque JA, Matorras R, Minguez JA: Pregnancy in 20 patients with bioprosthetic valve replacement. Chest 1983;84(1):26–28.

140. Odell JA: Calcification of porcine bioprostheses in children. In Cohn LH, Gallucci V (eds): Cardiac Bio-

prostheses: Proceedings of the Second International Symposium. New York, Yorke Medical Books, 1982, pp 231–237.

141. Sanders SP, Levy RJ, Freed MD, Norwood WI, Castaneda AR: Use of Hancock porcine xenografts in children and adolescents. Am J Cardiol 1980;46(3):429–438.

142. Silver MM, Pollock J, Silver MD, Williams WG, Trusler GA: Calcification in porcine xenograft valves in children. Am J Cardiol 1980;45:685–689.

143. Thandroyen FT, Whitton IN, Pirie D, Rogers MA, Mitha AS: Severe calcification of glutaraldehyde-preserved porcine xenografts in children. Am J Cardiol 1980;45:690–696.

144. Villani M, Bianchi T, Vanini V, Tiraboschi R, Crupi GC, Pezzica E, Parenzan L: Bioprosthetic valve replacement in children. In Cohn LH, Gallucci L (eds): Cardiac Bioprostheses: Proceedings of the Second International Symposium. New York, Yorke Medical Books,1982, pp 248–255.

145. Williams DB, Danielson GK, McGoon DC, Puga FJ, Mair DD, Edwards WD: Porcine heterograft valve replacement in children. J Thorac Cardiovasc Surg 1982;84:446–450.

146. Williams WG, Pollock JC, Geiss DM, Trusler GA, Fowler RS: Experience with aortic and mitral valve replacement in children. J Thorac Cardiovasc Surg 1981;81:326–333.

147. Odell JA, Gillmer G, Whitton ID, Vythilingum SP, Vanker EA: Calcification of tissue valves in children: Occurrence in porcine and bovine pericardial bioprosthetic valves. In Bodnar E, Jacoub M (eds): Biologic and Bioprosthetic Valves: Proceedings of the Third International Symposium. New York, Yorke Medical Books, 1986, pp 259–270.

148. Antunes MJ: Bioprosthetic valve replacement in children—long-term follow-up of 135 isolated mitral valve implantations. Eur Heart J 1984;5(11)913–918.

149. Fishbein MC, Gissen SA, Collins JJ Jr, Barsamian EM, Cohn LH: Pathologic findings after cardiac valve replacement with glutaraldehyde-fixed porcine valves. Am J Cardiol 1977;40:331–335.

150. Forfar JC, Cotter L, Morritt GN: Severe and early stenosis of porcine heterograft mitral valve. Br Heart J 1978;40:1184–1187.

151. Goffin YA, Bartik MA: Porcine aortic versus bovine pericardial valves: A comparative study of unimplanted and from patient explanted bioprostheses. Life Supp Syst 1987;5:127–143.

152. Ishihara T, Ferrans VJ, Boyce SW, Jones M, Roberts WC: Structure and classification of cuspal tears and perforation in porcine bioprosthetic cardiac valves implanted in patients. In Cohn LH, Gallucci V (eds): Cardiac Bioprostheses: Proceedings of the Second International Symposium. New York, Yorke Medical Books, 1982, pp 362–377.

153. Riddle JM, Jennings JJ, Stein PD, Magilligan DJ Jr: A morphologic overview of the porcine bioprosthetic valve—Before and after its degeneration. J Scan Electron Microsc 1984;(pt 1):207–214.

154. Thiene G, Bortolotti U, Panizzon G, Milano A, Gallucci V: Pathological substrates of thrombus formation after heart valve replacement with the Hancock bioprosthesis. J Thorac Cardiovasc Surg 1980;80:414–423.

155. Spray TL, Roberts WC: Structural changes in Hancock porcine xenograft cardiac valve bioprostheses. Adv Cardiol 1978;22:241–251.

156. Spray TL, Roberts WC: Structural changes in porcine xenografts used as substitute cardiac valves. Gross and histologic observations in 51 glutaraldehyde-preserved Hancock valves in 41 patients. Am J Cardiol 1977;40:319–330.

157. Ferrans VJ, Spray TL, Billingham ME, Roberts WC: Structural changes in glutaraldehyde-treated porcine heterografts used as substitute cardiac valves. Transmission and scanning electron microscopic observations in 12 patients. Am J Cardiol 1978;41:1591.

158. Bortolotti U, Gallucci V, Casarotto D, Thiene G: Fibrous tissue overgrowth on Hancock mitral xenograft: A cause of late prosthetic stenosis. Thorac Cardiovasc Surg 1979;27:281–344.

159. Bortolotti U, Milano A, Thiene G, Valente M, Mazzucco A, Gallucci V: Evidence of impending embolization of a calcific cusp fragment from a mitral porcine xenograft. Thorac Cardiovasc Surg 1982;30:405–406.

160. Thiene G, Arbustini E, Bortolotti U, Talenti E, Milano A, Valente N, Molin G, Gallucci V: Pathologic substrates of porcine valve dysfunction. In Cohn LH, Gallucci V (eds): Cardiac Bioprostheses. New York, Yorke Medical Books, 1982, pp 378–400.

161. Thiene G, Bortolotti U: Infected porcine valve xenografts. Int J Cardiol 1984;6:733–735.

162. Valente M, Arbustini E, Bortolotti U, Talenti E, Thiene G: Perforation of muscle shelf of right coronary cusp causing acute regurgitation of mitral xenograft. Am Heart J 1984;108:180–183.

163. Valente M, Bortolotti U, Arbustini E, Talenti E, Thiene G, Gallucci V: Glutaraldehyde-preserved porcine bioprosthesis—Factors affecting performance as determined by pathologic studies. Chest 1983;83:607–611.

164. Valente M, Bortolotti U, Thiene G: Ultrastructural substrates of dystrophic calcification in porcine bioprosthetic valve failure. Am J Pathol 1985;119:12–21.

165. Bortolotti U, Thiene G, Casarotto D, Mazzucco A, Gallucci V: Left ventricular rupture following mitral valve replacement with a Hancock bioprosthesis. Chest 1980;77(2):235–237.

166. Brown JW, Dunn JM, Spooner E, Kirsh MM: Late spontaneous disruption of a porcine xenograft mitral

valve: Clinical, hemodynamic, echocardiographic, and pathological findings. J Thorac Cardiovasc Surg 1977;75(4):606–611.

167. Dark JH, Bain WH: Rupture of posterior wall of left ventricle after mitral valve replacement. Thorax 1984;39:905–911.

168. Nunez L, Gil-Aguado M, Cerron M, Celemin P: Delayed rupture of the left ventricle after mitral valve replacement with bioprosthesis. Ann Thorac Surg 1979;27:465.

169. Bortolotti U, Thiene G, Milano A, Panizzon G, Valente M, Gallucci V: Pathological study of infective endocarditis on Hancock porcine bioprostheses. J Thorac Cardiovasc Surg 1981;81:934–942.

170. Thiene G, Bortolotti U, Talenti E, Guerra F, Valente M, Milano A, Mazzucco A, Gallucci V: Dissecting cuspal hematomas. A rare form of porcine bioprosthetic valve dysfunction. Arch Pathol Lab Med 1987;111:964–967.

171. Arbustini E, Bortolotti U, Valente M, Milano A, Gallucci V, Pennelli N, Thiene G: Cusp disruption by massive lipid infiltration. J Thorac Cardiovasc Surg 1982;84:738–743.

172. Salomon NW, Copeland JG, Goldman S, Larson DF: Unusual complication of the Hancock porcine heterograft: Strut compression in the aortic root. J Thorac Cardiovasc Surg 1979;77(2):294–296.

173. Valente M, Bortolotti U, Thiene G, Arbustini E, Milano A, Mazzucco A, Gallucci V: Post bending of the polypropylene flexible stent in mitral Hancock bioprosthesis. Eur J Cardiothorac Surg 1987;1:134–138.

Bodnar, E. and Frater, R. W. M., editors
(1991) *Replacement Cardiac Valves,*
Pergamon Press, Inc. (New York), pp. 277–285
Printed in the United States of America

CHAPTER 11

THE PERICARDIAL HEART VALVE: AN OPEN QUESTION

CARLOS G. DURAN

The tissue valve alternative to replacement with a mechanical valve has followed three different patterns. Initially it was the homograft aortic valve (1) followed by the heterograft (2). The third alternative was the use of nonvalvular tissue of auto-, allo- or xenogeneic origin. Typical examples were the use of autologous fascia lata (3), cadaver dura mater (4), and more recently, bovine pericardium (5).

This third possibility, bovine pericardium, seemed to possess the advantage of the cadaver and porcine valves over the mechanical valve, in terms of a lower thrombogenicity. Its availability made it more convenient than the homografts. Its ease of construction on unobstructive stents, and therefore better hemodynamics than the porcine valve, pointed toward a very promising venue. However, the unsatisfactory results of the previously used tissues, fascia and dura mater, and the recent reports on the incidence of tissue failure with the Ionescu-Shiley valves, have cast very serious doubts on the advisability of its continued use.

THE PERICARDIAL VALVE

So far all the pericardial valves commercially available have been made of glutaraldehyde-treated bovine pericardium, mounted on a stent.

1. *The Ionescu-Shiley valve* was the first and most widely used model. In 1966, Marian I. Ionescu and G. Wooler from Leeds, England, developed a titanium stent for the support of formalin-fixed heterografts that were used clinically during 1967. Two years later, Ionescu tried a series of autologous fascia lata mounted on that three-legged stent covered inside and out with Dacron velour. In 1970, given the poor results with fascia, he mounted glutaraldehyde-fixed bovine pericardium on this stent with its posts slightly splayed outward to provide a full orifice. The first valves constructed at the hospital were used between March 1971 and February 1976. From then on the valves were made at Shiley Laboratories and commercialized under the trade name Ionescu-Shiley pericardial valve. For "aesthetic reasons the sutures along the stent posts were covered with Dacron cloth" (6).

In 1981, a "low-profile" model that differed in some important aspects from the standard valve was released. The support frame was made of Delrin with radiopaque Elgiloy markers to make it flexible and reduce stress. The 9° splay of the stent was eliminated. The total valve height was reduced by 35%. The new model was claimed to be considerably more durable than the standard model in the in vitro mechanical fatigue tester. Unfortunately its limited clinical use showed a much earlier rate of failure than the standard Ionescu valve. Half of the patients presented as emergencies, and all of these had a torn cusp from apex to base (7). A further model III was implanted clinically before Shiley decided to cease the production of pericardial valves in October 1987.

2. *The Mitroflow Pericardial Valve* was designed by R. Siegel and R. Totten, previously at Hancock Laboratories, and commercialized by Mitral Medical. It is made of a single piece of pericardium wrapped around a Delrin stent covered with Dacron. Unlike the Ionescu model, it has no commissural sutures, and each valve is individually tested before release. The first clinical implantation was done in Santander, Spain, in March 1982 (8). The valve is now commercialized by Symbion.

3. *The Carpentier-Edwards Pericardial Valve* has the characteristic of having three pieces of pericardium mounted completely within the Elgiloy wire stent to reduce potential abrasion between the Dacron-covered frame and the pericardial leaflets. The pericardium is not fixed by holding sutures but retained inside the stent by a Mylar button. Its clinical implantation was started in Paris, France, in July 1980 (9).

Unlike the documentation of other pericardial valves, there are very few publications on the behavior of this valve. Pelletier and associates (10) have recently reported a very low incidence of tissue failure with 96% freedom at 6 years.

4. The sudden popularity of the pericardial valves during the late 1970s determined a spurt of new models either commercially available or hospital-made. The Hancock (Vascor) pericardial valve is the best known and probably of the shortest life span, since it was made available in 1981 and has already been discontinued in 1987 (11). The latest is the Bioflow, implanted since February 1987 in Glasgow, Scotland. This valve incorporates, among other features, a pericardial-covered support frame to reduce abrasion of the leaflets in their flexion over the frame (12).

A completely novel design developed by S. Gabbay and manufactured by Meadox Medical has a single pericardial monocusp that in closing meets a pericardium-covered Delrin stent (13, 14). Although sparsely used, its early clinical results have not been encouraging, and as far as we know, its production has been discontinued.

PERSONAL EXPERIENCE

Our personal experience with pericardial valves has been limited to the standard Ionescu-Shiley and Mitroflow valves. The former was used between August 1977 and October 1984, exclusively in the aortic position. An early and small experience with this valve in the mitral position showed a prohibitive incidence of left ventricular rupture ($\frac{5}{25}$) and such use was soon abandoned. The Mitroflow was used between March 1982 and March 1988 in all positions.

Ionescu-Shiley Experience

We implanted 244 pericardial bioprostheses in 241 patients with an average age of 50.8 years (range 15–78 years). By age group there were 15 patients less than 30 years of age, 51 patients from 30 to 45, 116 patients from 46 to 60, and 59 patients more than 60 years of age. The causes were rheumatic (69.7%), prosthetic valve failure (12.8%), infective endocarditis (7.05%), degenerative (4.9%), congenital (4.1%) and unknown (1.2%). Preoperatively, 52 patients (21.5%) were in NYHA functional classes I to II, 151 patients (62.7%) in class III, and 38 patients (15.8%) in class IV. Before surgery 159 patients (65.9%) were in sinus rhythm, 76 (31.6%) in atrial fibrillation and 6 (2.5%) in complete

AV block; 2 of them had a permanent pacemaker. Twenty-seven patients (11.2%) referred a preoperative thromboembolic episode.

Isolated aortic valve replacement was carried out in 121 cases (50.2%) and associated cardiac surgery in 120 (49.8%). Widening of the aortic root with a rhomboidal patch in the noncoronary sinus was necessary in three patients.

All patients with isolated aortic valve replacement received antiplatelet drugs (Persantin 300 mg per day, and aspirin 125 mg per day) for 3 months, like the mitroaortic patients in sinus rhythms. When associated cardiac surgery was performed, the mitroaortic patients in atrial fibrillation were anticoagulated for 3 months or permanently when a giant left atrium or massive atrial thrombus was present.

Results

The last month of follow-up was February 1988. Five patients (2.07%) were lost to follow-up. The maximum follow-up period was 10.5 years, with a cumulative total of 1260.08 patient years (mean follow-up of 5.16 patient years). There were 26 hospital deaths (10.7%) due to low cardiac output (14), infection (6), dysrhythmia (3), hemorrhage (1), neurologic complications (1), and left ventricular rupture (1). Twenty-three of the nonsurviving patients had concomitant cardiac surgery ($^{23}/_{120}$, or 18% mortality), while the other three hospital deaths were isolated aortic valve replacements ($^3/_{121}$, or 2.48% mortality). None of these hospital deaths were related to the aortic bioprosthesis.

There were 15 late deaths in this series (6.9% or 1.19% per patient year). Most of these late deaths occurred at home of unknown origin (8 cases). Five patients died at reoperation for valve failure 37 to 104 months after the first operation (average of 70 months). The remaining two patients died 4 and 42 months after valve replacement due to infective endocarditis and respiratory failure, respectively. Twelve late deaths occurred among patients with associated cardiac surgery.

The expected 10.5-year survival rate is 82% ± 2.9%. This figure is 90% ± 3.3% for patients with isolated aortic valve replacement, and for patients with concomitant cardiac surgery it is 74% ± 4.9% (Fig. 11–1).

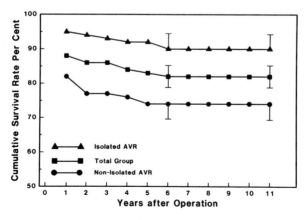

FIG. 11–1. Long-term survival after Ionescu-Shiley valve implantation.

Postoperatively, no patient was assigned to NYHA functional class IV, three patients (1.3%) were in class III, and 37 (17%) were in class II, and the remaining surviving patients are asymptomatic.

Valve-related complications There were 12 embolic episodes in seven patients (2.9%) (seven central and five peripheral); eight of them occurred in patients with associated cardiac surgery. Six events occurred within the first 5 postoperative years, and six events between the 5th and 10th postoperative years. The linearized incidence of thromboembolism was 0.95% per patient year; 0.32% for patients with isolated aortic valve replacement and 0.63% for patients with concomitant cardiac surgery. Freedom from embolic events at 10.5 years was 73% ± 12% (72% ± 10.9% for patients with isolated aortic valve replacement, and 74% ± 14.3% for patients with concomitant cardiac surgery) (Fig. 11–2).

Two cases of valve thrombosis occurred 2 and 20 months after implantation (0.8%, or 0.15% per patient year), one in a patient with isolated aortic valve replacement and the other in a patient who required additional mitral and tricuspid valve surgery. At reoperation, both pericardial bioprostheses showed massive thrombosis causing severe valve stenosis. These patients were not receiving antiplatelet or anticoagulant drugs at the time of the event.

Severe paravalvular leak was detected in seven patients (2.9%, or 0.55% per patient year). Four of them occurred within the first postoperative year, and three occurred 13, 19, and 102 months after surgery. All these patients required reoperation and survived it.

There were six cases of prosthetic valve endocarditis (2.48%, or 0.47% per patient year); three occurred within the first postoperative year, and the remaining three cases occurred 19, 84, and 102 months after valve implantation. Vegetations were present in all infected prostheses, and annular abscesses with extensive destruction of the aortic ring were found in three patients. Extensive infective tissue causing bioprosthesis stenosis was found in one patient.

Structural valve deterioration was found in 24 patients (9.95%, or 1.90% per patient year). Ten patients were under 40 years of age at the time of valve failure. All patients

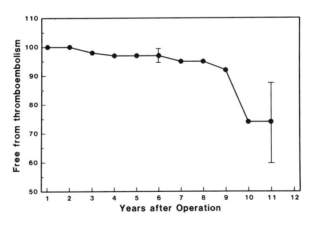

FIG. 11–2. Freedom from thromboembolism with Ionescu-Shiley valves in the aortic position.

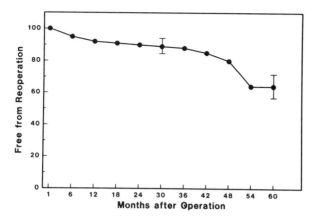

Fɪɢ. 11–3. Freedom from reoperation with Ionescu-Shiley valves in the aortic position.

required bioprosthetic explantation 13 to 108 months after surgery (mean 6.01 years); five patients died after reoperation.

Macroscopic examination of the explanted aortic pericardial valves showed cuspal tear in seven patients, calcification in five patients, rupture and calcification in 11 patients, and massive fibrous overgrowth invading the pericardial commissures and causing a severe valve incompetence in one valve 13 months after implantation.

The actuarial rate of freedom from prosthetic deterioration at 10.5 years follow-up was 77% ± 5.4%, and the actuarial projection of freedom from aortic valve-related reoperation at 10.5 years follow-up was 64% ± 6.0% (Fig. 11–3).

Mitroflow Experience

Since the first Mitroflow valve human implant was carried out in our unit in March 1982, until March 1988, 140 valves were implanted in 130 patients. There were 90 isolated aortic, 27 mitral, 3 tricuspid, and 10 mitroaortic replacements, and 27 patients (20.76%) had additional cardiac surgery.

Maximum follow-up was 7 years, with a mean of 52.8 months, and a cumulative of 572.67 patient years.

Overall hospital mortality was 2.30% (3 deaths). There were seven late deaths (5.51%), 1.22% per patient year. The actuarial survival curve was 89% ± 3.9%.

There were six embolic episodes in five patients (four mitral and one aortic) or 0.69% per patient year, and the actuarial thromboembolic-free rate was 94% ± 3.1%. An early aortic prosthetic endocarditis occurred.

Five valves developed primary tissue failure requiring explantation. Four were in the mitral position, showing tears in three and calcification in one. The dysfunctioning aortic valve had tears in one cusp. The incidence of primary tissue failure was 0.87% per patient year, and the actuarial freedom from valve deterioration was 86% ± 8.5% at 7 years.

A total of seven patients underwent reoperation (1.22% per patient year). The actuarial rate of freedom from reoperation was 85% ± 7.8%.

Comparative Study of Primary Tissue Failure Between Pericardial and Porcine Valves

In an attempt to know the difference in the incidence of primary tissue failure between these two types of valves, a comparative study was undertaken. All patients undergoing aortic valve replacement with an Ionescu-Shiley pericardial (I-S) and with a Hancock porcine valve operated at the same institution, by the same surgical team, and with a follow-up of 4 to 7 years were selected (15). Between August 1977 and June 1981, 221 Hancock and 133 I-S valves were implanted using a similar surgical technique.

Results

Two patients were lost to follow-up in the Hancock group. The 317 patients who were discharged form the hospital (118 in the I-S group and 199 in the Hancock group) were followed for 1 to 83 months (mean 55). Follow-up for the entire series was 1447 years, 973 and 474 patient years for the Hancock and I-S groups, respectively. There were 34 late deaths [20 patients (10%) in the Hancock group and 14 patients (12%) in the I-S group].

Eight instances of primary tissue failure occurred in the I-S group between 36 and 72 months after surgery. In the Hancock group, six valves failed between 24 and 83 months of follow-up. Linearized incidences were 0.61% failing valves per patient year in the Hancock group and 1.70% per patient year for the I-S group. The mean age of patients at the time of valve implantation was 38 years (range 25 to 55) in the Hancock group and 39 (range 15 to 62) in the I-S group. No significant difference in failure rates was found when size groups were compared among either Hancock or I-S recipients.

The actuarial rate of freedom from primary tissue valve failure was 93% $\pm$ 3.6% for the Hancock group and 80% $\pm$ 8% for the I-S group at 83 months follow-up. A statistically significant difference was observed at 6 and 7 years of follow-up.

The cause of valve failure in the I-S group was tear and calcification in six cases and calcification in two. Calcification of the pericardial tissue (from flat plaques to florid granulations) caused stenosis in two xenografts, and combined stenosis and regurgitation in six. Microscopically, all pericardial valves contained extensive areas with collagen degeneration and severe calcific deposits. Fibrillar pattern of collagen bundles was lost along the cusps. Collagen degeneration, calcification, and chronic inflammation areas with giant cells and polynuclear cells were observed in relation to tears of the pericardium.

Porcine bioprosthetic dysfunction was frequently associated with cuspal calcium deposits and calcium-related tears. Two prostheses had substantial cuspal defects associated with variable amounts of calcium in the cusps. Macroscopic lesions produced incompetence in two valves, stenosis in one and mixed lesions in three. Microscopically, all Hancock valves showed collagen degeneration and calcific deposits.

GENERAL OVERVIEW

The pericardial valve has enjoyed very high popularity for about 10 years. The overoptimistic initial reports necessarily followed by some negative reports have swung the pendulum toward rejection. However, the fact that a sizable number of new pericardial-based bioprostheses are being developed and used clinically today shows that there is still interest in this material which at least encourages the surgeon's inventiveness.

After review of our personal experience together with the available literature, we have come to several tentative conclusions.

Hemodynamics

The pericardial valve is superior to the porcine valve in terms of hemodynamic performance.

Pericardium offers design possibilities far superior to those of porcine valves. It has made possible the development of trileaflet stent-mounted bioprostheses with very low transannular gradients.

Wheatley's group in Glasgow (16), testing in vitro six different types of tissue valves and six mechanical valves, has shown that the porcine valves have much higher forward flow pressure gradients than pericardial, tilting disk, or bileaflet mechanical valves. However, the porcine valves showed least regurgitation, with pericardial valves having less regurgitation than mechanical ones.

Intraoperative hemodynamic studies performed with the Carpentier-Edwards pericardial valve in the aortic position, have shown gradients that range from 23 ± 7.8 mmHg for size 19 to 2.1 ± 0.7 mmHg for size 25. The authors concluded that it is less obstructive than the porcine valves (17).

Lesbre et al. from Montreal (18), in a very elegant Doppler study on 108 patients with Ionescu-Shiley, Carpentier-Edwards, and Mitroflow valves, have shown a significant superiority of the Mitroflow in the aortic position and of the Ionescu and Mitroflow at mitral level. They also clearly showed that the determining factors in the transvalvular gradients are not only type and size of valve but also the age of the bioprosthesis.

It can be said that the pericardial valve is a good alternative for aortic replacement, particularly in small aortic roots (19).

Thromboembolism

Rates of thromboembolism are difficult to establish, and even more so are attempts at comparison between series. Ionescu (20) has reported rates of 0.55% per patient year for implanted mitral and 0.62% per patient year for multiple replacement without permanent anticoagulation. He states that no single case of valve thrombosis occurred in this series. Cooley (21) reported in a very large series of 2701 patients a rate of 2.76% per patient year thromboembolism for mitral replacements, with 46% of them under anticoagulation.

Our incidence of thromboembolism for isolated aortic replacement is 0.32% per patient year, but two patients (0.15% per patient year) had severe valve thrombosis that required reoperation. It seems that thromboembolism does not constitute a major problem with this type of bioprosthesis, and it might have a lower thrombogenicity than the porcine valves.

Tissue Failure

Our comparative data of the incidence of primary tissue failure between the Hancock porcine and the Ionescu-Shiley valves are very valid since both (1) have the same time frame, (2) are implanted by the same surgical team and therefore with a similar technique, (3) are implanted to the same type of population, and (4) are followed up and reviewed at the same institution. The results of this study show at a statistically significant level that the pericardial valve deteriorates sooner and more frequently than the porcine one. The study of Odell and associates from South Africa (22), who reported the behaviour of the porcine and bovine bioprosthesis in a population of 270 children below 15 years of age, is, in our opinion, essential. These authors report an actuarial valve survival in the mitral position at 4 years of 32.5% for the porcine and 2.3% for the Ionescu-Shiley valve. It is now universally accepted that the rate of calcification, and therefore valve longevity, are strongly related to age.

The mode of failure of the pericardial valve has been widely reported. Experimental studies with subcutaneous implants in the rat have shown mineralization as early as 48 h post implantation (23). In our laboratory (24), studies in which porcine and pericardial valves were implanted in weaning sheep have also shown a higher degree of calcification of the bovine than of the porcine valve.

The glutaraldehyde-treated pericardium has a clear tendency toward calcification. However, stress probably plays a very important role in valve deterioration. The macroscopic analysis of the explanted prosthesis shows in all cases a fibrous covering of the leaflets that is more prominent on the outflow aspect whether aortic or mitral. This layer is often the site of extreme calcification. Ruptures without obvious macroscopic calcification occur far more often in the pericardial than in the porcine valves. These ruptures are basically located either parallel and close to the stent or at the base of the leaflet resulting from abrasion between tissue and stent.

Furthermore, in general, failures occur sooner in the mitral than in the aortic position, and different models of pericardial valves fail differently and at different times (25–28).

It can be concluded that the bovine pericardial tissue is an ideal material for valve construction. However, when treated with glutaraldehyde, calcification will result. The actual design that determines the amount and localization of the stresses can modify the wear and tear that inevitably will eventually destroy it.

The ideal tissue valve is not yet with us.

REFERENCES

1. Ross DN: Homograft replacement of the aortic valve. Lancet 1982;2:487.
2. Binet JP, Duran CMG, Carpentier A, Langlois J: Heterologous aortic valve transplantation. Lancet 1965;2:1275.
3. Senning A: Fascia lata replacement of aortic valves. J Thorac Cardiovasc Surg 1967;56:465–470.
4. Zerbini EJ, Puig LB: Experience with dura-mater allograft. Long term results. In: Sebening F et al (eds): Bioprosthetic Cardiac Valves. Munich, Deutsches Herzzentrum, 1979, pp 179–190.
5. Ionescu MI, Tandon AP, Mary DAS, Abid A: Heart valve replacement with the Ionescu-Shiley pericardial xenograft. J Thorac Cardiovasc Surg 1977;73:31–42.
6. Ionescu MI, Silverton NP, Tandon AP: The pericardial xenograft valve in the mitral position. In: Ionescu M, Cohn LH (eds): Mitral Valve Disease. London, Butterworths, 1985, pp 253–269.
7. Revichandran PS, Kay PH, Kollar A, Murday AJ: Ionescu-Shiley Legacy. In: Bodnar E (ed): Surgery for Heart Valve Disease. London, ICR Publishers, 1990, pp 715–724.
8. Anderson DR, Deverall PB, Revuelta JM, Gometza B, Duran CG: Early results of the Mitroflow valve. In: Bodnar E, Yacoub M (eds): Biologic & Bioprosthetic Valves. New York, Yorke Medical Books, 1986, pp 725–730.
9. Relland J, Perier P, Lecointe B: The third generation Carpentier-Edwards "bioprosthesis": Early results. J Am Coll Cardiol 1985;6:1149–1154.
10. Pelletier LC, Leclerc Y, Bonan R, Dyrda I: The Carpentier-Edwards bovine pericardial bioprosthesis: Clinical experience with 301 valve replacements. In Bodnar E (ed): Surgery for Heart Valve Disease. London, ICR Publishers, 1990, pp 691–701.

11. Bortolotti V, Milano A, Thiene G, Guerra F, Maezzucco A, Valente M, Talente F, Gallucci V: Early mechanical failures of the Hancock pericardial xenograft. J Thorac Cardiovasc Surg 1987;94:200–207.

12. Fisher J, Wheatley DJ: An improved pericardial bioprosthetic heart valve: Design and laboratory evaluation. Eur J Cardiothorac Surg 1987;1:71–79.

13. Gabbay S, Frater RWM: The unileaflet heart valve bioprosthesis: New concept. In: Cohn LH, Gallucci V (eds): Cardiac Bioprosthesis. New York, Yorke Medical Books, 1982, pp 411–424.

14. Gaddi O, Manari A, Brandi L, Guiducci U: Malfunctioning of the Meadox Bioprosthesis placed in the mitral position. Description of two clinical cases. G Ital Cardiol 1987;17:538–542.

15. Nistal F, Carcia-Satue E, Artinano E, Duran CMG, Gallo I: Comparative study of primary tissue valve failure between Ionescu-Shiley pericardial and Hancock porcine valves in the aortic position. Am J Cardiol 1986;57:161–164.

16. Fisher J, Reece IJ, Wheatley DJ: In vitro evaluation of six mechanical and six bioprosthetic valves. Thorac Cardiovasc Surg 1986;34:157–162.

17. Cosgrove DM, Lytle BW, Williams GW: Hemodynamic performance of the Carpentier-Edwards pericardial valve in the aortic position. Circulation 1985;72:II 146–152.

18. Lesbre JP, Chassat C, Lesperance J, Petitclerc R, Bonan R, Dyrda R, Pasternak A, Bourassa M: Evaluation of new pericardial bioprostheses by pulsed and continuous Doppler ultrasound. Arch Mal Coeur 1986; 79:1439–1448.

19. Revuelta JM, Garcia RG, Johnson RH, Bonnington L, Ubago JL, Duran CG: The Ionescu-Shiley valve: A solution for the small aortic root. J Thorac Cardiovasc Surg 1984;88:234–237.

20. Ionescu MI, Tandon AP, Silverton NP, Chindambaram M: Long term durability of the pericardial valve. In: Bodnar E, Yacoub M (eds): Biologic and Bioprosthetic Valves. New York, Yorke Medical Books, 1986, pp 163–164.

21. Cooley DA, Ott DA, Reul Jr GJ, Duncan JM, Frazier OH, Livesay JJ: Ionescu-Shiley bovine pericardial bioprosthesis, critical results in 2,701 patients. In: Bodnar E, Yacoub M (eds): Biologic and Bioprosthetic Valves. New York, Yorke Medical Books, 1986, pp 165–176.

22. Odell JA, Gillmer D, Whitton ID, Vythilingum SP, Vanker EA. Calcification of tissue valves in children: Occurrence in porcine and bovine pericardial bioprosthetic valves. In: Bodnar E, Yacoub M (eds): Biologic and Bioprosthetic Valves. New York, Yorke Medical Books, 1986, pp 259–270.

23. Schoen FJ, Tsao JW, Levy RJ: Calcification of bovine pericardium used in cardiac valve bioprosthesis. Implications for the mechanisms of bioprosthetic tissue mineralization. Am J Pathol 1986;123:135–145.

24. Gallo I, Nistal F, Artinano E, Fernandez D, Cayon R, Carrion M, Garcia Martinez V: The behaviour of pericardial versus porcine valve xenografts in the growing sheep model. J Thorac Cardiovasc Surg 1987;93:281–290.

25. Wheatley DJ, Fisher J, Reece IJ, Spyt T, Breeze P. Primary tissue failure in pericardial heart valves. J Thorac Cardiovasc Surg 1987;94:367–374.

26. Gabbay S, Bortolotti V, Wasserman F, Factor S, Strom J, Frater RWM: Fatigue-induced failure of the Ionescu-Shiley pericardial xenograft in the mitral position. In vivo and in vitro correlation and a proposed classification. J Thorac Cardiovasc Surg 1984;87:836–844.

27. Walley VM, Keon WJ: Patterns of failure in Ionescu-Shiley bovine pericardial bioprosthetic valves. J Thorac Cardiovasc Surg 1987;93:925–933.

28. Gabbay S, Kadam P, Factor S, Cheung TK: Do heart valve bioprostheses degenerate for metabolic or mechanical reasons? J Thorac Cardiovasc Surg 1988;95:208–215.

Bodnar, E. and Frater, R. W. M., editors
(1991) *Replacement Cardiac Valves,*
Pergamon Press, Inc. (New York), pp. 287–306
Printed in the United States of America

CHAPTER 12

VALVULAR HOMOGRAFTS

ENDRE BODNAR AND DONALD N. ROSS

Experimental, as well as clinical, implantation of homologous cardiac valves was preceded by documented success in the preservation and reimplantation of homologous vascular material in animal experiments by Alexis Carrel in 1908 and clinically by Robert Gross in 1948 (1, 2).

The first known successful implantation of a homologous cardiac valve, namely a canine valve into another dog's descending thoracic aorta, was carried out by Lamb and his colleagues in 1952 (3). The first true, orthotopic transplant of a valvular homograft, a canine tricuspid valve, was completed in Hungary by Francis Robicsek in 1953 (4).

Gordon Murray combined Gross's clinical experiences with preserved arterial grafts and Lamb's experimental success with heterotopically inserted aortic valves in 1956 when he completed a series of clinical insertions of aortic homografts into the descending thoracic aorta for the relief of aortic insufficiency (5). Satisfactory function of these valves extending to up to 6 years was reported by Kerwin et al. in 1962 (6).

The replacement of the aortic valve by inserting an aortic homograft into the subcoronary position was proposed by Duran and Gunning and completed with full clinical success by Donald Ross in 1962 (7, 8). Brian Barratt-Boyes reported in 1964 that he, too, had started subcoronary insertions in 1962, only a few months later than Donald Ross and entirely independently (9).

The first clinical series were published on aortic valve replacement with homografts (10), but the use of these valves was soon extended to right ventricular outflow tract reconstruction (11), mitral and tricuspid valve replacement (12), and eventually to the replacement of the entire aortic root and valve (13).

The use of mitral and tricuspid homografts was proposed early, but the concept has never reached clinical acceptance (4). Pulmonary homografts for right-sided use were first suggested by Eguchi and Asano in 1968, and results with the first clinical series were presented by Kay et al. in 1986 (14, 15).

It is estimated that about 15,000 homografts have been implanted worldwide, half of them between 1962 and 1972, approximately 40% since 1985, and probably not more than 1500 between 1972 and 1985. The reasons for this grossly disproportionate distribution were

The lack of competition from other biological valves, as they were not available during the first period.

The sweeping success of porcine bioprostheses from the mid-1970s until the mid-1980s.

The commencement of Cryolife, Inc., a well-organized commerical operation, in 1985, which has been providing large numbers of good-quality homografts, mainly for U.S. surgeons since. Cryolife has also been instrumental in rekindling surgeons' awareness worldwide through the company's efforts and support for presenting apparently good long-term clinical results with homografts processed by in-house, hospital laboratories since 1962.

In the current world experience, the majority of aortic and pulmonary homografts are inserted as valved conduits on the right side of the heart. However, the number of aortic homografts used for aortic valve or aortic root replacement is on the increase again.

The accumulated and reported clinical experience with homologous heart valves is considerable. However, the presentation of the published data in comparative terms is extremely difficult if not impossible. The difficulties are due to the number of factors that are different in the individual clinical series, varying broadly from center to center and from time frame to time frame within the same center. Furthermore, details of those factors are not necessarily contained in the clinical reports. These particulars entail pertinent data on valve processing, or on surgical methods, or on patient population, or on all of these.

In the following an attempt will be made to give a set of definitions that will serve in the rest of this chapter as a basis on which further discussions and inferences will be made and which, would they become generally adopted, could make clinical and experimental studies more comprehensible with substantially more potential for comparison in the future.

DEFINITIONS

An *anatomic* definition should include a clear statement as to which valve of the donor heart was inserted into which position; for example, aortic homograft in aortic position, pulmonary homograft in mitral position, and so forth.

A *biological* definition should state whether the study relates to homovital, viable, or nonviable valves.

Homovital valves are collected during transplant procedures and do not necessarily undergo sterilization, preservation, or chemical/physical treatment. The elapsed time between the cessation of the donor's heartbeat and insertion of the valve should not exceed 48 h, during which period the valves should be kept at 4°C in Hartman's solution or in a tissue culture medium.

At the time of insertion, *viable* homograft valves contain not less than 50% of the fibroblasts originally present, as assessed by radiolabeled amino acid essay, tissue culture, or both. Whether correctly or incorrectly, only the presence of live fibroblasts is required by international consensus to declare a valve "viable."

Nonviable homografts do not contain live cellular components because these were lost during the elapsed time preceding harvesting or through the method of sterilization or preservation, or any combination of these factors.

Donor criteria should disclose age limits, sex, and the source of the material, whether from transplant procedures or from routine or forensic autopsies. Unacceptable causes of death, that is, heart valve disease, septicemia, malignant diseases, tuberculosis or other major infective disease, hepatitis, or AIDS, should be noted.

It should be stated whether the *method of harvesting* was sterile, clean but nonsterile, or routine autopsy method.

Elapsed time from the cessation of the donor's heartbeat until harvesting should be reported as none (homovital), less than 6 hours (may be considered homovital), less than 24, 48, 72 hours, or more than 72 hours, as appropriate.

A statement should be made on the *method of transportation to the processing laboratory,* whether it was sterile or nonsterile, at controlled or ambient temperature, and with or without a fluid medium.

The *method of dissection* should be described, whether it was sterile or nonsterile, and also how the moisture was maintained.

Sterilization procedure(s) should be reported in full detail, including concentration, time, and temperature as appropriate. If no sterilizing procedure was applied (homovital valves) it should be clearly stated. The recognized sterilizing procedures should be grouped for reporting purposes as follows:

Chemical
    a. β-Propiolactone
    b. Ethylene oxide
    c. Other chemical

Irradiation, with details given on
    a. Temperature during γ irradiation
    b. Duration of process h/min/s
    c. Total amount applied in mrad-s

Antibiotic solution with details given on
    a. Name and concentration of all antibiotics and antifungal drugs used
    b. Length of time in antibiotics
    c. Temperature at which the antibiotics were used

The method of *preservation* should be described in terms of whether it was freeze-drying, cryopreservation, or the use of a nutrient medium. For cryopreservation, the method of freezing (flash or controlled), the freezing medium, and final temperature (acetone/CO_2 mixture $= -70°C$, immersion in liquid nitrogen $= -196°C$, vapor phase of a liquid nitrogen container $= -174°C$) and full details of the solution used as a cryoprotectant should be reported. Similarly, full details of the nutrient solution are to be described if the valve was "wet" stored at 4° C.

The *surgical method of insertion* should be specified in terms of whether it was done

1. Free-hand aortic valve replacement
    a. Ross method (anatomic placement)
    b. Barratt-Boyes methods (120° anticlockwise rotation)

2. Without dissecting the valve
    a. Aortic root replacement
    b. Right-sided valved conduit

3. Mounted homograft
    a. On a stent
        i. Rigid
        ii. Flexible
    b. Inside a Dacron/Teflon tube

The report on pre- and postoperative *patient management* should include statements on ABO matching or other tissue typing, immunosupression if any, anticoagulation if any, and antibiotic prophylaxis if any.

The definition of homograft valve failure should follow the guidelines published by Edmunds et al. (16). We have been working along the same lines during the last 10 years. There are, however, two important points on which the guidelines do not provide an unequivocal answer to reporting data on homografts.

Surgical technical error causing late valve failure is a cause of valve failure specific to replacement with homografts. It should be denoted if the mistake made at insertion is clearly identifiable at reoperation or autopsy. In general, surgical technical error leads to clinically manifest valve failure within 3 years of surgery.

Valve failure can be defined in two different ways. One is contained in the Edmunds guidelines and has been used by us during the past 10 years, denoting valve failure if and when it makes the removal of the valve necessary or causes death. However, it is possible with homografts, and was done by us before 1981, to define valve failure when clinical signs and symptoms of valvular incompetence and/or stenosis, which were not present immediately after surgery, are first reported.

The difference in clinical results, depending on which definition is used for valve failure, is significant, and the consequences can be far reaching (see below). For practical purposes, and to produce comparative clinical information, there must be no alternative to the Edmunds guidelines. Therefore, it is proposed to reintroduce and generally adopt the term *valve dysfunction* or *valve malfunction* (17–19) to be used in addition to *valve failure*, which, in reality, defines the *ultimate failure of the valve*. The former should be reported when clinical signs and symptoms reveal abnormal function of the valve. It is postulated that it may become a more sensitive measure of long-term performances than the robustly black-or-white end points given by reoperation and/or death, especially when different types of homografts are to be compared. The deficiencies of using reoperation as a censoring point were discussed by Brian Barratt-Boyes in 1987 and again in 1989 (20, 21), and in his study published in 1987 he used *significant incompetence,* in other words valve dysfunction, to compare different types of homografts.

Before elaborating on the important subjects of viability and antigenicity, a summary is given of past and current methods used for processing and preserving homografts.

DONOR SELECTION CRITERIA

There has been a general consensus over the years that any and every kind of transmittable disease should disqualify potential donors. This category includes septicemia, all contagious diseases, and malignancies. Major viral infections, especially hepatitis and AIDS, disqualify automatically if they are known. In addition, serologic tests are carried out to exclude the presence of Australian as well as HIV antigens.

The age limit set for donors seems to vary from center to center and also within the same center from time to time. There was no age limit set at the National Heart Hospital during the 1960s (10); currently it is 55 years. Donor age as a continuous variable was found by Barratt-Boyes to appear as a statistically significant incremental risk factor predisposing to late valve failure. In addition, a definite cutoff point was ascertained by him for donors older than 50 years (20). In sharp contrast to this finding, Radley-Smith and Yacoub, using similar statistical methods, were able to eliminate donors' age altogether as a risk factor (22). The same authors, however, found female sex of the donor as an incremental risk factor of valve failure (22).

It is possible that the diameter of the homograft has an effect on long-term valve performance, but the available information does not appear to be enough to draw final conclusions. Brian Barratt-Boyes, using the Cox proportionate hazard model analysis, found the increasing donor aortic root diameter acting as an incremental risk factor, the effect being intensified for valves larger than 30 mm in diameter (20). Interestingly, our own assessment of patient- rather than donor-related risk factors identified aortic incompetence compared with stenosis as an incremental risk of valve failure (23).

These two experiences confirm each other, but they seem to confuse rather than clarify the true nature of the causative factor. It may well be that impaired durability is inherent in homografts of larger sizes, and that it was not aortic incompetence but the necessarily large size of the inserted valve that lead to earlier failure in our study (23). However, it is also possible that the underlying clinical diagnosis rather than the size of the valve was the cause of early failure in the Auckland study (20).

In Radley-Smith and Yacoub's experience the opposite was true; they found aortic stenosis rather than incompetence predisposing to early homograft failure (22). Unfortunately, the authors did not offer an explanation for their surprising result.

HARVESTING

The source of homograft valves was uniformly forensic or hospital autopsy material until 1985. The first report with a sketchy reference to the clinical use of homovital valves collected during cardiac transplant procedures was presented in 1986 (24). Cryolife, Inc., have restricted themselves from the outset of the company in 1985 to the exclusive use of valves procured in conjunction with transplant procedures.

Currently, the vast majority of hospital laboratories processing homografts still only use autopsy material. There are a few, having an active transplant program, that collect homovital valves. The main difference between these hospital laboratories and Cryolife, Inc., is that the former collect valves only from suitable heart transplant recipients' hearts, while the latter uses hearts, which were originally designated for organ transplant but could not be used as such, for valve dissection.

The concept of homovital valves alludes to cellular viability and will be discussed in detail in the section on the biological aspects of homografts (see below). Proponents of this method emphasize its perceived value as the presence of live fibroblasts at insertion. This may or may not be correct.

To the knowledge of the authors of this chapter, there are no published data in the medical literature that compare long-term performances of homograft valves collected during transplant as opposed to autopsy procedures. In practical terms autopsy material is more readily available, cheaper, and easier to harvest, and, at the time of this chapter going to press, creates fewer legal and ethical problems than homovital valves.

TRANSPORTATION

The method of transportation is attaining importance with the distance the removed heart (or valve) has to travel from the site of removal to the processing laboratory. Historically, all those involved in the early development of homograft valves relied upon in-house or neighboring mortuaries; hence the question of transportation was paid very little, if any, attention, and was omitted from the relevant publications.

It was not before the late 1970s that it became essential for the National Heart Hospital to extend the collection of hearts from London to the entire countries of England, Wales, and Scotland. The hearts are transported by rail or as air freight, depending on the distance, and reach the Homograft Laboratory of the National Heart Hospital within 6 hours of the completion of the autopsy.

Ambient temperature was found adequate for transportation under the English climate as assessed by radioactive thymidine uptake of the valves. There has been no alteration introduced in this respect over the years, mainly because of our philosophy turning further and further away from the concept and importance of high cellular viability.

An entirely different situation is facing Cryolife, Inc., who have to collect valves from a vast area of North America and preserve preferably 100% viability of the fibroblasts. To solve the problem they developed a highly controlled method applying special accessories (Cryopack®). Similar efforts, however, may not be necessary for others collecting only mortuary valves.

If one is to draft principles for homograft transportation from mortuary or operating room to processing laboratory, then most probably, the transport

Should not last longer than 12 h.

Should take place at controlled, 4°C temperature.

Should not introduce contamination of any kind.

Should provide the optimum milieu for cellular and noncellular structures of the valves.

It is yet to be decided by hard data what the optimum milieu is. If the heart was kept moist in its own blood, the potential risk is hemolytic plasma insudation. If it was transported in Hartman's solution, osmotic damage to the surface might occur.

This area is one of the uncertainties still surrounding the processing of homografts.

DISSECTION OF THE VALVE

Both the aortic and the pulmonary valves are currently dissected from each heart. This was introduced as a routine procedure during the early 1980s at the National Heart Hospital, London, and became accepted worldwide with the only exception being Auckland, New Zealand, to our knowledge. We found it impossible to achieve 100% results and produce two valves from each heart. One or the other might get damaged during dissection, or was originally cut during autopsy. On average, 100 hearts offering in theory 200 valves (100 aortic, 100 pulmonary) provide 170 clinically useful aortic and pulmonary homografts.

Three criteria have to be strictly observed during the dissection of valves of mortuary origin:

The valve must not suffer new contamination during the procedure.

The dissecting person must be protected from contamination coming from the valve.

The valve must be kept moist at all times.

The protection of the dissecting personnel is compulsory by law in the United Kingdom and in several other countries, and the procedure has to be carried out under a certified exhaust hood accordingly.

The quality assurance of the individual valves extends to macroscopic inspection for abnormal anatomy, calcific or atheromatous plaques, and possible inconspicuous lesions of the leaflets. It is at this stage when measurements are taken to include inflow and outflow diameters and the length of the aortic or pulmonary segment.

Serologic tests are carried out to exclude the presence of Australian antigen and HIV antigen. The sterility is ascertained after the chosen sterilizing treatment by culturing for aerobic, anaerobic, and fungal growth and for mycobacteria.

The dissection of a homovital valve is a strictly sterile procedure, and as such it has to be done either in a class A environment or in a class B environment using a class A workstation.

STERILIZATION

There is a general consensus that valves of mortuary origin are contaminated; they have to be sterilized and the sterility ascertained by a qualified microbiologist before the valves are released for clinical use. This follows from the fact that postmortem blood cultures were found positive in 95% of the cadavers investigated (25).

The question of sterility of the homovital valves, collected during transplant procedures, is somewhat more complicated. In theory they should be sterile. In practice it is not necessarily the case. Gonzalez-Lavin and his associates completed a study on 17 homovital aortic and pulmonary valves harvested from brain-dead, beating heart, multiorgan donors where the heart could not be transplanted because of prolonged period of hypotension, a significant amount of isotropic support, or the lack of a suitable recipient. Nine out of the 17 valves were bacteriologically positive, growing anaerobic diphtheroids, *Staphylococcus aureus,* or *Propionibacterium* (26).

This finding certainly raises an eyebrow, as a number of those hearts were not transplanted *only because a suitable recipient could not be found.* The same authors state in the quoted publication that valves dissected from recipient hearts always proved to be sterile, but, regrettably, supportive data or reference is not provided by them.

Early series of homografts inserted between 1962 and 1969 were sterilized by β-propiolactone, ethylene oxide, or γ irradiation (9, 10, 27). Sterlization by γ irradiation was proposed by Malm et al. in 1967 (27) and denounced by Beach and Malm in 1972 (28).

Having been dissatisfied with the midterm clinical results using chemically (ethylene oxide, β-propiolactone) sterilized homografts, Brian Barratt-Boyes introduced antibiotic sterilization in 1968 (20). Subsequently he reduced the concentration of the antibiotic mixture to decrease cytotoxicity (20). At Guy's Hospital and the National Heart Hospital, London, ethylene oxide was used between 1962 and 1967, γ irradiation between 1967 and 1970, and antibiotic solution since 1969. The approach to sterilization in antibiotics has been rather pragmatic over the years at the National Heart Hospital, and at least four different, consecutive mixtures were introduced to achieve maximum effect at all times (29). There are no published data available on sterilizing methods currently used by Cryolife, Inc.

The basic problem with sterilizing the homograft valves is that any method that is capable of reliably destroying contamination causes unavoidable damage to the cellular and/or the fibrous structure of the valve itself. This was the rationale for abandoning chemical sterilization and irradiation altogether and for decreasing the antibiotic concentration originally proposed by Brian Barratt-Boyes.

Unfortunately, rules of general authenticity can not be set and do not seem to apply in this respect. The rate of rejection for contamination has been around 3 to 4% at the National Heart Hospital during the last 17 years, using a high concentration of the antibiotics. When an attempt was made to introduce the low-concentration solution advocated by Brian Barratt-Boyes that achieves 98% sterility in Auckland, 62% of the samples remained unsterile (30). Moreover, it was established by toxicology studies that although the Auckland soluton was less cytotoxic than the one used in London, they were both within the same range. It is worth mentioning that similar problems were encountered by surgeons of the University of Washington who attempted to use the Auckland mixture and concentration of antibiotics but were unable to duplicate the results (31).

Some clinical information, emerging only recently, seems to add to the controversy surrounding homograft sterilization. It was generally held until last year that chemically sterilized or irradiated homografts produced inferior long-term performances compared with those immersed in antibiotics. This was the outcome of a retrospective, comparative assessment carried out by us (17), and subsequently Barratt-Boyes's elegant comparative study seemed to provide additional clinical evidence to prove this assertion (20). It appears, however, that the effect of widely different time frames was not properly accounted for in those clinical studies.

By 1989, 20 years of follow-up information was available on antibiotic-sterilized valves at the National Heart Hospital, and we compared the performances in the first 10 years with those of an identical time frame taken from information on valves sterilized by ethylene oxide or γ irradiation. To our greatest possible surprise, and contradicting our own, previous results (17), we could not ascertain any difference in primary tissue failure between valves sterilized chemically, by irradiation, or in an antibiotic-containing solution (32). (Figs. 12–1 and 12–2). In addition, a 94% actuarial freedom from primary tissue failure after 19 years at risk was found in a select group of irradiated homografts

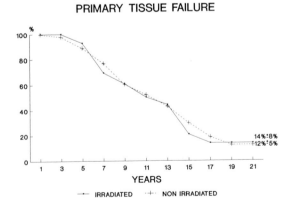

AORTIC HOMOGRAFTS
PRIMARY TISSUE FAILURE

FIG. 12–1. Comparison of freedom from primary tissue failure in homografts sterilized by γ irradiation versus other methods of sterilization. Reproduced with the publisher's permission from Bodnar E, Parker R, Davies J, Robles A, Ross DNR: Non-viable aortic homografts. In Bodnar E (ed): Surgery for Heart Valve Disease. London, ICR Publishers, 1990, p 494.

AORTIC HOMOGRAFTS
PRIMARY TISSUE FAILURE

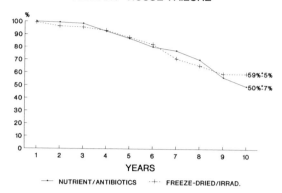

FIG. 12–2. Comparison of nutrient-antibiotic valves with freeze-dried and irradiated or ethylene oxide–sterilized valves. Reproduced with the publisher's permission from Bodnar E, Parker R, Davies J, Robles A, Ross DNR: Non-viable aortic homografts. In Bodnar E (ed): Surgery for Heart Valve Disease. London, ICR Publishers, 1990, p 494.

inserted into the right ventricular outflow tract position (Fig. 12–3). The importance of these results alludes to the cellular viability of the homologous valves and will be discussed later in this chapter (see below). The results, however, were found so convincing by us, that an experimental study has already been started to reevaluate γ irradiation of homologous valves. The preliminary results are encouraging (33).

All in all, it can be stated with confidence that, clinically, all types of homografts proved to be sterile irrespective of the method applied as attested by the lack of early endocarditis with these valves. The only exception to this general rule was the report by the Harefield team on a few cases of postoperative miliary tuberculosis attributed to aortic homografts (34). It was possible for them, however, to eliminate this complication by modifying the antibiotic mixture as well as the microbiological assessment of sterility.

IRRADIATED VALVES IN PULMONARY POSITION
PRIMARY TISSUE FAILURE

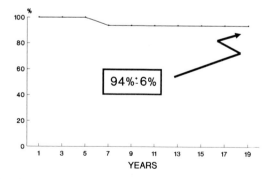

FIG. 12–3. Freedom from primary tissue failure in aortic homografts inserted into a normal pulmonary outflow tract (pulmonary autograft operation). Reproduced with the publisher's permission from Bodnar E, Parker R, Davies J, Robles A, Ross DNR: Non-viable aortic homografts. In Bodnar E (ed): Surgery for Heart Valve Disease. London, ICR Publishers, 1990, p 494.

PRESERVATION

If valvular homografts are to be made available in considerable numbers and not limited by the same factors as cardiac transplant procedures are, they have to be preserved from the time of harvesting until the clinical need emerges. Historically, and dictated only by intuition, of the first two valves ever inserted into the subcoronary position, one was freeze-dried (8) and the other a homovital valve (9).

The first large clinical series were completed with freeze-dried valves. Flash freezing in an acetone–carbon dioxide mixture ($-70°C$) or controlled freezing in liquid nitrogen ($-196°C$) were introduced in 1967. When the concept of cellular viability emerged, cryopreservation was abandoned and replaced by preservation in Hank's solution or in TC 199 tissue culture medium. Cryopreservation in liquid nitrogen was reinstituted by Marc O'Brien in Brisbane, Australia, and started on a large, commercial scale by Cryolife, Inc., in 1985 (35). Currently, the majority of homograft valves are cryopreserved; some hospital laboratories still use nutrient solution, and a few centers, actively involved in a heart transplant program, insert homovital, and hence unpreserved and untreated valves.

There has never been a prospective, randomized clinical trial to compare different methods of preservation and/or sterilization of homograft valves, and there are only three published clinical series comparing different methods of preservation by retrospective assessment of long-term performances experienced within the same surgical center.

The first such comparison was carried out by us in 1979 (17). It revealed a higher freedom from primary tissue failure with nutrient- and antibiotic–stored valves than with those freeze-dried or cryopreserved. However, and it is easy to state now with hindsight, we did not realize the importance of the existence of different time frames nor did we, or others in those days, clearly understand the effect of time-related changes in hazard functions. Hence the uncertain nature of the 1980 comparison; a 10-year period was the *shortest* potential follow-up for freeze-dried and cryopreserved valves still at risk, but it was the *longest* potential follow-up for valves stored in nutrient-antibiotics.

The second retrospective comparison was completed and published by O'Brien et al. in 1987 (36, 37). They compared long-term performances of nutrient-antibiotic–stored valves (series I) with those of cryopreserved valves (series II) and found a much higher freedom from primary tissue failure with the latter; 88 versus 99%, respectively, at year 10. However, the median follow-up for series I was 13.7 years, but it was not more than 4.3 years for series II. A period of 12.3 years was the shortest follow-up for series I, and it was the longest for series II, resembling the same problem we were experiencing in 1980 (17) (see above).

The third, and to our knowledge the last, comparison was made again by ourselves in 1989 (38), by which time the length of the potential follow-up period with the nutrient-antibiotic valves was 19 years, roughly twice as long as it was in 1980. *We compared the first, decisive 10-year time frame with freeze-dried, cryopreserved, and nutrient-antibiotic homografts and were not able to show any difference whatsoever in the rate of primary tissue failure with these three types of aortic homografts.*

Our own efforts, therefore, remain inconclusive, and our results do not permit a critical judgment favoring any one of the methods proposed and used for homograft preservation. If one applies the same cautions and criticism to Marc O'Brien's results as we did to ours from 1980, the conclusive nature of his study could similarly be questioned. For mere practical reasons we reintroduced cryopreservation at the National Heart Hospital in 1983 and made it the exclusive method 3 years ago.

There seems to be no reason why storage in a nutrient solution should not remain the method of choice for those who are experienced in performing it and can cope with the limited storage period permitted by this method. However, there is no clear-cut answer as to how limited this storage period is.

The rationale for introducing storage in a nutrient medium was to maintain cellular viability. The first efforts to define the length of permitted storage period without losing a significant proportion of viable cells were based on the assessment of decrease of cellular viability with elapsed time in a nutrient medium, using radiolabeled thymidine uptake as an indicator (39). It was found that valves could be kept at 4°C in Hartman's solution for 3 weeks and in TC 199 medium enriched by 10% fetal calf serum for up to 8 weeks (40). These results were contradicted by McGregor and Wheatley, who found virtually no viable cells left after 21 days of storage in nutrient medium as assessed by tissue culture (41). Similar findings led Marc O'Brien to reintroduce cryopreservation in 1975 (35).

We made two attempts to relate long-term clinical performances to the length of period from valve dissection to clinical implantation. The first study ascertained an apparent cutoff point after 21 days of storage, and the second failed to confirm these results (17, 23). *However, there was a substantial difference between these two studies in the definition of valve failure.* In the first study, valve failure was denoted when a diastolic murmur, which was not present at discharge from hospital, was first reported. In the second study valve failure was defined as an event leading to reoperation or causing death, corresponding to the generally adopted terminology (see above).

VIABILITY AND ANTIGENICITY OF THE HOMOGRAFT VALVES

It is remarkable that the most important single rationale for the introduction and continued use of heart valves of human cadaveric origin could not be validated by a clinical experience extending to more than 25 years. The existence of a normal or near-normal cellular and/or extracellular tissue turnover in the functioning homograft valves had been postulated by many, but proved to be true by none. The difficulties were made worse by the fact that animal experimental results could not have a direct application to clinical surgery.

First it was assumed that the inserted homograft, nonviable in those days, would act as an ideal frame and it would be repopulated by host cells that would maintain a normal fiber structure. The definition of *primary tissue failure* was not conceived then, and when the first examples of degeneration were found in explanted homografts together with complete or almost complete acellularity, it was assumed, but only assumed, that the continuing presence of fibroblasts would have prevented the degeneration from occurring.

As the theory of cellular repopulation was defeated, the concept of cellular viability has emerged (42). It was assumed this time that by sustaining the presence of living fibroblasts in the homograft valves, late degeneration could be eliminated or its incidence significantly reduced. The implicit assumption was, and it seems to be the case even today, that the presence of living fibroblasts in a valve at the time of insertion renders it "normal." Viabililty, therefore, as per definition, equals normal valve.

Viable valves, however, are not necessarily normal. Fibroblasts do not produce collagen, they produce only procollagen, and a normal extra- and intracellular environment is necessary in turn for the collagen fibers to develop. The essential role of the muco-polysaccharides and proteoglycans is ignored by the current definition of viability, as fibroblasts are not known to produce those vitally important macromolecules. Fibro-blasts do not produce elastin, either. Finally, the presence or absence of endothelial cells is not even searched for when the so-called cellular viability of a homograft is assessed. Indeed, those valves do not have endothelium.

In this context it is hardly surprising that we could not ascertain any difference in the long-term performances of aortic homografts in the subcoronary position whether they were "viable" or not (38), preserved by freeze-drying, cryopreservation, or in a nutrient solution at 4° C. The importance of this observation is emphasized by the fact that the freeze-dried valves did not contain viable cells. The other groups were, and the cryopre-served valves still are, declared and generally accepted as containing viable cells. The consequence is a simple conclusion:

Cellular viability is not preserved permanently by any one of the methods assessed.

or

Permanent cellular viability does not have any effect on long-term performances of the homologous heart valves.

or

Both of the above are true.

If results of long-term comparative assessment of the Auckland clinical experience with β-propiolactone or ethylene oxide versus antibiotic-sterilized homografts are reviewed with close scrutiny, they seem to confirm the above conclusions (20, 43). As Brian Barratt-Boyes stated: "Freedom from significant incompetence with the antibiotic preparation is much greater than with the chemical preparation during the first 9–10 years of follow-up, and thereafter the two curves become almost parallel" (20). It is apparent from reviewing this comparison that after 7 years at risk, the slope of the two actuarial curves, and therefore the rates of hazard of valve failure had they been calcu-lated, were identical for chemically sterilized, that is, definitely nonviable, and for anti-biotic-sterilized, that is, supposedly viable, valves. Hence viability (or the lack of it) does not appear to be an important factor determining long-term performance in either of the two largest and longest clinical series with homografts inserted in London and in Auckland.

Our own laboratory results as well as those of others have demonstrated a high per-centage of viable fibroblasts in valves of cadaveric origin (39, 40). The great many efforts over the years were only aiming at the preservation of the viability present 24 to 72 hours after death. It may well be the case that all those efforts have failed, as suggested by the results of McGregor, Wheatley, and associates, who found a total disappearance of cel-lular viability within 21 days in valves stored in nutrient-antibiotics (41).

However, the same authors completed an elegant series of animal experiments that provided strong evidence that the homovital valves with a demonstrably high cellular viability provoke a strong immunologic reaction and deteriorate faster than the nonvi-able valves (44). More recent studies using histocompatibility assays concluded that the antigen expression of the human valvular tissue is mainly localized to the endothelium and it declines rapidly during the first 48 h after death (45).

It would appear from recently emerged clinical experience that homograft valves with a well-preseved, high cellular viability can provoke acute immunologic rejection that causes early and rapid valve failure (46, 47). All rejected valves reported in the quoted references were processed and supplied by Cryolife, Inc., and the rejection was ascertained by specific immunologic tests carried out on the valves. *It is significant in this respect that all the cryopreserved valves published by Marc O'Brien were collected from mortuaries rather than transplant procedures.*

These observations lead us as well as others (48) to the conclusion that high cellular viability, if it was indeed preserved, might introduce immunologic problems that have so far been unknown. As the introduction of mandatory immunosupression would defeat the principles of using biological valves, it may well be that high cellular viability will prove to be an undesirable feature of valvular homografts.

AORTIC VALVE REPLACEMENT WITH A FREE-HAND INSERTED HOMOGRAFT

Replacement of the aortic valve with a homograft is now an accepted surgical procedure of proven value, and the technical details of the insertion are easily mastered.

The sizing of the valve is relatively simple, because for practical reasons homografts can be graded into three groups, 19 to 21 mm (small), 21 to 23 mm (medium), and 23 to 25 mm (large). Thus medium corresponds roughly to the average build while small relates to young people and lightly built females. Large valves are for a well-built man. Outside these, one can have very small valves for very young children (when a pulmonary autograft would be more applicable) and very large, 24 to 26 mm, for abnormal roots when a restraining ring would probably be incorporated.

Helpful guidelines are to be found in the general build of the patient and the echocardiogram and aortogram if available. The aortic orifice will of course be measured at operation, and one must keep in mind that the given homograft size represent its internal diameter, so that 2 to 4 mm should be added for wall thickness.

The initial aortic incision is vertical, and, once the valve is visualized, it is swung right well above the right coronary orifice and deeply into the base of the noncoronary sinus. The edges of the incision are retracted with 2/0 stay sutures; hand-held retractors are avoided. Bilateral coronary perfusion with soft balloon-tipped catheters is instituted, and with the heart beating, a functional view of the root and particularly the subvalvar muscle is achieved. Before inserting the homograft, cardioplegic solution is administered down the same coronary catheters (Fig. 12–4).

The valve remnants and all calcium are meticulously removed, leaving a flexible bed for the homograft-fixing sutures. During this time the homograft is thawed if it was frozen or decanted if fresh. The muscle remnant and the lower margin of the homograft are trimmed as necessary to reduce their bulk. No attempt is made to tailor the sinuses at this stage.

There has been some discussion with regard to orientation of the homograft in the aortic root. We believe firmly that it should be inserted in exact anatomic position with the shallower right cusp within the right sinus and the deeper commissure between the left and the noncoronary cusp in its corresponding position within the valve ring.

The lower margin of the homograft is trimmed horizontally between the bases of the sinuses, but no attempt is made at this stage to trim the aortic wall down into the sinuses. This provides a useful segment to hold in a soft clamp during insertion. About 1 to 2 mm of muscle and endocardial tissue is left to extend beyond the base of the sinuses.

Three primary interrupted through-and-through sutures (usually 4/0 Prolene) are now inserted at the base of the sinus remnants of the recipient heart, brought up through the

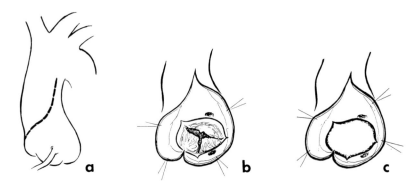

FIG. 12–4. Surgical exposure and removal of the aortic valve. (a) Recommended line of the aortotomy; (b) retraction of the aortic wall by stay sutures; (c) aortic annulus prepared for homograft insertion.

tough tissue at the base of the homograft cusp insertions, and held with rubber-shod clamps. The homograft is held in a position about 15 cm above the valve ring until all the lower interrupted sutures are in place.

The alternative technique of sewing the homograft in position by inverting it into the left ventricle invariably gives rise to a bulky lower suture line and a double layer of tissue once the valve is pulled back from the ventricle and the inside-out situation is reversed (Fig. 12–5).

About seven interrupted sutures are now placed between each of the three primary sutures and held loosely in the assistant's hand. They are inserted in a straight line between the bases of the sinuses and pick up a good bite of tissue. The subaortic curtain of the mitral valve is picked up by the sutures between the base of the left and noncoronary sinuses. The orientation of the His bundle should be kept in mind between the noncoronary and the right coronary sinus.

When the 24 sutures are in place, the homograft is gently eased down into position and the sutures are tied—all knots being outside the homograft (Fig. 12–5).

Three commissural (3/0 Prolene) sutures are now placed in position. These are mattress sutures passed through the homograft just above the commissural attachments and through the wall of the patient's aorta. The point of attachment to the latter is of great importance. It should be in the line of the original commissure but 1 to 1.5 cm higher so that the homograft will be attached under medium tension to prevent prolapse and regurgitation from that source. These sutures are not tied at this stage but act as a guide during the placement of the upper suture line.

Viewed from above it is now easy to see the position of the left and right coronary orifices—the left is usually near the midpoint of the left sinus and the right is often eccentric and positioned toward the commissure adjacent to the noncoronary cusp. This is the time to tailor the upper margin of the homograft with the three suspending sutures retracted under moderate tension. Enough of the left and right coronary sinus tissue of the homograft is excised to expose the two coronary orifices. The noncoronary sinus is not excised as it will be incorporated in the aortotomy closure.

A double-ended 4/0 Prolene suture is inserted at the lowest point of the excised sinus tissue and through the adjacent part of the recipient's aortic sinus wall. As this stuture approaches the suspending suture, it is brought out through the aortic wall, and after the suspending suture is tied, it is locked to this stitch (Fig. 12–6).

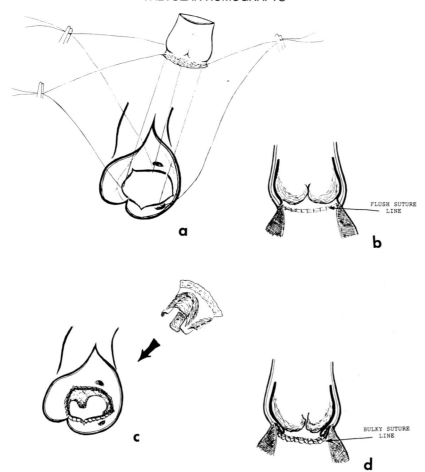

FIG. 12–5. Alternative methods of placing the proximal suture lines (a, b) with interrupted sutures and (c, d) continuously running suture by everting the homograft and lowering it into the left ventricle. Note the difference in valve adaptation at completion.

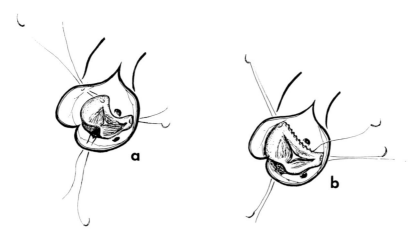

FIG. 12–6. Concluding steps of free-hand homograft insertion. (a) Commissural stitches; (b) continuously running distal suture line.

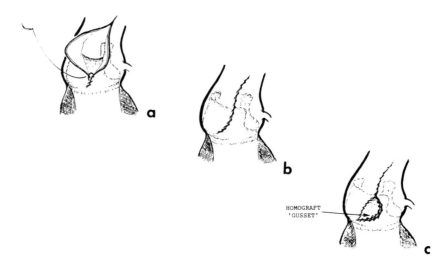

FIG. 12–7. (a) Closure of the aortotomy to incorporate the intact noncoronary sinus. (b) Completed suture line. (c) Incorporation of the noncoronary sinus of the homograft as a gusset to avoid distortion.

A similar maneuver is adopted with the remaining arc of the sinus, and an exactly similar procedure brings the excised homograft wall into opposition with the right aortic wall sinus.

When the edges of the aortotomy incision are brought gently together over the homograft, the correct line to follow in the closure will be apparent. The aortotomy is closed by sewing the edges of the incision to the underlying noncoronary sinus of the homograft. The first 4/0 suture passes through the lower point of the aortotomy and the adjacent homograft sinus near the base of the cusp. It returns as a mattress suture out through the aortic wall.

The closure proceeds with each stitch picking up half-thickness of the adjacent noncoronary sinus wall and following the line of the aortotomy closure as previously determined. In practice the suture line usually veers toward the right commissure.

Once the top of the sinus has been reached, a running 4/0 Prolene suture is inserted between the adjacent 3/0 suspending sutures to obliterate the space between the top of the homograft sinus and the aortic wall (Fig. 12–7). Additional mattress sutures can be added to obliterate any dead space. Rewarming proceeds during this phase of the operation.

Competence of the homograft is judged by noting if there is a significant drop of perfusion pressure on opening the aortic clamp and also by monitoring whether there is reflux into the left ventricle. An accurate assessment is provided by intraesophageal or epicardial echocardiography.

CLINICAL RESULTS

The immediate and short-term results are extremely good in experienced hands. The bypass time necessary for a free-hand homograft insertion into the aortic position is somewhat longer than would be necessary for inserting a manufactured replacement valve, but it is more than compensated for by the normal hemodynamics offered by the homograft. The total energy loss across a free-hand inserted homograft is not more than that across the normally functioning, natural aortic valve. This is in sharp contrast to the immediate postoperative behavior of mechanical prostheses, where the energy loss can be prohibitive with low cardiac output because of the disproportionately high reflux under those conditions (see Chap. 1). The ease of weaning the patient off bypass is the first reward for homograft users, especially if arrhythmia coexists with the aortic valve disease.

It is rare, almost exceptional, that gross valve failure develops during the early postoperative period. In the past it was invariably due to tissue deterioration in β-propiolactone, or more likely to surgical error at insertion. Currently, and for those using homovital or other highly viable valves, the possibility of early acute rejection should be borne in mind (*vide supra*).

Surgical technical error, however, at least according to our experience, cannot be completely eliminated with free-hand homografts. About 5 to 6% of these valves are likely to fail and have to be replaced during the first 3 to 5 postoperative years because of one or other type of technical error. The actuarial freedom from technical error is more than 90% at 10 years of follow-up and beyond.

The characteristic behavior of long-term overall performances is depicted in Fig. 12–8. The clinical material used for constructing the survival curves was a combined set of 639 homografts sterilized by ethylene oxide, irradiation, or antibiotics and preserved by freeze-drying, or cryopreservation, or in nutrient solution (32). To our knowledge, this is the largest series of aortic homografts in the aortic position with the longest follow-up information published so far.

It is apparent from Fig. 12–8 that more than 50% of the operative survivors who had isolated aortic valve replacement with a homograft survive longer than 20 years. It is also apparent that during the same period more than two-thirds of the patients remain free of valve-related death. However, only 9% of the valves originally inserted can be expected to function without complications beyond 20 years.

The nature of complications with homografts is limited to technical errors already mentioned, endocarditis on the inserted valve (equivalent of "prosthetic endocarditis"), and primary tissue failure.

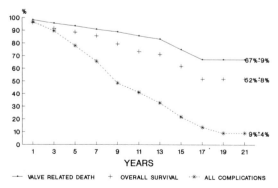

AORTIC HOMOGRAFTS
OVERALL PERFORMANCE INDICES

— VALVE RELATED DEATH   + OVERALL SURVIVAL   ···*··· ALL COMPLICATIONS

Fig. 12–8. Actuarial estimate of overall performance indices with 639 aortic homografts. Reproduced with the publisher's permission from Bodnar E, Parker R, Davies J, Robles A, Ross DNR: Non-viable aortic homografts. In Bodnar E (ed): Surgery for Heart Valve Disease. London, ICR Publishers, 1990, p 494.

Valve thrombosis and/or peripheral embolism remain unknown complications of homografts at the National Heart Hospital, London. Identical results were reported from Auckland (20). However, O'Brien et al. found a 97% freedom from embolism after 10, and 96% after 15 years (36), but the median age of their patients was almost 60 years, creating a high potential for background noise factor of stroke, which is more common in the elderly population.

Anticoagulant and/or antiplatelet treatment is unnecessary with homografts and is never applied. Bleeding due to anticoagulation, therefore, does not exist with these valves.

The lack of thrombosis, embolism, and bleeding, the unrestricted lifestyle, the restoration of valve function to normal, and the freedom of mind while the function remains normal are the great advantages of homograft valves. The price to pay is the reoperation if and when it becomes necessary.

The indications for the removal of an aortic homograft are endocarditis and ultimate valve failure.

Late endocarditis appears to be unavoidable with any type of replacement valve, including homografts. Its rate is in the range of 0.5 to 1% per annum, and it reacts only seldom to antibiotic treatment.

The ultimate failure of the valve may be caused by surgical technical error (see above), but in the vast majority of cases it is the consequence of primary tissue failure. Primary tissue failure in an aortic homograft includes tear, wear, attenuation, rupture, extrinsic and/or intrinsic calcification, and occasionally shrinkage of one or more cusps.

The cause of primary tissue failure is still not known, and the reader is referred to previous parts of this chapter as well as to relevant parts of Chaps. 5 and 6 for an outline of the complex nature of the problem.

Aortic and pulmonary homografts appear as the best valved conduits in the right side of the heart (11). In a recent series published by the German Heart Center, Munich, not more than four reoperations were necessary in a group of 186 homografts used as right-sided extracardiac conduits and followed for a mean of 3.8 years (48). The Hospital for Sick Children, London, reported a 93% freedom from obstruction after 10 years for a select group of homografts used as extracardiac conduits (49). The main reason for the excellent results is most probably the absence of peel, the major single cause of obstruction with other valved conduits. The wall of the aortic homograft may calcify in some cases, but it does not necessarily cause obstruction, nor does it interfere with the function of the valve cusps.

The replacement of the entire aortic root and valve with a homograft for infective endocarditis and aortic root abscess was first completed in 1972 (50). Later the indication was extended to complex left ventricular outflow tract obstruction (51). With low operative risk in elective cases and extremely good long-term results, this procedure emerges as the method of choice for aortic valve replacement, paving the road to achieve further improvements of the long-term clinical results with aortic and pulmonary homografts.

REFERENCES

1. Carrell A: Results of the transplantation of blood vessels, organs and limbs. JAMA 1908;51:1662.
2. Gross RE, Hurwitt EJ, Bill AH Jr, Peirce EC II: Preliminary observations on the use of human arterial grafts in the treatment of certain cardiovascular defects. N Engl J Med 1948;239:578–580.
3. Lamb CR, Aram HH, Mennell ER: An experimental study of aortic valve homografts. Surg Gynecol Obstet 1952;94:129–131.

4. Robicsek F: Transplantation of heart valves. Orvosi Hétilap 1953;25:1–4.
5. Murray G: Homologous aortic valve segment transplants as surgical treatment for aortic and mitral insufficiency. Angiology 1956;7:446–451.
6. Kerwin AG, Lenkei SC, Wilson DR: Aortic valve homograft in the treatment of aortic insufficiency: Report of nine cases, with one followed for six years. N Engl J Med 1962;266:852–854.
7. Duran CG, Gunning AJ: A method for placing a total homologous aortic valve into the subcoronary position. Lancet 1962;2:488.
8. Ross DN: Homograft replacement of the aortic valve. Lancet 1962;2:447.
9. Barrat-Boyes BG: Homograft aortic valve replacement in aortic incompetence and stenosis. Thorax 1964;19:131–135.
10. Davies H, Missen GAK, Blandford G, Roberts CI, Lessof MH, Ross DN: Homograft replacement of the aortic valve. Am J Cardiol 1968;22:195–202.
11. Ross DN, Somerville J: Correction of pulmonary atresia with a homograft aortic valve. Lancet 1966;2:1446–1447.
12. Ross DN, Somerville J: Mitral valve replacement with stored, inverted pulmonary homografts. Thorax 1972;27:583–586.
13. Lao GKH, Robles A, Cherian A, Ross DN: Surgical treatment of prosthetic endocarditis. J Thorac Cardiovasc Surg 1984;87:712–715.
14. Eguchi S, Asano KI: Homograft of pulmonary artery or ascending aorta with valve as right ventricular outflow. J Thorac Cardiovasc Surg 1968;56:413–415.
15. Kay PH, Livi U, Robles A, Ross DN: Pulmonary Homografts. In Bodnar E, Yacoub M (eds): Biologic and Biprosthetic Heart Valves. New York, Yorke Medical Books, 1986, p 58–63.
16. Edmunds LH, Clark RE, Cohn LH, Miller DG, Weisel RD: Guidelines for reporting morbidity and mortality after cardiac valvular operations. J Thorac Cardiovasc Surg 1988;96:331–353.
17. Bodnar E, Wain WH, Martelli V, Ross DN: Long term performance of 580 homograft and autograft valves used for aortic valve replacement. Thorac Cardiovasc Surg 1979;27:31–38.
18. Bodnar E, Haberman S, Wain WH: Comparative method of actuarial analysis of cardiac valve replacements. Br Heart J 1979;42:541–550.
19. Bodnar E, Wain WH, Haberman S: Assessment and comparison of the performance of cardiac valves. Ann Thorac Surg 1982;34:146–152.
20. Barratt-Boyes BG: 25 years' clinical experience of allograft surgery—a time for reflection. In Yankah AC, Hetzer R, Miller DC, Ross DN, Somerville J, Yacoub MH (eds): Cardiac Valve Allografts 1962–1987. New York, Springer, 1987, pp 347–358.
21. Barratt-Boyes BG: Discussion. In Bodnar E (ed): Surgery for heart valve disease. London, ICR Publishers, 1990, p 503.
22. Radley-Smith R, Yacoub MH: Long term results of antibiotic-treated aortic allografts in subcoronary position. In Yankah AC, Hetzer R, Miller DC, Ross DN, Somerville J, Yacoub MH (eds): Cardiac valve allografts 1962–1987. New York, Springer, 1987, p 265–269.
23. Matsuki O, Robles A, Gibbs S, Bodnar E, Ross DN: Long-term performance of 555 aortic homografts in the aortic position. Ann Thorac Surg 1988;46:187–191.
24. Dhalla N, Khaghani A, Radley-Smith R, Yacoub M: Early and long term performance of aortic root replacement. In Bodnar E, Yacoub M: Biologic and Bioprosthetic Valves. New York, Yorke Medical Books, 1986, pp 7–13.
25. Yacoub M, Kittle C: Sterilization of valve homografts by antibiotic solutions. Circulation 1970;(Suppl II)42:29.
26. Gonzalez-Lavin L, McGrath L, Alvarez M, Graf D: Antibiotic sterilization in the preparation of homovital homograft valves: Is it necessary? In Yankah AC, Hetzer R, Miller DC, Ross DN, Somerville J, Yacoub MH (eds): Cardiac Valve Allografts 1962–1987. New York, Springer, 1987, pp 17–24.
27. Malm JR, Bowman FO, Harris PD, Kovalik ATW: An evaluation of aortic valve homografts sterilized by electron-beam energy. J Thorac Cardiovasc Surg 1967;54:471–475.
28. Beach PM, Malm JR: Homologous aortic valve replacement. In Ionescu MI, Ross DN, Wooler GH (eds): Biological Tissue in Heart Valve Replacement. London, Butterworths, 1972, pp 31–43.
29. Wain WH, Pearce HM, Riddel RW, Ross DN: A re-evaluation of antibiotic sterilisation of heart valve allografts. Thorax 1977;32:740–745.
30. Bodnar E: Discussion in Yankah AC, Hetzer R, Miller DC, Ross DN, Somerville J, Yacoub MH (eds): Cardiac Valve Allografts 1962–1987. New York, Springer, 1987, p 379.
31. Mohri H, Reichenbach DD, Merendino KA: Biology of homologous and heterologous aortic valves. In Ionescu MI, Ross DN, Wooler GH (eds): Biological Tissue in Heart Valve Replacement. London, Butterworths, 1972, pp 137–156.
32. Bodnar E, Parker R, Davies J, Robles A, Ross DN: Non viable aortic homografts. In Bodnar E (ed): Surgery for Heart Valve Disease. London, ICR Publishers, 1990, pp 494–500.
33. Bodnar E: Discussion. In Bodnar E (ed): Surgery for Heart Valve Disease. London, ICR Publishers, 1990, p 506.
34. Anyanwu CH, Nassau E, Yacoub M: Miliary tuberculosis following homograft valve replacement. Thorax 1976;31:101–106.

35. Watts LK, Duffy P, Field RB, Stafford EG, O'Brien MF: Establishment of a viable homograft cardiac valve bank: A rapid method of determining homograft viability. Ann Thorac Surg 1976;21:230–234.

36. O'Brien MF, Stafford EG, Gardner MA, Pohler PG, McGiffin DC: A comparison of aortic valve replacement with viable cryopreserved and fresh allograft valves with a note on chromosomal studies. J Thorac Cardiovasc Surg 1987;94:812–817.

37. O'Brien MF, Stafford EG, Gardner MA, Pohler PG, McGiffin DC, Johnston N, Tesar P, Brosnan A, Duffy P: Cryopreserved viable aortic valves. In Yankah AC, Hetzer R, Miller DC, Ross DN, Somerville J, Yacoub MH (eds): Cardiac Valve Allografts 1962–1987. New York, Springer, 1987, pp 311–317.

38. Bodnar E, Matsuki O, Parker R, Ross DN: Viable and non viable aortic homografts in the subcoronary position: A comparative study. Ann Thorac Cardiovasc Surg 1989;47:799–804.

39. Al-Janabi N, Gibson K, Rose J, Ross DNR: Protein synthesis in fresh aortic and pulmonary allografts as an additional test for viability. Cardiovasc Res 1973;7:247–249.

40. Al-Janabi N, Ross DNR: Enhanced viability of fresh aortic homografts stored in nutrient medium. Cardiovasc Res 1973;7:814–817.

41. McGregor CGA, Bradley JF, McGee GO'D, Wheatley DJ: Tissue culture, collagen and protein synthesis in antibiotic sterilised heart valves. Cardiovasc Res 1976;10:389–395.

42. Stinson EB, Angell WW, Iben AB, Shumway NE: Aortic valve replacement with the fresh valve homograft. Am J Surg 1968;116:204–211.

43. Barrat-Boyes BG, Roche AHG, Subramanyan R, Pemberton JR, Whitlock RML: Long term follow up of patients with the antibiotic sterilised aortic homograft valve inserted freehand in the aortic position. Circulation 1987;75:768–775.

44. Wheatley DJ, McGregor GA: Influence of viability of canine allograft heart valve structure and function. J Cardiovasc Res 1977;11:2738.

45. Yacoub MH, Suitters A, Khagani A, Rose M: Localization of major histocompatibility complex (HLA, ABC and DR) antigens in aortic homografts. In Bodnar E, Yacoub M (eds): Biologic and Bioprosthetic Valves. New York, Yorke Medical Books, 1986, pp 65–72.

46. Campbell DN, Clarke DR, Bishop DA, Shaffer E: Extended aortic root replacement. In Bodnar E (ed): Surgery for Heart Valve Disease. London, ICR Publishers, 1990, pp 463–71.

47. Ziemer G: Discussion. In Bodnar E (ed): Surgery for Heart Valve Disease. London, ICR Publishers, 1990, p 472.

48. Kloevekorn WP, Meisner H, Paek SU, Sebening F: The use of porcine and allograft conduits for right ventricular outflow tract reconstruction. In Bodnar E (ed): Surgery for heart valve disease. London, ICR Publishers, 1990, pp 482–486.

49. Almeida RS, Wyse RKH, de Leval MR, Elliott MJ, Stark J: Long-term results of homograft valves in extracardiac conduits. Europ J Cardithorac Surg 1989;3:488–493.

50. Lau JKH, Robles A, Cherian A, Ross DN: Surgical treatment of prosthetic endocarditis. Aortic root replacement using a homograft. J Thorac Cardiovasc Surg 1984;87:712–717.

51. Sommerville J, Ross DN: Homograft replacement of aortic root with reimplantation of coronary arteries. Br Heart Jr 1988;47:473–477.

Bodnar, E. and Frater, R. W. M., editors
(1991) *Replacement Cardiac Valves,*
Pergamon Press, Inc. (New York), pp. 307–332
Printed in the United States of America

CHAPTER 13

"EXTINCT" CARDIAC VALVE PROSTHESES

BENSON B. ROE

The cardiac surgical literature of the late 1950s contains glowing descriptions—artistically illustrated—of surgical maneuvers to restore diseased malfunctioning valves. During this period surgical mortality was high for all open-heart procedures, patient selection tended to be limited to those with advanced functional disease, and long-term follow-up evaluation was minimal. It soon became evident, however, that the clinical results of reparative surgery were disappointing, and visual experience with the pathologic anatomy led to recognizing that diseased valves were usually unsalvageable. Replacement thus appeared to be the only realistic solution. Consequently, at the end of that decade numerous cardiac surgeons almost simultaneously directed their attention to developing valve devices suitable for intracardiac implantation.

The formidable obstacles associated with inserting and maintaining a safe and reliable mechanical foreign body in the bloodstream were approached in a sea of ignorance. The need was urgent, the science was nonexistent, and the only familiar tool was technical resourcefulness. True to the surgical personality, this vast and complex project was not initiated on the drawing boards of hydraulic engineers or developed by tedious testing in commercial laboratories. Instead, a variety of mechanical devices emerged from the "basement engineering" of surgeons and their technicians, who learned by trial and error about the magnitude of the problem and the multitude of unforseen obstacles. Those of us who sought assistance from supposed experts in hydrodynamics and biocompatible materials were usually disappointed to find very little authoritative information that was applicable to this particular objective. More often we progressed from guesswork, ingenuity, luck, failure, or serendipity.

The scenario of that pioneering era would be impossible to duplicate in the modern climate imposed by the Food and Drug Administration's control of all prosthetic devices. Very few of the early devices underwent prolonged rigorous fatigue testing or performance analysis in a pulse-duplicating apparatus. When such testing did become available there was considerable question about its clinical relevance. For some time it was extremely difficult to get animals to survive mere extracorporial perfusion, so large-scale long-term valve implantations in animals were virtually out of the question. With few exceptions the devices described hereinafter were simply implanted in human subjects with little reliable knowledge of their functional efficiency, durability, thrombogenicity, or biocompatibility.

The moral justification for a seemingly cavalier decision to undertake what amounted to human experimentation was based on the lack of any reasonable alternative for patients with advanced valvular dysfunction who were dying of their disease. The circumstances surrounding this decision were sometimes contradictory because in many institutions the only patients referred for such unproven and hazardous surgery were those in the terminal stages of heart failure. This understandable selection was counter-productive for the kind of results that would help to promote acceptance of a new modal-ity. High surgical mortalities often were attributed to the performance of the prosthetic valve, which may not itself have contributed to the outcome. On the other hand, some centers were more supportive of surgical objectives and helped to promote the reputation of open heart procedures by recommending them to more favorable candidates. Valve replacement results in these institutions were good, but to what extent those results reflected exceptional surgical skill and management will never be known. Another factor that influenced the popularity and acceptability of a given device was the reputed skill and reputation of the surgeon who used and recommended it on the basis of a large successful series. Intrinsic qualities or physiologic characteristics of the device may have been a relatively minor factor in its apparent performance.

Not until long-term follow-up results were obtainable was it possible to assess pros-thetic performance objectively. Even then those results had reason to be influenced by unmeasured variables other than the intrinsic characteristics of the valve itself. Inappro-priate intraoperative handling of the device could initiate structural damage, poppet wear, or thrombogenesis. Faulty methods of applying fixation sutures could promote thrombosis, impede poppet motion, or induce disruption (1). Improper size selection could lead to impeded flow, suboptimal fixation, or impaired ventricular contractility. Techniques for excising or retaining the diseased valve can precipitate cardiac dysfunc-tion or prosthetic failure. Perfusion methods and other aspects of operative management (i.e., anesthesia) can influence the clinical outcome. And the thromboembolic compli-cation rate is intimately related to the success of postoperative anticoagulation manage-ment. Each of these important factors can have a negative influence on the apparent clinical performance of any prosthetic valve, even if it were theoretically ideal.

Since the beginning of this endeavor in the late 1950s, a plethora of devices have been developed, implanted, and marketed. Each was presumed to be an improvement over the deficiencies of its predecessors, but most have succumbed to the attrition of time. Innovative features of each new valve covered a wide range. While some introduced fun-damental improvements in flow characteristics, antithrombogenicity, fixation, or mechanical performance, others offered only alternative materials or minor change in configuration. The objective of this chapter is to present a selected series of those devices no longer in clinical use and to determine, if possible, why they did not survive. Of some 300 devices collected by Barbara Tyrell of Baxter Laboratories, only a notable few can be included herein. Excluded are (1) experimental models that never reached human implantation, (2) current models still in clinical use and thus not "extinct," and (3) mod-els about which insufficient information was available (Burakovsky, Duplessis).

The reader will note a general commonality in design principle, materials, and prob-lems throughout this series. Explanations for why each device was discontinued are often unclear. As suggested above, the true merits—or deficiencies—of the valve itself fre-quently were not the principal explanation for the clinical success and consequent pop-ularity ultimately associated with it. The unmeasurable role of careful patient selection, skillful implantation techniques, and follow-up (anticoagulation) management undoubt-edly influenced the outcome as much or more than the performance of the device itself. These factors are rarely mentioned in the reports of clinical experience, which usually convey a strong implication that the results reflect only the comparative merits of the prosthesis. It is this author's impression that the popularity and survival of a prosthesis has been heavily influenced by market forces.

The first valve successfully implanted in the bloodstream was Charles Hufnagel's acrylic ball and housing device, which he inserted between a divided segment of the descending aorta. This large and noisy mechanism served only to reduce the volume of regurgitant flow in aortic valve insufficiency. While its physiologic benefit was limited, its successful presence in the bloodstream was a landmark event that led the way for subsequent intracardiac devices.

The year 1960 was a landmark in the history of intracardiac prosthetic valve implantation in humans. Among those initial "inventors" and "human experimenters" were Henry Bahnson of Baltimore, Dwight Harken of Boston, Earle B. Kay of Cleveland, C. Walton Lillehei of Minneapolis, Dwight McGoon of Rochester, Andrew Morrow of Bethesda, William H. Muller of Los Angeles, Albert Starr of Portland, and this author in San Francisco. With the exception of Starr's caged-ball valve, none of these early experimental devices became commercially available and widely used. Indeed, it was the commercial quality control and wide marketing of the Starr valve that was the principal impetus for others to cease using their relatively crude homemade devices.

These prosthetic valves can be grouped into three broad mechanism classifications of (1) flexible leaflet, (2) simple poppet, and (3) tilting disk (see Table 13–1). Subdivisions reflect the efforts to overcome both theoretical and demonstrated deficiencies of early models.

FLEXIBLE LEAFLET VALVES

Among the earliest efforts to replace diseased cardiac valves were implantations of cloth or plastic materials to mimic or substitute for the destroyed or removed native tissue.

C. Walton Lillehei of Minneapolis developed a flap valve of flexible Silastic that he first implanted in October 1958 to treat aortic valve regurgitation.

Henry Bahnson, then in Baltimore, developed individual molded cusps of Dacron mesh impregnated with Silastic monomer that were individually sutured in place in the aortic position beginning in 1959.

Earle B. Kay, in Cleveland, similarly fashioned a variety of polyester cloth cusps for the aortic valve and also experimented with mitral cloth leaflets.

David Moore, working with this author, developed a series of compression molds from which monomer castings were made of a three-cusp aortic valve replica, the first of which was implanted clinically in 1960. It is interesting that this flexible leaflet valve functioned very efficiently and reliably with suggestive evidence of potential durability and low thrombogenicity. No interest has yet been shown in marketing a device of this nature.

Charles Hufnagel, of Washington, D.C., in 1965 developed individual cusp valves that were similar to those of Bahnson, and later a composite three-cusp model similar to the Roe-Moore valve.

POPPET VALVES

The ancient mechanism of a caged ball to arrest retrograde flow was and remains a popular concept because of its simplicity and reliability. Variations on its theme have been to (1) reduce the thrombogenic surface of the cage by narrowing the strut diameter and by reducing from four struts (Harken) to three (Starr) (the latter incidentally permitted (1) removing and replacing the ball between struts); (2) leave the apex of the cage open (Harken) (Smeloff); and (3) reduce ball size to fit inside the orifice and obliterate

TABLE 13–1. *Classification of Mechanical Cardiac Prostheses*

A. FLEXIBLE LEAFLET
    1. *Cloth Leaflets:* Silicone-impregnated—surface-molded

Lillehei—flap valve (aortic)	1958*
Bahnson cusp (aortic)	1959
Kay (Earle) leaflet (mitral and aortic)	1959
Muller (aortic)	1960
[compressed Ivalon sponge, 1958]	
Braunwald-Morrow leaflet (mitral)	1960
McGoon (knitted Teflon "windsock")	1960
Hufnagel cusp (aortic)	1965

    2. *Compression Casting:*

Roe-Moore (3 cusp unitized) (GE elastomer)	1960

B. POPPET
    1. *Ball and Cage:*
      a) Ball Seats *on* Orifice:

Harken	1960
Starr-Edwards	1960
Cross (experimental)	
Magovern	1962
DeBakey	1968
Braunwald	1970

      b) Ball Seats *in* Orifice, *on* Countercage:

Smeloff-Cutter	1963

    2. *Disk and Cage:* (Low-Profile)
      a) Disk Seats *on* Orifice:

Cross-Jones	1965
Kay-Shiley	1965
Beall	1967, 1969
Harken	1968

      b) Disk Seats *in* Orifice, *on* Countercage:

Cooley-Cutter (biconical)	1971

    3. *Disk Without Cage:*

Capetown mitral	1962
Hammersmith-Alvarez	1963
Davila	1966

    4. *Spindle Poppet:*

Capetown aortic	1962

C. TILTING DISK (Central Flow)
    1. *Hinged Flaps:*

Gott-Daggett	1963
Wada-Cutter	1970
St. Jude†	1977

    2. *Floating Disk:*

Lillehei-Kaster	1967
Björk-Shiley†	1969
Medtronic-Hall†	1974

*Dates indicate initial clinical use.

†Valves remaining in use and marketed as of 1988.

the impact of the poppet on rim surface (this required the addition of an upstream countercage to prevent ball escape) (Smeloff).

The ball valve functioned very satisfactorily as long as the anatomic compartment it occupied did not impede the flow around the ball (in the aortic root) or did not become impaired by the cage (in the ventricle).

Initial mortalities for replacement of the mitral valve were significantly higher than those for the aortic valve—largely because a low-output syndrome frequently followed mitral replacement. An explanation for this life-threatening complication was postulated to be the trauma and contractual impairment caused by the presence of a large cage in the ventricle. Although later experimentally refuted by John Kirklin, this theory was widely prevalent and provoked the development of various *low-profile* poppet devices. Frederick Cross and his colleagues in Cleveland pioneered the development of a caged disk that was first implanted in September 1959. This same theme was later used by Jerome Kay (1965) and Arthur Beall and Charles Hufnagel (1965). The turbulent flow pattern around a flat poppet, the larger critical diameter of a disk to prevent its jamming in the orifice, and its propensity for being tilted (unseated) by an adjacent structure were all unfavorable characteristics of this generic group.

Other endeavors to achieve the low-profile objective while attempting to eliminate these disadvantages include the cageless skirted disk developed by Julio Davila (1966) and the collar button disk promoted by Christian Barnard at the University of Capetown in 1965. Somewhat later (1971) Denton Cooley developed a discoid valve with a flat biconical occluder that fitted inside a double-caged orifice. This design considerably improved the flow characteristics, obviated jamming, and reduced the tilting hazard.

THE TILTING DISK

The disadvantage of both ball and disk occluders was their path of motion in the axis of the orifice which diverted flow to traverse the periphery of the poppet. The contour and capacity of surrounding anatomic compartments frequently caused this flow to be impaired. This disadvantage promoted the objective of a central flow pattern which was achieved by having the occluder tilt away from the orifice.

The first prosthesis of this nature was the double "butterfly" leaflet developed by Vincent Gott and R. Daggett in 1966. While that initial device had limited success for structural reasons, the concept was sound, and one of the most popular prostheses in current use, the St. Jude valve, uses the hinged double-flap design.

There have been various approaches to a single tilting disk contained by ingenious mechanisms to avoid the problems of hinge action. This motif dominates most of the mechanical prostheses currently in use, including the Björk-Shiley, but included among the early models no longer available are the Lillehei-Kaster valve initiated in 1966 and the Wada valve introduced in 1967.

The following discontinued prosthetic valves represent only a small fraction of the prodigious development in that arena during the past three decades. Private communications added to the surgical literature indicated a multitude of devices that were built, tested, and discarded for a variety of reasons. A few may have had unreported human implantation, and many were merely variations of previous models. These have been selected because of their importance in the history of valve development. No attempt has been made to document the series of biological valves that have been discarded, the most notable of which was autogenous fascia. Also excluded are valves that remain on the current market.

HUFNAGEL

Charles Hufnagel provided a historical landmark in valve prostheses with his methyl methacrylate ball-and-chamber valve before the advent of open-heart surgery (2). This device—introduced into the descending thoracic aorta—provided partial arrest of systemic backflow in the presence of aortic insufficiency (Fig. 13–1).

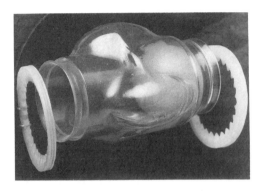

Fig. 13–1. Hufnagel acrylic ball-and-chamber valve for descending aorta.

Although its physiologic and clinical impact were not dramatic, it represented an important initial endeavor with sufficient success to demonstrate the feasibility of mechanical prostheses.

This early experience was a stepping-stone for a series of prosthetic devices that Hufnagel developed and used clinically. In 1965, he developed and used Silastic-impregnated cusps, which were very similar in appearance to those developed by Bahnson (Fig. 13–2).

The device that he developed in the same year and later implanted in several hundred patients was the caged plastic disk similar to that developed by Cross and Jones. Disk wear, cuff problems, and thromboembolic complications eventually led to abandoning its use (Fig. 13–3).

To do justice to Hufnagel's prolific productivity in prosthetic valve development would overload this chapter. Among his numerous models were (1) a Teflon cage and ball, (2) a double Silastic cusp in a polypropylene frame, (3) a polypropylene helical spring valve (Fig. 13–4), (4) a tilting disk of polypropylene, (5) a bicuspid Silicone-impregnated polypropylene cloth (Fig. 13–5), (6) a trileaflet valve of similar construction, and (7) multiple variations of the above. No information is available about the clinical experience with these valves.

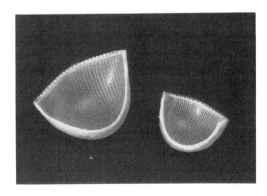

Fig. 13–2. Hufnagel single polypropylene cloth cusp.

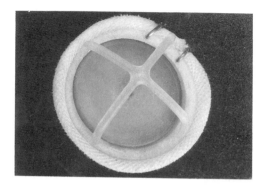

FIG. 13–3. Hufnagel experimental polypropylene disk valve.

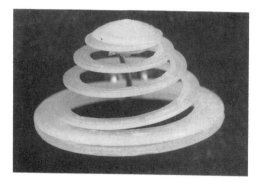

FIG. 13–4. Hufnagel experimental polypropylene helical spring valve.

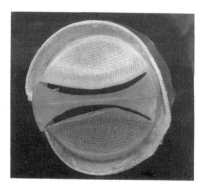

FIG. 13–5. Hufnagel experimental bicuspid polypropylene cloth valve.

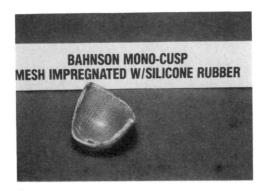

Fɪɢ. 13–6. Bahnson impregnated Dacron cloth single cusp. Provided through the courtesy of Baxter Museum of Heart Valve Design, Irvine, CA.

BAHNSON CUSP

Individual cusps were fashioned from Teflon cloth of 100-denier jersey knit and were heated on a cusp-shaped mold. The result was a reasonable facsimile of an aortic cusp, which held its shape but was moderately flexible to permit retraction (Fig. 13–6).

The first clinical application, on September 15, 1959, was a single-cusp replacement with good clinical result. A series of 47 patients had aortic cusps replaced between 1959 and October 1962. When a single cusp was replaced, results were generally successful, but when two or three cusps were replaced, the results were poor. Cusp retraction was probably minimal. Thickening and cusp fracture were commonly encountered (3).

The mechanism was eventually abandoned when better prostheses were available.

Collaborators in this project were Frank Spencer, Norman Jeckel, and Edward Busse.

EARLE B. KAY

Kay was one of the very earliest pioneers in prosthetic correctional surgery of diseased aortic valves. Beginning in 1958, he implanted in eight patients Teflon cloth leaflets coated with polyurethane foam. Variations of his original design included the incorporation of strings to be passed through the ventricular wall as artificial chordae tendineae (4).

Similar leaflet material was used to augment aortic cusps for treatment of aortic insufficiency. Unfortunately, illustrations of these valves are not available.

Leaflet material mounted in a rigid fixation ring provided a basis for relatively large scale clinical application (350 valves) between 1959 and 1963. Remarkably, these patients were not anticoagulated, and thrombus formation was not evident.

Long-term results were disappointing, but initial clinical success marked an important milestone in prosthetic history.

BRAUNWALD-MORROW

Nina Braunwald, in collaboration with Theodore Cooper and Andrew G. Morrow, developed a flexible (cloth) prosthesis to simulate the mitral valve structure. It was manufactured from polyurethane foam in steel molds developed from normal valve models

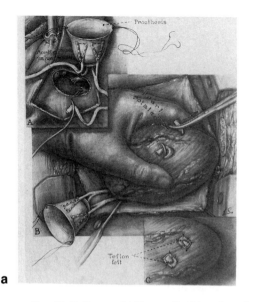
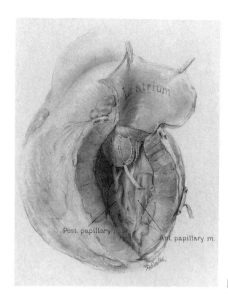

a

b

FIG. 13–7. Braunwald-Morrow flexible polyurethane leaflet valve. (a) Implantation technique. (b) In situ. Provided courtesy of Nina Braunwald, MD.

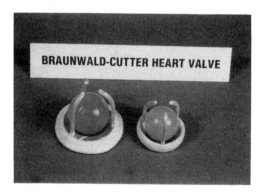

FIG. 13–8. Braunwald-Cutter cloth-covered ball valve. Provided through the courtesy of Baxter Museum of Heart Valve Design, Irvine, CA.

(Fig. 13–7). Thin knit Dacron fabric was stretched over one side of the mold and liquid polyurethane was poured over the other side as they were clamped together (5).

This device, which required precise tension on artificial chordae, had its first human implantation on March 11, 1960 (6).

Although a small clinical experience was successful, the device was abandoned because of the complex aspects of its implantation technique (7).

Braunwald also worked extensively with measures to prevent thrombogenesis by tissue ingrowth into cloth coverings on caged poppet valves. The commercial open-strutted ball valve that bears her name (Braunwald-Cutter) (Fig. 13–8) showed initial evidence of thromboembolic reduction (8). However, the product was later withdrawn from the market when abrasive action of the cloth covering resulted in erosion of the Silastic ball with size reduction that permitted it to escape from the cage. In addition there were instances

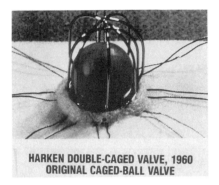

FIG. 13–9. Harken original ball valve. Provided through the courtesy of International Center for Artificial Organs, Cleveland, Ohio.

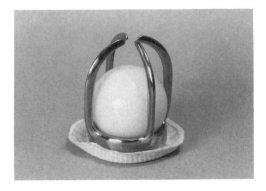

FIG. 13–10. Harken-Davila ball valve.

of erosion through the cloth with embolization of cloth fragments. This development resulted in its being withdrawn from the market and abandoning the temporarily popular concept of promoting tissue covering.

HARKEN

Dwight Harken was a prolific pioneer in prosthetic valves (9). His first clinical effort was after experimentation with the original multistrut double stainless steel cage and Silastic ball (Fig. 13–9). This device was implanted in a small series of patients beginning in March 1960 with disappointing results (10). His next model, manufactured by Davol Company, consisted of a Silastic ball with a four-strut open top titanium cage and a trimable Dacron cloth skirt (Fig. 13–10). This was later abandoned because of thromboembolic complications and structural defects. Later development, the Harken-Surgitool low profile valve reported in 1968, was a Silastic disk within a four-strut titanium cage attached to a Dacron-velour fixation skirt (11). Again, thromboembolic complications led to disappointing results (12).

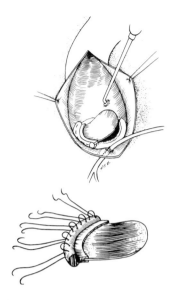

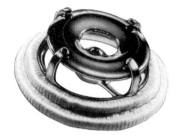

FIG. 13–11. Lillehei Silastic flap valve. Provided courtesy of C. Walton Lillehei, MD, PhD.

FIG. 13–12. Lillehei toroidal disk valve. Provided courtesy of C. Walton Lillehei, MD, PhD.

LILLEHEI

C. Walton Lillehei was one of the earliest pioneers in prosthetic valve development. His initial contribution was a Silastic flap valve, which he implanted in approximately 50 patients beginning October 31, 1958, and concluding in mid-1960 (13, 14). Initial results were very satisfactory, but material fatigue and disruption led to abandoning this model (Fig. 13–11).

He then developed a toroidal disk valve made of all titanium with a central hole and a controlling obturator (Fig. 13–12), manufactured by Washington Scientific Company.

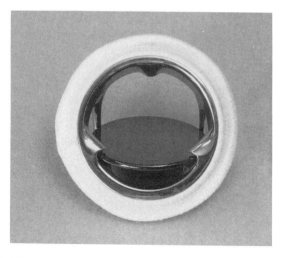

FIG. 13–13. Lillehei-Kaster tilting disk valve. Provided through the courtesy of International Center for Artificial Organs and Transplantation, Cleveland, Ohio.

Some 12,000 of these valves were manufactured and implanted in various centers. Lillehei's experience consisted of approximately 300 patients with this valve implanted in both mitral and aortic positions. The design and manufacture were durable, and no structural failures were reported. However, troublesome thromboembolism eventually led to its being withdrawn.

The best-known valve that carried Lillehei's name was the Lillehei-Kaster pivoting disk valve with a central opening and 85° excursion of the disk (Fig. 13–13). This valve was introduced in 1967, had good clinical results, and was implanted in some 65,000 patients.

An improvement and extension on this principal, for which Lillehei may receive insufficient credit, is the currently popular double-hinged disk St. Jude valve—introduced in 1978—which recently marked its 270,000th implant.

MULLER

William H. Muller, in collaboration with James Littlefield and Frank Damman, performed perhaps the first total replacement of an aortic valve with two compressed Ivalon leaflets. This was achieved in two stages, 2 years apart (1958 and 1960). He later performed a series of 76 valve replacements using knitted Dacron leaflets as illustrated (Fig. 13–14).

*Editor note: The predecessor—one may say the prototype model—of the St. Jude valve was the Kalke-Lillehei hinged bileaflet valve. It never reached clinical application and therefore is outside the scope of this chapter.

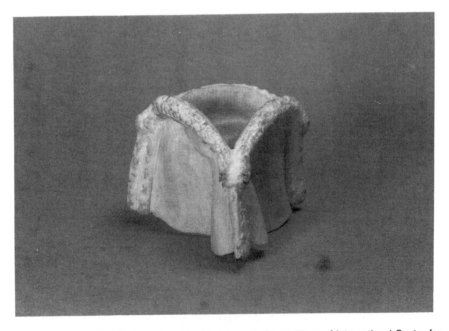

FIG. 13–14. Muller cloth leaflet valve. Provided through the courtesy of International Center for Artificial Organs and Transplantation, Cleveland, Ohio.

These devices survived as long as 9 years, but some were noted to develop holes in the leaflets after 1 year (William H. Muller, personal communication).

This series was abandoned because of variable results and the availability of a manufactured Starr-Edwards prosthesis.

McGOON

Dwight McGoon at the Mayo Clinic was one of the first to develop and implant a flexible leaflet prosthesis in a large series of patients. Beginning in August 1960, a series of 98 total replacements of the aortic valve took place over a 2-year period (15).

The prosthesis consisted of 200-denier Teflon cloth knitted into a round tube and fashioned into prosthetic cusps. Depending on the configuration of the diseased aortic root, the tube was fashioned into two or three cusps (Figs. 13–15 and 13–16). The cloth was

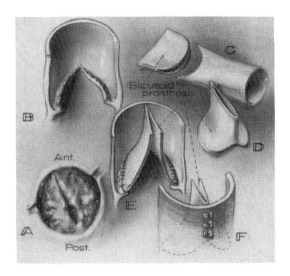

Fɪɢ. 13–15. McGoon tubular cloth aortic valve prosthesis—bicuspid model.

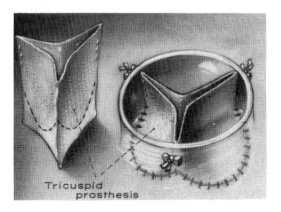

Fɪɢ. 13–16. McGoon tubular cloth aortic valve tricuspid model.

impregnated with polyurethane. The base of each cloth cusp was sutured along the attachment line of the resected anatomic valve. The dramatic consequences of a learning experience in this developmental period is demonstrated by an improvement in good results from 11% at the outset to 77% in the final period and a decline in hospital mortality from 55% at the outset and 15% in the final period (16).

Performance of the prosthesis was variable. Functional failure and disruption were common, but thromboembolism was notably minimal.

The ultimate course of events in this valve was usually deterioration of the Teflon cloth with stiffening and fracturing.

This method was abandoned in 1962 when the Starr-Edwards prosthesis became commercially available.

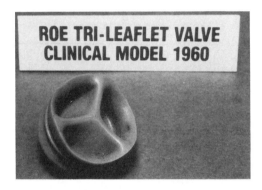

FIG. 13–17. Roe-Moore elastomer cast valve. Provided through the courtesy of Baxter Museum of Heart Valve Design, Irvine, CA.

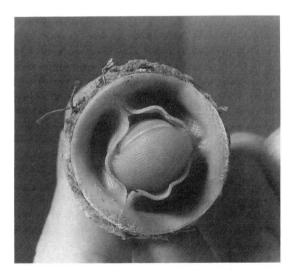

FIG. 13–18. Roe-Moore valve 6 years, 10 months postimplantation. Provided through the courtesy of Baxter Museum of Heart Valve Design, Irvine, CA.

ROE-MOORE

This author—along with an engineer, David Moore—developed a series of pressure-molded three-cusp aortic valve facsimiles (17). Progressive improvements in mold design were derived from pulse duplicator observations. Various materials were tested, including compressed Ivalon, polyvinyl chloride, and numerous elastomers (18). When optimal elastic and tensile characteristics were obtained in a GE elastomer, total competence was demonstrated at 600 mmHg pressure and all three cusps retracted equally and fully in forward flow (Figs., 13–17 and 13–18). Human models were molded with a Teflon mesh in the leaflets.

Only eight human implantations were performed (19). The longest survivor was 13 years without recovery of the prosthesis. But another patient who died at 6 years and 10 months proved to have a prosthesis with no evidence of thrombosis, unaltered leaflet excursion and flexibility, and only a 1-mm disruption of one cusp attachment (20).

The valve was never manufactured commercially.

MAGOVERN-CHROMIE

George Magovern developed a unique modification of the caged-ball valve with a mechanism for retracting and extending a double-circumferential row of clawlike fixation pins as part of the implantation process (Figs. 13–19 and 13–20) (21, 22). At the

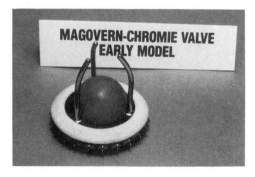

FIG. 13–19. Magovern-Chromie sutureless aortic valve (showing retractable "claws" extended for fixation). Provided through the courtesy of Baxter Museum of Heart Valve Design, Irvine, CA.

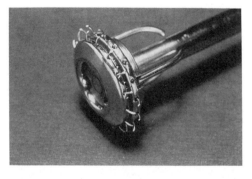

FIG. 13–20. Magovern-Chromie valve mounted on insertion tool, which controls retraction and extension of claws. Provided through the courtesy of Baxter Museum of Heart Valve Design, Irvine, CA.

time this device was introduced in March 1962, the speed factor of his implantation technique was an important consideration. The valve achieved considerable popularity, with perhaps 7000 having been implanted in the United States (23). Magovern's series of 700-odd patients had survival and complication rates that were comparable to those of other similar prostheses, and his longest human survivor is still alive at 25 years. Early models developed ball variance from hygroscopic swelling and splitting, but improved formulation of the elastomer eliminated this complication.

Early models of this valve had horizontal pins protruding and a closed-cage top, and a later model had a Silastic flange to cover the ring. A low-profile (disk) model was tried and abandoned. Magovern also tried various flexible cusp valves experimentally.

Although most of the surgeons have abandoned this clever device, Magovern continues to use it in the aortic position (24).

CAPETOWN (BARNARD-GOOSEN)

Christian Barnard and his group at the University of Capetown developed a series of poppet valves of unusual configuration. The principle was another variation on the attempt to control poppet escape without the use of a cage.

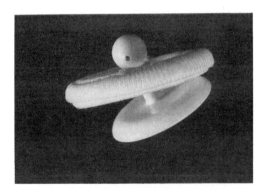

FIG. 13–21. Barnard-Capetown mitral valve.

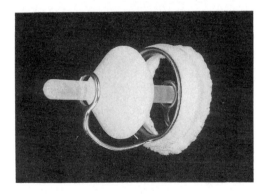

FIG. 13–22. Barnard-Capetown aortic valve.

The mitral version consisted of a Silastic poppet incorporating a shaft that passed through a ring on a single strut from the Ivalon-covered steel ring (Fig. 13–21) (25). The aortic version used a double-shafted spindle guided in both directions by a strut-supported ring extending in an arch from the suture ring (Fig. 13–22) (26).

This prosthesis was first implanted in September 1962 and discontinued in October 1968. During this period, 149 valves were implanted in the aortic area with a 21% 2-year mortality and 122 valves in the mitral area with a 46% 2-year mortality (27). The longest reported survival is 26 years (28).

The valve was discontinued because of a high incidence of embolism, troublesome hemolysis, and occasional poppet variance.

GOTT-DAGGETT

Vincent Gott, then at the University of Wisconsin, in collaboration with Ronald Daggett, professor of plastic engineering, and William P. Young, professor of cardiac surgery, developed the first hinged bileaflet ("butterfly wing") prosthetic valve, which had excellent flow characteristics. The carbon-coated valve housing was constructed of polycarbonate (Lexan) with two hinging leaflets constructed as a single wafer of silicone-impregnated Dacron fabric held in a cross-strut and supported on the upflow side with short

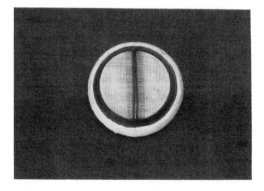

FIG. 13–23. Gott-Daggett butterfly leaflet valve (downstream view). Provided through the courtesy of International Center for Artificial Organs and Transplantation, Cleveland, Ohio.

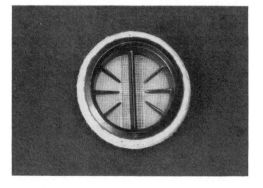

FIG. 13–24. Gott-Daggett butterfly leaflet valve (proximal view). Provided through the courtesy of International Center for Artificial Organs and Transplantation, Cleveland, Ohio.

prongs extending from the rim. The valve was coated with graphite-benzalkonium and heparin for thromboresistance. The suture ring was Telfon felt (Figs. 13–23 and 13–24).

The first clinical implant was in the aortic position in April 1963. Over a 3-year period from 1963 to 1966, Gott's series consisted of 48 aortic implants, 21 mitral implants, and three double implants (Vincent Gott, personal communication).

Early results were generally satisfactory, with 58 of the original 72 patients surviving 6 months or longer and at least 18 patients surviving for more than 10 years. The longest known survival was 22 years in 1986. Apparently approximately 600 of these valves were implanted around the world during a similar 3-year period (Vincent Gott, personal communication).

The valve was withdrawn from clinical use because of frequent thrombosis on the downstream side of the hinging leaflet, probably resulting from stasis between the leaflets and turbulence around the free edges. There was only one mechanical breakdown in Gott's series, but structural problems were not uncommon.

HAMMERSMITH-ALVAREZ

Dennis Melrose, Mark Bentall, and others, including M. Alvarez-Diaz, at Hammersmith Hospital in London developed a molded polypropylene valve with a hingeless tilting disk that was contained from escape by hooked legs extending to the opposite side of the orifice (Fig. 13–25). There was a series of designs with variations in the leg configuration intended to improve hydraulic characteristics and to reduce clot formation (29). The original Melrose version was implanted in the mitral position in a series of 15 patients in 1963 (30). In a similar time frame, nine patients had the Alvarez valve implanted at Leeds with good short-term results despite a high incidence of endocarditis (31).

The version of this valve that carries the Alvarez name was merely a modification developed by him after leaving Hammersmith and returning to Spain (Fig. 13–26). Clinical data and long-term follow-up information is minimal, but Gibbs reported that only 3 of the original 15 patients were alive at 10 years. He noted that erosive wear of the plastic legs caused late detachment of the disk from the valve ring (32).

Although ultimately unsuccessful, this prosthesis represented an important prototype of the central flow tilting disk which has become the standard of modern valves.

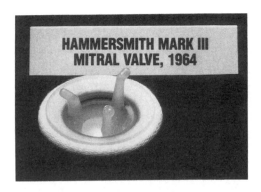

Fig. 13–25. Hammersmith Mark III mitral valve. Provided through the courtesy of Baxter Museum of Heart Valve Design, Irvine, CA.

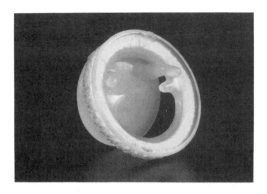

Fig. 13–26. Alvarez modification of Hammersmith valve. Provided through the courtesy of International Center for Artificial Organs and Transplantation, Cleveland, Ohio.

CROSS-JONES

Frederick Cross, working in collaboration with Richard Jones, was an early pioneer in prosthetic development. His initial clinical experience with the Bahnson flexible cusp was disappointing and led to the development of two experimental mitral valve prostheses, one a six-strutted Silastic caged-ball valve (Fig. 13–27) and the other a Silastic lenticular valve hinged on two arched flexible rods (Fig. 13–28) (33). These models were abandoned without clinical application because of their thrombogenicity. An important by-product of that project was the ability to study ball valve function fluoroscopically as a result of milling barium into the ball. They were, thus, the first to demonstrate impairment of ventricular function caused by the cage.

The clinical device that bears their name was developed specifically to address these problems. It is a three-strutted flat open cage, manufactured by PemCo, containing a lens-shaped poppet of silicone rubber reinforced with a thin titanium ring. A woven Teflon fixation flange was attached to the low-profile cage (Fig. 13–29) (34). Clinical application of this device began January 13, 1965, and a total of 230 valves were implanted (FS Cross, personal communication).

Despite reasonably good survival rates, clinical use was abandoned because better prostheses became available.

KAY-SHILEY

Jerome Harold Kay developed a low-profile disk valve, emulating the principles of the Cross-Jones valve, which were addressed to the concerns about a large (ball) cage in the ventricle. The device consisted of a Stellite (cobalt base alloy) double-strut cage with a fabricated Teflon cloth suture ring. His early models used a molded Silastic disk that was later replaced by a molded Delrin disk (Fig. 13–30) (35). Cloth-covered muscle guards were later added to prevent impairment of disk excursion by impingement on the ventricular wall (36).

This device was used by Kay in all positions, but it was particularly adapted to the atrioventricular valves.

The first human implantation was in February 1965. A total of 640 valves have been implanted, with the longest survivor at 21 years at the time of writing.

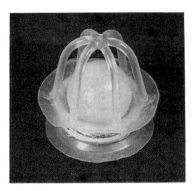

FIG. 13-27. Cross experimental Silastic caged-ball valve. Provided through the courtesy of Baxter Museum of Heart Valve Design, Irvine, CA.

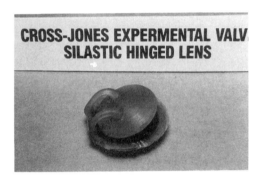

FIG. 13-28. Cross-Jones experimental hinged lenticular valve. Provided through the courtesy of Baxter Museum of Heart Valve Design, Irvine, CA.

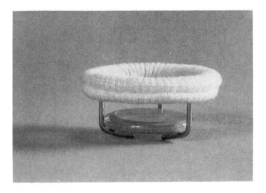

FIG. 13-29. Cross-Jones Pemco low-profile disk valve. Provided through the courtesy of International Center for Artificial Organs and Transplantation, Cleveland, Ohio.

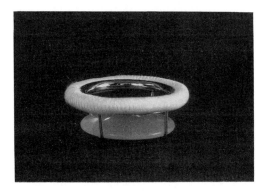

Fig. 13–30. Kay-Shiley disk valve. Provided through the courtesy of International Center for Artificial Organs and Transplantation, Cleveland, Ohio.

Kay reported that improved features of more recently available valves were the principal reason for discontinuing it, although he still uses it in the tricuspid position (personal communication, unpublished report, 1989).

DAVILA

Julio Davila initiated the development and implantation of a discoid prothesis that seated on a cloth-covered fixation ring without an attached cage. Poppet escape was prevented by an open plastic skirt or hoop attached to the disk, which caught on the underside of the cloth ring in the open position (Figs. 13–31 and 13–32) (37).

This prosthesis was first implanted in July 1966 in only 18 patients (38). Satisfactory hemodynamic function was unfortunately associated with either thrombosis or hemolysis, which led to discontinuing it (J. Davila, personal communication).

The principle of this prosthesis was attractive, with its limited excursion and lack of cage, but the results were disappointing for unknown reasons that probably were not related to the design.

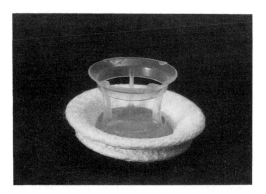

Fig. 13–31. Davila cageless mitral valve (closed position). Provided through the courtesy of International Center for Artificial Organs and Transplantation, Cleveland, Ohio.

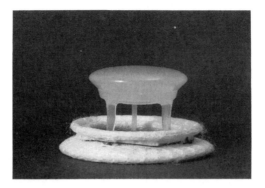

Fɪɢ. 13–32. Davila cageless mitral valve (open position). Provided through the courtesy of International Center for Artificial Organs and Transplantation, Cleveland, Ohio.

BEALL-SURGITOOL

Arthur Beall, Jr., joined the trend toward low-profile prostheses and developed a disk valve (model 103) that featured a cloth-covered ring to which were attached Teflon-covered "staples" to encage a Delrin disk, which seated on the top of a smaller orifice (Fig. 13–33).

This version was later replaced by a similar design with a Dacron velour–covered base and sewing ring, attached to which were struts covered with Pyrolite carbon and containing a Pyrolite disk (model 106) (Fig. 13–34).

The first Beall valve was implanted in 1966, and the inventor believes that several thousand were implanted. The longest known survivor was over 20 years at the time of writing (A. Beall, personal communication).

Problems associated with the model 103 were disk variance (grooving in the Delrin ring) in the form of *cold flow.* In the Pyrolite model there was a small incidence of cracked struts. The valve was eventually withdrawn from the market for fear of product liability when Surgitool was bought out (A. Beall, personal communication).

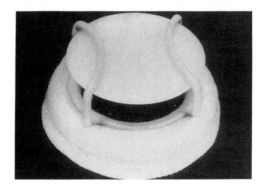

Fɪɢ. 13–33. Beall disk valve model 103. Provided through the courtesy of Arthur C. Beall, Jr., MD.

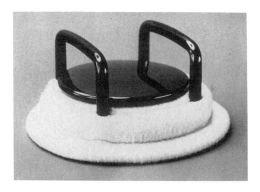

FIG. 13–34. Beall Disk valve model 106. Provided through the courtesy of Arthur C. Beall, Jr., MD.

DeBAKEY-SURGITOOL

Michael DeBakey's contribution to the prosthetic valve competition was largely an attempt to improve on the already established Starr-Edwards valve.

His ball valve—designed for implantation in the aortic position—was distinctive for a hollow-ball occluder coated with Pyrolite carbon. The valve frame and one-piece cage were made of titanium with a Dacron velour sewing ring (Fig. 13–35). Pyrolite was selected for its impermeability, wear resistance, and low thrombogenicity.

The valve was first used clinically in 1968, and the results of 345 consecutive patients were reported by DeBakey in 1978 (39). These patients were part of a larger series of 623 patients, many of whom had multiple procedures.

Overall results were gratifying, with a thromboembolic rate of 1.7% per year in coumadinized patients and a 5-year survival probability of 74%. Three valves developed strut failure at the point of attachment to the titanium ring. No other mechanical problems were encountered.

The valve was discontinued when the manufacturer, Surgitool, was bought out and the new owner decided to withdraw from the valve market.

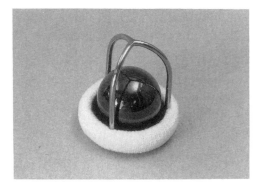

FIG. 13–35. DeBakey-Surgitool Pyrolite aortic ball valve. Provided through the courtesy of International Center for Artificial Organs and Transplantation, Cleveland, Ohio.

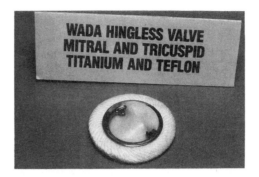

FIG. 13–36. Wada tilting disk valve. Provided through the courtesy of Baxter Museum of Heart Valve Design, Irvine, CA.

WADA-CUTTER

Juro Wada, in Sapporo, Japan, addressed the issue of overcoming the impaired flow around floating poppets. He mounted a hard Teflon disk in a titanium ring with a mechanism that permitted the valve to open by tilting the disk but prevented it from escaping (Fig. 13–36) (40, 41). The mechanism worked well, and he implanted some 200 over a 13-year period with excellent survival rates (J. Wada, personal communication).

The valve was eventually abandoned when it was demonstrated that cold flow of the Teflon disk at its anchor point resulted in its escape and embolization in a few instances (42).

This precursor to modern tilting disks had excellent hemodynamic performance, and the device may well have survived and achieved modern popularity had a Pyrolite carbon disk been available.

COOLEY-CUTTER

Denton Cooley, working with engineers at Cutter Laboratories, designed a valve that incorporated proven virtues from earlier types and theoretical improvements derived from his clinical observations.

Cooley had brief experimental and clinical experience with two precursors that he developed. The first was a Stellite ball in a cloth-covered three-pronged open cage that was reported in 1967, and the second was a four-pronged plastic disk valve seating on a cloth-covered ring. The latter of these was associated with a 38% short-term thromboembolic incidence including six fatal strokes. Also, the relatively soft poppets sustained disk edge wear, and the valve was discontinued in 1968.

The revised Cooley-Cutter valve was introduced in 1971. It used two sets of titanium struts to contain a flat biconical occluder of Pyrolite carbon. In keeping with the principle of the Smeloff-Cutter valve, the poppet seated *inside* the orifice and thus was slightly smaller than the orifice diameter. These two features provided for optimal flow characteristics. The titanium ring had a Teflon cloth sewing ring attached to it (Fig. 13–37).

This valve was first implanted in August 1971 and was successfully used by Cooley in a total of 3275 patients (1786 aortic and 1475 mitral) with excellent clinical results over a 10-year period (43).

The valve was discontinued by the manufacturer because of a desire to avoid product liability exposure in the valve manufacturing business.

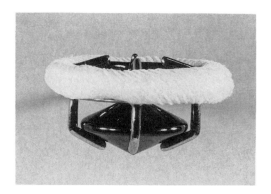

Fig. 13–37. Cooley-Cutter biconical intraorifice disk valve.

CONCLUSION

The objective of this chapter was to document the history of prosthetic valves no longer in use and to ascertain why they had failed. That information remains largely obscure. Clearly, some were withdrawn from use because of performance deficiencies, whereas in others these deficiencies were met with modifications, which are not addressed in this material. It appears that the predominant basis for discontinuing a valve's use was the marketing of an apparently superior alternative along with the feeling that the continued use of an experimental device was no longer justified.

Of particular concern is the fact that several valves have disappeared from the market not because of any performance deficiency but rather because manufacturers have sought to avoid product liability risk. The implications of that attitude are a serious threat to progress in medical technology.

REFERENCES

1. Roe BB: Complications of cardiac valve replacement. In Cardell R, Ellison R (eds): Complications of Intrathoracic Surgery. Boston, Little Brown, 1980, pp 133–145.
2. Hufnagel CA: Aortic plastic valvular prosthesis. Bull Georgetown U Med Cent 1951;4:128.
3. Bahnson HT, Spencer FC, Busse EF, Davis FW Jr: Cusp replacement and coronary artery perfusion in operations on the aortic valve. Ann Surg (Sept) 1960;152:494–505.
4. Kay EB, Suzuki A, Postigo J, Nogulera C: Prosthetic replacement of the mitral valve. In Merendino KA (ed): Prosthetic Valves for Cardiac Surgery. Springfield, IL, Charles C Thomas, 1961, pp 402–425.
5. Braunwald NS, Cooper TL, Morrow AG: Experimental replacement of the mitral valve with a flexible polyurethane foam prosthesis. Trans Am Soc Artif Intern Org 1960;6:312–322.
6. Braunwald NS, Cooper TL, Morrow AG: Complete replacement of the mitral valve. Successful clinical application of a flexible polyurethane prosthesis. J Thorac Cardiovasc Surg July 1960;40:1–11.
7. Braunwald NS, Morrow AG: A late evaluation of flexible Teflon prostheses utilized for total aortic valve replacement. J Thorac Cardiovasc Surg 1965;49:485.
8. Braunwald NS: Totally cloth covered valvular prostheses. Advances in Cardiovasc Surgery. Orlando, FL, Grune & Stratton, 1973, pp 147–158.
9. Harken DE, Lefemine AA: Surgery of Acquired Lesions of the Heart and Pericardium, vol 11, chap 12.
10. Harken DE, Soroff HS, Taylor WJ, Lefemine AA, Gupta SK, Lunzer S: Partial and complete prostheses in aortic insufficiency. J Thorac Cardiovasc Surg 1960;40:744–762.
11. Harken DE, Matloff JM, Zuckerman W, Chaux A: A new mitral valve. J Thorac Cardiovasc Surg 1968;55:369–382.
12. Gray RJ, Czer LSC, Chaux A, Sethna D, DeRobertis M, Raymond M, Matloff JM: Harken caged-disc mitral valve replacement, 1969–1975: Analysis of late mortality, thromboembolism, and valve failure. Texas Ht Inst J 1987;14:411–417.

13. Long DM Jr, Sterns LP, DeRiemer RH, Warden HE, Lillehei CW: Subtotal and total replacement of the aortic valve with plastic valve prostheses: Experimental investigation and successful clinical application utilizing selective cardiac hypothermia. Surg Forum 1960;10:660–665.
14. Lillehei CW et al: Aortic valve reconstruction and replacement by total valve prostheses. In Thomas CC (ed): Prosthetic Valves for Cardiac Surgery. Springfield, IL, Charles C Thomas, 1961, p 527.
15. McGoon DC: Prosthetic reconstruction of the aortic valve. Staff Proceedings Mayo Clinic. Feb 1961;36:88–96.
16. McGoon DC, Moffitt E: Total prosthetic reconstruction of the aortic valve. J Thorac Cardiovasc Surg Aug 1963;46:162–173.
17. Roe BB, Owsley JW, Boudoures PC: Experimental results with a prosthetic aortic valve. J Thorac Cardiovasc Surg 1958;36:563.
18. Roe BB, Moore D: Design and fabrication of prosthetic valves. Exper Med Surg 1958;16:177.
19. Roe BB, Burke MF, Zehner H Jr: The subcoronary implantation of a flexible tricuspid aortic valve prosthesis. J Thorac Surg 1960;40:561–567.
20. Roe BB: Late follow-up studies on flexible leaflet prosthetic valves. J Thorac Cardiovasc Surg 1964;58:59.
21. Magovern GJ, Kent EM, Cromie HW: Sutureless prosthetic heart valves. Circulation 1963;27:784.
22. Magovern GJ, Cromie HW: Sutureless prosthetic heart valves. J Thorac Cardiovasc Surg 1963;46:726.
23. Magovern GJ, Kent EM, Cushing WJ, Scott S: Sutureless aortic and mitral prosthetic valves: Clinical results and operative technique on sixty patients. J Thorac Cardiovasc Surg 1964;48:346.
24. Magovern GJ, Liebler GA, Cushing WJ, Park SB, Burkholder JA: A thirteen-year review of the Magovern-Cromie aortic valve. J Thorac Cardiovasc Surg Jan 1977;73:64–74.
25. Barnard CN, Goosen CC, Holgren LV, Schrire V: Prosthetic replacement of the mitral valve. Lancet 1962;2:1087.
26. Barnard CN, Schrire V, Goosen CC: Total aortic valve replacement. Lancet 1963;2:856.
27. Barnard MS, Barnard CN: Thrombo-embolic complications following total mitral valve replacement with the UCT lenticular mitral prosthesis. S African Med J 1966;43:263.
28. Schrire V, Beck W, Hewitson RP, Barnard CN: Immediate and long-term results of aortic valve replacement with University of Cape Town aortic valve prosthesis. Br Heart J 1970;32:255.
29. Raftery EB, Dayem MKA, Melrose DG: Mechanical performance of Hammersmith mitral valve prothesis. Brit Heart J 1968;30:666–675.
30. Melrose, Bentall, McMillan, Flege, Alvarez-Diaz, Nahas, Fautley, Carson: The evolution of a mitral valve prosthesis. Lancet 1964;2:623.
31. Edmunds LH Jr, Wooler GH, Watson DA: Clinical experience with the Alvarez and Starr-Edwards prosthetic mitral valves. J Thorac Cardiovasc Surg 1966;51:185–194.
32. Gibbs JL, Davies GA, Schofield A, Wharton GA, Watson DA, Gerlis LM: Mechanism of late failure of the Alvarez disk valve prosthesis. Br Heart J 1985;53:510–514.
33. Cross FS, Gerein AN, Jones RD: Evaluation of two prostheses for total replacement of the mitral valve. J Thorac Cardiovasc Surg Dec 1963;46:719–725.
34. Cross FS, Jones RD: A caged-lens prosthesis for replacement of the aortic and mitral valves. Ann Thorac Surg June 1966;2:499–507.
35. Kay JH, Kawashima Y, Yuzuru T, Kagawa M, Tsuji HJ, Redington JV: Experimental mitral valve replacement with a new disc valve. Ann Thorac Surg July 1966;2(4):485–498.
36. Mori T, Kitamura S, Verruno E, Kenaan G, Kay JH: Tricuspid valve replacement. A comparative experimental study with Starr-Edwards ball valve, Beall disc valve, and Kay-Shiley disc valve with muscle guard. J Thorac Cardiovasc Surg July 1974;68:30–36.
37. Davila JC, Amongero F, Sethi RS, Rincon NL, Palmer TE, Lautsch EV: The prevention of thrombosis in artificial cardiac valves. Ann Thorac Surg Sept 1966;2:714–741.
38. Davila JC: Initial clinical trials of a new, nonthrombogenic mitral-valve prosthesis. Ann Thorac Surg Aug 1968;6:99–118.
39. DeBakey E, Lawrie GM: DeBakey-Surgitool pyrolite aortic valve: Results of isolated replacement in 345 patients followed up to 13 years after operation. In Hilger HH, Hombach V, Rashkind WJ (eds): Invasive Cardiovascular Therapy. Dordrecht, Martinus Nijhoff, 1987, pp 77–92.
40. Wada J: Knotless suture method and Wada hingeless valve. Jpn Thorac Surg 1967;15:88.
41. Wada J: Wada hingeless valve. In Brewer LA (ed): Prosthetic Heart Valves. Springfield, Ill, Charles C Thomas, 1967.
42. Roe BB, Fishman NH, Hutchinson JC, Goodenough SH: Occluder disruption of Wada-Cutter valve prosthesis. Ann Thor Surg 1975;20:256.
43. Cooley DEA, Okies JE, Wukasch DC, Sandiford FM, Hallman GL: Ten year experience with cardiac replacement: Results with a new mitral prosthesis. Ann Surg June 1973;177:818–826.

Bodnar, E. and Frater, R. W. M., editors
(1991) *Replacement Cardiac Valves,*
Pergamon Press, Inc. (New York), pp. 333–355
Printed in the United States of America

CHAPTER 14

TRENDS IN PROSTHETIC HEART VALVE DESIGN

JACK C. BOKROS, AXEL D. HAUBOLD, ROBERT J. AKINS, L. ANDY CAMPBELL, CHARLES D. GRIFFIN, AND ERNEST LANE

CURRENT STATUS OF TISSUE AND MECHANICAL HEART VALVE PROSTHESES

Two important advances in materials technology in the late 1960s (Refs. 12–46 in Chapter 2) made possible a variety of mechanical and bioprosthetic cardiac valves that offer viable clinical alternatives for different patient populations.

Mechanical valve replacements that use carbon in their construction usually offer durability for the normal life span of any patient, but require anticoagulation therapy with the associated risk of hemorrhage (Refs. 49, 77–95 in Chapter 2). Bioprostheses offer thromboresistance suitable for patients that cannot safely be maintained on anticoagulants but lack durability so that, except for the oldest patients, reoperation must be anticipated especially for the young. The attendant risk is significant when failure is sudden and emergency reoperation must be performed (Refs. 53–72 in Chapter 2).

As a result of the continuing improvements in both types of prostheses, the risk to benefit ratio of the two has varied with time. In the mid to late 1970s usage of the two types was about equal; but, starting in the early 1980s, with the introduction of the all-carbon St. Jude prosthesis, the trend has been toward the use of mechanical devices. Currently the usage is about two to one in favor of mechanical prostheses (Ref. 53 in Chapter 2). This is because comparative in vivo results for mechanical valves and bioprostheses accumulated during the mid to late 1970s and 1980s are now being reported. These reports quantitatively identify the shortcomings of contemporary prosthetic cardiac valves and show the directions that future developments must take (Ref. 60 in Chapter 2; and Refs. 1–14).

Comprehensive reviews (15–22) have put the problem of thrombotic and bleeding complications in perspective. Such complications account for about 50% of valve related complications in patients with bioprostheses and about 75% of the complications in patients with mechanical valves. Further, the rate of both thrombotic and bleeding complications in patients with aortic bioprostheses is about half that for aortic mechanical valves (2% versus 4%), but is about equal for both bioprostheses and mechanical valves in the mitral position (approximately 4%). Fatal thrombotic and bleeding events, however, are two to four times higher in patients with mechanical prostheses (15).

Although the patient populations are not the same (excluding the use of bioprostheses in young patients and thus biasing toward older patients) the short-term results (<5 years) favor bioprostheses. In the period beyond five years, and increasingly at 10 years, mechanical devices are favored because of their durability and due to the increasing awareness of the true hazard of reoperation for failing bioprostheses (Refs. 53–72 in Chapter 2).

The direction of future development is obvious. Bioprostheses must be made more durable through improvements in tissue properties and by developing designs that distribute the stresses more favorably. Mechanical prostheses must be made more thromboresistant through the use of more compatible materials and by using designs that improve the quality of flow by reducing turbulence, shear, and stasis, thus avoiding hemolytic and thrombotic complications.

MECHANICAL VALVES

The improvement of mechanical cardiac valve replacements has been by a gradual evolutionary process coupled with a few, revolutionary advances. The development of the Björk-Shiley prosthesis is a good example (Refs. 78–80, 223 and 224 in Chapter 2; and Ref. 23). Because Björk-Shiley valves with Delrin® disks carried a high risk of valve thrombosis and other problems (Refs. 226–232 in Chapter 2), the standard Pyrolite® carbon (PYC) disk was introduced. The valve was further refined to provide better flow and washing through the introduction of the PYC convexoconcave disk occluder. Finally, motivated in part by strut failures, the introduction of the monostrut concept improved the quality of flow by making the orifice less obstructive, thus reducing hemodynamically related complications. As a consequence of the design and material changes, the performance of the Björk-Shiley prosthesis progressively improved. (See Fig. 7 of Ref. 78 in Chapter 2.)

The introduction of the all-carbon bileaflet concept represents a revolutionary step in the development of mechanical prosthetic heart valves. The bileaflet design with fixed pivots in itself was not new. The Wada design (Ref. 39 in Chapter 2) used a fixed pivot in a monoleaflet concept; the Kalke (24) concept used fixed pivots in a bileaflet design. The first was not viable at the time, because no material was sufficiently durable to survive the abrasive abuse of a fixed pivot; the second suffered from the same durability problem, compounded by the fact that no available material was sufficiently thromboresistant to survive clotting in the pivot recess.

The durability of PYC (Chapter 2), together with its remarkable blood compatibility, has made it possible to consider designs that previously were not viable. The biocompatibility of PYC is well documented (Refs. 233–235 in Chapter 2; Ref. 25). One obscure, but noteworthy example is as follows: Hill and Horres (26) perfused rats with powdered charcoal in physiologic solution (the maximum dose actually colored the rats' blood black). They compared the body weights of these rats over a two year period with those of control rats. The results are shown in Fig. 14–1. The rats with the highest level of powdered carbon in their blood did as well as the controls in both weight gain and survival rate.

In the following sections, the current trend of mechanical heart valve developments are listed. These developments focus on all-carbon designs that exploit the durability and compatibility of PYC and strive to improve the quality of flow (primarily through the improved design of hinge mechanisms), thus reducing thrombotic complications. The aim of these designs is to achieve a device that requires, at a minimum, a reduced level of anticoagulant therapy and, ultimately, no anticoagulant therapy at all.

Thromboresistance of Mechanical Valves

Conceptually, the trend of valve design is toward the elimination of obstructions caused by struts that protrude into the valve orifice. Even if contemporary designs using metallic orifices with struts could be fabricated using carbon technology, such devices

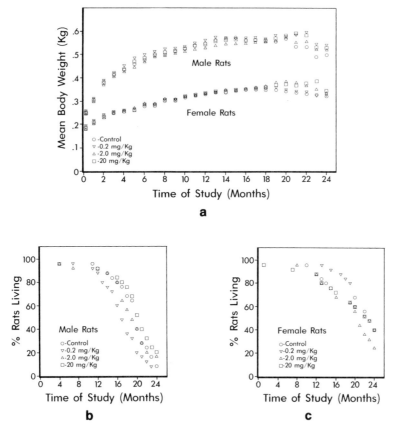

FIG. 14-1. (a) Survival versus time for male and female rats. (b) Weight gain for male rats. (c) Weight gain for female rats perfused with various amounts of powdered charcoal in physiologic solution compared to control rates (data from Ref. 26).

would suffer from turbulence and stasis created by such strut obstruction, and would result in an inferior flow quality. The only obstruction in the orifice should be the occluder itself. This observation also applies to approaches that attempt to promote endothelial growth on wires and struts by the use of a porous metal coating (27), an idea that is not new (Refs. 73–76 in Chapter 2; and Ref. 28).

The St. Jude valve, a so-called new generation valve, has demonstrated improved performance with respect to hemodynamics, thrombotic complication, and anticoagulation related hemorrhage (Refs. 90–95 in Chapter 2; and Refs. 2–4, 20–22, 29–53). Comparison of the Björk-Shiley with the St. Jude valve indicates that the latter has superior hemodynamics, a lower thromboembolic rate, and decreased risk of thrombosis (42, 52–54).

The St. Jude valve is the most widely used valve in the world today, but it is clearly not ideal. For example, although some reports seem to justify the use of the St. Jude prosthesis in children without postoperative anticoagulation (55–58), most suggest a more conservative approach (Ref. 55 in Chapter 2; and Refs. 21, 22, 59–67). It is pertinent to note, however, that for young patients in developing countries, a prosthetic valve less than ideal for western populations may perform better due to an apparent higher tolerance of mechanical prostheses by this patient group with respect to thromboembolism and thrombotic obstruction (Ref. 80 in Chapter 2; and Refs. 68–74).

It is also increasingly recognized that, just as early contentions that the replacement of a failing bioprosthesis could always be elective and thus carried a low operative risk if performed early were unfounded (Refs. 53–72 in Chapter 2), so is the contention that valve failure with bileaflet mechanical devices is always fatally catastrophic (Refs. 88, 108, 166, 167, 175–178 in Chapter 2; and Refs. 75–82).

Yoganathan et. al (29, 40, 46) have carried out in vitro studies identifying the velocity and turbulent shear stress fields in the immediate vicinity of the St. Jude valve using laser Doppler anemometry. The measurements show the peak velocities of the two side jets to be higher than that of the central jet, and that there is a large region of separation on either side of the jet next to the valve pivoting mechanism. Further, the flow through the two side channels is not equal, suggesting asynchronous motion of the leaflets, a behavior that has been reported clinically (Refs. 126, 127 in Chapter 2; and Refs. 29, 83–85).

The peak levels of shear stresses, 760 and 2,000 dynes/cm² for the mitral and aortic positions, respectively, are believed to be sufficient to damage blood elements (86). It was suggested that the mild to moderate hemolysis often reported (Ref. 91 in Chapter 2; and Refs. 46, 50, 52, 84, 87–90) for the St. Jude prosthesis could be the result of these shear stresses. It was also suggested that flow separation, together with elevated shear stresses in close proximity to the pivot mechanism, could lead to tissue overgrowth and/or thrombus formation that can cause leaflet dysfunction (Refs. 88, 89, 95, and 108 in Chapter 2; and Refs. 29, 76–79, 81, 82, 91–94).

During forward flow, most of the blood flow in the St. Jude prosthesis is centralized, with reduced flow next to the walls, especially in the vicinity of the pivot mechanism (Fig. 11 in Ref. 73, Chapter 2; and Ref. 40). Accordingly, the principal washing of the hinge mechanism occurs when the valve is closed and the leaflets support the highest differential pressure. The washing is accomplished by a scouring backward purge through the clearance allowed in the hinge, an action that has been suggested to minimize the number of coagulation elements activated by synthetic surface contact (15, 95). This backflow localized in the hinge of the St. Jude valve is depicted schematically in Fig. 14–2.

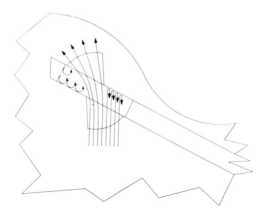

FIG. 14–2. Schematic diagram showing backflushing of the St. Jude prosthesis.

The backward flushing of the St. Jude hinge is most effective through the path open to flow which is shown in Fig. 14–2. The two regions identified by the shaded area in Fig. 14–2 are regions of reduced flow where minuscule thrombi can form and lead to hemolysis secondary to leaflet malfunction or lockup. The close-clearance perpendicularity requirement for lockup of the St. Jude valve leaflet occurs at all angular positions so that the mechanism can lock up in the open or closed position and in all positions in between, as clinical observations have shown (Refs. 88, 89, 95, 108, and 167 in Chapter 2; and Refs. 29, 75–79, 81, 82, 91–94, 96). Poor radiographic visibility compounds the problem because it makes it difficult to detect leaflet malfunction (Ref. 130 in Chapter 2; and Refs. 97–102).

In the remaining paragraphs, the backflow through the hinge, depicted in Fig. 14–2 for the St. Jude valve, will be compared to that of other all-carbon, new generation valves.

The Duromedics bileaflet prosthesis uses a unique hinge design comprised of a ball on the leaflet that engages an elongated recess in the orifice. When functioning, the ball travels along the length of the pivot slot effectively "pumping" blood in or out of the depression. When the valve is closed and the pressure differential across the valve is maximum, the leaflet sits on a lip so that the ball is free from contact within the engaging socket. The purging backflow through the hinge is unobstructed so that the hinge can be completely washed (103). Like the St. Jude prosthesis, both in vitro (104) and in vivo (105–108) macrohemodynamic characteristics of the Duromedics prosthesis are clinically adequate even in small sizes, and have been reported to be superior to those of the Björk-Shiley monostrut prosthesis (42, 52–54, 104). The effective washing (Fig. 14–3) of the hinge of the Duromedics valve is probably responsible for the low thromboembolic rates that have been reported for this valve (109–115).

The Omnicarbon® monoleaflet all-PYC device uses the same unloading principle as the Duromedics valve. In the closed position, the leaflet comes to rest on a seating lip, thus providing an unobstructed path for backflushing of the pivot areas (Fig. 14–4). A report, for a small number of patients followed for 221 patient years (mean 22 months), and who received no anticoagulant therapy, indicated no episodes of thromboembolism or valve thrombosis and only three transient ischemic events (116).

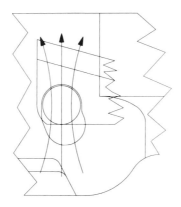

FIG. 14–3. Schematic diagram showing backflushing of the Duromedics prosthesis.

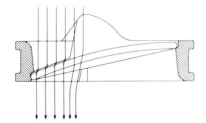

Fig. 14–4. Schematic diagram showing backflushing of the Omnicarbon® prosthesis.

When the hinge configuration of the CarboMedics valve, (Ref. 264 in Chapter 2) depicted in Fig. 14–5, is compared with that of the St. Jude valve (Fig. 14–2), it is seen that the regions obstructed to backflushing when the St. Jude valve is closed have been opened in the CarboMedics valve so that washing is possible. A stagnation point remains where the leaflet and the downstream pivot are in contact when the valve is closed; this region is washed during the initial stages of opening and the final stage of closing.

The newer Tascon bileaflet cardiac prosthesis (Fig. 14–6) uses the Carpentier hinge configuration (Ref. 266 in Chapter 2) that avoids the use of a recessed pivot socket. Like

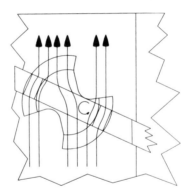

Fig. 14–5. Schematic diagram showing backflushing of the CardoMedics 226 prosthesis.

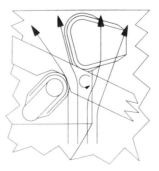

Fig. 14–6. Schematic diagram showing backflushing of the Tascon prosthesis.

the CarboMedics pivot, a stagnation point remains that is fully exposed for washing during the opening and closing cycle.

The Sorensen-Woien valve (Ref. 267 in Chapter 2) is a novel design. When closed, it sits on a seating lip so that the pivot region is clear with no contact; thus washing can be complete (see Fig. 2–10).

The Bramie valve is a bileaflet all-carbon device with a hinge similar to that of the CarboMedics design. The leaflets and orifice of this valve are contoured to promote washing on all surfaces. The special contours were optimized empirically by testing a large number of contours using a novel flow apparatus (117).

The Sorensen-Woien, Tascon, and Bramie concepts are in preclinical testing. All have solid PYC orifices with metallic stiffener rings and rotatable sewing rings.

Hemolysis Caused by Mechanical Valves

Just as rough surfaces and turbulent flow with high shear stresses promote thrombosis, they also cause hemolysis; the two processes are fundamentally related. Although the chemical nature of foreign surfaces has been reported to influence hemolysis (118), it is generally recognized that mechanical mechanisms such as pressure fluctuations, shear stresses, and other forms of energy dissipation are the primary factors responsible for the blood damage caused by prosthetic heart valves (41, 119–121). Accordingly, quantitative measurements of hemolysis as indicated by the elevation of lactate dehydrogenase (LDH) and the depression of serum haptoglobin are used as indicators of the extent of hemodynamic disturbances caused by a prosthesis (84).

Early ball valves covered with cloth have been reported to be hemolytic (39, 122), especially when the cloth is worn and the surface becomes very rough (123–125). Similarly, disk valves of the nontilting type were chronically hemolytic because of the shear effects associated with high velocity and turbulent flow through such valves, and were severely hemolytic when malfunction and improper seating occurred (Ref. 202 in Chapter 2). Even with modern tilting disk valves, which are only mildly hemolytic (Ref. 227 in Chapter 2; and Refs. 126–130), a leak caused by, for example, impingement can cause severe hemolysis similar to that reported for nontilting disk valves (131).

Although chronic hemolysis caused by the normally functioning St. Jude valve is typically of no clinical importance (Refs. 90–94 and 128 in Chapter 2; and Refs. 42–53, 84, 87–90, 132–134), there have been a number of isolated reports of very high rates of hemolysis without clear evidence of malfunction or perivalvular leak (Ref. 93 in Chapter 2; and 83, 84, 114, 133–141).

Horstkotte et al. (84), as well as Woo and Yoganathan (40), have suggested the asynchronous closure of the leaflets might be somehow related to at least some of isolated reports of severe hemolysis of the St. Jude prosthesis. In any event, the function of bileaflet mechanical prostheses is much more complex than that of prostheses that use only one leaflet. The precision required to assure the proper location of four hinges in an orifice so that leaflet engagement results in the required clearances at the circumferential perimeter, as well as at the leaflet's central contact, is beyond practical manufacturing capabilities. Therefore, individual leaflets and orifices must be computer selected from a large population of precisely measured components so that precise matching is achieved. It is possible that faulty matching occurs allowing gaps (leaks) that, like a perivalvular leak, cause hemolysis.

Improper seating caused by a combination of borderline matching and aggravated by

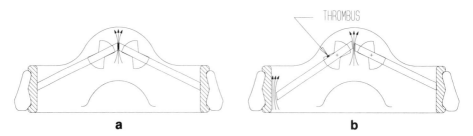

F_{IG}. 14–7. Schematic diagrams showing (a) hemolytic leak caused by fit of small leaflets in a large orifice of the St. Jude prosthesis, and (b) hemolytic leak caused by a minuscule thrombus in the hinge of a St. Jude prosthesis.

asynchronous leaflet closure, is suggested as a possible cause of leaks that are hemolytic. For example, Kotler et al. (139) reported a severe case of hemolysis and mitral regurgitation that was presumed to be due to abnormal seating with separation of the two leaflets during closure. Such an occurrence might result from two leaflets on the lower end of a radial tolerance band being fitted into an orifice on the high end of the diametrical tolerance band such that when the leaflets were at the full closed excursion allowed by the pivot, they did not meet at their central contact edge (Fig. 14–7). Alternately, it is possible that a "microthrombus" such as those described by Yamashita et al. (136), Morishita et al. (137), Yoganathan et al. (29), and Ziemer et al. (Ref. 166 in Chapter 2), could limit leaflet excursion and cause a hemolytic leak.

Results reported for the Duromedics valve (110–114, 142–144) indicate no clinically significant hemolysis of the sort indicated above for the St. Jude valve. This may be due to the fact that the number of St. Jude valves implanted is more than an order of magnitude greater than the number of Duromedics valves.

Blood data submitted to the United States Food and Drug Administration (FDA) by Medical, Inc. in support of a premarket approval application (Ref. 261 in Chapter 2) for the Omnicarbon® valve, indicate that the LDH values late post operatively are in the normal range, and that haptoglobin levels are depressed by about one-third in the late post-operative period. These data show that the Omnicarbon® valve causes less trauma to blood than bileaflet valves. This might be expected because the Omnicarbon® valve has a smaller total occluder perimeter than do bileaflet valves and the matching process (fitting a circular disk into a circular orifice) is much more straightforward so that chances for mismatch are minimal.

Prosthetic Valve Attachment

All prosthetic valves use an unnatural, rigid sewing ring. The junction between the new tissue formed on the sewing ring and the rigid prosthesis housing has been a major obstacle in the development of an ideal prosthesis. This is compounded by the fact that the rigid housing does not allow the normal valve support structure to deform with myocardial action.

Davila and collaborators (Refs. 73–76 in Chapter 2) have studied the healing process at the fixation perimeter and concluded that the best solution was to eliminate the junction by designing valves whose supporting frame would become completely encapsulated by healthy endothelialized scar tissue. For this purpose, valves were employed that were completely covered by cloth or a thin layer or porous metal to which endothelialized tissue could adhere. This approach has been reactivated and is showing some degree of success in a variant of the Björk-Shiley concept tested in goats (27). The problem, of course, is to ensure the formation of a tissue encapsulation that is stable and will not ultimately proliferate to embolize or interfere with occluder action.

An ideal tissue–prosthesis juncture, such as the one suggested by Nitter-Hauge and Dale (145), would maintain maximum shear stresses at all points around the fixation juncture in the critical range necessary for endothelial cell erosion to prevent tissue overgrowth (400 to 900 dynes/cm^2, reported by Fry (146, 147)). Such a condition is generally not achievable clinically because of flow variations that occur between patients. Accordingly, current thinking favors another concept described by Davila (148) in which the rim of the orifice is designed to stand proud of the sewing ring so that a centripetally contracting scar effectively seals the junction and stops proliferation (Fig. 350 in Ref. 148). Application of this concept depends on using a biologically inert material, such as carbon, at the junction so that a foreign body reaction that causes excessive tissue proliferation is avoided.

BIOPROSTHESES

The long-term clinical durability of bioprosthetic valves is currently a major impediment to their usage (149, 150). Before long-term durability data became available, improvement of hemodynamic performance was the focus of development (151–154). The clinical introduction of the bovine pericardial valve solved the hemodynamic problem, and such valves exhibit hemodynamics better than or equal to some mechanical prostheses (155–159).

As the number of the bioprostheses implanted for over five years increased, particularly certain bovine pericardial bioprostheses (160–163) and some longer term porcine implants (149–150), deficiencies in long-term durability became the paramount problem. The failure rates were often enhanced by calcification and this in turn appeared to be associated with stress concentrations. The association of calcification with regions of localized high stresses suggests that the failure rate could, at least in part, be alleviated through design.

The role of biochemical preservatives as a factor in tissue degeneration and the nature of calcification processes are both poorly understood and controversial (164–168). Clearly, the presence of elemental calcium in any quantity in the leaflet tissue markedly accelerates the degenerative process (169, 170). Whether tissue degeneration is initiated by calcium formation or mechanical stress needs resolution (171). In any event, in order to increase the long-term durability of bioprosthetic valves, simultaneous improvements in tissue preservation and mechanical design are required.

Most agree that unless regeneration of host tissue is possible, all materials used in bioprosthetic valves will eventually fail due to fatigue. Accordingly, as a first step, stress concentrations in the valve leaflets must be minimized through improvements in design.

Porcine Bioprostheses

Commissure Posts

The region of leaflet attachment at the commissure posts of the porcine prosthetic stent is stiffer than the natural attachment, so stresses are concentrated at these points. In some cases, the commissure posts of porcine bioprosthetic valves tested in a pulsatile chamber

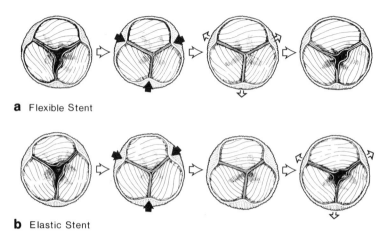

a Flexible Stent

b Elastic Stent

Fig. 14–8. Deflection of commissure posts during valve closing. (a) Abrupt return of the commissure posts of a flexible stent. (b) Smooth return of the commissure posts of an elastic stent.

in vitro, exhibit deflections of about one millimeter, which is in the same order as the deflection of natural aortic valves in vivo (172, 173). However, instead of deflecting inwardly and returning smoothly during closing, the commissure posts of bioprostheses spring back abruptly (Fig. 14–8). The sudden reversal in motion of the commissure posts creates undesirable dynamic stresses in the leaflets, particularly near the region of commissure attachment.

The design of a flexible valve stent is a difficult problem. This is because the speed at which the commissure posts return to their original position depends on the dynamic stiffness of the entire valve structure, and as the layer of host tissue develops and thickens, its presence affects the movement of the commissure posts. Accordingly, the proper elasticity of the commissure posts must be assessed under dynamic conditions in a pulsatile flow chamber while recognizing that changes in properties will occur in vivo. Using flexible commissure posts with limited deflection reduces stress concentrations at the leaflet attachment. Such designs also reduce the tendency for leaflet prolapse and disruption. The latter is one of the most common modes of valve failure and, because of the concomitant high, localized stress, is usually accompanied by calcification (164).

Commissure Height

It is important to keep the commissure height of the aortic porcine valve as close to that of the natural valve as possible. Stretching the aorta longitudinally, either with fluid or mechanical pressure, increases the height of the commissure (Fig. 14–9a), whereas dilating the aortic valve at the sinus of Valsalva region reduces the commissure height (Fig. 14–9b).

Using commissure heights higher than that of the natural aortic valve, tends to intensify the stress at the flexion zone (174) (Fig. 14–10). Commissure heights lower than the original height of the natural aortic valve cause a reduction in the coaptation surface between the leaflets and increase the stresses at the free edges of the leaflets. Therefore, it is necessary to maintain the natural commissure height of the porcine aortic valve. It should also be noted that the natural commissure height can vary for a given annulus

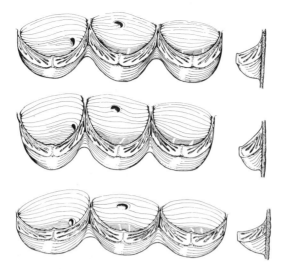

FIG. 14–9. Geometric alteration of the porcine aortic valve through chemical processing. (a) Geometry of a natural porcine aortic valve. (b) Geometry of a longitudinally stretched porcine aortic valve. (c) Geometry of a circumferentially stretched porcine aortic valve.

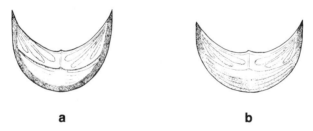

a   b

FIG. 14–10. The effect of the porcine aortic valve height on the flexion zone. (a) More intense and narrower flexion zone for a longitudinally stretched valve. (b) Wide and diffused flexion zone for a shorter aortic valve.

diameter, so simple proportioning is not possible and special care must be exercised to maintain the original height.

Right Coronary Muscle Shelf

The interventricular septal shelf at the right coronary leaflet of the porcine aortic valve is a natural part of the valve that some designers have tried to eliminate or reduce (175, 176). If the muscle shelf is left intact in the valve orifice, the orifice area is reduced; but, if the muscle shelf is reduced to increase orifice area, it is important that the natural geometry of the right coronary cusp and the cuspal attachment is not also altered.

Abnormalities caused by altering the right coronary septal region can only be detected by functionally testing each and every completed valve. Accordingly, functional quality control must be an integral part of manufacturing to assure reliable durability.

Mechanical Properties

Although glutaraldehyde fixation has been the most effective process used to preserve biomaterials for cardiac valves, the mechanical properties of the glutaraldehyde treated porcine aortic valves currently being produced are not ideal, and further improvements in the fixation process are required.

The introduction of low pressure (less than 4mm Hg) glutaraldehyde fixation has improved the durability of porcine aortic valves (177), but shortcomings remain. Unlike fresh valves, the valves fixed in low pressure glutaraldehyde become set in the processing position. Typically, this is the closed position. Thubrikar et al. called this position the neutral position (174). In contrast, the ease with which fresh valve leaflets move suggests that the stress in natural leaflets is very low throughout the entire cardiac cycle, so that fresh valve leaflets have no definite neutral position. This means that the fixation process should not set the leaflets; instead they should be pliable and move freely at all positions in the cardiac cycle.

In addition to pliability, the viscoelastic characteristics of the valve tissue are important to its durability. Unfortunately, the relationships between viscoelasticity and durability are complex and poorly understood.

Suaren et al. (178) studied the viscoelastic behavior of the porcine aortic tissues, and Rousseau et al. (179) reported the elastic and viscoelastic characteristics of fresh and glutaraldehyde treated porcine aortic valve tissue. Rousseau found that although tissues may possess similar elastic constants, they can have quite different viscoelastic characteristics. It should be noted that since the leaflets are viscoelastic, their properties are rate sensitive and the dynamic motion of the porcine leaflets is affected by the rate at which they move. Accordingly, caution is required in the interpretation of results from accelerated testing.

Bovine Pericardial Prostheses

Bovine pericardial bioprosthetic valves have been in wide clinical use. Although all are trileaflet, variations using one or two leaflets are currently under clinical investigation. The geometry of the leaflets in the monocuspid (180) and bicuspid valves are similar to the individual leaflets in a trileaflet valve (Fig. 14–11), so the discussion of all such valves can be combined.

Leaflet Attachment

Unlike the leaflets in trileaflet valve designs, the leaflet(s) of monocuspid and bicuspid bovine pericardial valves close against the stent. To assure durability, the leaflets must attach in the following manner:

the leaflets must not rub against any abrasive surface during the cardiac cycle

the leaflet attachment line must be a smooth and continuous curve

the region of attachment must have no points of stress concentration.

It has been reported that neointima does not always encapsulate all the valves implanted (181, 182). Accordingly, valves that depend on the deposition of host tissue to cover the cloth cannot be considered reliable (Fig. 14–12a).

Wear can be reduced by stretching pericardial tissue locally, making it stiff where the

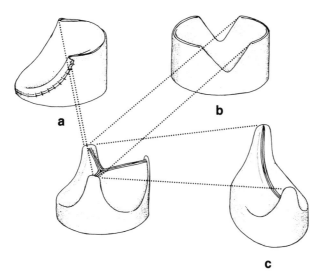

FIG. 14–11. Similarities among leaflet valves. A single cusp of a trileaflet valve may be considered as the basic building block for (a) a monocuspid valve, or (b, c) bicuspid valves.

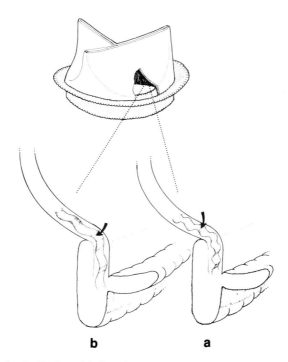

FIG. 14–12. Localized stiffening minimizes tissue abrasion. (a) More abrasion occurs when the tissue is soft and elastic. (b) Less abrasion occurs when the tissue is stiff.

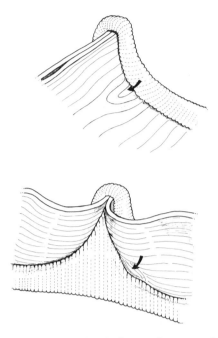

Fɪɢ. 14–13. Unevenness in the curvature of the leaflet attachment margin causes creases to form in the tissue.

leaflet rubs against the stent (Fig. 14–12b). This stiffening of setting process reduces the abrasive rubbing of the leaflet tissue against the stent or its cloth covering.

Any unevenness or discontinuity in the curvature of the leaflet attachment line usually produces creases or folds in the leaflet during the cardiac cycle (Fig. 14–13). This repeated folding of the leaflet can cause rupture by a fatigue mechanism. Folds or creases that form in the leaflets as it functions can only be observed during testing under physiological conditions. Obviously, the geometry and the fluid field around the valve during the natural cardiac cycle must be duplicated in functional testing, and reliability depends on thorough (100%) quality control during manufacture.

Stress concentrations can be reduced by sewing the valve leaflets to the stent with pledgets; however, the added bulk will limit the motion of the leaflets and reduce the size of the orifice. Attaching the valve leaflets to the stent with bare sutures, especially at the commissure tip area, can cause wear and lead to tears in the leaflets (181). Accordingly, the method of leaflet attachment is not straightforward, but rather a complex compromise.

Coaptation Surfaces

The durability of a valve with leaflets that seal against a soft, smooth support on the stent is not known; however, experience has shown that the durability of a valve with leaflets that coapt with each other is good. A smooth, fixed sealing surface, with cushioning, will not roll with the motion of the closing leaflets, nor will it have the necessary area of leaflet contact during the closing of the valve (Fig. 14–14). Although the magni-

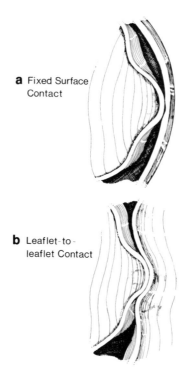

a Fixed Surface
Contact

b Leaflet-to-
leaflet Contact

FIG. 14–14. Effect of different coaptation surfaces on durability. (a) Fixed surface contact produces more stress. (b) Leaflet-to-leaflet contact produces minimum stress.

tude of the stresses at coaptation is small, cumulative effects of these stresses are thought to affect long-term durability.

Commissure Attachment

It is desirable to have an adequate amount of coaptation surface at the region of commissure attachment to avoid short-term leaks and long-term leaflet prolapse (Fig. 14–15). The placement of only buttress sutures to hold the leaflets closed together at the commissure region is expected to introduce high shear stresses and cause tears in the cusps (183). Again, the mechanical durability of the commissure attachment of the bovine pericardial valve design must be assessed in durability tests and maintained with functional tests in quality control.

Commissure Posts

Stress induced calcification initiated at the region of commissure attachment in the bovine pericardial valve has been reported (165, 184). Regardless of the mechanism, it is clear that localized stresses at the commissure attachment must be minimized by design without sacrificing the performance of the valve. The preferred commissure structure is one that is elastic, so that localized stresses in the leaflets are avoided. Since the bovine pericardial valve is fabricated from a membrane heart sac having its own inherent

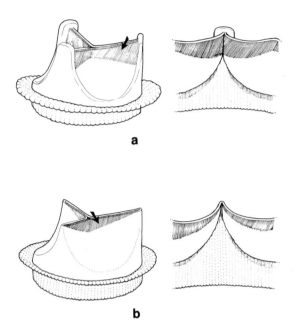

FIG. 14–15. The long term effect of coaptation surface area at the commissures on valve stability. (a) Stable design. (b) Less desirable design.

properties that differ from fixed aortic valve tissue, the dynamic characteristics of stent components properly designed for pericardial valves must also differ from the dynamic characteristics of properly designed stents used in porcine bioprostheses.

Mechanical Properties

Bovine pericardium tissue used in cardiac bioprostheses has been reported to have better mechanical durability than the leaflet tissue of porcine bioprostheses, so that the tears and disruption of the first generation of bovine pericardial bioprostheses documented in clinical reports are thought to be due to shortcomings in design. This suggests that properly designed bovine pericardial bioprostheses with little or no stress concentrations can be expected to provide better durability than porcine bioprostheses.

CURRENT DESIGN TRENDS

Marked improvements in porcine aortic valve durability can be realized by making incremental improvements in every component of the valve through design and processing advances. The benefit of such advances can only be realized through strict and appropriate quality control.

The long-term durability of bovine cardiac bioprostheses can be improved through innovative stent designs that minimize stress concentrations, and these stress concentrations must be reduced through improved processing that yields more pliable tissue.

If these challenges are met, so that bioprostheses can be produced that are durable and are at the same time capable of maintaining a sufficiently high level of thromboresistance that anticoagulation therapy is not required, there will probably be another cyclic swing toward increased use of bioprostheses. Whether research yields bioprostheses with improved durability, or mechanical prostheses that are thromboresistant, or some other solution, it is hoped that improvements will not be long in coming.

REFERENCES

1. Marshall WG Jr, Kouchoukos NT, Karp RB, Williams JB: Late results after mitral valve replacement with the Björk-Shiley and porcine prostheses. J Thorac Cardiovasc Surg 1983;85:902–910.
2. Joyce LD, Nelson RM: Comparison of porcine valve xenografts with mechanical prostheses. J Thorac Cardiovasc Surg 1984;88:102–113.
3. Kawachi Y, Tokunaga K, Watanabe Y, Nose Y, Nakamura M: In vivo hemodynamics of prosthetic St. Jude Medical and Ionescu-Shiley heart valves analyzed by computer. Ann Thorac Surg 1985;39:456–461.
4. Gray RJ, Chaux A, Matloff JM, DeRobertis M, Raymond M, Stewart M, Yoganathan AP: Bileaflet, tilting disc and porcine substitutes: in vivo hydrodynamic characteristics. J Am Coll Cardiol 1984;3:321–327.
5. Miller HC, Bloomfield P, Kitchin AH, Wheatley DJ, Walbaum PR, Lutz W: A prospective evaluation of the Björk-Shiley, Hancock, and Carpentier-Edwards heart valve prostheses. Circulation 1986;73:1213–1222.
6. Douglas PS, Hirschfeld JW Jr, Edie RN, Harken AH, Stephenson LW, Edmunds LH Jr: Clinical comparison of the St. Jude and porcine aortic valve prostheses. Valv Heart Dis 1985;72(suppl 2):135–139.
7. Martinell J, Fraile J, Artiz V, Moreno J, Rabago G: Long-term comparative analysis of the Björk-Shiley and Hancock valves implanted in 1975. J Thorac Cardiovasc Surg 1985;90:741–749.
8. Cohn LH, Allred EN, Cohn LA, Austin JC, Sabik J, DiSesa VJ, Shemin RJ, Collins JJ: Early and late risk of mitral valve replacements: a 12 year concomitant comparison of the porcine bioprosthetic and prosthetic disc mitral valves. J Thorac Cardiovasc Surg 1985;90:872–881.
9. Cohn LH, Allred EN, DiSesa VJ, Sawtelle K, Shemin RJ, Collins JJ: Early and late risk of aortic valve replacement: a 12 year concomitant comparison of the porcine bioprosthetic and prosthetic disc aortic valves. J Thorac Cardiovasc Surg 1984;88:695–705.
10. Jamieson WRE: Bioprostheses are superior to mechanical prostheses. Z Kardiol 1986;75(suppl 2):258–271.
11. Cobanoglu A, Brockman SK: Selection of a prosthetic heart valve. Cardiovasc Clin 1986;16:399–414.
12. Bonchek LI: Basis for selecting a valve prosthesis. Cardiovasc Clin 1987;17:107–125.
13. Nashef SAM, Sethia B, Turner MA, Davidson KG, Lewis S, Bain WH: Björk-Shiley and Carpentier-Edwards valves. J Thorac Cardiovasc Surg 1987;93:394–404.
14. Hammond GL, Geha AS, Kopf GS, Hashim SW: Biological versus mechanical valves: analysis of 1116 valves inserted in 1012 adult patients with 4818 patient-year and a 5327 valve follow up. J Thorac Cardiovasc Surg 1987;93:182–198.
15. Edmunds LH Jr: Thrombotic and bleeding complications of prosthetic heart valves. Ann Thorac Surg 1987;44:430–445.
16. Cohn LH: Thromboembolism in different anatomical positions: aortic, mitral, and multiple valves. In Rabago G, Cooley DA (eds): Heart Valve Replacement and Future Trends in Cardiac Surgery. Mount Kisco NY, Futura Publishing, 1987, pp 259–270.
17. Edmunds LH Jr: Thromboembolic and bleeding complications of prosthetic heart valves. In Rabago G, Cooley DA (eds): Heart Valve Replacement and Future Trends in Cardiac Surgery. Mount Kisco NY, Futura Publishing, 1987, pp 271–284.
18. Deviri E, Levinsky L, Schachner A, Nili M, Levy J: Thromboembolism and anticoagulant treatment in patients with heart valve prostheses. In Rabago G, Cooley DA (eds): Heart Valve Replacement and Future Trends in Cardiac Surgery. Mount Kisco NY, Futura Publishing, 1987, pp 285–296.
19. Thulin LI, Luhrs CH, Schuller HLA, Olin CL: Anticoagulation therapy in patients with mechanical heart valves. In Rabago G, Cooley DA (eds): Heart Valve Replacement and Future Trends in Cardiac Surgery. Mount Kisco NY, Futura Publishing, 1987, pp 297–306.
20. Antunes MJ: Thromboembolic complications and anticoagulants: compliant versus noncompliant patient populations. In Rabago G, Cooley DA (eds): Heart Valve Replacement and Future Trends in Cardiac Surgery. Mount Kisco NY, Futura Publishing, 1987, pp 307–317.
21. Duveau D: Anticoagulation is necessary in all patients with mechanical prostheses in sinus rhythm. Z Kardiol 1986;75(suppl 2):326–331.
22. Dale J, Nitter-Hauge S: Do all patients with mechanical heart valve prostheses need anticoagulant therapy? Z Kardiol 1986;75(suppl 2):332–337.
23. Lindblom D, Lindblom U, Henze A, Björk VO, Semb KH: Three year clinical results with the monostrut Björk-Shiley prosthesis. J Thorac Cardiovasc Surg 1987;94:34–43.
24. Kalke BR, Mantini EL, Kaster RL, Carlson RG, Lillehei CW: Hemodynamic features of a double-leaflet prosthetic heart valve of new design. Trans Am Soc Artif Intern Organs 1967;13:105–110.

25. Bruck SD: Properties of Biomaterials in the Physiological Environment. Boca Raton FL, CRC Press, 1980, pp 24, 51–56.
26. Hill JB, Horres CR: The BD hemodetoxifier: particulate release and its significance. In Briggs G (ed): Proceedings of Seminar on "How To" on Premarket Clearance of New Devices and Diagnostics. Chicago, Health Industry Manufacturers Association, 1977, Chapter 6.
27. Björk VO, Sternlieb J: Artificial heart valve testing in goats. Scand J Thorac Cardiovasc Surg 1986;20:97–102.
28. Kaster RL, Tanaka S, Carlson RG, Lillehei CW: Initial laboratory development and evaluation of the cageless free-floating pivoting-disc prosthetic heart valve. In Nose Y (ed): Cardiac Engineering. New York, John Wiley and Sons, 1970, pp 261–271.
29. Yoganathan AP, Chaux A, Gray RJ, Woo YN, DeRobertis M, Williams FP, Matloff R: Bileaflet, tilting disc and porcine aortic valve substitutes: in vitro hydrodynamics characteristics. J Am Coll Cardiol 1984;3:313–320.
30. Heiliger R: Hydrodynamic advantages and disadvantages of mechanical bileaflet valves and tilting disc valve No. 29. Engineering Medicine 1987;16:77–85.
31. Yoganathan AP, Corcoran WH, Harrison EC, Carl JR: The Björk-Shiley aortic prosthesis: flow characteristics, thrombus formation, and tissue overgrowth. Circulation 1978;58:70–76.
32. Moreno-Cabral RJ, McNamara JJ, Mamiya RT, Brainard SC, Chung GKT: Acute thrombotic obstruction with Björk-Shiley valves: diagnostic and surgical considerations. J Thorac Cardiovasc Surg 1978;75:321–330.
33. Wright JO, Hiratzka LF, Brandt B III, Doty DB: Thrombosis of the Björk-Shiley prosthesis. J Thorac Cardiovasc Surg 1982;84:138–144.
34. Kohler J: In vitro hemodynamics of 33 technical and biological valve prostheses. Life Support Syst 1985;3(suppl 1):172–176.
35. Fisher J, Reece IJ, Wheatley DJ: In vitro evaluation of six mechanical and six bioprosthetic valves. Thorac Cardiovasc Surg 1986;34:157–162.
36. Gabbay S, Yellin EL, Frishman WH, Frater RW: In vitro hemodynamic comparison of St. Jude, Björk-Shiley and Hall-Kaster valves. Trans Am Soc Artif Intern Organs 1980;26:231–235.
37. Yoganathan AP, Reamer HH: The Björk-Shiley aortic prosthesis: flow characteristics of the present model vs the convexo-concave model. Scand J Thorac Cardiovasc Surg 1980;14:1–8.
38. Yoganathan AP, Woo YN, Williams FP, Stevenson DM, Franck RH, Harrison EC: In vitro fluid dynamics characteristics of Ionescu-Shiley and Carpentier-Edwards tissue bioprostheses. Artif Organ 1983;7:459–469.
39. Yoganathan AP, Reamer HH, Corcoran WH, Harrison EC, Shulman IA, Parnassuc W: The Starr-Edwards aortic ball valve: flow characteristics, thrombus formation, and tissue overgrowth. Artif Organ 1981;5:6–17.
40. Woo YR, Yoganathan AP: Pulsatile flow velocity and shear stress measurements on the St. Jude bileaflet valve prosthesis. Scand J Cardiovasc Surg 1986;20:15–28.
41. Schoen FJ: Cardiac valve prostheses: pathological and bioengineering considerations. J Cardiovasc Surg 1987;2:65–108.
42. Horstkotte D, Korfer R, Seipel L, Bircks W, Loogen F: Late complications in patients with Björk-Shiley and St. Jude Medical heart valve replacement. Circulation 1983;68(suppl 2):175–184.
43. Arom KV, Nicoloff DM, Kersten TE, Northrup WF, Lindsay WG: Six years of experience with the St. Jude Medical valvular prosthesis. Circulation 1985;72(suppl 2):153–158.
44. D'Angelo GJ, Kish GF, Sardesai PG, Tan WS: Clinical assessment of the St. Jude Medical cardiac prosthesis; a 5 year experience. Am Surg 1986;52:101–104.
45. Chaux A, Czer LSC, Matloff JM, DeRobertis MA, Stewart ME, Bateman TM, Kass RM, Lee ME, Gray RJ: The St. Jude Medical bileaflet valve prosthesis. J Thorac Cardiovasc Surg 1984;88:706–717.
46. Yoganathan AP, Chaux A, Gray RJ, DeRobertis M, Matloff JM: Flow characteristics of the St. Jude prosthetic valve: an in vitro and in vivo study. Artif Organ 1982;6:288–294.
47. Nicoloff DM, Emery RW, Arom KV: Clinical and hemodynamic results with the St. Jude Medical cardiac valve prosthesis: a three-year experience. J Thorac Cardiovasc Surg 1981;82:674–677.
48. Duveau D, Michaud JL, Despins P, Dupon H: Mitral valve replacement with St. Jude Medical prosthesis: incidence of thromboembolic event in 349 patients. Eur Heart J 1984;5:49–52.
49. Horstkotte D, Korfer R, Budde T, Haerten K, Schulte HD, Bircks W, Loogen F: Late complications following Björk-Shiley and St. Jude Medical heart valve replacement. Z Kardiol 1983;72:251–261.
50. Leclerc JL, Wellens F, Deuvaert FE, Premo G: Long term results with St. Jude Medical valve. In DeBakey ME (ed): Advances in Cardiac Valves. New York, Yorke, 1983, pp 33–40.
51. DeBakey ME, Lawrie GM, Morris GC, Crawford ES, Howell JF: Experience with 366 St. Jude valve prostheses in 346 patients. In DeBakey ME (ed): Advances in Cardiac Valves. New York, Yorke, 1983, pp 14–21.
52. Horstkotte D, Korfer R: The influence of prosthetic valve replacement on the natural history of severe acquired heart valve lesions. In DeBakey ME (ed): Advances in Cardiac Valves. New York, Yorke, 1983, pp 47–86.

53. Kopf GS, Hammond GL, Geha AS: Long term performance of the St. Jude Medical valve: low incidence of thromboembolism and hemorrhagic complications with modest doses of warfarin. Circulation 1987;76:(suppl 3):131–147.
54. Horstkotte D: Late complications in patients with Björk-Shiley and St. Jude Medical prostheses. In Matloff JM (ed): Cardiac Valve Replacement. Boston, Martinus Nijhoff Publishing, 1984, pp 225–231.
55. Pass HI, Sade RM, Crawford FA Jr, Hohn AR: Cardiac valve prosthesis in children without anticoagulation. J Thorac Cardiovasc Surg 1984;87:832–835.
56. Sade RM, Crawford FA Jr, Pass HI, Kratz JM: Pediatric use of the St. Jude Medical prosthesis. In Matloff JM (ed). Cardiac Valve Replacement. Boston, Martinus Nijhoff Publishing, 1984, pp 137–140.
57. Cornish EM, Human DG, deMoor MMA, Hassoulas J, Sanchez HE, Sprenger KJ, Reichart BA: Valve replacement in children. Thorac Cardiovasc Surgeon 1987;35:176–179.
58. Ilbawi MN, Idriss FS, DeLeon SY, Muster AJ, Duffy CE, Gidding SS, Paul MH: Valve replacement in children: guidelines for selection of prosthesis and timing of surgical intervention. Ann Thorac Surg 1987;44:398–403.
59. Deviri E, Levinsky L, Schachner A, Nili M, Levy MJ: Thromboembolism and anticoagulant treatment in patients with heart valve prostheses. In Rabago G, Cooley DA (eds): Heart Valve Replacement. Mount Kisco NY, Futura Publishing, 1987, pp 285–296.
60. Borkon AM, Reitz BA, Donahro JS, Gardner TJ: St. Jude Medical valve replacement in infants and children. In Rabago G, Cooley DA (eds): Heart Valve Replacement. Mount Kisco NY, Futura Publishing, 1987, pp 129–135.
61. Subramanian S: Use of the St. Jude Medical prosthesis in children. In DeBakey ME (ed): Advances in Cardiac Valves. New York, Yorke, 1983, pp 129–137.
62. Bradley LM, Midgley FM, Watson DC, Getson PR, Scott LP: Anticoagulation therapy in children with mechanical prosthetic cardiac valves. Am J Cardiol 1985;56:533–535.
63. Schaff HV, Danielson GK: Current status of valve replacement in children. Cardiovasc Clin 1986;16:427–436.
64. Stewart S, Cianciotta D, Alexson C, Manning J: The long term risk of warfarin solium therapy and the incidence of thromboembolism in children after prosthetic cardiac valve replacement. J Thorac Cardiovasc Surg 1987;93:551–554.
65. Schaffer MS, Clarke DR, Campbell DN, Madigan CK, Wiggins JW Jr, Wolfe RR: The St. Jude Medical cardiac valve in infants and children: role of anticoagulation therapy. J Am Coll Cardiol 1987;9:235–239.
66. McGrath LB, Gonzalez-Lavin L, Eldridge WJ, Colombi M, Restrepo D: thromboembolic and other events following valve replacement in a pediatric population treated with antiplatelet agents. Ann Thorac Surg 1987;43:285–287.
67. Serra AJS, McNicholas KW, Olivier HF Jr, Boe SL, Lemole GM: The choice of anticoagulation in pediatric patients with the St. Jude Medical valve prosthesis. J Cardiovasc Surg 1987;28:588–591.
68. Kinsley RH: Valve replacements in the third world. J Thorac Cardiovasc Surg 1984;88:638.
69. John S: Valve replacements in the third world. J Thorac Cardiovasc Surg 1984;88:638–639.
70. John S, Bashi VV, Jairaj PS, Muralidharan S: Mitral valve replacement in the young patient with rheumatic heart disease. J Thorac Cardiovasc Surg 1983;86:209–216.
71. John S, Bashi VV, Jairaj PS, Muralidharan S, Ravikumar E, Rajarajeswari T, Krishnaswami S, Sukumar IP, Sundar Rao PSS: Closed mitral valvotomy. Early results and long-term followup of 3726 consecutive patients. Circulation 1983;68:891–896.
72. Baker C, Brock RC, Campbell M, Wood P: Valvotomy for mitral stenosis. A further report on 100 cases. Br Med J 1952;1:1043–1055.
73. John S, Munsh SC, Gupta RP, Ramachandran V, Milledge JS, Sukumar IP, Cherian G: Results of mitral valve replacements in young patients with rheumatic heart disease. J Thorac Cardiovasc Surg 1973;66:255–264.
74. Venugopal P, Iyer KS, Kaul U, Reddy KS: Letter to the Editor. J Thorac Cardiovasc Surg 1986;92:965–966.
75. Anagnostopoulos C: In discussion: Chaux A, Czer LSC, Matloff JM, DeRobertis MA, Stewart ME, Bateman TM, Kass RM, Lee ME, Gray RJ: The St. Jude Medical bileaflet valve prosthesis. J Thorac Cardiovasc Surg 1984;88:706–717.
76. Donzeau-Gouge P, N'Guyen A, Touchot B, Dunica S, Weber S, Guerin F, Piwnica A: Thrombose aigue d'une prothese aortique de St. Jude Medical chez une femme enceinte de quatre mois. Ann Chir 1986;40:548–550.
77. Ilbawi MN, Lockhart CG, Idriss FS, DeLeon SY, Muster AJ, Duffy E, Paul MH: Experience with St. Jude Medical valve prosthesis in children. J Thorac Cardiovasc Surg 1987;93:73–79.
78. Bowen TE, Tri TB, Wortham DC: Thrombosis of a St. Jude Medical tricuspid prosthesis. J Thorac Cardiovasc Surg 1981;82:257–262.
79. Donzeau-Gouge P, N'Guyen A, Touchot B, Dunica S, Weber S, Guerin F, Piwnica A: Acute thrombosis of a St. Jude Medical prosthesis in a pregnant woman. Thorac Cardiovasc Surg 1985;33:248–249.
80. Bradley LM, Perry LW, Watson DC: Failure of St. Jude Medical mitral prosthesis diagnosed by two-dimensional echocardiography. Am J Cardiol 1984;54:1385.

81. Turinetto B, Cahsai G, Dozza F, Marinelli G, Pierangeli A: Early thrombosis of an aortic St. Jude valve in spite of effective anticoagulation treatment. J Cardiovasc Surg 1984;25:182–184.

82. Moulton AL, Singleton RT, Oster WF, Bosley J, Mergner W: Fatal thrombosis of an aortic St. Jude Medical valve despite adequate anticoagulants. J Thorac Cardiovasc Surg 1982;83:472–473.

83. Pandis IP, Ren JF, Kotler MN, Mintz GS, Mundth ED, Goel IP, Ross J: Clinical and echocardiographic evaluation of the St. Jude cardiac valve prosthesis: followup of 126 patients. J Am Coll Cardiol 1984;4:454–462.

84. Horstkotte D, Curtius JM, Bircks W, Loogen F: Noninvasive evaluation of prosthetic heart valves. In Rabago G, Cooley DA (eds): Heart Valve Replacements and Future Trending Cardiac Surgery. Mount Kisco NY, Futura Publishing, 1987, pp 349–373.

85. Feldman H, Gray R, Chaux A: Non invasive in vivo and in vitro study of the St. Jude mitral valve. Am J Cardiol 1982;49:1101–1109.

86. Blackshear PL: Hemolysis at prosthetic surfaces. In Hair ML (ed): Chemistry of Biosurfaces. New York, Marcel Dekker, 1972, vol 2, pp 523–562.

87. Lillehei CW: Worldwide experience with the St. Jude Medical valve prosthesis: clinical and hemodynamic results. Contemp Surg 1982;20:17–31.

88. Koja K, Kusaba A, Yara I, Kina M, Vesato T, Kuniyoshi Y, Iha K: Five year clinical evaluation of the St. Jude Medical valve prosthesis in 136 patients. Jap J Surg 1985;15:177–183.

89. Nicoloff MD, Emery RW: Current status of the St. Jude cardiac valve prosthesis. Contemp Surg 1979;45:11–13.

90. Sezai Y: Experience with the St. Jude Medical prosthesis: studies on cinefluorography, hemolysis, and tricuspid replacement. In DeBakey ME (ed): Advances in Cardiac Valves. New York, Yorke, 1983, pp 87–102.

91. Ross EM, Roberts WC: A precaution when using the St. Jude Medical prosthesis in the aortic position. Am J Cardiol 1984;54:231–233.

92. Bradley LM, Perry LW, Watson DC: Failure of St. Jude Medical mitral prosthesis diagnosed by two dimensional echocardiography. Am J Cardiol 1984;54:1385–1388.

93. Commerford PJ, Lloyd EA, DeNobrega JA: Thrombosis of St. Jude Medical cardiac valve in the mitral position. Chest 1981;80:326–327.

94. Sharma A, Johnson DC, Cartmill TB: Entrapment of St. Jude Medical aortic valve prosthesis in a child. J Thorac Cardiovasc Surg 1983;86:453–454.

95. Kohanna FH, Salzman EW: Thromboembolic complications of cardiac and vascular prostheses. In Sabiston DC Jr, Spencer FC (eds): Gibbon's Surgery of the Chest. Philadelphia, W B Saunders, 1983, p 1267.

96. Baeza O: Potential for immobilization of the valve occluder in various valve prostheses. In Matloff JM (ed): Cardiac Valve Replacement. Boston, Martinus Nijhoff Publishing, 1984, pp 281–284.

97. Czer LSC, Weiss M, Bateman TM, Pfaff JM, DeRobertis M, Eigler N, Vas R, Matloff JM: Fibrinolytic therapy of St. Jude valve thrombosis under guidance of digital cinefluoroscopy. J Am Coll Cardiol 1985;5:1244–1249.

98. Crawford FA Jr, Kratz JM, Sade RM, Stroud MR, Bartles DM: Aortic and mitral valve replacement with the St. Jude Medical prosthesis. Ann Surg 1984;199:753–761.

99. Amann FW, Burckhardt D, Hasse J, Gradel E: Echocardiographic feature of the correctly functioning St. Jude Medical valve prosthesis. Am Heart J 1981;101:45–51.

100. Hidajat HC, Gottwik MG, Thormann J, Schlepper M: Echocardiographic identification and analysis of function of the St. Jude Medical heart valve prosthesis. Eur J Cardiol 1980;12:167–176.

101. Hehrlein FW, Gottwik M, Mulch J, Walter P, Fraedrich G: Heart valve replacement with the new all-pyrolytic bi-leaflet St. Jude Medical prosthesis. J Cardiovasc Surg 1980;21:395–398.

102. Mehlman DJ: Radiographic and cineradiographic evaluation of heart valve prostheses. In Rabago G, Cooley DA (eds): Heart Valve Replacement. Mount Kisco NY, Futura Publishing, 1987, pp 337–348.

103. Klawitter JJ: Design and in vitro testing of the Duromedics bileaflet valve. Proceedings First International Hemex Symposium on the Duromedics Bileaflet Valve, Austin TX, January 23–27, 1985. Austin TX, Hemex Scientific, 1985, pp 9–15.

104. Heiliger R, Geks J, Mittermayer C: Results of a comparative in vitro study of Duromedics and Björk-Shiley monostrut mitral heart valve prostheses. J Biomed Eng 1987;9:128–133.

105. Pomar JL, Pare C, Cardona M, Mestres C, Barriuso C, Hearas M, Bosch X, Mulet J, Betriu A: Hemodynamic evaluation of the Duromedics bileaflet heart valve—continuous and pulsed weave doppler and cardiac catheterization studies. Proceedings Second International Hemex Symposium on the Duromedics Bileaflet Valve, Austin TX, January 31–February 1, 1986. Austin TX, Hemex Scientific, 1986, pp 71–76.

106. Jamieson MPG, Cleland J, Bain WH, Faichney A: The Duromedics valve—late non-evasive hemodynamic evaluation. Proceedings Second International Hemex Symposium on the Duromedics Bileaflet Valve. Austin TX, January 31–February 1, 1986. Austin TX, Hemex Scientific, 1986, pp 77–80.

107. Dimitri W, Carey K, Webb-Peploe MM, Williams BT: Postoperative hemodynamic characteristics of the Duromedics prosthesis: comparative doppler echocardiographic studies. Proceedings Second International Hemex Symposium on the Duromedics Bileaflet Valve. Austin TX, January 31–February 1, 1986. Austin TX, Hemex Scientific, 1986, 81–92.

108. Lepage G, Bonan R: The Montreal Heart Institute experience with 76 Duromedics valves. Proceedings Second International Hemex Symposium on the Duromedics Bileaflet Valve. Austin TX, January 31– February 1, 1986. Austin TX, Hemex Scientific, 1986, pp 93–98.

109. Fontan F, Roques X, Baudet E, Deville C, Fernandez G: Is the Edwards-Duromedics bileaflet prosthesis the least thrombogenic mechanical cardiac valve. Proceedings of the Third International Symposium on the Edwards-Duromedics Bileaflet Valve. Santa Ana CA, Baxter Healthcare, 1987, pp 9–19.

110. del Vencovo A, Bertoletti G, Rabitti G, Creazzo V, Pogany G, Nesi F, D'Alessandro LC: Preliminary clinical results after valve replacement with a new bileaflet all-carbon prosthetic valve—a series of 121 patients. Proceedings of the Third International Symposium on the Edwards-Duromedics Bileaflet Valve. Santa Ana CA, Baxter Healthcare, 1987, pp 21–34.

111. Stahl E, Albrechtsson U, Olin C, Kurc HH: Clinical and cineradiographic evaluation of the Edwards-Duromedics heart valve prosthesis. Proceedings of the Third International Symposium on the Edwards-Duromedics Bileaflet Valves. Santa Ana CA, Baxter Healthcare, 1987, pp 47–53.

112. Kreuzer EK: Hemodynamic and hemolytic data of the Edwards-Duromedics bileaflet heart valve in the aortic position. Proceedings of the Third International Symposium on the Edwards-Duromedics Bileaflet Valves. Santa Ana CA, Baxter Healthcare, 1987, pp 67–76.

113. Watson DA, Dimitri WR, Jamieson M: The Edwards-Duromedics bileaflet pyrolytic carbon valve—a three center study. Proceedings of the Third International Symposium on the Edwards-Duromedics Bileaflet Valves. Santa Ana CA, Baxter Healthcare, 1987, 77–86.

114. Deuvaert FE, Van Nooten G, DePaepe J, Dernovoi B, Primo G: St. Jude Medical versus Edwards-Duromedics. Proceedings of the Third International Symposium on the Edwards-Duromedics Bileaflet Valves. Santa Ana CA, Baxter Healthcare, 1987, pp 99–115.

115. Klepetko W, Moritz A, Khunl-Brady G, Schreiner W, Schlick W, Mlczoch J, Kronik G, Wolner E: Implantation of the Duromedics bileaflet cardiac valve prosthesis in 400 patients. Ann Thorac Surg 1987;44:303–309.

116. Thevenet A, Albat B, Thevenet E: Clinical experience with the Omnicarbon® cardiac valve prosthesis. In Proceedings, 37th Congress of the European Society for Cardiovascular Surgery. Helsinki, Finland, August 3–6, 1988.

117. Brami B, Acar J, Carpentier A: Flow through mechanical heart valves and thrombosis. European Heart Journal 1983;4(Suppl.1):4.

118. Stewart JW, Sturridge MF: Haemolysis caused by tubing in extracorporeal circulation. Lancet 1959;1:340.

119. Yoganathan AP, Corcoran WH, Harrison EC: In vitro measurements in the vicinity of aortic prosthesis. J Biomechanics 1979;12:135–152.

120. Roberts WC, Morrow AG: Renal hemosiderosis in patients with prosthetic aortic valves. Circulation 1966;33:390–397.

121. Roschke EJ, Harrison EC: Fluid shear stress in prosthetic heart valves. J Biomechanics 1977;10:299–311.

122. Myhre E, Dale J, Rasmussen K: Erythrocyte destruction in different types of Starr-Edwards aortic ball valves. Circulation 1970;42:515–519.

123. Schotterfeld M, Wisheart JD, Ross JK, Lincoln JCR, Ross DN: Cloth destruction and haemolysis with totally cloth-covered Starr-Edwards prostheses. Thorax 1971;26:159–162.

124. Wukasch DC, Sandiford FM, Reul GJ, Hallman GL, Cooley DA: Complication of cloth-covered prosthetic valves: results with a new mitral prosthesis. J Thorac Cardiovasc Surg 1975;69:107–116.

125. Ahmad R, Manohitharajah SM, Deverall PB, Watson DA: Chronic hemolysis following mitral valve replacement. J Thorac Cardiovasc Surg 1976;71:212–217.

126. Lillehei CCW, Kaster RL, Coleman M, Bloch JH: Heart valve replacement with the Lillehei-Kaster pivoting disc prosthesis. NY State J Med 1974;74:1426–1438.

127. Slater SD, Sallam IH, Bain WH, Turner MA, Lawrie TDV: Haemoloysis with Björk-Shiley and Starr-Edwards prosthetic heart valves: a comparative study. Thorax 1974;29:624–632.

128. Nitter-Hauge S, Sommerfelt SC, Hall KV, Froysaker T, Efskind L: Chronic introvascular haemolysis after aortic disc valve replacement. Br Heart J 1974;36:781–785.

129. Nitter-Hauge S: Haemolysis after mitral valve replacement with the Björk-Shiley and the Lillehei-Kaster disc valve prosthesis. Brit Heart J 1976;38:977–980.

130. Henze A, Fortune RL: Regurgitation and haemolysis in artificial heart valves. Scand J Thorac Cardiovasc Surg 1974;8:167–175.

131. Moisey CU, Manohitharajah SM, Tovey LAD, Deverall PB: Haemolytic anemia in a child in association with congenital mitral valve disease. J Thorac Cardiovasc Surg 1972;63:765–769.

132. Goy JJ, Grec V, Payot M, Fischer A, Morin D, Maendly R, Sigwart U, Sadeghi H: St. Jude Medical prostheses in patients over 65 years of age. Arch Mal Couer 1985;78:1377–1382.

133. Arom KV, Nicoloff DM, Kersten TE, Lindsay WG, Northrup WF: St. Jude Medical prosthesis: valve-related death and complications. Ann Thorac Surg 1987;43:591–598.

134. Czer LSC, Matloff JM, Chaux A, DeRobertis M, Stewart ME, Gray RJ: An eight year experience with the St. Jude valve. In Rabago G, Cooley DA (eds): Heart Valve Replacement and Future Trends in Cardiac Surgery. Mount Kisco NY, Futura Publishing, 1987, pp 153–166.

135. Chiba Y, Ishihara H, Ihaya A, Kobayashi A, Akita T, Muraoka R, Yamasato A, Tatsuta N: Chronic

hemolysis after mechanical valve replacement: comparative study between St. Jude Medical valve and Omniscience valve prostheses. Nippon Kyobu Geka Gukkai Zasshi 1987;35:161–167.

136. Yamashita M, Saigenji H, Shimokawa S, Arikawa K, Morishita Y, Taira A: Severe mechanical hemolysis after valve replacement with St. Jude Medical valve—a report of five cases. Nippon Kyobu Geka Gukkai Zasshi 1986;34:2142–2146.

137. Morishita Y, Arikawa K, Yamashita M, Yuda T, Shimokawa S, Saigenji H, Hashiguchi M, Taira A: Fatal hemolysis due to unidentified cause following mitral valve replacement with bileaflet tilting disc valve prosthesis. Heart Vessels 1987;3:100–103.

138. Yoshida K, Takenchi E, Murase M, Yasuura K, Hibi M, Ogawa K, Maeda M, Abe T: Two cases of severe intravascular hemolysis after valve replacement. Kyoku Geka 1987;40:539–541.

139. Kotler MN, Mintz GS, Paeidis F, Morganroth J, Segal BL, Ross J: Noninvasive evaluation of normal and abnormal prosthetic valve function. J Am Coll Cardiol 1983;2:151–173.

140. Jones EJ: St. Jude Medical prosthesis. J Thorac Cardiovasc Surg 1981;81:642–644.

141. Narducci C, Russo L, Battaglia L, Angelica G, Giovannini E, D'Alessandro V: Dysfunction of double disc valvular prosthesis: report on five cases. Life Support Syst 1986;4(suppl 2):160–162.

142. Wolner E, Wollinek G: Hematologic alternations following valve prosthesis with Duromedics bileaflet heart valves. Proceedings Second International Hemex Symposium on the Duromedics Bileaflet Valve. Austin TX, January 31–February 1, 1986. Austin TX, Hemex Scientific, 1986, pp 9–15.

143. Watson DA, Crow MJ, Rajah SM: Intravascular hemolysis following heart valve implantation—a comparative study. Proceedings of the Second International Hemex Symposium on the Duromedics Bileaflet Valve. Austin, TX, January 31–February 1, 1986. Austin, TX, Hemex Scientific, 1986, pp 17–20.

144. Mohiuddin SM, Schultz RD, Hilleman DE, Peetz DJ Jr, Schluetar WJ, Sketch MH: Prosthetic cardiac valves: effect on blood components. Proceedings of the Second International Hemex Symposium on the Duromedics Bileaflet Valve. Austin, TX, January 31–February 1, 1986. Austin, TX, Hemex Scientific, 1986, pp 21–32.

145. Nitter-Hauge S, Dale J: High complication and failure rates of anticoagulant therapy are unavoidable. Z Kardiol 1986;75(suppl 2):293–297.

146. Fry DL: Acute vascular endothelial changes associated with increase blood velocity gradients. Circ Res 1968;22:165–197.

147. Fry DL: Certain histological and chemical responses of the vascular interface to acutely induced mechanical stresses in the aorta of the dog. Circ Res 1969;24:93–108.

148. Davila JC: Where do we go from here? In Merendino KA, Morrow AG, Lillehei CW, Muller WH (eds): Prosthetic Valves for Cardiac Surgery. Springfield IL, Charles C Thomas, 1961, pp 846–854.

149. Foster AH, Greenberg GJ, Underhill DJ, et al: Intrinsic failure of Hancock mitral bioprostheses: 10-to-15 year experience. Ann Thorac Surg 1987;44:568–577.

150. Galucci V, Bortolotti U, Milano A, et al: Isolated mitral valve replacement with the Hancock bioprothesis: a 13-year appraisal. Ann Thorac Surg 1984;38:571–578.

151. Pelletier C, Chaitman BR, Baillot R, et al: Clinical and hemodynamic results with the Carpentier porcine bioprosthesis. Am Thorac Surg 1982;34:612–624.

152. Lurie AH, Miller PR, Maxwell KS, et al: Hemodynamic assessment of the glutaraldehyde-preserved porcine heterograft in the aortic and mitral positions. Circulation 1977;56(suppl 2):104–110.

153. Ubago JL, Figueroa A, Colman T, et al: Hemodynamic factors that affect calculated orifice areas in the mitral Hancock xenograft valve. Circulation 1980;61:388–394.

154. Cotter L, Miller HC: Clinical and hemodynamic evaluation of mounted porcine heterograft in mitral position. Br Heart J 1979;41:412–417.

155. Scotten LN, Walker DK, Brownlee RT: The in vitro function of 19 mm bioprosthetic heart valves in the aortic position. Life Support Syst 1987;5:145–153.

156. Cosgrove DM, Lytte BW, Williams GW: Hemodynamic performance of the Carpentier-Edwards pericardial valve in the aortic position in vivo. Circulation 1985;72:146–152.

157. Relland J, Perier P, Lecointe B: The third generation Carpentier-Edwards bioprosthesis: early results. J Am College Cardiol 1985;6:1149–1154.

158. Wortham DC, Tri TB, Bowen TE: Hemodynamic evaluation of the St. Jude Medical valve prosthesis in the small aortic annulus. J Thorac Cardiovasc Surg 1981;81:615–620.

159. Cosgrove DM, Lytle BW, Gill CC, et al: In vivo hemodynamic comparison of porcine and pericardial valves. J Thorac Cardiovasc Surg 1985;89:358–368.

160. Gabbay S, Bortolotti U, Wasserman F, et al: Fatigue induced failure of the Ionescu-Shiley pericardial xenograft in the mitral position: in vivo and in vitro correlation and a proposed classification. J Thorac Cardiovasc Surg 1984;87:836–844.

161. Gabbay S, Factor SM, Strom J, et al: Sudden death due to cuspal dehiscence of the Ionescu-Shiley valve in the mitral position. J Thorac Cardiovasc Surg 1982;84:313–314.

162. Reul GJ, Cooley DA, Duncan JM, et al: Valve failure with the Ionescu-Shiley bovine pericardial bioprosthesis: analysis of 2680 patients. J Vasc Surg 1985;1:192–204.

163. Walley VM, Bedard P, Brais M, Keon WJ: Valve failure caused by cusp tears in low-profile Ionescu-Shiley bovine pericardial bioprosthetic valves. J Thorac Cardiovasc Surg 1987;93:583–586.

164. Ishihara T, Ferrans VJ, Boyce SW, et al: Structure and classification of cuspal tears and perforations in the porcine bioprosthetic cardiac valves implanted in patients. Am J Cardiol 1981;48:665–678.
165. Thubrika MJ, Deck JD, Aouad J, Nolan SP: Role of mechanical stress in calcification of aortic bioprosthetic valves. J Thorac Cardiovasc Surg 1983;86:115–125.
166. Webb CL, Benedict JJ, Schoen FJ, et al: Inhibition of bioprosthetic heart valve calcification with covalently bound aminopropanehydroxydiphosphonate. Trans Am Soc Artif Intern Organs 1987;33:592–595.
167. Schoen FJ, Levy RJ: Bioprosthetic heart valve failure: pathology and pathogenesis. Cardiology Clin 1984;2:717–739.
168. Levy RJ, Schoen FJ, Howard SL: Mechanism of calcification of porcine bioprosthetic aortic valve cusps: role of T-lymphocytes. Am J Cardiol 1983;52:629–631.
169. Ishihara T, Ferrans VJ, Jones M, et al: Calcific deposits developing in a bovine pericardial bioprosthetic valve 3 days after implantation. Circulation 1981;63:718.
170. Forfar JC, Cotter L, Morritt GN: Severe and early stenosis of porcine heterograft mitral valve. Br Heart J 1978;40:1184.
171. Gabbay S, Kadam P, Factor S, Cheung TK: Do heart valve bioprostheses degenerate for metabolic or mechanical reasons? J Thorac Cardiovasc Surg 1988;95:208–215.
172. Thomson FJ: Progress report on the development of a flexible stent for heart valve homograft. Report No. 132 M76/5, School of Engineering, University of Auckland, New Zealand, 1976.
173. Thubrikar M, Bosher LP, Nolan SP: The mechanism of opening of the aortic valve. J Thorac Cardiovasc Surg 1979;77:867–870.
174. Thubrikar M, Piepgrass WC, Deck JD, Nolan SP: Stresses of natural versus prosthetic aortic valve leaflets in vivo. Ann Thorac Surg 1980;30:230–239.
175. Morse D, Steiner RM: Cardiac valve identification atlas and guide. In Morse D (ed): Guide to Prosthetic Cardiac Valves. New York, Springer-Verlag, 1985, pp 292, 294–297, 330–331.
176. Fernandez J: Surgical aspects of valve implantation. In Morse D (ed): Guide to Prosthetic Cardiac Valves. New York, Springer-Verlag, 1985, pp 138–143, 147–150.
177. Broom ND, Thomson FJ: Influence of fixation conditions on the performance of glutaraldehyde-treated porcine aortic valves: towards a more scientific basis. Thorax 1979;34:166–176.
178. Sauren AAHJ, van Hout MC, van Steenhaven AA, Veldpaus FE, Janssen JD: The mechanical properties of porcine aortic valve tissue. J Biomechanics 1983;16:327–337.
179. Rousseau EPM, Sauren AAHJ, van Hout MC, van Steenhaven AA: Elastic and viscoelastic material behavior of fresh and glutaraldehyde-treated porcine aortic valve tissue. J Biomechanics 1983;16:339–348.
180. Gabbay S, Bortolotti U, Cipolletti G, Wasserman F, Frater RWM, Factor SM: The Meadox unicusp pericardial bioprosthetic heart valve: new concept. Ann Thorac Surg 1984;37:448–456.
181. Wheatley DJ, Fisher J, Reece IJ, Spyt T, Breeze P: Primary tissue failure in pericardial heart valves. J Thorac Cardiovasc Surg 1987;94:367–374.
182. Walley VM, Keon WJ: Patterns of failure in Ionescu-Shiley bovine pericardial bioprosthetic valves. J Thorac Cardiovasc Surg 1987;93:925–933.
183. Rainer WG: In discussion: Cosgrove DM, Lytle BW, Gill CC, et al: In vivo hemodynamic comparison of porcine and pericardial valves. J Thorac Cardiovasc Surg 1985;89:358–368.
184. Goffin YA, Bartik MA: Porcine aortic versus bovine pericardial valves: a comparative study of unimplanted and from patient explanted bioprostheses. Life Support Syst 1987;5:127–143.

Bodnar, E. and Frater, R. W. M., editors
(1991) *Replacement Cardiac Valves,*
Pergamon Press, Inc. (New York), pp. 357–381
Printed in the United States of America

CHAPTER 15

MATERIALS CONSIDERATIONS FOR IMPROVED CARDIAC VALVE PROSTHESES

FREDERICK J. SCHOEN, ROBERT J. LEVY, BUDDY D. RATNER, MICHAEL D. LELAH, AND GRANT W. CHRISTIE

This chapter summarizes some evolving issues related to the biomaterials that compose present heart valve prostheses and those under consideration. The objective is to provide both the foundation for understanding observed and potential complications of biological and synthetic prostheses and principles to guide development of improved and novel valve materials and designs.

BIOLOGICAL TISSUE

Structure and Function of the Native Aortic Valve

The natural aortic valve allows the unidirectional passage of blood with optimal hemodynamics (no obstruction or regurgitation) without causing areas of localized stress concentration within the tissue, trauma to molecular or formed blood elements, or thrombotic complications. Aortic valve cusps must also close under minimal reverse pressure to ensure that the closed valve is fully competent throughout diastole. Although the pressure differential across the closed valve induces a large load on the leaflets, the fibrous arrangement within the leaflets assists in transferring the resultant stresses to the aortic annulus.

The aortic valve achieves the basic requirements of valvular function by means of a highly specialized and complex structure. There are three major layers: (a) the *fibrosa* on the outflow side, composed predominantly of circumferentially aligned, microscopically crimped collagen fibers, (b) the *ventricularis* on the inflow side, composed predominantly of elastin and collagen, without any distinct directional alignment, and (c) the *spongiosa,* between the two fibrous layers, which has a large content of mucopolysaccharide (1–3). The spongiosa has only negligible structural strength but appears to perform important roles in minimizing mechanical interaction (i.e., lubricating relative movement) between the two fibrous layers, and dissipating energy during closure. Aortic valve cusps have highly anisotropic material properties in the plane of the tissue (i.e., the properties are not the same in all directions); this reflects an oriented leaflet tissue architecture (4). A consistently observable feature of fibrosa morphology is the presence of corrugations that produce a grossly visible surface rippling, whose function is unknown but probably significant. The ridges of the corrugations are approximately parallel to the collagen fiber bundles in the fibrosa. The fibrosa and spongiosa have approximately equal cell density (5).

The major stresses in the aortic valve cusps are circumferential, as determined by detailed stress analysis (6–8). Collagen crimp, whose ridges are perpendicular to the long axis of the collagen bundles, enables the leaflets to be extremely soft and pliable when unloaded but virtually inextensible when pressure is applied; exaggerated sag of the leaflet centers is prevented when the valve is shut, thereby preserving maximum coaptation. Straightening of the crimp accounts for the majority of circumferential compliance. The tissue compliance in the radial direction (i.e., perpendicular to the free margin) is very much greater than that in the circumferential direction (i.e., fibrosa offers little mechanical resistance to radial extension) (2). The stresses in the radial direction during normal valve function are very small; the large radial stretches in excess of those that could be accounted for by collagen crimp are derived from the soft but highly and reversibly compliant elastin (6). Elastin in the ventricularis enables the leaflet to have minimal surface area when the valve is open but still stretch to form a large coaptation area when back pressure is applied.

The coaptation area of the natural aortic valve represents approximately 50% of the loaded leaflet surface area (9). The coaptation area of the leaflet is structurally weaker, is physically thinner (except close to the central nodulus Aranti at the free edge, which is thickened by repeated compression), and has less collagen than the load-bearing area (2). The circumferential alignment of the collagen fiber array in the fibrosa ensures that excessive stress is not concentrated at the commissures, provided that normal coaptation is maintained. However, the stresses in the cusps at the valve commissures increase sharply with decreasing coaptation area, or with decreasing anisotropy of the leaflet material (tending toward isotropic, i.e., same properties in all directions), as discussed below (6).

Fixation with Glutaraldehyde

Chemical Effects

The goals of aldehyde pretreatment of bioprosthetic tissue are enhanced material stability and decreased antigenicity, with maintained thromboresistance and preserved antimicrobial sterility. Glutaraldehyde (1,5-pentanedialdehyde) has been used since antiquity for the tanning of leather and more recently as a fixative in the preparation of tissues for electron microscopy (10). Studies of the chemical reactions of glutaraldehyde and formaldehyde with tissues led to the use of aortic valve xenografts pretreated with these reagents as cardiac bioprosthetic valves (11–13). However, formaldehyde-pretreated bioprostheses frequently developed primary material failures (14, 15), presumably due to the instability of formaldehyde-derived, methylene-based cross-links (16). Therefore, glutaraldehyde has replaced formaldehyde for bioprosthesis preparation, chiefly because of the superior stability of glutaraldehyde-pretreated bioprosthetic tissue.

Chemical reactions of glutaraldehyde with tissue result in the cross-linking of proteins, especially collagen (17, 18), the most abundant structural protein of both porcine aortic valves (19) and bovine pericardium (20). In both tissues, type I collagen predominates, with lesser amounts of type III also present (19, 20). The chemical interactions of glutaraldehyde with collagen and other proteins involve reactions of the aldehyde functions with protein-bound amines, yielding inter- and intramolecular cross-links (16–18). Glutaraldehyde reacts rapidly with tissue proteins; after only 30 min, half the maximal amount of glutaraldehyde is incorporated, while plateau levels are reached by 18 h (20). Maximal thermal stability is noted by 4 h of incubation (16). Moreover, in contrast to formaldehyde-induced cross-links, glutaraldehyde–tissue protein reaction products are stable after long-term storage (16, 21). Interestingly, glutaraldehyde pretreatment of bioprosthetic tissue appears to potentiate cuspal calcification (22, 23), but the mechanism responsible for this effect is incompletely understood. Since homograft valves that are not chemically cross-linked also calcify, the specific role of glutaraldehyde is uncertain (24).

There has been little research into bioprosthetic tissue preservatives alternative to aldehydes. Glycerol, a compound previously used to preserve erythrocytes and spermatozoa during frozen storage (25), has been used to prepare homologous dura mater valves (26, 27). However, failure rates have been high, particularly due to cuspal tears and endocarditis (28, 29). Interestingly, pathologic examination suggests that not only is calcification of dura less than that of other bioprosthetic materials, but also that remodeling of glycerol-preserved dura may take place. However, it is possible that glycerol treatment does not maintain complete sterilization at room temperature. Polyepoxy compounds have recently been considered for use as xenograft tissue cross-linking agents and are purported to reduce antigenicity without altering mechanical properties (30).

Mechanical Effects

The functional and mechanical characteristics of the natural aortic valve and other tissues used in bioprostheses are altered by glutaraldehyde cross-linking procedures (Fig. 15-1) (31–35). Fixed tissue has different mechanical properties than fresh tissue. Nevertheless, while some studies suggest that freely fixed aortic valve tissue has diminished compliance relative to fresh tissue (2), other studies suggest that both porcine valve (34) and bovine pericardial tissue (35) have increased distensibility following fixation.

Moreover, during glutaraldehyde-induced cross-linking, the aortic valve is usually preloaded by a hydrostatic back pressure, which locks the valve structure into a geometric

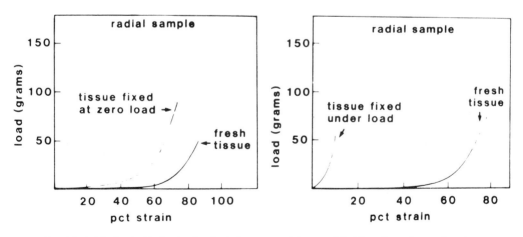

FIG. 15–1. Mechanical behavior (load–strain response) from radial strips of porcine aortic valve cusps before and following fixation (left) in fully relaxed state and (right) in loaded state. Reproduced with permission from Broom N, Christie GW: The structure–function relationship of fresh and glutaraldehyde fixed aortic valve leaflets. In Cohn LH, Gallucci V (eds): Cardiac Bioprostheses. New York, Yorke Medical Publishers, 1983, pp 476–491.

configuration characteristic of diastole. When the fibrosa is loaded with back pressure, the crimp waveform in the circumferential direction is fully straightened (31, 32). Locking the fibrosa in this position by fixation maintains the leaflet in its fully extended state thereafter, virtually without elastic extensibility. Thus, following fixation under back pressure, the natural collagen crimp is permanently lost and the leaflet surface area is near maximal even when the load is removed. Porcine valve or bovine pericardial leaflets fixed under load are relatively stiff and inflexible and have poor hemodynamic function and high propensity toward tissue fatigue at points of sharp bending (31, 33, 34).

The effects of glutaraldehyde interactions with elastin and ground-substance components are not certain, but evidence suggests that although the mechanical properties of elastin-rich tissues are altered by glutaraldehyde, some elasticity is retained (36–38). It may be expected, therefore, that fixation of aortic valves with glutaraldehyde under a hydrostatic back pressure, even at pressures as low as 2 mmHg, completely fixes the collagen component of the leaflet in a fully stretched state, but partially retains elasticity (39). The mechanical properties of the leaflets are improved when fixation occurs without any back pressure (31, 39).

Tissue mechanical properties may be further altered during function in vivo. Tissue obtained from explanted pericardial valves is thicker and less extensible than unimplanted tissue (40). The chemical and mechanical effects of interactions of blood with bioprosthetic tissue are largely unknown.

Prevention of Calcification of Bioprosthetic Valves

Calcification is the major pathologic feature contributory to clinical bioprosthetic valve failure (41, 42). Therefore, considerable work is being directed toward elucidation of mechanisms of bioprosthetic valve mineralization and methods for eliminating this problem.

The clinical implications and pathobiology of bioprosthetic valve calcification are discussed in detail elsewhere in this volume (24). Key characteristics of valve mineralization relevant to the potential prevention of calcification-associated valve failures include the following: (1) Calcification begins primarily in cells and cell fragments residual in the bioprosthetic tissue, while collagen involvement occurs subsequently (43, 44). (2) The phosphorus necessary for nucleation of calcific crystals is probably initially present in the bioprosthetic tissue. (3) Calcification occurs in a complex environment whose critical elements include only a susceptible substrate in a permissive chemical milieu; thus, alterations in these influences (implant and host factors) could be beneficial. (4) Functional mechanical deformation potentiates but is not a prerequisite for calcification. These four pathologic features give direction to efforts toward inhibiting bioprosthetic valve calcification. Moreover, since almost all valves removed for calcific failure have at least 10 to 20 times the amount of calcium present in normal bioprosthetic valve tissue (45), less than absolute prevention of accumulation of calcific deposits could make a significant clinical impact.

The several approaches under investigation to reduce the problem of calcific bioprosthetic valve failure focus on one or more of the host, implant, and mechanical determinants of the mineralization process. One strategy is to understand critical early events and ongoing steps in the mineralization process, and subsequently to block one or more of these processes. Although considerable insight has been gained by directed research into pathogenesis, useful direct application of this concept awaits the further elucidation of the earliest key pathophysiologic phenomena.

Design changes have been purported to enhance durability through lowering mechanical stress (46–48). Moreover, pretreatment of bioprosthetic valve leaflets with detergent compounds may inhibit their calcification by removing nucleation sites from the substrate. Pretreatment for 24 h in a 1% sodium dodecyl sulfate (SDS) solution, which removes over 80% of tissue phospholipids, considered to be related to initial membrane-based nucleation sites (24, 49), also significantly inhibits calcification of porcine valve tissue implanted subcutaneously in rats (50). However, other experimental results using orthotopic and conduit-mounted valve replacements treated with various surfactants have shown inconsistent efficacy (51–56). This is possibly due to reaccumulation of blood-borne components, which could negate the advantage of phospholipid extraction or charge modification, the probable modes of calcification inhibition by detergents such as SDS. Some studies suggest that this approach might be useful for porcine valves, but not for valves fabricated from bovine pericardium (53, 56). Moreover, the extent to which cuspal structural integrity could be compromised by detergent exposure has not been carefully studied. Nevertheless, SDS pretreatment is used in the preparation of porcine valves (Hancock II, Medtronic, Inc.), now in clinical trials. Cuspal incorporation of polyacrylamide (52) and charge modification by protamine (57) have also been investigated.

An alternative strategy employs exogenous mineralization inhibitors. Diphosphonate compounds are potent inhibitors of physiologic and pathologic calcification, which act through retardation of calcium-phosphate crystal growth, and are therefore used for the therapy of metabolic bone disease (50, 58). However, these compounds can have severe and irreversible adverse effects on bone and calcium metabolism, including growth inhibition and disruption of bone architecture, when circulating concentrations are high (58–61). Thus, although mineralization of bovine pericardial valves implanted in calves and porcine aortic valve cusps subcutaneously implanted in growing rats is inhibited by systemically administered ethanehydroxy diphosphonate (EHDP), retarded bone and somatic growth complicate the therapy. A dose of 10 mg of EHDP per kilogram per day in rats yields significant inhibition of calcification (approximately 15% of control in 21 days) with an absence of adverse effects, but doses necessary for complete inhibition produce skeletal growth disturbance (Fig. 15–2) (61). Delayed-onset therapy is not effective unless initiated within 48 h of implantation and maintained indefinitely (61). Therapy begun following 1 week of implantation is totally ineffective (61).

Alternatively, incorporation of EHDP into controlled-release drug delivery polymers, such as ethylene vinylacetate or polydimethylsiloxane [both highly compatible polymers approved by the Food and Drug Administration (FDA) for clinical use], results in slow-release drug delivery systems that, when implanted adjacent to an experimental bioprosthetic leaflet implant, profoundly inhibit leaflet calcification with no adverse effects (Table 15–1) (62–64). By using mixtures of the highly soluble sodium and less-soluble calcium salts of EHDP, it has been possible to achieve extrapolated release durations exceeding 30 years. Using this direct route, the total amount of drug required to inhibit valve calcification is 100 times less than that needed by daily injection. In ongoing work with EHDP drug delivery systems, a modified bioprosthetic valve sewing ring configuration incorporating a drug release matrix is being investigated in mitral valve replacements in sheep (Fig. 15–3). The drug release matrix would be seated adjacent to and in contact with the lateral aortic wall of the prosthesis; it would not extend to the portion

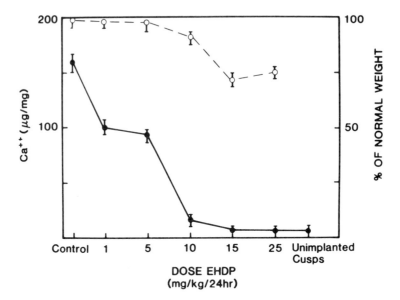

FIG. 15-2. The ethanehydroxy diphosphonate (EHDP) dose-response relationship for the inhibition of calcification of rat (21-day-old males) subcutaneous implants (21 days duration) of bovine pericardium used in bioprosthetic heart valves. Calcium concentration is plotted as mean ± SEM. The EHDP effects on growth are plotted as percentage of normal weight comparing EHDP-treated mean weights (± SEM) when the rat was killed with those of the corresponding control group. Reproduced with permission from Levy RJ, Schoen FJ, Lund SA, Smith MS: Prevention of leaflet calcification of bioprosthetic heart valves with diphosphonate injection therapy. Experimental studies of optimal doses and therapeutic durations. J Thorac Cardiovasc Surg 1987;94:551–557. Copyright 1987, CV Mosby Company.

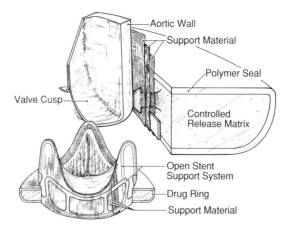

FIG. 15-3. Schematic diagram of proposed porcine aortic valve bioprosthesis incorporating local drug release of diphosphonates or other efficacious compounds by a controlled-release matrix.

TABLE 15–1. *Inhibition of Bioprosthetic Tissue Calcification by EHDP Controlled Release from Biocompatible Matrices**

	Calcium, μg/mg
20% EHDP in ethylene vinyl acetate	1.0 ± 0.1‡
No EHDP in ethylene vinyl acetate (control)	169.8 ± 8.7
30% EHDP in Silastic 382	
All-sodium EHDP	2.3 ± 0.5
50:50, sodium EHDP:calcium EHDP	4.2 ± 0.9
All-calcium EHDP	34.7 ± 14.5
No EHDP in Silastic 382 (control)	160.0 ± 9.1

*60-day subcutaneous implants of bovine pericardium adjacent to controlled-release matrix. EHDP = 1,1-hydroxyethylidene diphosphonate (ethanehydroxy diphosphonate).

†Mean ± SEM, n = 10.

‡Data from Ref. 63 and 64.

of the sewing ring that would be punctured by sutures used to seat the valve in the annulus. Studies intended to optimize the drug-matrix system are in progress, with particular attention directed toward (1) concentration and molecular form of the drug in the polymer matrix necessary for efficacy, (2) optimization and control of release rate and duration, (3) matrix mechanical stability during washout, and (4) blood–material interactions and other local and systemic biocompatibility concerns.

Cuspal preloading of anticalcification agents may provide an important adjunct to localized controlled-release therapy. Aminopropanehydroxydiphosphonate (APDP) inhibits bioprosthetic valve leaflet calcification when covalently bound to residual aldehyde functions in cuspal tissue. Calcification inhibition is directly related to the amount of APDP incorporated, with mineralization less than 15% of control (in 21 days) when >30 nm of bound APDP per milligram of tissue is present (Fig. 15–4) (65). No adverse

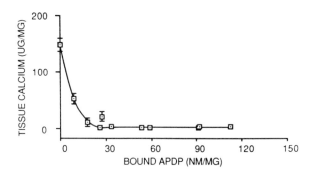

FIG. 15–4. Anticalcification effects of bound APDP. As higher levels of APDP were bound, calcification of 21-day-old rat (3-week-old male CD) subdermal bioprosthetic leaflet implants was inhibited to a greater degree. At ≥ 30 nmol/mg bound APDP, levels of tissue calcium were equivalent to those of unimplanted tissue. APDP = aminopropanehydroxy diphosphonate. NM/MG = nanomoles per milligram; UG/MG = micrograms per milligram. Reproduced with permission from Webb CL, Benedict JJ, Schoen FJ, Linden JA, Levy RJ: Inhibition of bioprosthetic heart valve calcification with aminodiphosphonate covalently bound to residual aldehyde groups. Ann Thorac Surg 1988;46:309–316.

TABLE 15–2. *Chemical Approaches to Inhibit Bioprosthetic Valve Calcification*

Specific approach*	References
Systemic diphosphonates (EHDP)	59–61
Cuspal modification	
Detergents (SDS and Tween 80)	50–56
Protamine	57
Cuspal Incorporation	
Diphosphonates (EHDP and APDP)	60,66
Aluminum	68
Localized Therapy	
Osmotic minipumps releasing diphosphonates (EHDP)	59
Controlled-release matrices loaded with diphosphonates (EHDP)	62–64

*EHDP = ethanehydroxy diphosphonate; SDS = sodium dodecyl sulfate; APDP = aminopropanehydroxy diphosphonate.

effects related to cuspal diphosphonates have been noted. Moreover, calcification is inhibited in bioprosthetic tissue preloaded with EHDP by precipitating this compound within the tissue as the calcium salt (66).

It has recently been discovered that cuspal incubation in solutions of the trivalent ion of aluminum (Al^{3+}), an element associated with osteomalacia in renal dialysis patients (67), markedly inhibits calcification of subcutaneously implanted bioprosthetic tissue in the rat at extremely low preincubation concentrations (0.001 M) (68). Calcification of non-glutaraldehyde-treated rat homograft aorta (which, in contrast to porcine valve, bovine pericardium, and purified type I collagen preparations, calcifies in subcutaneous implants without glutaraldehyde pretreatment) is also prevented by incubation in either $AlCl_3$ or APDP. Furthermore, cuspal pretreatment with Al^{3+} is not associated with any detectable aluminum-related adverse effects. It is conceivable that limited-duration Al^{3+} exposure may suffice for long-term inhibition of bioprosthetic tissue calcification.

Chemical approaches toward prevention of bioprosthetic valve calcification that have been studied are summarized in Table 15–2. The most potent and practical single method appears to be controlled-release disphosphonate therapy. An optimally effective strategy could use combinations of inhibitory effects, which might typically involve either diphosphonate, detergent, or aluminum cuspal pretreatment, in conjunction with long-term localized controlled release of diphosphonates. Furthermore, a future goal of research in this area would be therapeutic interventions that could arrest or reverse ongoing pathologic calcification in conventional bioprosthetic valves implanted prior to the availability of inhibitory therapies.

Pericardial Tissue as Leaflet Material

Pericardial tissue, used as a material for the construction of bioprosthetic heart valve leaflets, differs from aortic valve leaflet material in that (1) it has approximately isotropic elastic properties in the plane of the tissue, and (2) the cross-section is not as clearly differentiated into distinct structural layers that have different mechanical properties (69). Since, as previously discussed, highly anisotropic elasticity is the major structural property of aortic valve leaflets that promotes leaflet coaptation, anatomically appropriate leaflet shape is not in itself sufficient to ensure good coaptation, uniform distribution of stress, and satisfactory valve function (2, 6). In general, pericardial tissue with uniform thickness, uniform fibrous organization, and high-percentage collagen content is considered most desirable for use as valve leaflets.

Stress can be transmitted in any direction in isotropic, homogeneous pericardial leaflets, in contrast to anisotropic aortic leaflets, in which stress is transmitted primarily along the circumferentially aligned collagen fibers. Therefore, stress in pericardial leaflet valves will be directed toward the natural mechanical focal point, the commissures, leading to high stress concentrations at that site not encountered in the natural valve. Maximizing the coaptation area will reduce, but not eliminate, the intensity of commissural stress concentrations. Thus, decreasing the high ratio of radial to circumferential compliance normally existing in the aortic valve (i.e., tending toward a more isotropic material) leads to a decreased coaptation area and an increased stress magnitude near the commissures. Introduction of holes in the tissue at sutures used for commissural tissue coaptation and attachment (i.e., alignment sutures) exacerbates stress concentrations that occur during leaflet flexure. Therefore, it is not surprising that cuspal tearing at the top of the stent post is a common mode of pericardial valve failure (70–72). These considerations of leaflet attachment and the functional role of cuspal isotropy are also relevant to polymeric leaflet valves and other isotropic fibrous tissues considered for valves (e.g., fascia lata, dura mater). Moreover, pericardial valves calcify similarly to porcine valves (20). Biological valves constructed of other isotropic collagenous tissues, including variously treated fascia lata and dura mater, have not been successful because of cuspal tearing, and, in some cases, calcification and fibrosis, with shrinkage and loss of pliability (73–75).

Pericardium also has the property that repeated loading causes *dynamic creep* of this viscoelastic material, progressively stretching the tissue and leading to permanent leaflet deformation (which has been called *sagging*), which can contribute to valvular incompetence (Fig. 15–5). The effect of tissue elongation on leaflet geometry and coaptation

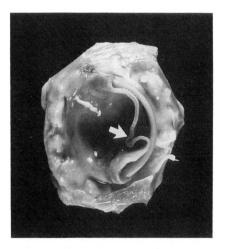

FIG. 15–5. Severe cuspal stretching and redundancy of pericardium (arrow) in novel unileaflet pericardial bioprosthetic valve implanted in sheep. Reproduced by permission from Schemin RJ, Schoen FJ, Hein R, Austin J, Cohn LH: Hemodynamic and pathologic evaluation of a unileaflet pericardial bioprosthetic valve. J Thorac Cardiovasc Surg 1988;95:912–919. Copyright 1988, CV Mosby Company.

must be considered in the design development of pericardial valves. Neither the cause nor the potential clinical importance of pericardial stretching is known. However, a recent study demonstrated heterogeneity in mechanical properties of tissue among sites within a pericardial sac; one particular site had both increased distensibility and a reduced content of elastic tissue (35). Although the role of elastin in the mechanical properties of pericardium is unknown, such studies raise important issues related to tissue selection for bioprosthetic valves.

The results of an experimental study of a novel unileaflet pericardial bioprosthesis (the Meadox-Gabbay unileaflet bioprosthesis, characterized by a single large pericardial cusp that in closing meets a pericardium-covered flexible Delrin stent), implanted as mitral and tricuspid replacements in sheep for 3 to 5 months, emphasize the progressive degradative processes that can occur in pericardial valves (76). Intrinsic cuspal calcification was prominent, particularly at the linear attachments of the mobile cusp to the fixed strut. The stationary pericardial covering of the fixed strut had minimal and focal intrinsic microscopic calcification, primarily limited to sites of compression of the tissue adjacent to sutures anchoring the covering to the plastic frame. Almost all valves had some degree of stretching and redundancy of the mobile cusp, particularly at its free edge, more prominently in mitral than in tricuspid replacements. In some cases, cuspal deformation was probably sufficient to cause valvular incompetence, without prolapse of the mobile cusp. This study, as others, suggests that the limitations to the durability of glutaraldehyde-pretreated pericardial valves are multifactorial, including generalized functional stresses, predisposition to high mechanical stresses near the stent posts, specific design inadequacies, underlying material characteristics, and changes induced by the host environment, including fluid insudation, evolving mechanical properties, and calcification. This study, as well as others (50), demonstrated that pericardial tissue can undergo deep penetration by inflammatory cells and subsequent inflammatory architectural destruction, particularly at the edges of pericardium cut during valve fabrication. The significance of noninfective inflammation is unknown.

The superimposition of mechanical and biological factors in valve deterioration suggests that in vitro accelerated testing, although highlighting some specific modes of failure and design flaws, will virtually always overestimate the fatigue life of a bioprosthetic valve. Moreover, such studies potentially fail to reveal the nature of important mechanisms of dysfunction due to materials degeneration that depend on an interaction with host biological processes.

SYNTHETIC MATERIALS

The wide range of manufactured materials that have been used in heart valve prostheses is listed in Table 15–3. This section summarizes considerations related to the most widely used synthetic materials and proposals for improved valve materials.

Pyrolytic Carbon Valves

Most mechanical heart valve prostheses currently in use have carbon occluders, and some have both carbon occluders and carbon cage components. Thromboresistance, high strength, wear resistance, and ability to be fabricated into a wide variety of shapes render pyrolytic carbon advantageous as a material for construction of heart valve components (77–79). The wide use of pyrolytic carbon as an occluder and strut-covering

TABLE 15–3. *Materials Used in Synthetic Heart Valve Prostheses*

Rigid Mechanical Valves
    Stellite 21 (alloy of Co, Cr, Mo, and Ni)
    Titanium
    Stainless steel
    Ceramic (alumina)
    Silicone rubber
    Delrin (polyoxymethylene)
    Polytetrafluoroethylene (Teflon)
    Polyester (Dacron)
    Pyrolytic carbon coatings
Flexible Trileaflet Valves
    Polyurethanes
    Polypropylene
    Polytetrafluoroethylene (Teflon)
    Silicone rubber
    Hexsyn (copolymer of 1-hexene and methyl hexadiene)
    Composite materials

material for mechanical valve prostheses has virtually eliminated abrasive wear as a long-term complication of cardiac valve replacement. Contemporary tilting disk designs (either single disk or double hemidisk) with pyrolytic carbon have generally good durability with minimal abrasion of metallic or carbon occluder cage components, but rare fractures of valve components have been reported (42). The following is a brief discussion of the relevant materials science of carbons, intended to highlight the advantages and limitations of this unique class of materials.

Carbon occurs naturally in organic molecules, as relatively amorphous coal, as partially crystalline graphite, and as more highly crystalline diamond. Poorly crystalline carbons may be synthesized by three major processes: (1) by decomposing a gaseous hydrocarbon at elevated temperatures in a specialized furnace (the fluidized bed) leading to the type of pyrolytic carbons used in clinical heart valves, (2) by baking a preformed polymeric body to drive off all noncarbonaceous elements (a process that forms vitreous or glassy carbon), or (3) by deposition of a carbon vapor in a vacuum at ambient temperatures. Pyrolytic carbons have achieved the most widespread clinical use, largely because the structure and properties of these materials may be carefully tailored to yield favorable biological and physical properties.

Pyrolytic carbon is generally deposited as a coating on heat-resistant substrates, such as graphite or metal, preformed to the desired configuration. Thus, pyrolytic carbon components of medical devices are usually composite structures, consisting of a substrate material with a carbon coating less than 1 mm thick (Fig. 15–6). Control of the conditions of deposition leads to a predictable structure and properties of the carbon deposit; moreover, introduction of other elements into the gas and their codeposition with carbon, (e.g., silicon) enhances the mechanical properties (80). Although the as-deposited surface of pyrolytic carbon is rough, because of the deposition mechanism, which involves precipitation of carbon droplets from the gas, cardiovascular application generally requires a smooth surface; thus, most carbon device components are polished.

The bulk structure of pyrolytic carbon is best understood by comparing and contrasting it with that of graphite crystals (77, 79). In graphite, the carbon atoms are linked together by strong covalent bonds to form large, planar, hexagonal arrays, with nearly

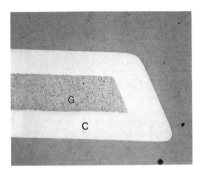

FIG. 15-6. Cross-section of pyrolytic carbon disk of bileaflet tilting disk valve. This illustration shows that pyrolytic carbon (C) is applied as a coating to a graphite (G) substrate. Magnification approximately 50×. Illustration courtesy of CarboMedics, Inc., Austin, TX.

perfect three-dimensional orientation of the layers. The overall structure and resultant properties are highly anisotropic. In contrast, pyrolytic carbon is composed of microscopic crystallites with imperfect layer planes facilitating cross-links among layers and groups of layers. The crystallites are randomly oriented; thus, the aggregate has almost completely isotropic properties.

Carbons have an unusual combination of mechanical properties: high fracture strength with relatively low modulus of elasticity (i.e., stiffness), and high toughness (77–79). Unlike deterioration of metals, polymers, and some ceramics, progressive deterioration of pyrolytic carbon does not occur on cyclic loading (i.e., carbons do not fail in fatigue (81–83). Wear resistance is excellent; carbon-bearing-on-carbon systems, especially for the hardest carbon surfaces (strongest carbons), have superior wear resistance to that obtained with carbon-metal systems (84).

Smooth, polished pyrolytic carbons have excellent blood compatibility and high thromboresistance (85, 86). Studies indicate that many surfaces that are compatible with blood have low surface energies (< 30 dyn/cm) (87) (such low energy surfaces are called *hydrophobic,* since they do not wet easily). Despite its relatively high surface energy in the freshly prepared, clean, polished state (approximately 50 dyn/cm), carbon develops an altered surface that has a surface energy of 30 dyn/cm following exposure to blood for a short period of time (86). Thus, the interaction of a smooth, polished pyrolytic carbon with blood generates a low-reactivity blood–material interface, by a mechanism as yet poorly understood.

Fabrication or cost constraints may discourage the use of pyrolytic carbons under certain circumstances. For example, the relatively high temperatures required for deposition of conventional pyrolytic carbons (> 1000°C) prevent the use of this material as a coating for polymeric substrates for flexible valve prostheses. Nevertheless, by the use of vacuum techniques, structurally analogous carbons may be deposited onto a substrate that is maintained at relatively low, near-ambient temperatures, and tailored to give useful structures. The coatings are generally very thin (0.5–1.0 μm) (88). Nevertheless, some vapor-deposited coatings have properties equivalent to those of the typical pyrolytic carbons, including favorable thromboresistance (89). While such coatings have not yet been used on polymeric heart valves, they have been used to coat clinical heart valve sewing rings and experimental vascular grafts (90).

Porous Metal Surfaces

Original attempts to reduce the thromboembolic complications of caged-poppet heart valve prostheses by covering the stents with porous material that would encourage the progressive formation of a thromboresistant endothelialized tissue layer led to unfavorable results, because of cloth fragmentation, particularly in the harsh mechanical environment of the aortic valve location (91). On the other hand, tilting disk valve struts with a microporous metallic alloy (Haynes 25) coating support the formation of a smooth, stable tissue covering that resists fragmentation (92). Recent studies using mitral orthotopic tilting disk valves in goats yielded favorable results, suggesting further consideration of this concept.

Ceramics in Cardiac Valves

The most promising ceramic for use in heart valve prostheses is alumina (aluminum oxide, Al_2O_3), because of its strength, fracture toughness, and ability to support a stable, adherent tissue covering under some circumstances (93). A twin-flap mitral valve was constructed from a porous alumina frame and Delrin hemidisk (93). The alumina of the valve housing was essentially the same as that used in hip joint prostheses, previously demonstrated to develop an adherent tissue coating. The porosity of the ceramic was augmented by including short strands of an organic flock filler with the alumina powder to be sintered. On firing, these strands were burned away, leaving long, randomly connected pores, intended to enhance tissue adherence. Prototype valves of this type implanted in minipigs failed because of thrombotic complications initiated on the Delrin, while the ceramic supported a fine, firmly fibrous adherent tissue layer. This tissue was noted to be similar to other types of fibrous tissue overgrowth on valves. A later study, using a modification of this valve with alumina occluders as well as housing yielded results favorable to those of a control Björk-Shiley valve (93). Nevertheless, the long-term performance of alumina valves remains to be determined. Although ordinary higher-density medical-grade alumina supports static tissue overgrowth, whether tissue adhesion can withstand the shear stresses in the vicinity of a valve prosthesis is unknown. Dense alumina has good wear resistance, but that of porous alumina is less good (94). A tilting disk ceramic valve with a single crystal alumina disk and titanium nitride (TiN) cage has shown good blood compatibility, durability, and hemodynamics in preliminary in vitro and in vivo studies (95).

Polymers for Flexible Leaflet Valves

Heart valve constructions with polymeric leaflets having functional characteristics similar to those of natural human cardiac valves are appealing for use as low-cost and efficient orthotopic replacement valves as well as valves for total artificial heart or ventricular assist systems. However, near-anatomic, central-flow trileaflet prostheses using synthetic polymers, developed originally more than two decades ago, were not successful due to tearing and calcification of the cusps (96–100). More recently, as a result of major developments in the technology of polymeric materials, and better understanding of the interaction of polymeric materials with biological tissue, there has been a reconsideration of the use of polymeric leaflet heart valves (Fig. 15–7). The polyurethanes, in particular, allow considerable latitude in design and construction. The use of polymeric leaflets in

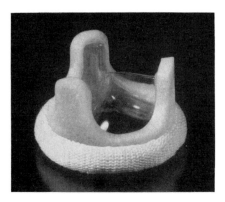

FIG. 15–7. Prototype polyurethane flexible trileaflet synthetic heart valve prosthesis. Illustration courtesy of Biocontrol Technology, Indiana, Pa.

cardiac valve construction will be examined below, with particular emphasis on the role of material characteristics on performance.

Polyurethanes

Polyurethanes have been investigated in numerous heart valve configurations (101–110) and have been used widely in other medical devices, including pacemaker leads, total artificial hearts, and heart-assist devices, catheters, and experimental vascular prostheses (111–115). The interest in polyurethanes for trileaflet heart valves stems largely from the favorable mechanical properties of these materials, especially their elastomeric behavior and their high tensile strength, low stress relaxation, and their resistance to fatigue failure, despite long-term cyclic loading. However, the resistance to biodegradation, calcification, and blood compatibility of polyurethanes are important current problematic issues that impair rapid progress toward clinically useful flexible leaflet valves.

The general scheme for the synthesis of polyurethanes of the type commonly used in biomedical applications is shown in Fig. 15–8. The mechanical properties of the thermoplastic elastomeric polyurethanes derive from a phase separation (domain formation), which divides the polymer into *soft segments* (polyester, polyether, or polyalkyldiol) contributing to the elastomeric behavior, and *hard segments* (urethane or urethane-urea), which noncovalently cross-link the polymer and add mechanical strength and toughness. These segments form a two-phase microstructure with the hard segment dispersed into domains 5 to 10 nm in size, in a matrix of soft segments (Fig. 15–9). The soft and hard segments combine to form a virtually infinite family of block copolymers of molecular weight about 20,000 to 1,000,000 (Fig. 15–10). The hard domains act as multifunctional cross-linking sites, and as reinforcing fillers. Within the large range of molecular weight and molar ratios of reactants possible for each segment, a broad range of physical properties can be engineered.

Many types of polymers can be classified under the generic name *polyurethane*. The materials of most interest for biomedical applications are segmented block copolyurethanes with polyether and urethane components (*polyetherurethanes,* PEUs). A wide range of polymers can be classified under the PEU designation and have been specifically investigated for medical applications (Table 15–4). Commercial medical PEUs (and their

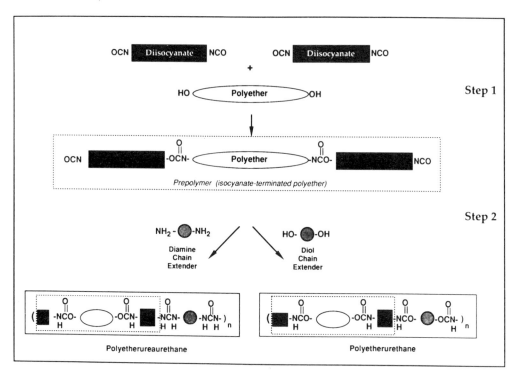

FIG. 15–8. Scheme for synthesis of polyether urea urethanes and polyether urethanes.

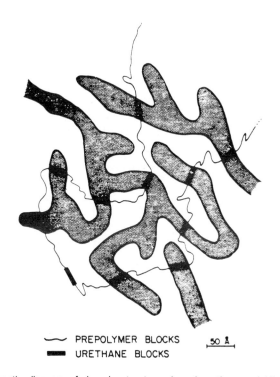

PREPOLYMER BLOCKS

URETHANE BLOCKS

50 Å

FIG. 15–9. Schematic diagram of domain structures in polyurethanes yielding hard and soft segments.

371

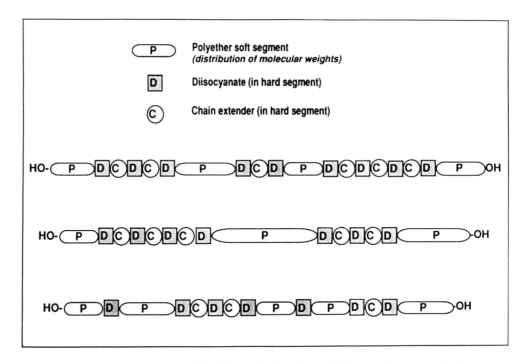

FIG. 15–10. The three basic building blocks of polyurethanes (diisocyanates, chain extenders, and polyethers) combine to form a large number of possible molecular structures. Three examples are presented here.

TABLE 15–4. *Types of Polyurethanes**

Conventional
  MDI-PTMG-ED (Biomer, Mitrathane, Lycra)
  MDI-PTMG-BD (Pellethane)
  HMDI-PTMG-ED (Tecoflex)
  MDI-PPG-ED (SRI)
Unconventional
  MDI-PEG-ED (Hydrogel)
  Bioelectric (carbon-filled)
  Alkyl-derivatized
  Alkyl soft segment
  PEU-PDMS (Avcothane, Cardiothane)
  Heparinized
  Radiation-grafted
  Surface-active additives in conventional PEUs
  Cross-linked

---

*MDI = methylene bisphenyl diisocyanate; PTMG = poly(tetramethylene glycol); PPG = poly(propylene glycol); PEG = poly(ethylene glycol); HMDI = methylene dicyclohexyl diisocyanate; PDMS = poly(dimethyl siloxane); ED = ethylene diamine; BD = butanediol.

manufacturers) include Biomer (Ethicon), Pellethane (Upjohn), Cardiothane (Kontron), Tecoflex (Thermedics), Mitrathane (Mitral Medical), and TM-3 (Toyobo). Each of these trade names may itself represent a family of materials and, in some cases, may be a blend, for example, polyurethane and silicone in Cardiothane (formerly Avcothane).

With high mechanical strength and toughness, attributed to the high cohesive energies that can be realized between the many polar functional groups in this type of polymer, PEUs are well suited for trileaflet heart valves. For example, the cohesive energy of inter-action between urethane groups has been estimated at three times that of energy for the carboxyl functionalities in polyesters (e.g., Dacron). Also, PEUs typically exhibit low stress relaxation (i.e., creep). A number of evaluation schemes have been developed to assess long-term durability and fatigue life under conditions relevant to their application in a flexing cardiovascular device. Under the test conditions used, PEUs have performed well compared with other materials, but predictions of which PEU would exhibit the best long-term mechanical stability are inconsistent among studies.

Polyurethanes have a long history of use in contact with blood and other biological fluids (111–114, 116). In general, polyurethanes are nonimmunogenic, are nontoxic, and cause relatively little foreign body reaction. Although the choice of polyurethanes for valve and artificial heart applications and for other blood-contacting devices was largely based upon published studies suggesting good blood compatibility for this class of mate-rials, there is much controversy over the interpretation and significance of the published data.

One of the major concerns that must be addressed in order to understand the blood compatibility of polyurethanes is the definition of blood compatibility. This definition is complex and in itself the subject of some controversy (117–119). For example, different coagulation mechanisms predominate in shear (arterial) blood flow or in low-shear (venous) flow. A material that performs well in one flow environment (i.e., that would be labeled blood-compatible) may perform poorly in another site in the bloodstream. Also, studies that compare accumulation of thrombus at the surface of a material in contact with blood often do not agree with studies that measure either the systemic pro-cess of blood element destruction or the production of emboli, since "accumulation" studies cannot accurately distinguish between materials that are nonthrombogenic and those that are reactive but nonthromboadhesive. Other considerations that will influence apparent blood compatibility include the time scale of measurement (short-term reaction versus longer-term or steady-state reaction), the animal model used, and the geometry of the evaluation system.

Studies based upon measurement of platelet or fibrin accumulation have attributed good blood compatibility to PEUs (115, 122), while others, including artificial heart implantations in humans, have raised concern (120, 121). Morphologic and chemical factors that have been implicated in the blood compatibility of PEUs include microphase separation (122–125), ionomer content (126), hydrophilicity (127–129), and surface hydrocarbon content (130–133). Since many methods are available for the surface mod-ification of these materials, it is likely that development of a mechanically suitable poly-urethane heart valve prosthesis will be accompanied by adjustment of the surface prop-erties to yield the desired blood interaction characteristics.

Results of chronic in vivo evaluations suggest that calcification could be a major lim-itation to long-term function of the PEU device. The cusps of polyurethane valves implanted in juvenile sheep for 17 to 21 weeks had extrinsic calcification associated with surface microthrombi or fibrous sheaths and intrinsic plaque-like deposits (134), uniformly distributed over the leaflet surface, that appeared to be independent of structural defects. The relationships of the rate and extent of PEU calcification to physicochemical parameters are under investigation (135, 136). The use of specific calcification inhibitors in conjunction with PEU valves is also being considered (115).

The biostability of polyurethanes has been the subject of much study, largely because of degradation associated with PEU insulation on some clinical pacemaker leads (137–140) and with coverings on breast implants (141). Polyesterurethanes have high biodegradation potential. In contrast, PEUs are susceptible to low-level hydrolysis, oxidative degradation, discoloration (due to absorption of lipids), or enzymatic degradation. In addition, the penetration of lipids into the hard segment of certain PEUs impairs fatigue strength (142). Polyurethane biodegradation leads to loss of fatigue resistance, flexural strength, and elastic modulus; reduced crack propagation resistance; and environmental stress cracking. Biodegradation is variable among formulations and can be minimized through careful choice of the composition purity, reaction conditions, and fabrication of PEU components (139, 140, 143–148).

Physical and chemical factors implicated in PEU degradation include water and lipid sorption, extraction by biological fluids, enzymatic polymer chain cleavage, and oxidative polyether cleavage. Upon immersion in aqueous media, most PEUs absorb 1% or more water, which can act as a plasticizer and reduce mechanical properties, or provide access to the polymer chains by enzymes. Lipid uptake swells, plasticizes, and can initiate microcracks in PEUs (149). Bilirubin absorption into PEU vascular grafts has been observed (150). Plasma and other proteinaceous fluids have a surfactant-like quality because of the amphophilic nature of proteins. Soaps and organic liquids have been seen to extract low-molecular-weight material from PEUs leading to the formation of voids and surface irregularities (151). Although there are no known enzymes associated with the foreign body reaction that are specific for the urethane chemical linkage, nonspecific limited enzymatic attack probably does occur. Peroxide and strong oxidizing compounds produced by macrophages have been implicated in the in vivo breakdown of the polyether portion of PEUs (152). These factors can act synergistically to produce the degradation reactions observed. For example, extraction or lipid uptake might generate surface microdefects that could serve as points of stress concentration leading to failure during flexing. Flexing opens more surface area to attack. Alternatively, enzymatic breakdown might lead to increased water uptake that may, in turn, lead to microcracking or to enhanced access of low-molecular-weight materials into the bulk of the polyurethane. Moreover, fungal degeneration of polyurethanes could occur (153). Nevertheless, the successful long-term implant performance of most polyurethane pacemaker leads suggests that degradation-resistant PEUs can be developed.

Silicone Elastomer

Silicone elastomers (Fig. 15–11) generally have good biostability and high blood compatibility. The long history of use of silicone rubber poppets in mechanical heart valves encourages their application for trileaflet valves.

In early studies, problems were reported with thrombosis (96, 154). In 1974, Dacron-reinforced Silastic tricuspid valves had over 2 years of good performance after implantation in calves (102). Results with a polypropylene trileaflet valve coated with silicone rubber implanted in 20 patients were generally poor using this valve design, with major

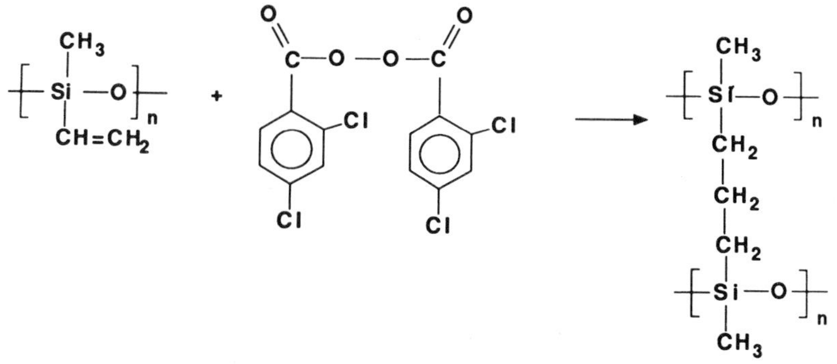

FIG. 15–11. A thermal vulcanizing silicone elastomer. Poly(dimethylsiloxane) units are interspersed between the cross-link units.

problems associated with leaflet fracture and thrombosis (100). Approaches to reducing the thrombogenicity of silicone rubber have been described (155). Lipid uptake can also be expected, but fabrication protocols for reducing this problem have been described (156). Studies also report problems with fluid uptake (157) or mechanical failure (158). Durability will probably continue to be the most significant problem with silicone elastomer trileaflet heart valves (159, 160). Silicone rubber has low tear strength and thus needs reinforcement. Other polymer combinations including silicone rubber with polyester fabric reinforcement and Teflon fabric–reinforced silicone rubber (161) have been tried without success; the long-term durability of the boundary between the silicone rubber and the reinforcement is poor.

Other Materials

Solid polytetrafluoroethylene (PTFE, Teflon) materials have been used extensively in cardiovascular applications, because of their relative inertness and stability. Porous PTFE materials have also been used satisfactorily in cardiovascular applications (e.g., expanded PTFE vascular grafts). Leaflets constructed from jersey-knit Teflon, both plain and coated with Teflon dispersions, have been used in tricuspid Muller-Littlefield valves and Bahnson bileaflet and trileaflet designs (99). Early clinical and hemodynamic results were good; however, at later postoperative periods (1–2 years), the leaflets stiffened with mild to moderate stenosis, followed by fracture and fenestrations leading to regurgitation. The fabric was thickened and stiffened by tissue overgrowth and calcification.

A few reports have appeared in the literature on Teflon trileaflet valves (162, 163). Valves fabricated with a laminate of Gore-Tex expanded PTFE had generally good function in 12 out of 20 dogs for up to 15 months (162). The thickness of the laminate was implicated as a key factor in the mechanical performance of the valve. Calcification was not reported.

Other polymers have been used experimentally as leaflets for replacement heart valves. In particular, valves fabricated from Hexsyn, a copolymer of 1-hexene and methyl hexadiene cross-linked with sulfur, showed promise in one study (164). The mechanical properties and durability of this elastomer are good, and little thrombus deposition was noted compared with PEU valves after 3 weeks of implantation in calves.

REFERENCES

1. Broom ND, Christie GW: The structure, function relationship of fresh and glutaraldehyde-fixed aortic valve leaflets. In Cohn LH, Gallucci V (eds): Cardiac Bioprostheses. New York, Yorke Medical Books, 1982, pp 476–491.
2. Ferrans VJ, Spray TL, Billingham ME, Roberts WC; Structural changes in glutaraldehyde-treated porcine heterografts used as substitute cardiac valves. Transmission and scanning electron microscopic observations in 12 patients. Am J Cardiol 1978;41:1159–1184.
3. Lee JM, Courtman DW, Boughner DR: The glutaraldehyde-stabilized porcine aortic valve xenograft: I. Tensile viscoelastic properties of the fresh leaflet material. J Biomed Mater Res 1984;18:61–77.
4. Broom ND: The observation of collagen and elastin structures in wet whole mounts of pulmonary and aortic leaflets. J Thorac Cardiovasc Surg 1978;75:121–130.
5. Schoen FJ, Levy RJ, Nelson AC, Bernhard WF, Nashef A, Hawley M: Onset and progression of experimental bioprosthetic heart valve calcification. Lab Invest 1985;52:523–532.
6. Christie GW: An analysis of the mechanics of bioprosthetic heart valves. Doctoral dissertation, University of Auckland, New Zealand, 1982.
7. Christie GW, Medland IC: A non-linear stress analysis of bioprosthetic heart valves. In Gallagher RH, Simons BR, Johnson PC, Gross JF (eds): Finite Elements in Biomechanics. New York, John Wiley, 1982.
8. Thubrikar MJ, Nolan SP, Aouad J, Deck JD: Stress sharing between the sinus and leaflets of canine aortic valve. Ann Thorac Surg 1986;42:434–440.
9. Broom ND, Marra D: Effect of glutaraldehyde fixation and valve constraint conditions on porcine aortic valve coaptation. Thorax 1982;37:620–626.
10. Hayat MA (ed): Fixation for Electron Microscopy. New York, Academic Press, 1981.
11. Carpentier A, Lemaigre G, Robert L, et al: Biological factors affecting long-term results of valvular heterografts. J Thorac Cardiovasc Surg 1969;58:467–482.
12. Carpentier A, Deloche A, Relland J, et al: Six year follow-up of glutaraldehyde preserved heterografts: With particular reference to the treatment of congenital valve malformation. J Thorac Cardiovasc Surg 1974;68:771–782.
13. Carpentier A, Dubost C, Lane E, Nashef A, Carpentier S, Relland J, Deloche A, Fabiani JN, Chauvaud S, Perier P, Maxwell S: Continuing improvements in valvular bioprostheses. J Thorac Cardiovasc Surg 1982;83:27–42.
14. Rose AG: Pathology of the formalin-treated heterograft porcine aortic valve in the mitral position. Thorax 1972;27:401–409.
15. Stephens BJ, O'Brien MF: Pathology of xenografts in aortic valve replacement. Pathology 1972;4:167–173.
16. Woodroof EA: The chemistry and biology of aldehyde treated tissue heart valve xenografts. In Ionescu MI (ed): Tissue Heart Valves. London. Butterworths, 1979, pp. 347–362.
17. Cheung DT, Nimni ME: Mechanisms of crosslinking of proteins by glutaraldehyde: II. Reaction with monomeric and polymeric collagen. Connect Tissue Res 1982;10:201.
18. Cheung DT, Perelman N, Ko EC, Nimni ME: Mechanism of crosslinking of proteins by glutaraldehyde: III. Reaction with collagen in tissues. Connect Tissue Res 1985;13:109–115.
19. Mannschott P, Herbage D, Weiss M, et al: Collagen heterogeneity in pig heart valves. Biochem Biophys Acta 1976;434:177–183.
20. Schoen FJ, Tsao JW, Levy RJ: Calcification of bovine pericardium used in cardiac valve bioprostheses. Implications for the mechanisms of bioprosthetic tissue mineralization. Am J Pathol 1986;123:134–145.
21. Bowes JH, Cater CW: The interaction of aldehydes with collagen. Biochim Biophys Acta 1968;168:341–352.
22. Levy RJ, Schoen FJ, Levy JT, Nelson AC, Howard SL, Oshry LJ: Biologic determinants of dystrophic calcification and osteocalcin deposition in glutaraldehyde preserved porcine aortic valve leaflets implanted subcutaneously in rats. Am J Pathol 1983;113:143–155.
23. Golomb G, Schoen FJ, Smith MS, Linden J, Dixon M, Levy RJ: The role of glutaraldehyde-induced cross-links in calcification of bovine pericardium used in cardiac valve bioprostheses. Am J Pathol 1987;127:122–130.
24. Schoen FJ, Levy RJ: Calcification of bioprosthetic heart valves. In Bodnar E, Frater R (eds): Replacement Cardiac Valves. Elmsford, New York, Pergamon Press, 1991, pp. 125–148.
25. Lovelock JE: Mechanism of the protective action of glycerol against haemolysis by freezing and thawing. Biochem Biophys Acta 1953;11:28–36.
26. Zerbini EJ: Results of replacement of cardiac valves by homologous dura mater valves. Chest 1975;67:706–710.
27. Puig LB, Verginelli G, Kawabe L, Melo R, Concelcao A, Bittencourt D, Zerbini EJ: Four years experience with dura mater cardiac valves. J Cardiovasc Surg 1977;18:247–255.
28. Permanyer-Miralde G, Soler-Soler J, Casan-Cava JM, Tornos-Mas MP: Medium term fate of dura mater valvular bioprostheses. Eur Heart J 1980;1:195–199.
29. Allen DJ, Highison GJ, DiDio LJ, Zerbini EJ, Puig LB: Evidence of remodeling in dura mater cardiac valves. J Thorac Cardiovasc Surg 1982;84:267–281.

30. Murayama Y, Satoh S, Oka T, Imanishi J, Noishiki Y: Reduction of the antigenicity of xenografts by a new cross-linking reagent. Trans Am Soc Artif Organs 1988;32.
31. Broom ND, Thomson FJ: Influence of fixation conditions on the performance of glutaraldehyde-treated porcine aortic valves—Towards a more scientific basis. Thorax 1979;34:166–176.
32. Broom ND: Simultaneous morphological and stress/strain studies on the fibrous components in wet heart valve tissue. Conn Tissue Res 1978;6:37–50.
33. Reece IJ, van Noort R, Martin TRP, Black MM: The physical properties of bovine pericardium: A study of the effects of stretching during chemical treatment in glutaraldehyde. Ann Thorac Surg 1982;33:481–485.
34. Lee JM, Boughner DR, Courtman DW: The glutaraldehyde-stabilized porcine aortic valve xenograft: II. Effect of fixation with or without pressure on the tensile viscoelastic properties of the leaflet material. J Biomed Mater Res 1984;18:79–98.
35. Trowbridge EA, Roberts KM, Crofts CE, Lawford PV: Pericardial heterografts. Toward quality control of the mechanical properties of glutaraldehyde-fixed leaflets. J Thorac Cardiovasc Surg 1986;92:21–28.
36. Fung YC: Biomechanics—Mechanical Properties of Living Tissue. New York, Springer-Verlag, 1981, chap 7.
37. Sobin SS, Fung YC, Tremer HM: The effect of incomplete fixation of elastin on the appearance of lung alveoli. Trans ASME 1982;104:68–71.
38. Fung YC, Sobin SS: The retained elasticity of elastin under fixation agents. J Biomech Eng 1981;103:121–122.
39. Mayne ASD, Christie GW, Smaill BH, Hunter PJ, Barratt-Boyes BG: An assessment of the mechanical properties of leaflets from four second-generation porcine bioprostheses using biaxial testing techniques. J Thorac Cardiovasc Surg 1989;98:170–180.
40. Trowbridge EA, Lawford PV, Crofts CE, Roberts KM: Pericardial heterografts: Why do these valves fail? J Thorac Cardiovasc Surg 1988;95:577–585.
41. Schoen FJ: Cardiac valve prostheses: Pathological and bioengineering considerations. J Cardiac Surg 1987;2:65–108.
42. Schoen FJ: Modes of failure and other pathology of mechanical and tissue heart valve prostheses. In Bodnar E, Frater R (eds): Replacement Cardiac Valves. Elmsford, New York, Pergamon Press, 1991, pp. 99–124.
43. Ferrans VJ, Boyce SW, Billingham ME, Jones M, Ishihara T, Roberts WC: Calcific deposits in porcine bioprostheses: Structure and pathogenesis. Am J Cardiol 1980;46:721–734.
44. Valente M, Bortolotti U, Thiene G: Ultrastructural substrates of dystrophic calcification in porcine bioprosthetic valve failure. Am J Pathol 1985;119:12–21.
45. Schoen FJ, Kujovich JL, Webb CL, Levy RJ: Chemically determined mineral content of explanted porcine aortic valve bioprostheses: Correlation with radiographic assessment of calcification and clinical data. Circulation 1987;76:1061–1066.
46. Wright JTM, Eberhardt CE, Gibbs ML, Saul GT, Gilpin CB: Hancock II—An improved bioprosthesis. In Cohn LR, Gallucci V (eds): Cardiac Bioprostheses. New York, Yorke Medical Books, 1982, pp. 425–444.
47. Broom ND: Fatigue-induced damage in glutaraldehyde-preserved heart valve tissue. J Thorac Cardiovasc Surg 1978;76:202–211.
48. Bodnar E, Bowden NL, Drury PJ, et al: Bicuspid mitral bioprosthesis. Thorax 1981;36:45–51.
49. Schoen FJ, Harasaki H, Kim KM, Anderson HC, Levy RJ: Biomaterial-associated calcification: Pathology, mechanisms, and strategies for prevention. J Biomed Mater Res: Applied Biomater 1988;22(A1):11–36.
50. Levy RJ, Schoen FJ, Golomb G: Bioprosthetic heart valve calcification: Clinical features, pathobiology, and prospects for prevention. CRC Crit Rev Biocompat 1986;2:147–187.
51. Lentz DJ, Pollock EM, Olsen DB, Andrews EJ: Prevention of intrinsic calcification in porcine and bovine xenograft materials. Trans Am Soc Artif Intern Organs 1982;28:494–497.
52. Thubrikar MJ, Nolan SP, Deck JD, Aouad J, Levitt LC: Intrinsic calcification of T6-processed and control porcine and bovine bioprostheses in calves. Trans Am Soc Artif Intern Organs 1983;29:245–249.
53. Arbustini EI, Jones M, Moses RD, et al: Modification by the Hancock T6 process of calcification of bioprosthetic cardiac valves implanted in sheep. Am J Cardiol 1984;53:1388–1396.
54. Carpentier A, Nashef A, Carpentier S, Ahmed A, Goussef N: Techniques for prevention of calcification of valvular bioprostheses. Circulation 1984;70(suppl 1):I-165–I-168.
55. Jones M, Eidbo EE, Hilbert SL, Ferrans VJ, Clark RE: Anti-calcification treatments of bioprosthetic heart valves: In vivo studies in sheep. J Cardiac Surg 1989;4:69–73.
56. Gallo I, Nistal F, Artinano E, Fernandez D, Cayon R, Carrion M, Garcia-Martinez V: The behavior of pericardial versus porcine valve xenografts in the growing sheep model. J Thorac Cardiovasc Surg 1987;93:281–290.
57. Golomb G, Ezra V: Prevention of bioprosthetic heart valve tissue calcification by charge modification: Effects of protamine binding by formaldehyde. J Biomed Mater Res 1991;25:85–98.
58. Fleisch H: Diphosphonates: History and mechanisms of actions. Metabol Bone Dis Rel Res 1981;4–5:279–288.

59. Levy RJ, Hawley MA, Schoen FJ, Lund SA, Liu PY: Inhibition by diphosphonate compounds of calcification of porcine bioprosthetic heart valve cusps implanted subcutaneously in rats. Circulation 1985;71:349–356.

60. Dewanjee MK, Solis E, Mackey ST, Lenker J, Edwards WD, Didisheim P, Chesbro JH, Zollman PE, Kaye MP: Quantification of regional platelet and calcium deposition on pericardial tissue valve prostheses in calves and effect of hydroxyethylene diphosphonate. J Thorac Cardiovasc Surg 1986;92:337–348.

61. Levy RJ, Schoen FJ, Lund SA, Smith MS: Prevention of leaflet calcification of bioprosthetic heart valves with diphosphonate injection therapy. Experimental studies of optimal dosages and therapeutic durations. J Thorac Cardiovasc Surg 1987;94:551–557.

62. Levy RJ, Wolfrum J, Schoen FJ, Hawley MA, Lund SA, Langer R: Inhibition of calcification of bioprosthetic heart valves by local controlled-released diphosphonate. Science 1985;227:190–192.

63. Golomb G, Langer R, Schoen FJ, Smith MS, Choi YM, Levy RJ: Controlled release of diphosphonate to inhibit bioprosthetic heart valve calcification: Dose-response and mechanistic studies. J Control Rel 1986;4:181–194.

64. Golomb G, Dixon M, Smith MS, Schoen FJ, Levy RJ: Controlled release drug delivery of diphosphonates to inhibit bioprosthetic heart valve calcification: Release rate modulation with silicone matrices via drug solubility and membrane coating. J Pharm Sci 1987;76:271–276.

65. Webb CL, Benedict JJ, Schoen FJ, Linden JA, Levy RJ: Inhibition of bioprosthetic heart valve calcification with aminodiphosphonate covalently bound to residual aldehyde groups. Ann Thorac Surg 1988;46:309–316.

66. Johnston TP, Schoen FJ, Levy RJ: Prevention of calcification of bioprosthetic heart valve leaflets by Ca^{++} diphosphonate pretreatment. J Pharm Sci (in press).

67. Parfitt AM: The localization of aluminum in bone: Implications for the mechanisms of fixation and for the pathogenesis of aluminum-related bone disease. Int J Artif Org 1988;11:79–90.

68. Webb CL, Schoen FJ, Flowers WE, Alfrey AC, Horton C, Levy RJ: Inhibition of mineralization of glutaraldehyde-pretreated bovine pericardium by $AlCl_3$: Mechanisms and comparisons with $FeCl_3$, $LaCl_3$, and Ga $(NO_3)_3$ in rat subdermal model studies. Am J Pathol 1991;138:971–981.

69. Ishihara T, Ferrans VJ, Jones M, Boyes SW, Roberts WC: Structure of bovine parietal pericardium and of unimplanted Ionescu-Shiley pericardial valvular bioprostheses. J Thorac Cardiovasc Surg 1981;81:747–757.

70. Walley VM, Keon WJ: Patterns of failure in Ionescu-Shiley bovine pericardial bioprosthetic valves. J Thorac Cardiovasc Surg 1987;93:925–933.

71. Schoen FJ, Fernandez J, Gonzalez-Lavin L, Cernaianu A: Causes of failure and pathologic findings in surgically removed Ionescu-Shiley standard bovine pericardial heart valve bioprostheses: Emphasis on progressive structural deterioration. Circulation 1987;76:618–627.

72. Wheatley DJ, Fisher J, Reece IJ, Spyt T, Breeze P: Primary tissue failure in pericardial heart valves. J Thorac Cardiovasc Surg 1987;94:367–374.

73. McEnany MT, Ross DN, Yates AK: Valve failure in seventy-two frame supported autologous fascia lata mitral valves. Two-year follow-up. J Thorac Cardiovasc Surg 1972;63:199–214.

74. Yarbrough JW, Roberts WC, Reis RL: Structural alterations in tissue cardiac valves implanted in patients and in calves. J Thorac Cardiovasc Surg 1973;65:364–378.

75. Silver MD, Hudson RED, Trimble AS: Morphologic observations on heart valve prostheses made of fascia lata. J Thorac Cardiovasc Surg 1975;70:360–366.

76. Shemin RJ, Schoen FJ, Hein R, Austin J, Cohn LH: Hemodynamic and pathological evaluation of a unileaflet pericardial bioprosthetic valve. J Thorac Cardiovasc Surg 1988;95:912–919.

77. Bokros JC, LaGrange LD, Schoen FH: Control of structure of carbon for use in bioengineering. In Walker P, Thrower P (eds): Chemistry and Physics of Carbon. New York, Marcel Dekker, 1973, vol 9, pp 103–171.

78. Haubold AD, Shim HS, Bokros JC: Carbon in medical devices. In Williams DF (ed): Biocompatibility of Clinical Implant Materials. Boca Raton, FL, CRC Press, 1981, pp 4–44.

79. Schoen FJ: Carbon in heart valve prostheses: Foundations and clinical performance. In Szycher ML (ed): Biocompatible Polymers, Metals and Ceramics: Science and Technology. Westport, CT, Technamic Publishing, 1983, pp 239–261.

80. Kaae JL, Gulden TD: Structure and mechanical properties of codeposited pyrolytic C-SiC alloys. J Am Ceram Soc 1971;54:605–609.

81. Kaae JL: Structure and mechanical properties of isotropic pyrolytic carbons deposited below 1600C. J Nucl Mater 1971;38:42–50.

82. Schoen FJ: On the fatigue behavior of pyrolytic carbon. Carbon 1973;11:413–414.

83. Shim HS; The behavior of isotropic pyrolytic carbons under cyclic loading. Biomater Med Dev Art Org 1974;2:55–65.

84. Shim HS, Schoen FJ: The wear resistance of pure and silicon-alloyed isotropic carbons. Biomat Med Dev Art Org 1974;2:103–118.

85. Baier RE: Key events in blood interactions at nonphysiologic interfaces—A personal primer. Artif Organs 1978;2:422–426.

86. Bokros JC, La Grange LD, Fadali AM, Vos KD, Ramos MD: Correlations between blood compatibility and heparin adsorptivity for an impermeable isotropic pyrolytic carbon. J Biomed Mater Res 1969;3:497–528.

87. Hanson SR, Harker LA, Ratner BD, Hoffman AS: In-vivo evaluation of artificial surfaces with a non-human primate model of arterial thrombosis. J Lab Clin Med 1980;289–304.

88. Haubold AD, Shim HS, Bokros JC: Carbon cardiovascular devices. In Unger F (ed): Assisted Circulation. New York, Springer-Verlag, 1979, pp 520–532.

89. Schultz JS, Goddard JD, Ciankowski A, Penner JA, Lindenauer SM: An ex-vivo method for the evaluation of biomaterials in contact with blood. Ann NY Acad Sci 1977;283:494–523.

90. Aebischer P, Goddard MB, Sasken HF, Hunter TJ, Galletti PM: Tissue reaction to fabrics coated with turbostratic carbon: Subcutaneous versus vascular implants. Biomaterials 1988;9:80–85.

91. Schoen FJ, Goodenough SH, Ionescu MI, Braunwald NS: Implications of late morphology of Braunwald-Cutter mitral heart valve prosthesis. J Thorac Cardiovasc Surg 1984; 88:208–216.

92. Bjork VO, Wilson GJ, Sternlieb JJ, Kaminsky DB: The porous metal-surfaced heart valve. Long-term study without long-term anticoagulation in mitral position in goats. J Thorac Cardiovasc Surg 1988;95:1067–1082.

93. Gentle CR: The use of ceramics in prosthetic heart valves. Engin Med 1987;16:115–117.

94. Gentle CR, Juden H: Wear tests on alumina for application in heart valve prostheses. Engin Med 1984;13:79–82.

95. Mitamura Y, Mikami T, Yuta T, Matsumoto T, Shimooka T, Okamoto E, Eizuka N, Yamaguchi K: Development of a fine ceramic heart valve for use as a cardiac prosthesis. Trans Am Soc Artif Intern Organs 1986;32:444–448.

96. Akutsu T, Dreyer B, Kolff WJ: Polyurethane artificial heart valves in animals. J Appl Physiol 1959;14:1045–1048.

97. Bjork VO, Cullhed I, Lodin H: Aortic valve prostheses (Teflon): Two year follow-up. J Thorac Cardiovasc Surg 1963;45:635–644.

98. Larson RE, Kirklin JW: Early and late results of partial and total replacement of the aortic valve with individual Teflon cusps. J Thorac Cardiovasc Surg 1964;47:720–724.

99. Braunwald NS, Morrow AG: A late evaluation of flexible Teflon prostheses utilized for total aortic valve replacement. J Thorac Cardiovasc Surg 1965;49:485–496.

100. Fishbein MC, Roberts WC, Golden A, Hufnagel CA: Cardiac pathology after aortic valve replacement using Hufnagel trileaflet prostheses: A study of 20 necropsy patients. Am Heart J 1975;89:443–448.

101. Moulopoulos SD, Anthopoulos L, Stamatelopoulos S, Stefadouros M: Catheter-mounted aortic valves. Ann Thorac Surg 1971;11:423–430.

102. Gerring EL, Bellhouse BJ, Bellhouse FH, Haworth WS: Long-term animal trials of the Oxford aortic/pulmonary valve prosthesis without anticoagulants. Trans Am Soc Artif Intern Organs 1974;20:703–707.

103. Sawyer PN, Stanczewski B, Srinivasan S, Stempack JG, Kammlott GW: Implantation characteristics of metal-backed polymer-coated heart valves: Biophysical scanning and transmission electron microscopic studies. Trans Am Soc Artif Intern Organs 1974;20:692–702.

104. Davies H, Christopher RA, Walker L: In-vitro flow characteristics of a completely flexible prosthetic heart valve. Biomed Sci Instrum 1975;11:141–144.

105. Phillips SJ, Ciborski M, Freed PS, Cascade PH, Jaron D: A temporary catheter-tip aortic valve: Hemodynamic effects on experimental acute aortic insufficiency. Ann Thorac Surg 1976;21:134–137.

106. Rennekamp F, Clevert HD, Henning E, Bucherl ES: A paracorporeal pump with new valves for atrio-aortic left heart assist. Trans Am Soc Artif Intern Organs 1979;25:249–253.

107. Kolff J, Hershgold EJ, Hadfield C, Olsen DB, Lawson J, Kolff WJ: The improving hematologic picture in long-term surviving calves with total artificial hearts. Artif Organs 1979;3:97–103.

108. Wisman CB, Pierce WS, Donachy JH, Pae WE, Myers JL, Prophet GA: A polyurethane trileaflet cardiac valve prostheses: In-vitro and in-vivo studies. Trans Am Soc Artif Intern Organs 1982;18:164–168.

109. Herold M, Lo HB, Reul H, Muckter H, Taguchi K, Gievsiepen M, Birkle G, Hollweg G, Rau G, Messer BJ: The Helmholtz-Institute-Tri-Leaflet-Polyurethane-Heart Valve Prosthesis: Design, manufacturing and first in-vitro and in-vivo results. In Planck H, Syre I, Dauner M, Egbers G (eds): Polyurethanes in Biomedical Engineering II. Amsterdam, Elsevier, 1987, pp 231–256.

110. Bos WJW, Mohammad SF, Yu LS, Olsen DB, Kolff WJ: Comparison of tilting disc and polyurethane tricusp semilunar valves in high blood flow—In-vitro model. Am Soc Artif Organs Abstr 1988;p 44.

111. Planck H, Egbers G, Syre I: Polyurethanes in Biomedial Engineering. Amsterdam, Elsevier, 1984, vol 1, Progress in Biomedical Engineering.

112. Lelah MD, Cooper SL: Polyurethanes in Medicine, Boca Raton, FL, CRC Press, 1986.

113. Planck H, Syre I, Dauner M, Egbers G: Polyurethanes in Biomedical Engineering II. Amsterdam, Elsevier, 1987.

114. Grasel TG: Polyurethanes in biomedical applications. Biomed Polymers 1987;3:1–6.

115. Szycher M, Poirier VL: Synthetic polymers in artificial hearts: A progress report. Ind Eng Chem Prod Res Dev 1983;22:588–593.

116. Ito Y: Antithrombogenic heparin-bound polyurethane. J Biomat Appl 1987;2:235–265.

117. McIntire LV, Addonizio VP, Coleman DL, Eskin SG, Harker LA, Kardos JL, Ratner BD, Schoen FJ, Sefton MV, Pitlick FA: Guidelines for Blood–Material Interactions. NIH Publication No. 85-2185, revised July 1985. Devices and Technology Branch, Division of Heart and Vascular Diseases, National Heart, Lung and Blood Institute, US Department of Health and Human Services.
118. Williams DF: Definitions in Biomedicals. Amsterdam, Elsevier, 1987, pp 1–72.
119. Ratner BD: Evaluation of the blood compatibility of synthetic polymers: Consensus and significance. In Boretos JW, Eden M (eds): Contemporary Biomaterials: Material and Host Response, Clinical Applications, New Technology and Legal Aspects. Park Ridge, NJ, Noyes Publications, 1984, pp 193–204.
120. DeVries WC: The permanent artificial heart: Four case reports. JAMA 1988;259:849–859.
121. Akutsu T, Dreyer B, Kolff WJ: Polyurethane artificial heart valves in animals. J Appl Physiol 1959;14:1045–1048.
122. Nojima K, Sanui K, Ogata N, Yui N, Kataoka K, Sakurai Y: Material characterization of segmented polyether poly(urethane-urea-amide)s and its implication in blood compatibility. Polymer 1987;28:1017–1024.
123. Grasel TG, Cooper SL: Surface properties and blood compatibility of polyurethaneureas. Biomaterials 1986;7:315–328.
124. Takahara A, Tashita J, Kajiyama T, Takayanagi M, MacKnight W: Microphase separated structure, surface composition and blood compatibility of segmented poly(urethaneureas) with various soft segment components. Polymer 1985;26:987–996.
125. Lelah MD, Grasel TG, Pierce JA, Cooper SC: Ex-vivo interactions and surface property relationships for polyetherurethanes. J Biomed Mater Res 1986;20:433–468.
126. Lelah MD, Pierce JA, Lambrecht LK, Cooper SL: Polyether-urethane ionomers: Surface property/ex vivo blood compatibility relationships. J Coll Interf Sci 1985;104:422–439.
127. Sa Da Costa V, Brier-Russell D, Salzman EW, Merrill EW: ESCA studies of polyurethanes: Blood platelet activation in relation to surface composition. J Coll Interf Sci 1981;80:445–452.
128. Egboh SHO: Graft copolymerization of unsaturated segmented polyurethanes with 2-hydroxethyl methacrylate. Angew Makromol Chem 1987;148:79–86.
129. Gnanou Y, Hild G, Rempp P: Hydrophilic polyurethane networks based on poly(ethylene oxide): Synthesis, characterization, and properties. Potential applications as biomaterials. Macromolecules 1984;17:945–952.
130. Grasel TG, Pierce JA, Cooper SL: Effects of alkyl grafting on surface properties and blood compatibility of polyurethane block copolymers. J Biomed Mater Res 1987;21:815–842.
131. Pitt WG, Grasel TG, Cooper SL: Albumin adsorption on alkyl chain derivatized polyurethanes: II. The effect of alkyl chain length. Biomaterials 1988;9:36–46.
132. Ratner BD, Yoon SC, Kaul A, Rahman R: Control of polyurethane surface structure by synthesis and additives: Implications for blood interactions. In Planck H, Syre I, Dauner M, Egbers G (eds): Polyurethanes in Biomedical Engineering II. Amsterdam, Elsevier, 1987, pp 213–228.
133. Munro MS, Quattrone AJ, Ellsworth SR, Kulkarni P, Eberhart RC: Alkyl substituted polymers with enhanced albumin affinity. Trans Am Soc Artif Intern Organs 1981;27:499–503.
134. Hilbert SL, Ferrans VJ, Tomita Y, Eidbo EE, Jones M: Evaluation of explanted polyurethane trileaflet cardiac valve prostheses. J Thorac Cardiovasc Surg 1987;94:410–429.
135. Glasmacher B, Reul H, Rau G, Erckes C, Wieland J: In-vitro investigation of the calcification behavior of polyurethane biomaterials. In Planck H, Syre I, Dauner M, Egber G (eds): Polyurethanes in Biomedical Engineering II, Amsterdam, Elsevier, 1987, pp 151–168.
136. Wouters LHG, Rousseau EPM, Van Steenhoven AA, German AL: An experimental set-up for the in-vitro analysis of polyurethane calcification. In Planck H, Syre I, Dauner M, Egbers G (eds): Polyurethanes in Biomedical Engineering II, Amsterdam, Elsevier, 1987, pp 169–182.
137. Hanson JS: Sixteen failures in a single model of bipolar polyurethane-insulated ventricular pacing lead: A 44-month experience. PACE 1984;7:389–394.
138. Byrd CL, McArthur W, Stokes K, Sivina M, Yahr WZ, Greenberg J: Implant experience with unipolar polyurethane pacing leads. PACE 1983;6:868–882.
139. Coury AJ, Stokes KB, Cahalan PT, Slaikeu PC: Biostability considerations for implantable polyurethanes. Life Sup Syst 1987;5:25–39.
140. Phillips R, Frey M, Martin RO: Long-term performance or polyurethane pacing leads: Mechanisms of design-related failures. PACE 1986;9:1166–1172.
141. Samhel J: Tissue reactions to breast implants coated with polyurethane. Plast Reconstr Surg 1978;61:80–85.
142. Takahara A, Tashita J, Kajiwara T, Takayanagi M: Effect of aggregation state and hard segment in segmented poly (urethane-ureas) on their fatigue behavior after interaction with blood components. J Biomed Mater Res 1985;19:13–34.
143. Boretos JW, Detmer DE, Donachy JH: Segmented polyurethane: A polyether polymer: II. Two year experience. J Biomed Mater Res 1971;5:373–387.
144. Hunter SK, Gregonis DE, Colman DL, Andrade JD, Kessler T: Molecular weight characterization of pre-

and post implant artificial heart polyurethane materials. Trans Am Soc Artif Intern Organs 1982;28:473–477.

145. Thoma RJ, Phillips RE: Studies of poly (ether) urethane pacemaker lead insulation oxidation. J Biomed Mater Res 1987;21:525–530.

146. Smith R, Williams DF, Oliver C: The biodegradation of poly(etherurethanes). J Biomed Mater Res 1987;21:1149–1166.

147. Marchant RE, Zhao Q, Anderson JM, Hiltner A: Degradation of a poly (ether urethane urea) elastomer: Infra-red and XPS studies. Polymer 1987;28:2032–2039.

148. Ratner BD, Gladhill KW, Horbett TA: Analysis of in-vitro enzymatic and oxidative degradation of polyurethanes. J Biomed Mater Res 1988;22:509–527.

149. Takahara A, Murakami A, Tashita J, Kajiyama T, Takayanagi M: Influence of lipid absorption on fatigue strength of segmented poly (urethaneureas). Rep Prog Polym Phys Japan 1982;25:849–852.

150. Martz H, Paynter R, Forest JC, Downs A, Guidoin R: Microporous hydrophilic polyurethane vascular grafts as substitutes in the abdominal aorta of dogs. Biomaterials 1987;8:3–11.

151. Ratner BD, Paynter RW: Polyurethane surfaces: The importance of molecular weight distribution, bulk chemistry and casting conditions. In Planck H, Egbers G, Syre I (eds): Polyurethanes in Biomedical Engineering. Progress in Biomedical Engineering. Amsterdam, Elseiver, 1984, vol 1, pp 41–68.

152. Coury AJ, Sliakeu PC, Stokes KB, Skorich SR, Coscio MR: Similarity of in vivo and in vitro oxidation of polyether urethanes. Trans Soc Biomat 1987;10:12.

153. Darby RT, Kaplan AM: Fungal susceptibility of polyurethanes. Appl Microbiol 1968;16:900–905.

154. Hessel EA, Mohri H, Nelson RJ, Anderson HN, Dillard DH, Merendino KA: Design and durability test of silastic trileaflet aortic valve prostheses. J Thorac Cardiovasc Surg 1973;65:576–582.

155. Kolobow T, Stool EW, Weathersby PK, Pierce J, Hayano F, Suaudeau J: Superior blood compatibility of silicone rubber free of silica filler in the membrane lung. Trans Am Soc Artif Intern Organs 1974;20:269–276.

156. Nyilas E, Kupski EL, Burnett P, Haag RM: Surface microstructural factors and the blood compatibility of a silicone rubber. J Biomed Mater Res 1970;4:369–432.

157. Mohri H, Hessel EA, Nelson RJ, Anderson HN, Dillard DH, Merendino KA: Design and durability test of silastic trileaflet aortic valve prostheses. J Thorac Cardiovasc Surg 1973;65:576–582.

158. Chetta GE, Lloyd JR: The design, fabrication and evaluation of a trileaflet prosthetic heart valve. J Biomech Eng 1980;102:34–41.

159. van Noort R, Black MM: Silicone rubbers for medical applications. In Williams DF (ed): Biocompatibility of Clinical Implant Materials. Boca Raton, CRC Press, 1981, vol 2, pp 70–99.

160. Cuddihy EF, Moacanin J, Roschke EJ, Harrison EC: In vivo degradation of silicone rubber poppets in prosthetic heart valves. J Biomed Mater Res 1976;10:471–476.

161. Gott VL, et al: The development of a prosthetic heart valve utilizing a rigid housing and a flexible butterfly-wing leaflet. Trans Am Soc Artif Intern Organs 1962;8:72–84.

162. Imamura E, Kay MP: Function of expanded-polytetrafluoroethylene laminated trileaflet valves in animals. Mayo Clin Proc 1977;52:770–775.

163. Braunwald NS, Morrow AG: A late evaluation of flexible Teflon prostheses utilized for total aortic valve replacement. J Thorac Cardiovasc Surg; 1965;44:485–496.

164. Kiraly R, Yozu R, Hillegass D, Harasaki H, Murabayashi S, Snow J, Nose Y: Hexsyn trileaflet valve: Application to temporary blood pumps. Artif Organs 1982;6:190–197.

Bodnar, E. and Frater, R. W. M., editors
(1991) *Replacement Cardiac Valves,*
Pergamon Press, Inc. (New York), pp. 383–390
Printed in the United States of America

CHAPTER 16

PREMARKET TESTING OF NEW ARTIFICIAL HEART VALVES

Robert W. M. Frater

In the early days, artificial heart valves were often made on a kitchen table (1) or in a "factory" set up impromptu in a garage. While imagination, creativity, and daring are no less needed than they used to be, the process from conception to clinical use is more orderly. It is governed by legitimate concerns about the prediction of performance and the protection, as far as possible, of the patient, who is the consumer par excellence of the product.

In the United States this process is governed by the Food and Drug Administration (2).* This came about as the result of efforts by surgeons, prominent among them being Dwight Harken, Arthur Beall and Theodore Cooper, to establish guidelines for the premarket development of heart valves. A conference held in 1969 by the Association for the Advancement of Medical Instrumentation (AAMI) established the concept that a properly devised governmental system could ensure the development of safe and efficient devices, allow this to take place without undue delay, and at the same time protect the interests of the public. Dr. Theodore Cooper who was, at that time, the Director of the Heart and Lung Institute, was appointed Chairman of a Department of Health Education and Welfare Task Force to help develop the appropriate legislation for such a regulatory process. The 1976 Amendments to the Food Drug and Cosmetic Act was the result of this activity. It established classes of devices. All heart valves are Class III devices which:

1. purport, or are represented, to be for use in supporting or sustaining human life or,

2. present a potential for serious risk to the health, safety or welfare of a subject.

The Act defines in detail the circumstances under which a Class III device must be tested, manufactured, and tried before being brought to regular commercial use. There is provision in the law for an individual physician to make and use a Class III device, without Federal permission, for a particular patient. However, as soon as it is planned to make and test a device with the ultimate intention that it be available for public use, it is the law that the permission of the FDA be obtained.

Approval is a two-stage process. The first stage is the Investigational Device Exemption (IDE). This defines the information that must be provided on the structure and testing of the device, and the format of the intended clinical trial. The FDA is required to respond in 30 days. If the information provided by the sponsor of the device is accepted, the device may then be shipped lawfully for the purpose of conducting investigations.

*Reference 2 contains all FDA regulations affecting medical devices.

When the sponsor has gathered the clinical data required to establish that it is a safe and effective device, this is submitted to the FDA for Premarket Approval (PMA). The FDA is required to respond within 180 days. At the heart of the process established by the 1976 amendments is review at a public meeting by an Advisory Panel of qualified experts in engineering, biology, physical science, and clinical medicine. The FDA need not accept the advice of the panel, but must inform the sponsor of its decision to approve or disapprove with explanations, before the time limit of 180 days has expired. In addition to the legally defined process embodied in the Act, the FDA has published guidelines for the premarket approval of artificial heart valves, setting out the standards expected to be followed by developers (3).

In summary, the system established in the United States for the evaluation before general public use of a new heart valve is well-defined, is open to public scrutiny, has the assistance of an independent panel of evaluators, and most important, has the authority of law. As the FDA process has been evolving over the last 16 years, standards for the development of artificial heart valves have voluntarily been developed by AAMI, and the International Standards Organization (ISO). The AAMI American Standard was published in 1982 (4) and the ISO version in 1984 (5). In both bodies there was a mix of manufacturers, academic bioengineers, and surgeons on the working committees. There was also representation from AAMI on the ISO committee. As a result the two documents are similar, and in fact the more specific and detailed ISO version may soon be adopted by AAMI.

Governmental bodies in some countries are beginning to formulate processes for approving devices. At the present time, in those countries that have begun to consider these issues, FDA, IDE, or PMA approval will assure the granting of an import license. In Canada (6) and the United Kingdom (7) there are already systems in operation for controlling the general use of new valves.

In Canada, the Health Protection Branch of the Bureau of Radiation and Medical Devices undertakes a premarket review of devices intended for implant. Such devices cannot be sold in Canada until a notice of compliance with the premarket review provisions has been obtained by the manufacturer.

In the United Kingdom, there is no product approval scheme in operation. However, the Department of Health and Social Services (DHSS) encourages suppliers of heart valves to comply with certain recommendations and in general to follow the British Standard (BS) for the Development of Heart Valves. This is in fact identical to the ISO Standard. For the hemodynamic and wear testing recommendation of the ISO/BS standard, manufacturers are encouraged to use the DHSS funded laboratory under the direction of Professor Martin Black of the University of Sheffield. The manufacturers are encouraged to register under the Manufacturer's Registration scheme. This requires the adherence to the Department's description of Good Manufacturing Practices (8). Registration will not be granted unless the establishment and its procedures pass an inspection by DHSS officials, the costs of which are borne by the manufacturer. None of these carries the force of law. However, purchasing officers of hospitals of the National Health Service will expect the DHSS recommendations to have been followed if a device is to be bought for use in their hospitals.

Once implantation starts, the DHSS expects clinical trials to be conducted according to ISO/BS Standards, and the data and all implant information to be passed on to the UK Heart Valve Registry.

COMPONENTS OF PREMARKET TESTING

The components of premarket testing are:

1. Design/material combination
2. Fluid dynamics testing
3. Wear testing
4. Animal testing
5. Establishment of manufacturing facility
6. Clinical testing.

Design and Choice of Materials

The FDA requires complete information on the raw materials to be used in the construction of a valve. This includes chemistry, biologic source, the thermal/mechanical/chemical condition in both raw and finished form, and, where applicable, a complete inventory of physical properties.

The design specifications must be described from an engineering point of view. A worst-case description of the status of all components of the valve, the effects of the manufacturing process on the response to those stresses, fatigue tests on all structural members, and determinations of the margins of safety are required.

These requirements have particular relevance to mechanical valves, but are required also for structural members of biological or polymer membrane devices.

The purpose is obviously to anticipate and avoid as far as possible design deficiencies that could lead to premature failure.

Fluid Dynamics Testing

Fluid dynamics testing is described precisely in all the standards. The FDA guidelines refer to the ISO standard for information on the requirements for the pulse duplicator and the test methods to be employed. The ISO specifies detailed characteristics of pulse duplicator performance, measuring equipment accuracy, test fluid, test method, and test report. For forward flow, root mean square volume flow is specified. Regurgitant volume is divided into closing volume and leakage volume. Data are required on three samples of each size as well as a reference valve.

Wear Testing

Both the FDA guidelines and the ISO standard acknowledge that the correlation between in vitro wear tests and clinical performance is not exact. The lack of correlation may be in either direction. For instance, porcine bioprosthetic valves tend to tear in the Shellhigh system at a number of cycles less than the Shiley pericardial valve, and yet in life they have, in the mitral position, lasted longer than the Shiley, and far longer than either valve in the wear tester (9).

Paradoxes of this kind reflect the difficulties of the subject. Wear testing is an evolving science. There is a variety of quite different systems currently in use. For example the

Rowan-Ash tester moves the valve within a fluid filled cylinder, while the Shellhigh system has the valve mounted in a compliant walled closed loop subject to intermittent compression. Each testing system has its own characteristics. All users acknowledge that the "tuning" or adjustment of a particular system has a crucial influence on the results of testing a valve. The number of cycles to failure can vary by a factor as large as 10 according to the way the testing machine is set to run. Mechanical and biological valves of the same mounting size require different settings to achieve proper wear testing, and the pressure wave forms are smooth with biological valves and erratic with mechanical valves (10).

The in vitro conditions of wear testing are obviously different from the in vivo conditions to which the valve will be subject after implantation. For biological valves which inevitably interact with their environment this means that only some forms of durability problems can be studied: tears due to abrasion wear are testable; tears at the junction of calcified and noncalcified tissue are not.

The minimum requirements of the wear-testing apparatus specified by the ISO and FDA are that there be full opening and closing during each cycle and that there be "simulated physiologic loading conditions" (FDA) or a closing pressure of at least 75 mm Hg (ISO). The Shellhigh equipment, first developed by Gabbay, also measures flow, thereby improving the capacity for sensitive tuning. The ISO standard requires the test to be run until 350 million cycles have been completed or failure has occurred and makes no distinction between types of valve. Three each of the largest, medium, and smallest sizes, and at least one reference valve, must be tested. The FDA recommends testing three of each size and six of the largest. For biological valves the requirement is 200 million cycles. At least one reference valve that is marketed in the United States must be tested.

The FDA also requires fatigue testing of components such as struts, stents, and pivots. The ISO standard also requires testing of components, but states that testing of the complete valve may satisfy the requirements for component testing.

In summary, the skilled and knowledgeable use of a wear tester is an indispensable part of the development and preclinical testing of a new artificial heart valve. It may not effectively predict the later clinical performance of a valve, but the failure to use this tool will inevitably increase the possibility of unexpected failure of even the most carefully designed valve.

Animal Testing

The requirements of the FDA, AAMI, and ISO standards are modest in numbers and period of observation. A minimum of five animals followed for 5 months is specified by the FDA. The ISO requirement is five animals for 3 months and the AAMI standard, as first written, did not define the number of animals to be studied. Although expressed in different terms the goals are the same:

1. Evaluation of in vivo hemodynamic performance
2. Evaluation of valve pathology after short-term use
3. Evaluation of hematologic consequences of implantation
4. Evaluation of abdominal solid organs for possible (embolic) effects of the prosthesis.

The animal model used is to be clearly defined and the rationale for choosing a particular animal must be given. If calcification is an issue the age of the animal must be given.

All animals surviving the prescribed minimum time are required to undergo hemodynamic and hematologic testing before sacrifice, and autopsy after sacrifice. The FDA requires that animals dying before 20 weeks must have the cause of death and the hematological and pathologic studies recorded.

The ISO does not provide details of the testing to be done. The FDA is precise, but the information required is generally what would be obtained by anyone attempting to meet the four goals listed above.

The ISO Standard states that the objective is "to aid in the evaluation of these valve performance characteristics which are not assessable by in-vitro testing", and the FDA that "the intent of this study is to provide initial in-vivo data on the ease of surgical implantation, hemodynamic performance, assessment of valve related deaths and valvular pathology resulting from short-term implantation." These statements indicate a level of uncertainty about the predictive value of animal results for the behavior of devices in humans. In general, most manufacturers will want to test more animals for longer periods especially during the evolution of a design. We have taken the position that it is useful to have a few animals surviving for a longer period of time in case unforeseen changes in structure or complications occur with longer interaction between device and host. However, it is quite possible that such interactions are specific to a particular host-device combination. It is certain that no number of experiments and no duration of study are known that will predict with certainty the subsequent long-term behavior of a new device in humans. It is equally certain that some animal testing of the whole device is essential.

Establishment of Manufacturing Facility

Both the FDA and the DHSS require or encourage that the devices to be used in a clinical trial be manufactured according to defined standards of Good Manufacturing Practices. Good Manufacturing Practices (GMP) are particularly clearly described in the DHSS Guide to GMP Sterile Medical Devices and Surgical Products; these are the sum of all activities needed to satisfy the consumer's need for maximal quality safety and performance. The achievement of GMP demands meticulous attention to detail. The DHSS guide lists nine basic principles:

1. An integrated system of manufacture and quality assurance
2. Separate management responsibilities for both production and quality assurance
3. Suitable premises, equipment, and materials
4. Trained personnel
5. Documented procedures for manufacture and quality assurance
6. Appropriate batch and product records
7. Adequate transport and storage
8. A recall system
9. A system for auditing the operation of GMP.

To satisfy each of these principles requires thoughtful and extensive planning. There must be:

1) a plan for every action needed to complete every phase of the valve

2) a system to check the quality of every material or component used

3) a system to check the quality of every process used and every test performed

4) a system to record and track all materials, all procedures, all tests so that it will be possible, at any time, to find any deviation from the highest possible standards of manufacture, and prevent defective products being released for use, or, if released for use, to be able to get to the source of the problem precisely and rapidly.

The Food and Drug Administration regulations pertaining to GMP are codified and published in part 820 of Title 21 Food and Drugs. In addition to the Code of Federal Regulations there are Manuals describing in detail what is expected of the manufacturer under these regulations (11). The FDA in its publications refers also to certain AAMI standards, manuals, and technical information reports as authoritative. Inevitably, with experience, both the Code and the Manuals undergo change. Inspection is a part of the process and, as with all bureaucratic processes, inspector and manufacturer may differ on their interpretations of the law. Partly as a result of this, and partly because of the sheer complexity and difficulty of the task of attempting to avoid all possible hazard in the production of an artificial heart valve, a secondary business has developed in the United States: the provision of consultation and advice on the subject of fulfilling FDA requirements. The consultants are commonly people who have worked as FDA employees or in the regulatory departments of corporations developing devices that need FDA approval.

Clinical Testing

Before human implantation is started the FDA, AAMI, and ISO specify exactly what data are required for the clinical trials and what form they should take. The DHSS requires the ISO standard to be followed. The FDA requires no less than three selected primary centers. All United States centers and all foreign centers listed in the IDE are regarded as primary centers. A common protocol for patient selection and treatment is stated to be highly desirable. With a common protocol each center is required to enter a minimum of 35 patients with aortic implants and 35 with mitral implants. For each location of implant they must include an adequate representation of all available sizes. If common protocols are not used, the minimum number of implants in aortic or mitral locations per institution is 50. Reporting can be pooled with a common protocol, but otherwise must be analysed separately. The most important provisions of the FDA regulations are: 1) All patients entered in the study must be accounted for; a patient not willing, or not able, to participate in follow-up studies must be excluded; and 2) the follow-up must involve direct contact with the investigators for interviews and the performance of tests. The ISO requires 150 recipients of each type of valve (i.e., aortic or mitral) and a minimum of 20 per institution.

The actual data required are similar in the FDA, AAMI, and ISO documents. It includes a complete description of the patient, the patient's history, the abnormal hemodynamics, and hematologic and biochemical blood studies preoperatively; the valvular and cardiac pathology seen at surgery; the details of the operative technique, the valve model size and serial number, and the nature of any operative complications.

Postoperatively, the data required include information about the treatment the patient receives (antiplatelet treatment and especially anticoagulation), the biochemical and hematologic status of the patient, evidence of hemolysis, and the occurrence of complications, (especially thromboembolic, hemorrhagic and valvular), and the condition of the artificial valve. The May 1990 revision of the FDA guidance document on Replacement Heart Valves has finally taken the major and very important step of accepting echocardiographic investigation for the follow-up of implanted devices. The techniques required are laid out precisely and in detail. The significant difficulty and burden of requiring well patients to undergo cardiac catheterization for the sole purpose of acquiring follow-up information has now been removed.

During the study period the manufacturer agrees to report postoperative progress— initially between three and six months, and then annually. While not specifically requested it would be wise to report the occurrence of a major structural failure as soon as data is available rather than at the next available follow-up period.

DISCUSSION

It has been fashionable to complain about the negative effect of FDA regulations on the development and bringing to market of new devices in the USA. However, the standards developed by government bureaucrats and their scientific advisors for the FDA, and by private organizations such as AAMI and ISO whose members include both academic scientists and a majority of representatives from the valve manufacturers, are in substantial agreement about what should be required before a new device is implanted. Looked at in another way, if a knowledgeable physician user and a knowledgeable engineer manufacturer were to set themselves the task of listing all the information on the design, in vitro testing, in vivo testing, manufacture, and plans for clinical testing that they would like to have in order to feel satisfied that they were providing the best possible product to the public, they would surely arrive at a list very little different from the standards discussed in this paper. In fact, in the area of Good Manufacturing Practices, and all its subsections, the guidance provided is a distillation of experience, and, even with careful forethought, not all of the provisions prescribed would be obvious to a new manufacturer. The presence of regulatory agencies must then result in better and safer products.

There is, however, a caveat to the last statement. Government agencies have two problems. The first is that they are, in democracies, answerable to many masters. There are the legislators who vote the funding and never miss an opportunity to try to seem heroes by criticizing a part of the bureaucracy for wasting governmental money, or for failing to protect the public, or for failing to provide the public with new advances quickly enough. The virtuecrats of many different consumer groups are equally assiduous from the other side of the fence, and manufacturers bemoan the time (and therefore the cost) of achieving compliance. For the government bureaucrat decision making is extremely difficult in this atmosphere and often the easiest answer to a problem is inaction or postponement of a decision. It is a common complaint of manufacturers that the requirements change during the approval process of a particular valve. There are times when the extra information asked for seems only remotely related to the actual risk of failure of a device. However, that the officials should take the most cautious position possible is inevitable in the system as described.

Alternative systems could involve a mix of industry and academic personnel, and consumers, and could be funded by government, or industry, or both. Such a scheme could work, but acceptance by government or industry would probably be difficult. For the time being, the system run by the FDA provides the best possibility that new heart valves will arrive on the market in the safest possible condition.

REFERENCES

1. Frater RWM: The flexible monocusp valve: the second and third successful mitral valve replacements. Ann Thorac Surg 1989;48:S96-97.
2. Code of Federal Regulations, Food and Drugs, Title 21, Parts 800 to 1299. Government Printing Office Stock Number 869-007-00013-1. Washington DC, Superintendent of Documents, U.S. Government Printing Office (telephone # 202-783-3238).
3. Replacement Heart Valves—Guidance for Data to be submitted to the Food and Drug Administration for Premarket Approval, May 1, 1990. FDA HF2-450, 1390 Picard Drive, Rockville, MD 20850 (telephone # 301-427-1200).
4. American National Standard for Cardiac Valve Prostheses. ANSI/AAMI CVP 32/82. Association for the Advancement of Medical Instrumentation, 1901 Ft. Myer Drive, Suite 602, Arlington, Va. 22209.
5. Implants for Surgery—Cardiovascular Implants—Cardiac Valve Prostheses. ISO 5840:1984. ISO Central, Secretariat 1 rue de Varembe, CH-1211, Geneva 20, Switzerland (telephone # 4122 734 1240).
6. Guide to the Preparation of a Submission Pursuant to Part V of The Medical Devices Regulations 84-END-107, 1984. Public Affairs Directorate, Department of National Health and Welfare, 5th floor, Brooke Claxton Building, Ottawa K2AOK9, Canada.
7. Requirements for Marketing Heart Valves in The U.K. Department of Health, Procurement Directonate, 14 Russel Square, London WC1B5EP (telephone #01 636 6811 ext. 3297).
8. Guide to Good Manufacturing Practice for Sterile Medical Devices and Surgical Products, 1981. HMSO Publications Centre, P.O. Box 276, London SW85DT. (telephone #01-622-3316).
9. Gabbay S, Bortolotti U, Josif M: Mechanical factors influencing the durability of heart valve pericardial bioprostheses. Trans Am Soc Artif Intern Org, 1986;23:282–287.
10. Gabbay S, Mueller E (eds): Clinical Predictive Value of In-vitro Accelerated Fatigue Testing of Heart Valve Bioprostheses. Transcript of Technical Session, 24th Annual Meeting, AAMI, St. Louis MO, May 16, 1989. Newark NJ, IACBI, Department of Cardiothoracic Surgery, New Jersey Medical Schools Medical Science Building, 100 Bergen St. G502, Newark, NJ, 07103.
11. Device Good Manufacturing Practices Manual U.S. Government Printing Office Stock Number 017-012-00330-3. Rockville, MD, FDA Center for Devices and Radiological Health, 1987.

Bodnar, E. and Frater, R. W. M., editors
(1991) *Replacement Cardiac Valves,*
Pergamon Press, Inc. (New York), pp. 391–434
Printed in the United States of America

CHAPTER 17

METHODS AND LIMITATIONS OF FOLLOW-UP ASSESSMENT OF REPLACEMENT HEART VALVES

Eugene H. Blackstone

Methods and limitations of follow-up assessment of replacement heart valves can be addressed in a general and well-rounded sense only by describing the general (basic) aspects of clinical studies of time-related events, of which follow-up assessment of replacement heart valves is but a specific subset. In fact, the information required by the title becomes nearly self-evident when the general aspects of these kinds of investigations are mastered. To assist in making the transition from the general to the specific, the examples in this chapter are chosen from the specific area of the replacement of heart valves.

PURPOSE AND METHODOLOGY

Purpose

Clinical studies are performed so as to develop inferences. These inferences relate to the efficacy of therapy, the correlates and causes of therapeutic failure, the nature of these causes of failure, and thereby suggestions as to methods for neutralizing them, and to predicting and comparing. In the specific setting, the inferences address such questions as

Does heart valve replacement favorably affect the predicted or observed survival of a group of patients in comparison with the predicted survival without valve replacement of an identical group?

Does it effect a cure; that is, does it provide a survivorship indistinguishable from that of the general population of the patient's age, race, and gender (1)?

If not, what are the modes of failure, and are they likely to be related to patient-specific factors or to valve replacement device factors?

What can be done to minimize or neutralize the effects of either of these, including the use of a different valve replacement device?

Appropriately derived inferences provide a quantitative basis for discussing expected outcome with patients and their families, for selecting the most appropriate device for a given patient, and for optimal timing of valve replacement that simultaneously minimizes the combined risks of progressive irreversible damage to the heart were the valve(s) not replaced and of early and late mortality and morbidity associated with valve replacement. Such inferences also provide a rational basis for programming the research and development required to minimize risks in the future.

Methodology

Inferences are developed in the setting of valve replacement operations by compiling information concerning all fatal and nonfatal (morbid) events happening to patients following their operation, including the time of occurrence of each event, and analyzing these events using methodology developed specifically for the study of time-related events. In this chapter, the events relevant to the clinical performance of prosthetic cardiac valves are defined and characterized, the methods for study of an event are presented, including those of data compilation, risk factor identification, prediction, and comparison, and the process by which inferences are developed is detailed. The chapter discusses methods in current use in cardiac surgery, but it also encompasses methods less commonly used than these, but ones more appropriate and comprehensive.

There has been a strong tendency in cardiac surgery to adopt and promote certain methods of assessing clinical experiences as standards to which all reports must conform at just the time when these methods are at risk of becoming obsolete. Cardiac surgeons above all should be familiar with this phenomenon of a vigorous, progressing discipline: not infrequently, by the time their surgical method is published they will have improved upon it! Yet, they do not always realize that methodology in the disciplines of data analysis and scientific inference is also changing, particularly in the dynamic area of the analysis of time-related events. Non-time-related logistic regression analysis of hospital deaths (2), nonparametric analysis of "late" events using the product-limit method of Kaplan and Meier (3), semiparametric Cox regression analysis of postdismissal events (4), and single-parameter patient-year assessment of events that may recur (5), while continuing to be of some value in the ultimate process of drawing inferences from longitudinal clinical studies, are being supplemented or even replaced by more comprehensive methodology.

Some of these alternative or supplemental methods will seem new to cardiac surgeons and even to some of their statistical advisors, and may be viewed with skepticism. However, they have been developed, tested, and used in such fields as the testing of industrial systems for reliability, testing of computer hardware and software for reliability, and the military. Some have been applied to the clinical field of oncology, just as the actuarial methods were first applied in a widespread fashion to that field after being relegated to demography for a couple of centuries. Statisticians have also performed important statistical research on published transplantation data, thereby developing and testing improved statistical methods. In the process they have evolved new knowledge about transplantation, but their papers have appeared in journals rarely read by surgeons. (Interestingly enough, and conversely, the area of risk factor assessment has developed largely within the medical discipline, and is just now beginning to penetrate the industrial arena (6).)

Unfortunately, in this and other fields, as the methods become better they also become more complex and more difficult to understand fully, and more difficult to use. Two undesirable extremes of response by cardiac surgeons to the complexities inherent in new methods for analyzing clinical data will emerge, judging from their responses to the introduction of complexities in their own field: (1) the surgeons will try to educate themselves to "do all their own analyses," but with rare exceptions will appear to professional statisticians as nonexperts attempting to wield quite powerful tools, or (2) the surgeons will throw up their hands, claim ignorance of "statistics," and drop their data on the desk of their friendly statistician, expecting the statistician, who is not personally participating in cardiac surgery, to analyze the data and develop surgically relevant inferences from them. Instead, experts in both cardiac surgery and in data analysis, each respecting the other's knowledge and expertise and willing to understand each other at a working level, need to work cooperatively in this serious endeavor that affects the lives and happiness of present and future patients. We and other groups have demonstrated the feasibility and productivity of this approach. With it, the inferences that result are usually simple and true.

Quick Guide to Terms and Methods

A number of the terms and methods that will be used in this chapter are briefly defined here before rigorously developing the ideas of the chapter.

Time-related event: An occurrence observed at a specific instant of time. Often this definition is an oversimplification of a process that occurs over a relatively brief time span or that becomes evident at a specific time. The technical term for an event so defined is a *stochastic point process* or *counting process.*

Terminating event: A time-related event beyond which the individual is no longer traced (e.g., death).

Repeating event: A time-related event that may recur repeatedly (e.g., episodes of thromboembolism).

Actuarial method(s): A large group of methods developed for portraying time-related events, all having the general properties of taking into account all available information (that is, they accommodate incomplete information or censoring), and being nonparametric. The method popularized by J. Berkson at the Mayo Clinic was adopted from that used by insurance actuaries.

Kaplan-Meier (product limit) method: One of the nonparametric (actuarial) methods for estimating the survivorship function (3). Generally, the method is used to position graphically each event at its time of occurrence and at the estimated freedom from the event. The method uses more fully (although not completely) the available information concerning the time relatedness of an event than methods that divide time into discrete (usually equally spaced) intervals (7).

Censored observation: An observation (in this context, a patient) that is removed from the set of observations remaining at risk of an event before the occurrence of an event. An *uncensored observation* denotes a patient experiencing the event.

Parametric, nonparametric, semiparametric, quasiparametric: An equation, developed to summarize parsimoniously the distribution of time intervals to an event, will be expressed in terms of a few constants, called parameters. The numerical values of these parameters are estimated from the data. A completely parametric method implies to this writer a method formed upon biomathematical models (distributional models, compartmental models). A *nonparametric* approach does not develop a parsimonious model of the distribution. A *semiparametric* method may be nonparametric in some respect (such as with respect to the underlying hazard function in the Cox proportional hazards methodology (4)) and parametric in other respects, such as in evaluating the effect of risk factors on the event. A *quasiparametric* method is a completely parametric method that is based on an empirical equation-built strategy without a biomathematical basis (for example, splines).

Survivorship function: The probability of surviving from time zero to a later time. The survivorship function is defined for terminating events (or morbid events treated as terminating ones). It is estimated by nonparametric (actuarial) methods or various parametric and quasiparametric methods.

Hazard function, force of mortality, conditional failure rate, Mill's ratio: The instantaneous time-related risk of an event (a rate, expressed in terms of events per unit time).

Cumulative hazard function: The time-related mathematical integral of the hazard function. It depicts the mean number of events per patient from time zero to a later time that is expected in an individual remaining at risk (that is, not yet experiencing the event). It is obtained as the area beneath the hazard function between time zero and that later time.

Cumulative event function: An analog of the cumulative hazard function for repeating events. It depicts the mean number of episodes of the event from time zero to a later time that is expected in an individual remaining at risk of further episodes. The difference lies in the fact that patients experiencing the event remain at risk of recurrence of the event.

Cumulative morbidity function: An analog of the cumulative event function whereby each episode is weighted by a numerical estimate of the severity of the morbidity. It depicts the mean severity of morbidity from time zero to a later time that is expected in an individual remaining at risk of the event.

Cox proportional hazards model: A semiparametric method to assess the influence of variables on a time-related event (4). The underlying hazard is not modeled but is, rather, assumed to give rise to a survivorship similar to that obtained by the Kaplan-Meier method. The risk factors are incorporated into the analysis as a log-linear model of hazard:

$$\ln[\lambda(t)] = \ln[\lambda(0)] + \beta_1 x_1 + \cdots + \beta_k x_k \tag{17-1}$$

where x_i are the risk factors, β_i are the regression coefficients, and $\ln[\lambda(0)]$ is the logarithm (ln) of the unknown underlying hazard. The model is a convenient and tractable one computationally and guarantees that $\lambda(t)$ will always be a positive value. The idea of proportional hazards arises as follows. Let us compare the hazard function under two conditions, namely with $x_1 = 0$ on the one hand and $x_1 = 1$ on the other:

$$\ln[\lambda(t|x_1 = 0)] = \ln[\lambda(0)] + c \tag{17-2}$$

and

$$\ln[\lambda(t|x_1 = 1)] = \ln[\lambda(0)] + c + \beta_1 \tag{17-3}$$

where $c = \beta_2 x_2 + \cdots + \beta_k x_k$. We can exponentiate these:

$$\lambda(t|x_1 = 0) = \lambda(0) \exp(c) \tag{17-4}$$

and

$$\lambda(t|x_1 = 1) = \lambda(0) \exp(c) \exp(\beta_1) \tag{17-5}$$

Now make the simple substitution:

$$\lambda(t|x_1 = 1) = \lambda(t|x_1 = 0) \cdot \exp(\beta_1) \tag{17-6}$$

Thus, the risk for $x_1 = 1$ is proportional to the risk for $x_1 = 0$ by the constant $\exp(\beta_1)$, that is, they are multiplicative. The two hazard functions will run in parallel. Tests can be made to verify the proportionality assumption (8).

Linearized rates (subject-year rate, Pearl index, constant hazard rate, exponential survival, Poisson rate, etc): A one-parameter estimate of the risk (hazard) of an event across time, estimated simply as the number of events divided by the total duration of all follow-up times. The calculation is a useful one only if the risk is constant (unchanging) over time, neither increasing nor decreasing. The estimate has been called by several names; in keeping with recent guidelines published for reporting time-related valve events, the term *linearized rate* will be used in this chapter (9).

Logistic regression: A set of methods for analyzing risk factors for a non-time-related event (generally, but not necessarily, a dichotomous or binary yes/no variable) and based upon the logistic equation

$$P(\text{event}|\mathbf{x}) = \{1 - \exp[-Z(\mathbf{x})]\}^{-1} \qquad (17\text{-}7)$$

where $Z(\mathbf{x}) = \beta_0 + \beta_1 x_1 + \cdots + \beta_k x_k$ and $P(\text{event})$ is the probability of an event (2). The method replaces linear discriminant analysis with its restriction on the distributional properties of the risk factors. The inherent medical rationale for its use has been described (1, 10). Its use in analyzing time-related events that can be considered to have occurred within a brief time interval (e.g., in-hospital events) may be valuable. However, if time-related follow-up information is available, this artificial limitation can be circumvented (11).

Sample size, n: The number n of individuals in a clinical study or in a subgroup analysis. In studies of non-time-related variables (such as postoperative blood loss or serum CK-MB levels), the information content is commonly directly proportional to some function of n (for example, the square root). In the study of time-related events, the determinants are (1) the number of events (rather than the number of subjects, although the degree of uncertainty is proportional to n) and (2) the duration of follow-up. The number of events places an upper limit on the number of parameters that can be estimated (any shaping parameter plus all regression coefficients). The duration of follow-up places a limit on the resolution or identifiability of the shape of late risk. Thus, one may amass 1000 patient years of information by a study of 50 patients over a mean follow-up duration of 20 years each, or of 1000 patients over a mean follow-up duration of 1 year each. The inferences potentially available from each of the two studies are quite different. The first would yield estimates of long-term risk, albeit with relatively wide confidence limits, while the latter would yield good short-term information with narrow confidence limits, but no long-term information. Concerns about a sample being "too small" are best handled by use of confidence limits whose width directly conveys the uncertainty associated with the data.

EVENTS AFTER VALVE REPLACEMENT

Death

The least controversial (from the standpoints of definition and adherence to the assumptions underlying methods commonly used for the analysis of time-related events) of the relevant events that can follow heart valve replacement is *death.* As soon as only a subset of all deaths is considered (such as "cardiac" deaths), the possibility exists for lack of objectivity. As nonspecific as it may seem as a measure of the clinical performance of heart valve replacement devices, the portrayal and analysis of all deaths remain highly relevant and reliable. Its dilution by apparently noncardiac-related factors such as cancer or trauma is not great, since the majority of patients dying after valve replacement do so under cardiac-related circumstances (12). Only after a thorough analysis of all deaths is it of possible value to increase the sensitivity of some analyses, or to draw inferences about the feasibility of preventing some types of premature deaths, by considering subsets of deaths, such as "cardiac deaths."

Assigning a *mode of death* (sometimes erroneously described as the "cause" of death) is the first step in identifying subsets of death. The mode of death is a simple description of the general circumstances associated with death, such as death in acute, subacute, or chronic heart failure, sudden death, or death during a documented arrhythmic episode, death from trauma, death from cancer, or neurologic death (1, 12). This descriptive categorization does not presume a specific mechanism or knowledge of the results of an often unavailable postmortem examination. Rather, assigning a mode of death organizes simple observations of the manner in which the patient died.

Assigning a *mechanism (cause) of death* is more controversial as a means of subsetting the deaths because it requires formulating an inference derived from interpretation of the circumstances surrounding the death. For example, a patient dying suddenly several years after valve replacement may be found at postmortem examination with the poppet of his replacement valve lodged at the bifurcation of his abdominal aorta. Poppet escape is inferred to be the mechanism (cause) of his death, with a high probability that this inference is correct. Another patient dying in a similar manner may undergo a postmortem examination limited to the heart, at which time no abnormality other than an intact replacement valve is found. The mechanism (cause) of death is inferred to be an arrhythmia, but this inference is made with lesser certainty (although a number of mechanisms, including poppet escape, are excluded). A third patient dies suddenly while on a trip, and no postmortem examination is performed. Again, it may be inferred that the patient died of an arrhythmia, but he or she could have experienced an escaped poppet or a pulmonary embolus, or an acutely thrombosed valve. So the inference concerning the mechanism (cause) of death in this patient has a yet lower probability of being correct.

Since identification of a causal relation between a mechanism and the death is an inference, we have found it helpful to draw yet another type of causal inference that can assist in individual and institutional efforts to improve results, namely to infer just two *causes of death:* (a) lack of scientific progress in preventing such a death and (b) human error in applying known information (1, 10). This means of subsetting deaths, despite its potential for controversy and its demand for openness and honesty, has been found in other areas of human endeavor (such as the analysis of airline or mining disasters (13–15)) to focus attention precisely on those areas in need of further research on the one hand, and on those requiring development on the other. Both are worthy and relevant scientific pursuits aimed, in the present context, at lowering the early and late mortality associated with replacement of cardiac valves.

Assigning a mode, drawing inferences about the possible mechanism, and attributing the cause to lack of scientific progress or human error is just as valuable a process for other morbid events as it is for the event death (16). A limitation of the process is that it is truly retrospective in the statistical meaning of the word [a study of patients experiencing an event followed backward in time toward a "cause," as distinguished from a prospective study of a defined group of patients followed forward in time toward an event; the denominator is unstated in a retrospective study, whereas it is the basis for a prospective study (17)]. Inferences and hypotheses formulated on the basis of a retrospective study should be tested prospectively.

Other Morbid Events and Their Consequences

In addition to death, other morbid events are of importance to patients and their doctors after cardiac valve replacement. Definitions of these events have been developed by the Ad Hoc Liaison Committee for Standardizing Definitions of Prosthetic Heart Valve Morbidity of the American Association for Thoracic Surgery and the Society for Thoracic Surgeons (9). The committee has categorized the events as either *morbid events* or as *consequences of a morbid event*. Brief definitions of the events, excerpted directly from the reporting guidelines, are as follows, along with only a few of the several detailed examples given for each by the committee.

Morbid Events

Structural deterioration: Any change in valve function due to an *intrinsic* abnormality causing stenosis or regurgitation (for example, wear, stress fracture, poppet escape, calcification of a tissue valve).

Nonstructural dysfunction: Any abnormality resulting in stenosis or regurgitation at the valve that is not intrinsic to the valve itself (for example, pannus or suture entrapment, paravalvular leak, or inappropriate sizing, but not thromboembolism or infection).

Thromboembolism: Valve thrombosis or embolus exclusive of infection [includes any new, permanent or transient, focal or global, neurologic deficit (exclusive of hemorrhage) and any peripheral arterial emboli].

Anticoagulant-related hemorrhage: Any episode of internal or external bleeding that causes death, stroke, operation, or hospitalization, or requires transfusion.

Prosthetic valve endocarditis: Any infection involving a heart valve substitute or a reconstructed native valve (diagnosed by customary clinical criteria including a combination of positive blood cultures, clinical signs, or histologic confirmation).

Consequences of Morbid Events

Reoperation: Any operation that repairs, alters, or replaces a previously placed prosthesis or repaired valve.

Valve-related mortality: Death caused by structural deterioration, nonstructural dysfunction, thromboembolism, anticoagulant-related bleeding, prosthetic endocarditis, or death at reoperation (including most sudden deaths, but not deaths in chronic heart failure).

Permanent valve-related impairment: A permanent functional deficit due to structural deterioration, nonstructural dysfunction, thromboembolism, anticoagulant-related bleeding, prosthetic endocarditis, or reoperation.

Combinations of morbid consequences: A variety of composite events is suggested, such as an event representing the earliest of valve-related mortality, operative deaths, and reoperation (several other examples are given by the committee).

CHARACTERISTICS OF EVENTS

An event should be characterized as to

Its importance

The reliability with which it can be identified

The time of its occurrence, including the possibility of uncertainty in that time

Its time-relatedness to the operation

Its inevitability and the possibility or not of its occurring more than once

The influence of a nonterminating event on the occurrence of subsequent events

Closely related to the characteristics of an event are the characteristics of so-called *censoring,* the term applied to the process by which a patient ceases to be traced as regards the event after a specific time point. Censoring should be characterized as to

Its type (for example, right censoring, interval censoring)

The mechanism responsible for it

The degree to which it is noninformative (lacks correlation with the event being considered)

Whether or not it represents incomplete information concerning patients still at risk of the event by the end of follow-up or represents individuals withdrawn from risk

The majority of analyses of time-related events following valve replacement have used methods that assume that (a) the event occurs at an instantaneous point in time (termed, therefore, a *point process*), (b) the event is inevitable and nonrecurring (terminating), (c) the data are *right censored* (patients are followed in time "to the right" from time zero to a date of follow-up, then untraced thereafter), (d) the censoring mechanism is noninformative, and (e) censored observations represent incomplete information (patients remain at risk at the end of their follow-up). These assumptions are fulfilled, in most studies, only by the event *death* at any time and in any mode.

Importance

Not all events that occur in the life history of patients following replacement of a cardiac valve have the same importance for assessing replacement heart valve performance. For example, death from any cause is reliably identified but is considered to be of limited value (low sensitivity) in comparing replacement heart valve devices because it predominantly reflects patient-specific factors. Nevertheless, it is an important event per se that exhibits a protracted and substantial early phase of risk followed by a risk well above that of the general population, both of which suggest that a substantial improvement is yet to be made in the prevention of premature death after cardiac valve replacement (18).

On the other hand, the equally reliably identified event *valve reoperation* poses substantial interpretive problems. The timing of the reoperation may reflect patient or physician-related factors, and the reoperation may be for a number of totally different indications (that is, it is one possible consequence of a number of different morbid events) (9, 12). Probably the individual morbid events themselves are the more important events to analyze and interpret than the event reoperation.

The formulation of some events, particularly composite events (such as the time-related depiction of the first valve event of any kind), places equal importance on clinically unequal events (such as death and a rapidly resolving transient ischemic episode). Repeating events such as thromboembolism may also result in highly variable morbidity. Only recently (see below) has the degree of importance of each episode been taken into account.

Reliability of Identification

Some events are reliably identified: death and reoperation are two. Others are identified less reliably for several reasons. There may be definitional differences (such as in the case of a thromboembolic event). There may be an apparent overlap between two events, reflecting a lack of scientific progress in clearly distinguishing between them (prosthetic valve endocarditis versus noninfected periprosthetic leakage). Some events may be missed, such as structural valve failure in the absence of complete autopsy information, or all thromboembolic episodes because of lack of obvious signs or their misinterpretation. The prevalence of morbid events may be underestimated in patients who have died, not so much because the events were not identified by the patient, but because they do not appear in a medical record and cannot be recalled by the family. Events may be missed because of faulty communication, either in the wording of the inquiry and its interpretation by the patient or his or her family or by failure of the investigator to ask the right question. The event may represent a process that only becomes evident at a recognizable time (such as degeneration of a bioprosthesis) or may represent an event occurring immediately but becoming evident after a variable delay that in part depends on the sensitivity of the patient to it or to the sensitivity of its detection (for example, some periprosthetic leaks).

The Time of Occurrence

Throughout most discussions of time-related events, it is assumed that an event is a highly localized phenomenon occurring at instances along the continuous time line. They are, therefore, analyzed as *stochastic point processes* (19) or *counting processes* (20, 21). In reality, most events are processes that extend over a finite period of time (such as the time of a reoperation). Considerable theory has been developed and some clinically relevant analyses have been made, particularly in oncology, of the time-related transitions of patients from one state of health to another, with specific rates of transition between these states and with specific residence times longer than an instant within each state (22–24). While some of these ideas will be developed in this chapter, the assumption will be made that the events following cardiac valve replacement are reasonably well represented as stochastic point processes.

The time of occurrence of the event is important if an analysis is to be made of the event as a time-related one. If the risk of an event is changing rapidly, the time resolution must be greater. For example, early after operation, when the risk of death is high, the interval between the end of the procedure (when the patient is first exposed to risk) and death should be expressed in terms of minutes or hours. Events beyond these first few days require less precise time resolution, and the intervals can be expressed adequately in terms of days.

Despite all attempts to establish the precise time of an event, it may only be known to have occurred within a finite time interval (for example, between September 1 and September 15). The analysis can proceed using techniques established for managing *interval censored data,* of which this situation is but one example (11, 25).

The time of an event may be associated with uncertainty because the event represents a time-related process rather than a point process (evident valvular stenosis, evident bioprosthesis degeneration). Usually information about the evolution of such an event over time is unknown if the patient has been asymptomatic and serial noninvasive studies have not been made.

The Time-Relatedness of an Event

Presentation of a time-related event after cardiac valve replacement simply as the number of events divided by the number of patients undergoing operation always underestimates the probability of the event. Such a presentation does not take into account the duration of follow-up, variations in the prevalence of events at various times after surgery, or the decreasing number of patients remaining at risk as time progresses. Recognition of these shortcomings of a simple presentation of results led investigators such as Berkson at the Mayo Clinic to recommend the use of *actuarial methods* (7) to portray and analyze events in a time-related manner.

There is not just one actuarial method; rather, a variety of methods has been developed. They differ from each other by (a) the amount of information they require or use and (b) their mathematical development, some being based strictly on intuition and others being based on statistical theory (26). Their popularity relative to one another is currently more related to their accessibility in widely available data analysis software systems than to their theoretical advantages or their use of all available data. None portrays "raw data"; they all *derive* estimates of survival or freedom from an event based upon the set of individual times of the event or of censoring that constitute the raw data.

From the very inception of portrayal of time-related events by Galton, at least two complementary aspects have been of interest: the probability of surviving from time zero to a later time (the survivorship function) and the instantaneous risk of the event (the hazard function, sometimes referred to as the *force of mortality*) (27, 28).

An intuitive appreciation of the mathematical interrelations between these two functions may be facilitated by using the familiar biological compartment analog (the model assumed for calculations of blood flow from indicator dilution curves). Suppose there is a compartment containing at time $t = 0$ a certain quantity of substrate, $S(0)$. The substrate is removed from this compartment unidirectionally with a reaction rate $\lambda(t)$ to form $F(t)$:

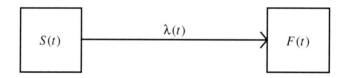

Suppose also that the decrease in $S(t)$ with time [denoted $\partial S(t)/\partial t$] depends also on the quantity of S remaining:

$$\partial S(t)/\partial t = -\lambda(t)S(t) \qquad (17\text{-}8)$$

(Elandt-Johnson and Johnson term rates that denote change per unit time per unit of substrate available *relative rates*, while those that are independent of substrate availability are *absolute rates*) (29). Rearrangement of Eq. 17-8 yields

$$\partial S(t)/S(t) = -\lambda(t)\,\partial t \qquad (17\text{-}9)$$

The term on the left side of the equals sign might be recalled as the derivative of a logarithmic (ln) term:

$$\partial \ln[S(t)] = -\lambda(t)\,\partial t \qquad (17\text{-}10)$$

Integrating both sides yields:

$$S(t) = S(0) \exp\left[-\int_0^t \lambda(u)\, du\right] \qquad (17\text{-}11)$$

where exp is e, the base of the natural logarithms.

In analyses of time-related events, the patients exposed to risk (sometimes called the *risk set*) correspond to $S(t)$ and the rate function $\lambda(t)$ is called the *hazard function*. The integral of the rate is the *cumulative hazard function* $\Lambda(t)$ (that is, the cumulative hazard function depicts the area beneath the hazard function from time = 0 to time = t). In our biochemical analog it is the amount of substance F that would be formed by time t if the substrate were being continuously refreshed (that is, equivalent to keeping a person at risk). In analyses of time-related events it is the mean number of events predicted by time t among patients remaining at risk:

$$\Lambda(t) = \int_0^t \lambda(u)\, du \qquad (17\text{-}12)$$

Since the cumulative hazard function is integrated over time, it is a nondecreasing function and is relatively "smooth" in comparison to its derivative (rate of change over time), the hazard function. Estimates of $\Lambda(t)$ are used extensively in industry (30–32). Since its slope at any time t is the hazard function $\lambda(t)$, a visual analysis of the slope of $\Lambda(t)$ will reveal the contour of $\lambda(t)$.

Since generally $S(0) = 1$ (all patients at risk) at $t = 0$ in Eq. 17-11, then:

$$S(t) = \exp[-\Lambda(t)] \qquad (17\text{-}13)$$

Of course, $F(t)$, the accumulation of biochemical product (or of events in analysis of time-related events), is the complement of $S(t)$:

$$F(t) = 1 - S(t) \qquad (17\text{-}14)$$

and the rate of its accumulation $\partial F(t)/\partial t$ or $f(t)$ is the *death density function*. By substitution and rearrangement of the various equations, one can verify that

$$\lambda(t) = f(t)/S(t) \qquad (17\text{-}15)$$
$$\lambda(t) = \partial \Lambda(t)/\partial t \qquad (17\text{-}16)$$

and

$$\Lambda(t) = -\ln[S(t)] \qquad (17\text{-}17)$$

The probability density function $f(t)$ is rarely used in drawing inferences about time-related events; rather, it is the basis for constructing maximum likelihood estimation functions used in obtaining parametric and semiparametric estimates (see below).

The estimation of these various "survival" functions from actual data is quite varied (26). In addition to differences related to the amount of information used and to the degree of formality of statistical underpinning, the methods also differ according to the function that was of most interest to the developers of the method. Most of the methods in use in cardiac surgery are ones developed for estimating the survivorship function. In industry the methods were developed with an emphasis on the hazard or cumulative hazard functions, with the object of determining the timing of taking a machine out of service after accumulation of the number of hours of use equivalent to some measure of average failure. Demographers have used the survivorship and hazard functions in parallel as the bases for their work. The latter workers, dealing with large populations, have not been concerned with the potential "roughness" of a rate (the hazard function) compared with the integral (survivorship function), but industry has had to deal with this. The thrust of newer methods of estimating these functions is to derive "smooth" (and therefore interpretable) estimates in all domains, particularly the hazard function domain.

The major complication of estimating survivorship functions is that the time of the event is unknown in some, and perhaps many, patients because the end of follow-up observation finds them as yet free of the event *(censored observations)*. Older life table methods (which should be considered obsolete) circumvented this problem by calculating, for example, 5-year survival only using that cohort of patients operated upon 5 years or more previously! All modern actuarial methods incorporate some mechanism for estimation in the face of incomplete information, using information on all patients operated upon at any time. (In our biochemical analogy one may think of censoring as a competing process that depletes the substrate available for reaction; actuarial methods adjust for this, yielding an $S(t)$ and $\lambda(t)$ as if no depletion by censoring had occurred.)

The Survivorship Function—Prevalence of an Event Across Time

The survivorship function is a generic term denoting the function representing the proportion of individuals free of an event starting from time zero to any given time; for example, the expected 5-year survival after valve replacement, or the freedom from a thromboembolic event. The most common nonparametric method used for estimating the survivorship function in cardiac surgery today is the *product-limit method of Kaplan and Meier* (3). By this method, each event is depicted actuarially positioned at the time of its occurrence. Details of the Kaplan and Meier method are given in *Cardiac Surgery* (1), including an exact method for calculating confidence limits of the estimates [a formulation by Greenwood (33) of an approximation to the variance of actuarial estimates, amenable to a desktop calculator, is still widely used today, despite the use of calculators and computers that make such approximations unnecessary].

The Kaplan and Meier method uses and depicts a larger proportion of the raw data than does the actuarial method used by Berkson (7) that generates only interval estimates (for example, at yearly intervals). However, except for determining the rank order of patients according to their follow-up interval, the Kaplan and Meier estimates incorporate no information about the exact duration of follow-up in its computations. Chiang was perhaps the first to advocate a piecewise parametric actuarial method that uses the *exact* follow-up interval for both uncensored and censored observations (26). His method will be described more completely below since it found immediate application in estimating the hazard function. To date his method has not been incorporated into widely available statistical software packages as a replacement for either the Kaplan and Meier or the Berkson actuarial methods for estimating the survivorship function.

Completely *parametric methods* may also be used to estimate the survivorship function. These methods have been in common use for decades in the industrial reliability discipline, having been initially developed for population trend studies (34). These methods express the distribution of times until events in terms of an *equation* whose *parameters* are estimated from the raw data. (An analogy is the expression of age at valve replacement by a mean value and a standard deviation. The mean and standard deviation are parameters of the "normal distribution" equation, and the parameter estimates are found using the data and simple estimating methods. The analogy is even more closely drawn if a number of the patients are known only to be older than some given age, corresponding to censored observations.) In this chapter we will make use of one such parametric method developed by us (11). The usefulness of having available a simple equation describing survival is illustrated by the desire of a patient who has survival for T years after valve replacement to know his or her probability of surviving another τ years. The conditional survival estimates are calculated as

$$S_c(\tau) = S(t)/S(T) \tag{7-18}$$

where T is the conditional time after operation, $S(T)$ is the survivorship to time T, τ is time after conditional time T, $S(t)$ is the overall survivorship, which may also be expressed as $S(T + \tau)$, and $S_c(\tau)$ is the conditional survivorship after T. With a parametric equation available, such calculations are simple solutions of the equation.

The Hazard Function—Rate of an Event (Incidence) Across Time

The *hazard function* is a rate, whereas the survivorship function is a prevalence (29). In common with all rates, it has units of inverse time (time^{-1}) and is commonly expressed as the mean number of events per individual at risk per unit time. It is probably the easiest time-related function for laypersons to understand, since most are aware of their own physiologic response to the increase and decrease in risk during everyday activities, such as the increased danger when stepping off a curb at a busy intersection or driving during a blinding rainstorm. It is not surprising that many of the events following valve replacement exhibit a time-varying hazard function as well (12).

The most common way that the hazard function for events following valve replacement has been presented is as a constant hazard rate per patient year or per 100 patients. This constant hazard rate has been called by many names, such as Pearl Index, but has been designated a *linearized rate* in the Edmunds reporting guidelines (9). The linearized rate is specifically appropriate, and is valid for predicting and comparing, when the risk of an event is constant, neither increasing nor decreasing over time or during a time interval of interest; it then corresponds to a linearly increasing cumulative hazard function and to an exponentially decreasing survivorship function (5, 35). Thus, death after the first few months of higher risk, late prosthetic valve endocarditis, and late periprosthetic leakage are examples of events after cardiac valve replacement that occur at a constant hazard rate (12). If the hazard function is increasing (as for bioprosthesis degeneration), or peaking (as in early prosthetic valve endocarditis, periprosthetic leakage, or valve thrombosis), or rapidly decreasing (as in death early after operation) then the overall linearized rate has little descriptive and predictive value and precludes inferences concerning the changing nature of the hazard function over time.

In spite of this, linearized rates have become commonplace in the cardiac surgery literature, in large part because of their ease of calculation rather than their appropriateness. The linearized rate is estimated by dividing the total number of events observed by the total duration of follow-up experienced by all the patients in the study group. For example, if 10 events were observed during 10,000 patient months of follow-up, the rate would be 0.001 events per patient at risk per month (or 0.1 events per 100 patients at risk). In mathematical form, this simple calculation can be written as

$$\hat{\lambda} = N_d \bigg/ \sum_{i=1}^{n} \tau_i \tag{17-19}$$

where $\hat{\lambda}$ is the linearized rate, N_d is the total number of events observed among n patients, and τ is the duration of follow-up for each of the patients. The denominator is simply the mathematical way to indicate the sum total duration of follow-up experienced by the n patients.

To assist in understanding the meaning of the linearized rate $\hat{\lambda}$, refer once again to the biochemical reaction example (Eqs. 17-1 to 17-6). The hazard function is not an absolute rate, so a $\lambda = 0.1$ per 100 patients at risk per month does not mean that after 120 months (10 years) 12 patients ($0.1 \cdot 120$) will experience the event. Fewer than 12 are predicted because as an individual experiences the event, he or she is removed from the *risk set,* thus reducing the *substrate.* In fact, using Eq. 17-13 and knowing that the integral of λ over time is simply $\lambda \cdot t$, one can calculate that of 100 patients free of the event at $t = 0$, 88.7% will be free of the event at 120 months $[-\exp(0.001 \cdot 120)]$, which translates to 11.3 events. (When there is the possibility that an event can be repeated, such as thromboembolism, and patients are not removed from the risk set at the time of their events, then the hazard rate is analogous to an absolute rate, and 12 events would be predicted by 120 months.)

Cox and Oakes suggest that asymmetric approximate confidence limits for $\hat{\lambda}$ may be obtained using the gamma distribution (36). A simple alternative is to consider the variability about λ to be lognormal in distribution. This consideration leads to a simple estimate of the variance of $\ln\hat{\lambda}$, namely $1/N_d$ where N_d is the number of events observed. Confidence limits (CL) equivalent to ± 1 standard deviation of $\hat{\lambda}$ are formulated in the logarithmic domain as

$$CL(\hat{\lambda}) = \exp[\ln(\hat{\lambda}) \pm (1/N_d)^{1/2}] \tag{17-20}$$

where exp means exponentiation to the base e. Such asymmetric confidence limits are to be preferred over the large-sample approximation to the standard deviation (SD) of λ, in particular for smaller data sets, namely:

$$SD(\hat{\lambda}) = \hat{\lambda}/N_d^{1/2} = N_d^{1/2} \bigg/ \sum_{i=1}^{n} \tau_i \tag{17-21}$$

and

$$CL(\hat{\lambda}) = \hat{\lambda} \pm SD \tag{17-22}$$

In the example given in Cox and Oaks, the 95% confidence limits for 9 events in 359 patient years ($\lambda = 0.025$) from the likelihood ratio are 0.0120 to 0.0452; from the gamma, 0.0115 to 0.0439; from the lognormal, 0.0130 to 0.0480; and from the symmetric method, 0.0087 to 0.0413.

If there is a strong desire to use linearized rates, the validity of assuming a constant hazard may be verified visually from a plot of the empirical cumulative hazard function (Eq. 17-17, minus the logarithm of the survivorship function, Fig. 17–1b). If the cumulative hazard is increasing at a constant rate (as it does in Fig. 17–1b only after about the first year of operation), then calculation of a linearized rate is appropriate. In other situations, the calculation may be valid for some interval of time (after a year in Fig. 17–1). If parametric estimation software is available (such as PROC LIFEREG (37) or PROC HAZARD (38) under SAS), then a direct test of the constant hazard assumption may be performed (for example, with a comparison to the Weibull function alternative).

In recognition that the hazard function may not be constant over time, *piecewise linear rates* have been calculated separately for a number of continuous intervals (for exam-

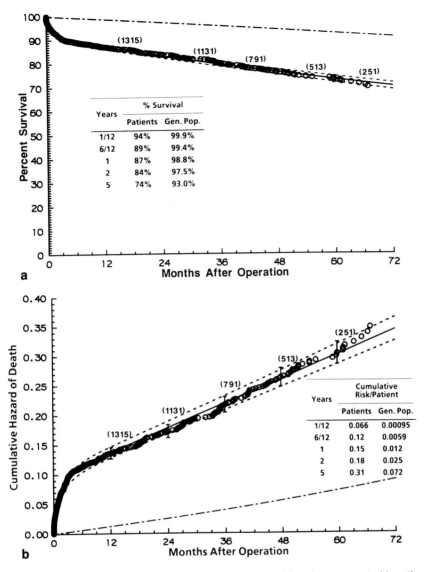

Years	% Survival	
	Patients	Gen. Pop.
1/12	94%	99.9%
6/12	89%	99.4%
1	87%	98.8%
2	84%	97.5%
5	74%	93.0%

a

Years	Cumulative Risk/Patient	
	Patients	Gen. Pop.
1/12	0.066	0.00095
6/12	0.12	0.0059
1	0.15	0.012
2	0.18	0.025
5	0.31	0.072

b

FIG. 17–1. Death after first-time valve replacement among 1533 patients presented in a time-related manner using both actuarial and parametric methods. (a) *Survival.* Each circle represents a death, positioned along the horizontal axis at the time of death and along the vertical axis actuarially. The asymmetric vertical bars about the point estimate indicate the number of patients remaining at risk across time. The solid line is an independently derived parametric estimate of survival, shown with its 70% confidence interval (dashed lines enclosing the equivalent of ±1 standard duration). The dash-dot-dash line represents the survival of a matched general population. The table presents parametric point estimates along the smooth line of survival at the indicated number of years after operation. Also depicted numerically is the survival of a matched general population. (b) *Cumulative hazard.* The format of the depiction is as in (a) except that the vertical axis is now in terms of mean number of events per patient at risk as a function of time after operation. Figure continued next page. (c) *Hazard function.* Two contrasting methods for determining the hazard function are depicted. The circles (presented without confidence intervals) are the estimates for each intraevent interval according to the method of Chiang (26). Notice their instability, with peaks and valleys representing, in part, the coarseness of the time scale (to the nearest day) for recording the time of each event. In contrast is the smooth model-based parsimonious parametric estimate shown by the solid line (38). (d) *Parametric hazard function.* Depiction of the solution of a parsimonious parametric equation for estimation of the hazard function, shown here without the unstable estimates. The dashed lines enclose the 70% confidence interval. The values in the table are point estimates along the smooth line.

405

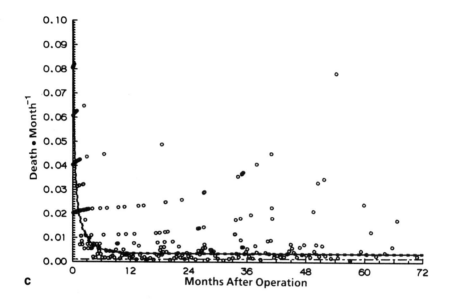

c

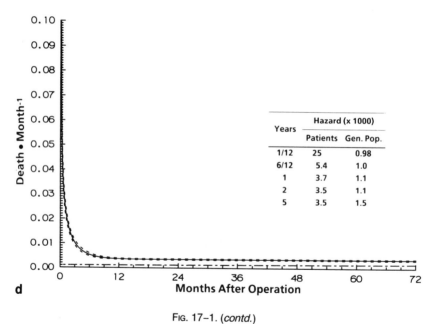

Years	Hazard (x 1000)	
	Patients	Gen. Pop.
1/12	25	0.98
6/12	5.4	1.0
1	3.7	1.1
2	3.5	1.1
5	3.5	1.5

d

FIG. 17-1. (contd.)

ple, at yearly intervals) as first suggested by Chiang (26). Specifically, the number of events in each interval is divided by the sum total of follow-up duration experienced by all individuals at risk *during that interval*. In mathematical notation, for the ith the interval

$$\hat{\lambda}(t_i) = n_{di} \bigg/ \sum_{j=1}^{n_i} \tau_j \tag{17-23}$$

where n_{di} = number of events in the interval t_{i-1} to t_i, n_i is the number of patients at risk during this same interval, and τ_j is the duration of follow-up time for each of the n_i patients at risk within the interval. This method is available in many of the readily available statistical software packages such as BMDP (39) and SAS (37). However, the estimates are difficult to interpret because they often have dips and valleys (instability) that one might suspect are highly data set–dependent, rather than reflecting the general trends so important in predicting and drawing inferences (Fig. 17–1c).

Because of the limitations for inferences of the methods just described, and because of the growing appreciation of the value of the hazard function for drawing inferences about time-related events, a great deal of attention is being focused upon the development of methods that portray stable (smooth) estimates of time-related hazard (Fig. 17–1d). Two approaches are being developed. One approach is to devise new *quasiparametric empiric methods* that yield stable hazard estimates. Examples of this approach are the recent work of Whittemore and Keller (40) and of Jarjoura (41), who propose the use of simple functions, such as splines, to smoothly estimate the hazard function. These methods make use of all the individual follow-up times and so use the available data efficiently, as does Chiang (26).

A second approach is to obtain stable estimates of the hazard function using *parsimonious parametric equations* as described in the section on the survivorship function. Since *parametric* can have various interpretations in statistics, by parametric equations we mean that the number of parameters is small (*low-order*, parsimonious) compared with the number of patients and number of events. Once a parametric equation is established for the distribution of events, any of the interrelated survivorship functions can be calculated as smooth interpretable functions. In our approach we have chosen equations that have an explicit derivative and integral form to simplify the calculations (11, 38).

These two divergent approaches can be compared. The more classic parametric methods that have developed over the past several hundred years use model-based equations, often having interpretable parameters, with their roots in biomathematics, biochemical kinetics, or probability distribution theory. The parametric method we have developed over the past 13 years, and now distributed by SAS Institute, Inc. (38), represents a broad generalization of this type of modeling effort. The more recent quasiparametric empiric methods use general low-order mathematical functions such as splines to build an equation (42, 43). This approach has general appeal since once computer software becomes available, relatively little decision making and computational work must be performed to obtain a smooth hazard function equation, although choosing the best position and number of knots for splines can be challenging. It remains to be seen, however, if meaningful incorporation of risk factors is possible using these strategies and if these methods yield prediction equations as robust as model-based parametric methods. A procedure to explore the possibilities of a spline model with concomitant variables (including time-varying covariates, to be discussed later) will shortly become generally distributed by SAS Institute, Inc. (44).

The Cumulative Hazard Function—Total Number of Events Across Time

The cumulative hazard function, like the survivorship function, is a time-related function, but instead of being a proportion bounded by the limits of 0 and 1, it depicts the mean number of events experienced up to a given point in time (or interval), usually expressed as events per individual (or per 100 individuals, per 1000 individuals, etc.). To repeat in different context the interrelations of the cumulative hazard function $\Lambda(t)$ with the survivorship $S(t)$ and hazard $\lambda(t)$ functions, recall that (Eqs. 17-17, 17-13, and 17-12):

$$\Lambda(t) = -\ln[S(t)]$$

or

$$S(t) = \exp[-\Lambda(t)]$$

and

$$\Lambda(t) = \int_0^t \lambda(u)du$$

The cumulative hazard function $\Lambda(t)$ has found little place in cardiac surgical literature, but it has often been used, perhaps unobtrusively, in the process of data analysis for visually estimating the shape of the hazard function (Fig. 17–1b) (11). On the other hand, it has been used commonly in the industrial setting as an aid for estimating the shape of the hazard function (30–32). Until recently, the cumulative hazard function was used exclusively for terminating events; it is now finding a unique place in the portrayal of repeated events where the number of events may exceed the number of individuals (45). Such a situation has no survivorship counterpart since it does not have a proper probability density function in the sense of a death density function.

The cumulative hazard function for a time-related event is estimated using the same actuarial, or more simply, counting methods as are used to obtain estimates of the survivorship function. Generally, in the medical sciences, it has been obtained from the survivorship estimates using the logarithmic transformation shown in Eq. 17-17. In industrial applications, the reverse is more common: the survivorship function is obtained from cumulative hazard estimates using the exponential transformation (Eq. 17-13).

There are as many procedures for estimating $\Lambda(t)$ as there are actuarial methods. However, only one of these, that of Nelson, will be presented (30). In the mathematical formulations it is assumed that the patients have been sorted according to their duration of follow-up, from shortest to longest. Although historically, and in all population demography, calculations are made over uniform time intervals, in cardiac surgery (and in most industrial applications) *calculations will be made at the time of each event*. We will denote the time of occurrence of the ith event as t_i and the time of the immediately preceding event as t_{i-1}; n_{di} events will have occurred at t_i (generally one, but if two or more patients experienced the event at exactly the same interval from operation, see the note below); n_i patients will be at risk (in common with other nonparametric methods, a patient who is censored at exactly t_i is considered at risk for the calculations made for the ith event). Using this notation, Nelson of the General Electric Company proposes a simple empiric estimate (30):

$$\Lambda(t_i) = \sum_{k=1}^{i} n_{dk} \Big/ n_{ik} \qquad (17\text{-}24)$$

with the important provision that n_{dk} be restricted to 1 (when the event is not a repeated one). This means that if three patients die at the same time t_i, the sum must be $1/n_{ik} + 1/(n_{ik} - 1) + 1/(n_{ik} - 2)$ for that interval.

Hazard estimates can be obtained as

$$\lambda(t_{mi}) = [\Lambda(t_i) - \Lambda(t_{i-1})]/(t_i - t_{i-1}) \qquad (17\text{-}25)$$

where t_{mi} indicates a midinterval estimate.

Terminating, Inevitable, and Recurring Events

An event is *terminating* if the patient is no longer traced after its occurrence. That is, the occurrence of the event simultaneously reduces the risk set, just as in the biochemical analogy leading to Eq. 17-8. The most usual example of a terminating event is death and the analysis of its various modes, mechanisms, and causes. Nearly all the readily available techniques for analyzing time-related events assume the event is a terminating one, since they were developed initially to analyze the event death (27, 28).

A further assumption of most methods for analyzing time-related events is that the event is *inevitable* (generally, given an infinitely long time as opposed to a specific time boundary (46)). Overall mortality is the prototypical, and perhaps only, example of such an event. Some actuarial methods, not in wide use, have been developed with the idea that not all individuals will experience the event (26). Such methods are of particular relevance to analysis of the competing risks of events, described below.

Nonfatal morbid events can occur *repeatedly* to the same patient. Examples include several episodes of thromboemboli, several episodes of important anticoagulant-related bleeding, and repeat valve reoperations. *Actuarial methods are not formulated to analyze repetition of an event.* Rather, uncensored observations (patients experiencing the event) are removed from the risk set and from all calculations for times later than that of an event's first occurrence. Because of this limitation, commonly only the first occurrence of the event is analyzed. Further follow-up concerning the patient is ignored, treating the event as if it were a terminating one. While this yields an important function, namely the probability of being completely free of the event, it underestimates the number of episodes of the event and may bias the risk factors for the event, possibly leading to incorrect inferences. For example, consider a morbid event that occurs in a large proportion of patients and is very prone to recur (an episode of rejection after cardiac transplantation is such an event). If only the time of first occurrence is analyzed as a terminating event, and if the event occurs in most patients shortly after time zero, the risk of the event may appear to decrease rapidly over time. However, the actual risk of the event in general, because of its recurring nature, may not be decreasing at all over time!

When repeating events have been considered, the most commonly used method in cardiac surgery for expressing the risk of all episodes of the event has been as a linearized rate (events per patient per year or events per 100 patients per year). Equation 17-23 is used, but all episodes are counted and the *total* follow-up time of each patient is used. The justification for this calculation is usually not given, but, in fact it is the correct maximum likelihood estimate for a constant hazard rate.

The intuitive basis for calculations of the time-related risk of a recurring event may be appreciated by referring again to a compartment analogy. Suppose that $R(t)$ is the substrate "at risk" at time t, that the reaction is $\lambda(t)$, and that events $E(t)$ are observed:

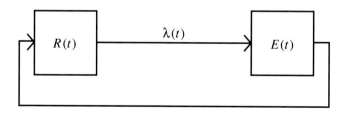

However, as soon as an event occurs and is counted, the substrate is "regenerated" instantaneously and is again at risk of reacting; there is instant feedback from $E(t)$ to

$R(t)$ as the arrows show. From the vantage point of analysis of recurring events, $E(t)$ represents a point process, and upon observing and counting the event, the patient is again at risk (in reality, he or she is never removed from risk). Now:

$$\partial E(t)/\partial t = \lambda(t)R(t) \tag{17-26}$$

But $R(t)$ remains constant (at 1 for example). Then, integrating both sides,

$$E(t) = \int_0^t \lambda(u)\,du \tag{17-27}$$

If $\lambda(t)$ is constant at $\hat{\lambda}$,

$$E(t) = \hat{\lambda}t \tag{17-28}$$

The Cumulative Event Function

Notice that $E(t)$, the *cumulative event function*, has the form of the cumulative hazard function (Eq. 7–12) and is expressed as mean number of events per patient at risk across time. In the system reliability literature, Eq. 17–27 describes a *nonhomogeneous Poisson process* and Eq. 17–28 a *homogeneous Poisson process* (19).

Nonparametric estimates of the cumulative event function are described by Nelson (who refers to the function as the "mean cumulative repair function") for repairs of industrial machinery (45). His estimation method parallels that of Eq. 17–24, except that patients remain at risk of repeating episodes after each event for as long as they remain at risk at all (they are censored only by death, removal of the valve being studied, or reaching the end of their study interval).

Approximate confidence limits for the cumulative event function have been derived assuming a lognormal distribution of variability (Turner ME Jr, Bartolucci AA, Naftel DC, Blackstone EH: Confidence limits for Nelson estimates assuming Poisson variation and approximating the distribution of the cumulative event function by an appropriate lognormal. Personal communication, 1989). Assuming Poisson variation:

$$\tilde{V}[\Lambda(t_i)] = \left(\sum_{k=1}^{i} 1/n_{rk}\right)\Lambda(t_i)/i \tag{17-29}$$

where $\tilde{V}[\Lambda(t_i)]$ is the variance of the cumulative event function for the ith event at time t_i and n_{rk} is the number of patients remaining at risk. The parameter estimates of the lognormal distribution are

$$\tilde{\eta}_i^2 = \tilde{V}[\Lambda(t_i)]/\Lambda(t_i)^2 \tag{17-30}$$
$$\tilde{\sigma}_i^2 = \ln[\tilde{\eta}_i^2 + 1] \tag{17-31}$$

and

$$\tilde{\mu}_i = \ln[\Lambda(t_i)] - (\tilde{\sigma}_i^2/2) \tag{17-32}$$

The confidence limits (CL) for the cumulative event function are:

$$\text{CL}[\Lambda(t_i)]_L = \exp(\tilde{\mu}_i - \alpha\tilde{\sigma}_i) \tag{17-33}$$

and

$$\text{CL}[\Lambda(t_i)]_U = \exp(\tilde{\mu}_i + \alpha\tilde{\sigma}_i) \tag{17-34}$$

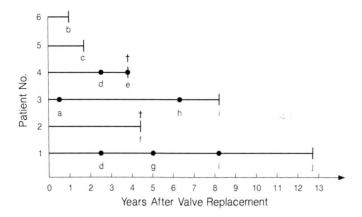

FIG. 17–2. Hypothetical thromboembolism history in six patients to illustrate methods of constructing the cumulative event function of a repeating event (see Table 17–1). A closed circle represents an event, a + represents a death, and a vertical bar denotes the end of follow-up. Each unique event and censoring time is marked by a letter that is keyed to the calculations in Table 17–1.

where α is the confidence coefficient (1 for "70%" confidence limits, 1.96 for 95% confidence limits, corresponding to 1 and 2 standard deviations, respectively). The method of calculating the cumulative event function and its confidence limits is illustrated in Fig. 17–2 and Table 17–1.

The interpretation of the cumulative event function is that by any given time t one would expect on the average $\Lambda(t)$ events per patient. The concept is illustrated in Fig. 17–3a, which depicts cumulative event functions across time for all thromboembolic events after cardiac valve replacement using a mixture of several mechanical devices. At present there is limited accessibility to computer software that provides stable parametric estimates of the instantaneous risk of a recurring event. However, one such estimate for the thromboembolic episodes depicted in Fig. 17–3a is shown in Fig. 17–3b.

TABLE 17–1. *Calculation of the Cumulative Event Function and Its Confidence Limits Based Upon the Assumption of Poisson Variation and Approximating the Distribution of $\Lambda(t)$ by an Appropriate Lognormal Distribution**

Time of event or censoring t	Event label on Fig. 17–2	Number of events n_d	Index of event times i	Number at risk n_r	$\dfrac{n_d}{n_r}$	Cumulative hazard estimate $\Lambda(t)$ (24)	Variance of $\Lambda(t)$ $\Sigma 1/n_r$	$V[\Lambda(t)]$ (29)	Lognormal distribution parameters $\bar{\eta}^2$ (30)	$\bar{\sigma}^2$ (31)	μ (32)	"70%" (1 SD equivalent) confidence limits (33) (34)
0.5	a	1	1	6	0.17	0.17	0.17	0.028	1.0	0.69	−2.1	0.051–0.27
1.0	b			5								
1.7	c			4								
2.5	d	2	2	4	0.50	0.67	0.42	0.14	0.31	0.27	−0.54	0.35–0.98
3.8	e	1	3	4	0.25	0.92	0.67	0.20	0.24	0.22	−0.20	0.52–1.3
4.4	f			3								
5.0	g	1	4	2	0.50	1.4	1.2	0.41	0.21	0.19	0.25	0.84–2.0
6.3	h	1	5	2	0.50	1.9	1.7	0.64	0.17	0.16	0.57	1.2–2.6
8.2	i	1	6	2	0.50	2.4	2.2	0.87	0.15	0.14	0.81	1.6–3.3
12.7	j			0								

*The notation and equations for each element in the table are given in the text. The numbers in parentheses beneath the column headings denote the equation number in the text from which the calculations were made.

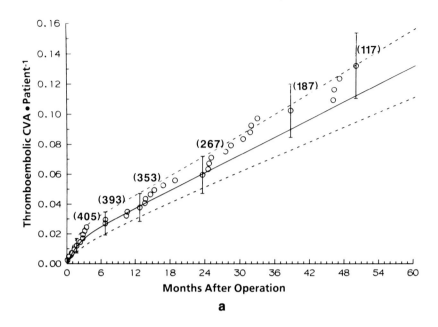

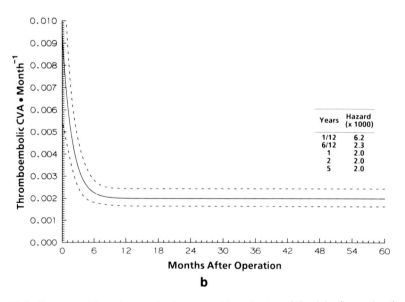

FIG. 17–3. Nonparametric and approximate parametric estimates of the risk of recurring thromboembolic events following mechanical heart valve prosthesis insertion. (a) Cumulative event function of all thromboembolic episodes. The circles represent each episode of the event in the same types of depiction as for Fig. 17–1, with each circle positioned according to the method of Nelson (45). The event may be in a different patient or in the same patient. All patients remain at risk until death or the end of follow-up. The solid curve and its 70% confidence limits represent the parametric estimates. Data kindly provided by Kuntze CEEE, Ebels TE, Eijgelaar A, van der Heide JHN. Academisch Ziekenhuis Groningen, Groningen, The Netherlands. (b) Parametric estimates of the instantaneous risk of a thromboembolic episode per patient per month.

The Cumulative Morbidity Function

An extension of the cumulative event function analysis of a repeating event is the *cumulative morbidity function* (*M*). In Nelson's formulation, each event may be weighted by a specific morbidity severity. Thus, Eq. 17-24 becomes

$$M(t_i) = \sum_{k=1}^{i} w_{ek} n_{ek} \Big/ n_{ik} \qquad (17\text{-}35)$$

where w_e is the morbidity severity of the events n_e (42). In the industrial arena, w_e is generally the financial cost of the repair. Thus Nelson calls the function *mean cumulative cost function.* He demonstrates that the rate of repairs may be constant or even decreasing while the rate of cost may be increasing. While financial costs may be considered in the morbidity function, generally an arbitrary scale of morbidity must be developed.

Purely to illustrate the ideas, we have considered the morbidity of thromboembolic events following mitral valve commissurotomy, censoring patients at valve replacement. Each thromboembolic episode was assigned a severity of morbidity index: 0 = no event, 1 = complete resolution of the effects of the event, 2 = permanent residual from the event, and 3 = death from the event. (Perhaps a power scale of 0, 1, 2, 4 would have been a more realistic choice.) The cumulative morbidity function so constructed is depicted in Fig. 17–4a, with estimates of its confidence limits and approximate parametric equivalent. The morbidity rate, or hazard, function is depicted in Fig. 17–4b.

A risk factor analysis for repeating events and for the severity of their morbidity is possible, but a specific limitation is that only variables available at $t = 0$, the time of original valve replacement, may be considered in the analysis. Any subsequent information, such as the number of episodes of the event or the intervals between episodes in a given patient, can be entered only if the analysis permits inclusion of *time-varying covariates* (to be discussed below). This limitation reflects an unstated assumption inherent in a general depiction of all episodes of a repeating event, namely that all episodes are treated independently. That is, no distinction is made between 10 repeating events occurring in one patient and 2 repeating events in five patients, nor between second and third episode of the event.

Comprehensive Analyses of Repeating Events

The above limitation has introduced the potential complexity of analyzing repeating events comprehensively. Therefore, further methods will be presented in the format of asking specific questions about the recurring events that may arise in assessing heart valve replacement data. Some of the methods are straightforward extensions of easily accessible and understandable methods. Others are more complex and are under intensive investigation in both medical and industrial arenas.

Does the first episode of an event predispose a patient to a second episode? To assess the conditional risk of a second episode, given the occurrence of a first episode of the event, the subset of patients that have experienced the first episode of the event can be analyzed, starting them at a new time zero corresponding to the time of the first occurrence of the event and following each patient from that time to the time of the next recurrence of the event or the end of follow-up (Fig. 17–5). Risk factors for this second occurrence can be determined, although the analysis will be limited by a smaller number of events, because the study subset includes a smaller number of patients. Among the

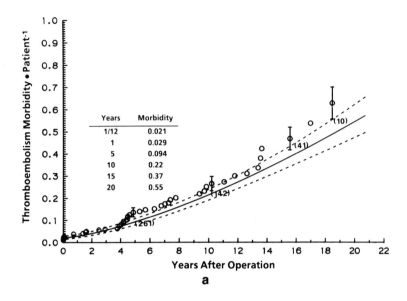

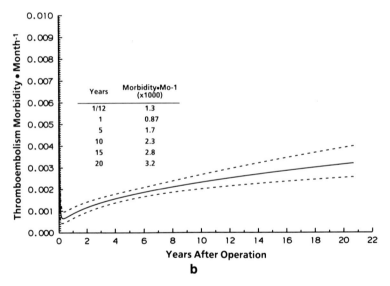

FIG. 17–4. Time-related morbidity from thromboembolic events after closed or open mitral valve commissurotomy. (a) Cumulative morbidity function. Each episode of thromboembolism has been assigned an arbitrary severity on the scale of 1 to 3 (1 = no residual; 2 = residual; 3 = death from the episode). The mean morbidity from thromboembolic events per patient over time was then constructed. The presentation is otherwise as in Fig. 17–3. (b) The mean rate of thromboembolism morbidity per patient per month is depicted parametrically.

risk factors that may be assessed is the interval from operation to the first event. Any other variable pertinent to the new time zero, as well as all the variables examined in the analysis of first occurrence, may be considered. This process can be repeated for all recurrences, resetting time 0 to the time after each preceding event.

In theory, a single comprehensive analysis can be done of the risk of each episode with

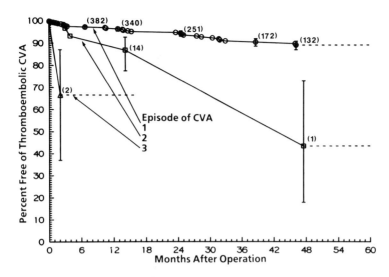

FIG. 17–5. Freedom from thromboembolism after cardiac valve replacement. The actuarially determined freedom from a first episode as a function of time after operation is shown by the open circles. Actuarial freedom from a second episode among patients already experiencing one episode is shown by open squares, time zero beginning at the time of the first episode. Freedom from a third episode among patients already experiencing two such episodes is shown by the open triangles, time zero beginning at the time of the second episode. Kindly provided by Kuntze CEEE, Ebels TE, Eijgelaar A, van der Heide JNH, Academisch Ziekenhuis Groningen, Groningen, The Netherlands.

the resetting of time to zero when each event occurs (interevent interval analysis with retention separately of the connectivity of these intervals for each patient). Then mathematical convolution techniques can be used to calculate the freedom from two or more, three or more, and so forth, episodes (22). Extensions of this type of analysis to include risk factors form the basis for a truly comprehensive parametric or semiparametric analysis of a repeated event. Details of a generalization of the Cox semiparametric risk factor methodology for this purpose have been presented and applied to time-related data concerning recurring infection episodes following bone marrow transplantation (47).

Since no explicit representation of the hazard function is necessary for the Cox model, its development has preceded that of a comprehensive parsimonious parametric method. However, it is reasonable to presume that simple relationships may be discovered among the individual hazard functions for each episode. The analysis would be thereby simplified and made more tractable by a reduction in the total number of parameters to be estimated. In analyzing the data, for example, for thromboembolism following mitral valve commissurotomy, such a simplification was found reasonable, as is shown by the parametric curves superimposed in Fig. 17–6a. Specifically, a new data set was constructed consisting of (a) the original cohort of patients, (b) the patients experiencing a first thromboembolic event, with time zero set to the time of first thromboembolism occurrence, and (c) the patients experiencing a second episode, with a new time zero set to the time of the second episode. An overall hazard function was determined for this augmented data set (Fig. 17–6b), and an analysis was made of the single variable *number of previous thromboembolic episodes* (0, 1, or 2). The analysis showed that after the early hazard phase, this linear ordered variable was highly predictive of subsequent episodes.

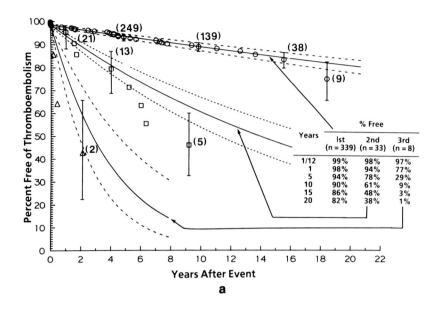

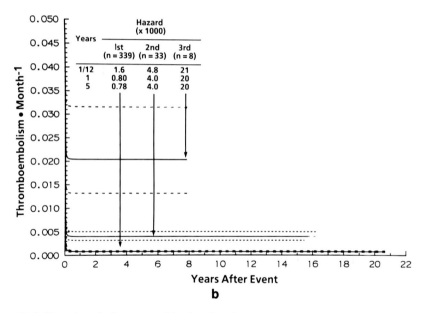

FIG. 17–6. Thromboembolism events following closed or open mitral valve commissurotomy illustrating that each thromboembolic episode increases the risk of a subsequent one. (a) Freedom from thromboembolic events according to number of previous episodes (0, 1, or 2). The depiction is as in Fig. 17–1. Time zero for the uppermost curve is the time of operation, for the second curve the time of the first thromboembolic event, and for the third curve the time of the second thromboembolic event. The parametric curves depicted by the solid lines with their 70% confidence intervals represent the solution of an equation generated by a univariate analysis of the variable *number of previous embolic events* (0, 1, or 2). (b) Parametric hazard function estimates of the time-related risk of the first, the second (after a first), and the third (after two previous episodes) thromboembolic event.

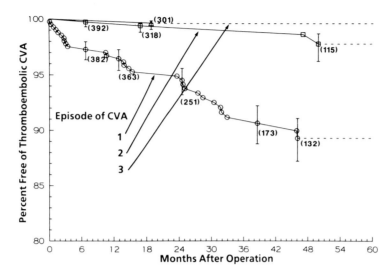

FIG. 17-7. Actuarial freedom from one or more (open circles), two or more (open squares), or three or more (open triangles) episodes of thromboembolism after cardiac valve replacement as a function of time after operation. All patients are followed from the date of operation (time zero) for each event. Each event is analyzed as if it were a terminating one. Data kindly provided by Kuntze CEEE, Ebels TE, Eijgelaar A, van der Heide JNH, Academisch Ziekenhuis Groningen, Groningen, The Netherlands.

Solutions to that univariate equation produced the smooth curves depicted in Fig. 17–6a.

This augmented data set, then, becomes the basis for further multivariate analysis. Because time zero is redefined for each episode, covariates relative to that episode, as well as all past historical data, may be entered into the risk factor analysis. Specifically, the number of previous episodes and the interval since the last episode may be entered along with other relevant variables.

What is the risk over time of at least two episodes of thromboembolism? One readily accessible way to assess the risk of a specified number of episodes of an event (such as the risk of at least two episodes of thromboembolism) involves defining each episode as a separate, terminating time-related event, each starting at the time of the original valve replacement (Fig. 17–7). At any point in time the risk of the second occurrence of the event will always be less than that of the first. Since all methods for analyzing a terminating event apply, risk factors for each specific occurrence can be determined. The analysis will be limited by (1) the progressively fewer number of events available for analysis and (2) the inappropriateness of incorporating any information about preceding episodes of the event (except as time-varying covariates, discussed later in this chapter). Convolution techniques can be used to estimate freedom from the *k*th episode of an event from the individual analyses of each recurrence as described above (22).

Influence of an Event on Subsequent Events (Time-varying Covariates)

The Committee for Standardizing Definitions of Prosthetic Heart Valve Morbidity recognized that some morbid events are the consequence of others (9). In the language used by the statisticians developing the theory and methods of analysis for time-related events, a morbid event that influences the occurrence of another event of the same or of a different variety is a *time-varying covariate*. At time zero the morbid event has not yet occurred, but at a specific, but variable, time thereafter it has; the variable representing that morbid event switches from being *no* to *yes* at that time.

It is desirable to incorporate time-varying covariates into an analysis of events to reduce the variability inherent in predicting the time of an event when changes occur in the condition of the patient. Methods are accessible to accommodate time-varying covariates as a generalization of the Cox methodology in the BMDP software package (48). It has been our experience that the computer time and resources to accomplish such an analysis are large. However, as powerful and very fast computers become increasingly prevalent, such so-called computationally intensive techniques become feasible. Interestingly enough, one form of accommodating time-varying covariates using completely parametric methods has been demonstrated by Herndon to consume computer resources only directly proportional to the number of transitions occurring in the time-varying covariates within the data set (44). The limitation of his method is that the *shape* of the underlying hazard curve is maintained at the time of a transition, the curve being merely shifted abruptly upward or downward. A more comprehensive analysis, just as for repeating events, would permit a new hazard function shape to be estimated at the time of transition. Simplification to that of merely scaling the original hazard function shape from its original time zero may be demonstrated. Clayton has recently reviewed the current state of progress and remaining challenges in analyzing complex "event history" data such as these (23).

Certain useful studies can be made of the consequences of events using accessible techniques by studying the subset of patients experiencing the morbid event, setting time zero to the time of the morbid event, and then determining the occurrence of subsequent events of either the same or a different nature (12). For example, the impact of prosthetic valve endocarditis on subsequent reoperation, periprosthetic leakage, or death can be analyzed. These analyses, conditional upon the occurrence of a morbid event, provide useful and relevant information to patients experiencing them. Among the risk factors that might be examined in such analyses are the number of preceding events and the interval from operation. In our analysis of 1533 primary valve replacements, 75 patients had a total of 103 reoperations during their follow-up (12). The 103 reoperations were entered as additional observations to assess the risk of *number of reoperations* on death.

Not all time-varying covariates of interest are morbid events. The functional status of the patient at various points in time is one such variable. When functional class has been assessed periodically, Herndon provides an example of how to incorporate these observations as time-varying covariates in a risk factor assessment (44). Here a word of caution is required, however. In many follow-up studies, functional status is assessed only once, namely, at the time of follow-up inquiry. The time of transition of a patient from say, class I to class II or from class II to class III is rarely determined. It may, nevertheless, be possible to draw inferences from cross-sectional follow-up information as to the time-related change in functional status of patients. Methods for analyzing time-related *ordinal* models are required for such an analysis. In ordinal models, the event variable can take on more than binary, yes or no, values; the "event" can be an ordered response variable such as NYHA class. Methods such as ordinal logistic regression may then be used (2, 49).

While changes of any variable can be incorporated into an analysis of time-varying covariates, there are a group of techniques being developed that specifically trace patients through recognizable changes of state of the patient (21–24). A patient's condition may worsen, get better for a time, and then worsen and lead to death. Data adequate to estimate the transition rates from state to state in such a comprehensive analysis are not often available for cardiac valve replacement. However, as medical information systems become more prevalent in the future, such analyses may be feasible and remove much of the uncertainty concerning predicted time until an event that is inherent in present-day analyses.

Censoring Considerations

In the development of most time-related analyses, it is assumed that censoring represents *incomplete information* concerning the time of an event and that the censoring mechanism is *noninformative* (50). Except for analyses of all deaths following valve replacement, censoring usually does not represent incomplete information of the kind for which the theory was developed, and the censoring may not be noninformative.

If a patient remains at risk of the event at the end of his period of follow-up, censoring represents incomplete information concerning the time of the event. This is the classic situation for which actuarial methods were developed (3, 7). However, if the event is *sudden death following valve replacement,* any patient dying in other modes of death is censored for the event *sudden death,* but that censoring mechanism is now *removal from the risk set.* If the patients were followed even 100 years until all patients died for one or another reason, the actuarial depiction of freedom from sudden death would never reach zero. In other words, the event *sudden death* is not considered to be an inevitable one, and there will be a finite freedom from the event as long as the patients are followed. In any analysis other than that for all deaths, considerable care must, therefore, be taken in determining just who is a censored patient, but still at risk, a censored patient, but no longer at risk and an uncensored patient who experiences the event (or in the case of repeated events, an uncensored patient remaining at risk of another episode of the event).

Patients being followed after valve replacement are likely to have accrued into the study rather uniformly over time. If the follow-up status of all the patients is assessed formally during a very short interval of time, the distribution of censoring will be uniform over the study period (51). The pattern of censoring would not be expected to affect the information concerning the event. This is called noninformative censoring. A large number of untraced patients represents an example of potentially informative censoring, for it is well established that untraced patients tend to have a very different distribution of death from the traced patients (52). When studying any event other than all deaths, the uniform pattern of censoring may be altered by the addition of censoring representing patients no longer at risk as discussed in the above paragraph. In the next section we will discuss how this may, under some specific circumstances, affect the analysis, particularly that of risk factors.

Influence of an Event on Censoring (Competing Risks of an Event)

The occurrence of some events precludes, by definition, the occurrence of other events. For example, death in chronic heart failure precludes sudden death, death from trauma, or death in any other mode. The censoring inherent in the analysis of mutually exclusive subset categories can influence the pattern of censoring and thereby even the risk factor analysis. A risk factor for chronic heart failure might be the preoperative New York functional class. If most patients in a high NYHA functional class die early after surgery in cardiac failure, an apparent inverse relationship between NYHA functional class and modes of death predominating at a later time could be found. Such a correlate might be spurious, arising from the censoring of most patients with a high NYHA class. This is known as the problem of *competing risks* of an event (53). That is, death in one mode is in competition with death in all other modes. Fortunately, events after valve replacement are rather rare (the degree of censoring is high), and although this makes the establishment of risk factors more difficult, it probably reduces the possibility that competing risks of an event will influence the analysis spuriously.

The problem of competing risks also applies to the separate analysis of various phases of risk for an event. For example, deaths after valve replacement tend to exhibit a period of very high risk for the first few months after operation, and thereafter a period of rather constant or increasing risk (Fig. 17–1d) (12). If the early death rate were very high (and fortunately it is not for valve replacement), the early deaths may alter the distribution of risk factors among surviving patients so as to make interpretation of an analysis difficult (54, 55).

A specific subset of competing risks of an event is the *decomposition of a composite event* into separate subevents. Analysis can be made of subsets of an event such as death (Fig. 17–8). Separate analyses of risk factors may then be made for each subevent. Such a decomposition is particularly valuable in examining an event such as reoperation after valve replacement that represents a final common pathway for several morbid events. Reoperation may be decomposed usefully into separate analyses of specific valve types, or of specific indications for reoperation (11, 12). Further, it may become apparent that it is more useful to analyze the primary morbid event such as all episodes of prosthetic endocarditis, all valve thromboses, or all periprosthetic leakages, rather than just reoperation for them. Of course, the decomposition reduces the number of events for each analysis. However, the risk factors that are identified may well be more relevant than those found in the general analysis of a fundamentally composite event.

STUDY OF AN EVENT

Data Requirements

To analyze time-related clinical events properly and usefully, their occurrence in time must be ascertained and compiled. This means that a serious study of replacement heart valve performance requires a formal follow-up of all relevant patients before commencing analysis.

Previously we have reviewed several methods for conducting the follow-up inquiry (51): the *anniversary method* (yearly contact on the anniversary of each patient's heart valve replacement), the *common closing date method* (cross-sectional follow-up of all patients as of a specified date), and *date of last report method* (Berkson method (56)). The common closing date method best meets the assumptions of the analytic methods in use today.

Recently, a fourth method of follow-up, the *passive method,* has been evaluated (57). In this method, no patient is actually contacted. Rather, at some point in time, a repository of mortality statistics is consulted (such as a national registry of vital statistics), and the mortality status of each patient ascertained. For large studies with death as the only end point, rather small discrepancies (in the order of 5%) have been found (patients who

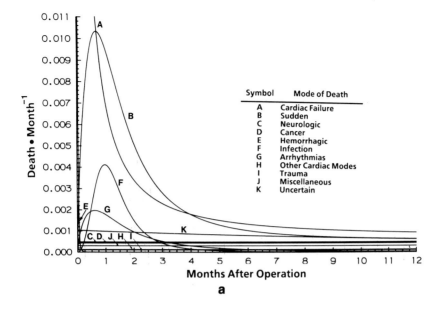

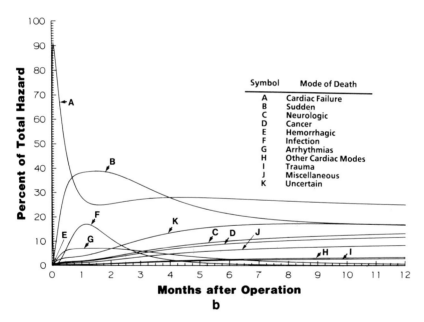

FIG. 17–8. Mode-specific hazard functions for death after heart valve replacement, illustrating competing risks for the event death. The sum of these mutually exclusive individual hazard functions yields an overall hazard function for death that is indistinguishable from that shown in Fig. 17–1d by the solid line. (a) Separate hazard functions for each of the modes of death. (b) Contribution at each moment in time of each mode of death is depicted as a percentage of the total hazard for the event death.

apparently never appear in the statistical registry), and some reasonable techniques for estimating the errors and taking them into account have been developed when the prevalence of death is high (57).

We suspect that cardiac surgical centers have very often used an *informal passive follow-up method,* whereby no rigorous attempt of any kind has been made to trace each patient; rather, only clinic visit records and occasional letters from referring physicians have been assembled. It has been well documented that such a follow-up "study" underestimates the number of events (52). Although such studies admittedly belong to the realm of *anecdotal information,* we have observed an interesting phenomenon with regard to the analysis of follow-up studies that have consisted of data obtained by this informal passive follow-up method. In four such experiences to date, the shape of the cumulative hazard function has appeared "ill behaved" (complex in shape), a behavior accentuated when attempting to model the distribution of events parametrically. In two of these instances, we were subsequently able to obtain a true cross-sectional assessment of all patients. The cumulative hazard curves were then well behaved (as they usually are with true cross-sectional follow-up), with a clear and simple shape, readily amenable to parametric analysis.

We infer that there is no place in serious follow-up studies for use of less than rigorous methods. It is our strong recommendation that a formal follow-up of all patients in a study be conducted over a brief period of time, using when available the growing cadre of individuals trained in the conduct of follow-up studies that has been a valuable spin-off of several multicenter studies, generally in ischemic heart disease.

Because of the large number of patients involved in a study of heart valves, it may not be possible to interview each patient (or his or her family if the patient has died) individually. Instead, a questionnaire is mailed to patients. This document must be short (preferably a single page), easily understood, and designed to elicit a positive response from the patient that can be discussed in more detail personally with the patient, the family, or primary physician later if necessary.

Risk Factor Analysis

The propensity of patients to experience events after cardiac valve replacement varies from one individual to another. Characteristics of the patient, his disease, his systemic response to his disease, the details of his operation, the subsequent progression of his underlying disease or development of other disease, and possibly the valve replacement device itself may be correlated with a greater or lesser risk of an event. Generally, risk factors are associations with the event and are not causes of it. Nevertheless, they should provide clues to the cause and thus stimulate research to find and neutralize the causes and thus neutralize the risk factor (1). Risk factors, such as the functional status and age of the patient, or the morphology of his or her valve lesion, may also provide information that is relevant to the optimal timing of intervention in the natural history of the patient's disease such that maximum benefit is obtained with a minimum of prosthesis-related risks. The one use of risk factors that we do not recommend is as a vehicle to exclude certain patients from operation unless the predicted risks exceed those of an alternative treatment or predict near certain death (for example, upper confidence limit for early survival below 5%).

The risk factors to be entered into an analysis must be selected with considerable care, preferably as a collaborative effort of the senior surgeon-investigator and his or her statistical colleagues (as we will describe later, the processes of establishing the "final" risk factor model and interpreting it are also collaborative efforts). In order for a variable to be entered, it must have been observed and recorded prospectively. This requires either an ongoing registry with expert data entry and verification or a disciplined approach to the daily routine recording of clinical observations for later review and collection. Subjective clinical indices (such as NYHA functional class) should be well defined, since one purpose of a clinical study is to communicate information applicable to other settings and to future patients.

Unless time-varying covariates are to be entered (and generally this would be done under selective circumstances), all variables should be those pertaining at *time zero*. These include preoperative variables and, when appropriate, operative details. As regards the latter, we caution against incorporation of cardiopulmonary bypass time as a risk factor candidate since longer times may result from a very poor hemodynamic state and efforts to improve it, rather than being the cause of that state; in addition, although global myocardial ischemic time as a risk factor is valuable in assessing myocardial protection modalities, it may not be a good variable in a model that is intended for general predictive use.

There is considerable controversy and discussion about how to establish a final multivariate risk factor model (58–60). If a stepwise computer algorithm is used, entering all the variables for possible selection that are possibly relevant, and with some criterion for retention of variables in a final model, it might be supposed that a single computer "run" should produce a final result (model). Unfortunately, this is not the case, nor should it be the case. The quality and success of a risk factor analysis depends, of course, on the availability, quality, and completeness of the variables being considered. However, different investigators working with the same set of data may each produce a different final model! This may be due to variability in cleverness, or failure to examine some interaction between variables, or a propensity of the person analyzing the data to work in isolation from his or her surgical colleagues, or from the pressures of a busy general "shop" that takes a superficial approach to a study to "get it out." Assuming, however, a really serious in-depth investigation of risk factors, one usually finds that the different models contain the same *types* of variables (surrogates for one another) that yield the same *inferential* model (60).

Some guidelines for conducting the analysis can be given that may reduce the variability between different analyzers of the data. As will be seen, the techniques rest heavily on organization of the variables and a thorough understanding of the variables in relationship to the event.

Organization and Characterization of Potential Risk Factor Variables

The variables being considered should be organized in several logical ways. The organization begins when the study is first devised. Variables might be organized according to their type (such as demographic, morphologic, physiologic, clinical assessment) or their source (such as angiographic, echocardiographic, operative) in order to gather the data efficiently. In the course of compiling the data, each variable should be categorized as to its completeness, its range (if the range is too narrow, the risk factor will lack discrimination), and its quality (is it a soft or a very accurately quantitated variable?). Considerable thought needs to be given to the *inferential* categorization of each variable (NYHA functional class as a reflection of an increasing degree of left ventricular functional deterioration, tricuspid annuloplasty as a reflection of right ventricular dysfunction, and so forth). Other statistical categorizations and characterizations are made during the course of examining the interrelations among variables (discussed below).

Descriptive Analysis of the Variables under Consideration

The association of the variables under consideration with the event being studied should then be examined by the person who will perform the risk factor analysis. The process includes constructing simple contingency tables for all categorical variables (often for arbitrary "phases" of risk such as death within 6 months, death beyond 6 months, and so forth, corresponding to obvious changes in the hazard function that has previously been established). Variables need not be considered further if they are associated with no, or perhaps only one, event in a small subgroup of patients, or if a substantial amount of data is missing, or if the variable is considered to be unreliable for a well-justified reason. If the variable is an ordered one (such as NYHA functional class) the effect of ordering is investigated using univariate logistic regression. Continuous variables are tested using a t test, but more importantly are examined univariately with logistic regression to reveal trends.

In addition, logistic scattergrams of the continuous variable are constructed to assist in identifying the need for transformations of the variable. This is accomplished as follows. The patients are divided into several groups of roughly equal number (5–10 groups is a good number). Within each group the proportion $\hat{p}$ experiencing the event is calculated. This quantity is converted to logit units:

$$\hat{z} = \ln[\hat{p}/(1 - \hat{p}] \tag{17-36}$$

A plot is then constructed with the continuous variable along the horizontal axis and logit units along the vertical axis. The individual $\hat{z}$'s are plotted at the mean or median value of the continuous variable within each group. The points should fall roughly along a straight line. If not, a transformation is made (logarithmic, a power, the inverse, a quadratic term). This step is important for making accurate inferences from the *shape* of the relation of a variable to the event.

The construction of cumulative distribution functions will reveal unusual extreme values in the data. These should be checked. If the data are found to have been recorded properly, the potential undue influence on the analysis of these extreme values must be borne in mind. For example, an analysis can be made with the patient having extreme values included, and again with that patient excluded. We have been surprised by how closely the analyses usually match, attesting to the resistance of many analyses to extreme values.

It is not necessary, nor often desirable, to convert a continuous variable into a discrete set of variables such as age <30, age 30 to 50, age >50. This common practice loses information, denies the continuity of nature, calls for "breakpoint" decisions, and clouds inferences. The prevalence of this undesirable practice may reflect a misunderstanding of the methods of estimation currently available to the investigator. Namely, maximum likelihood estimation techniques for time-related events permit any mixture of discrete, ordered categorical, and continuous variables to be analyzed stimultaneously.

In the descriptive stages of analysis the variables should be examined within their logical categories. It often becomes apparent that one or the other of several variables reflecting the same quantity (such as pulmonary wedge pressure, left atrial pressure, and left ventricular end diastolic pressure in patients with aortic valve disease) may have fewer missing data and be preferred for an analysis, or that similar variables might be combined into one index (such as augmentation of NYHA class by the addition of class V to designate a moribund condition of the patient at operation) (61).

Simple correlations between all the variables still remaining under consideration are calculated. These may reveal strong correlations that will affect the multivariate analysis. A more detailed examination of interrelations among variables will be made subsequently.

In order to preserve the full information content of the analysis, missing values may have to be replaced by the mean or median value for the group as a whole or for an appropriate subgroup (for example, mean global myocardial ischemic time within the subgroup of patients having cardioplegic myocardial protection). If the number of patients with missing values for a variable is large (that is, includes at least one event), then a *dummy variable* or flag variable should be created to indicate *missing value*. If the patients with missing values behave in all other respects as those with data available, this flag will have a value no more different from zero than expected by chance.

When these initial steps are completed, the investigators will have acquired an excellent knowledge of the variables, their relative quality, their prevalence, their potential role in the analysis ("If this variable were to enter into the analysis, would I understand why?"), and their appropriateness for a particular analysis. Variables that represent measurements or conditions pertaining after time zero, such as any postoperative ones, are discarded (they may be worthy events to study in and of themselves) unless time-varying covariate analyses are being contemplated. All relevant variables are then included in the analysis, not just those that univariately appear correlated with the event (for an example of the importance of retaining all relevant variables in the analysis, see Ref. 62).

Aids for Establishing a Risk Factor Model

The process of multivariate analysis now begins. It commences with a formal examination of the multivariate structure that is contained within the variables themselves. Generally, there is considerable sharing of information content among variables (height, weight, and body surface area, for instance). A procedure should be applied to the variables under consideration that clusters them into groupings according to the degree of information they share (for example, PROC VARCLUS under SAS to group variables according to their intercorrelations with one another (63)). The importance of this step is that (1) these closely related variables (some unexpectedly related, perhaps) provide similar information in the analysis, (2) one or the other of several variables in the group might be preferred in the model a priori (ease of interpretation, reliability of measurement, completeness of information, more related to a presumptive cause–effect relation) to the exclusion of the others, and (3) if one of the variables in a group enters, it is possible that another closely correlated variable will be selected to slightly adjust for the variable already in the model (often the sign of the regression coefficient will change), and this is to be avoided (perhaps by a more appropriate transformation in scale of the preferred variable). Probably the final model should have no more than one variable from each closely interrelated group of variables. Again, it is emphasized that categorizations and appropriate grouping of the variables is an indispensable key to the intensive intellectual process of establishing a risk factor model.

An alternative to this organizational strategy is the formation of principal components (or indices). These can be thought of as empirical variables formed by statistically weighting and combining ordinary variables (58). This method, however, does not provide a readily interpretable analysis, despite its parsimony and often demonstrated superior stability for prediction.

With all this information available, the multivariate risk factor analysis is ready to be undertaken. The now very highly organized and characterized variables are successively entered. While this procedure may be carried out in many different ways, most accessible methods employ an automatic *stepwise forward* procedure (variables are entered one by one in ascending order of P value or other entry criterion) or *stepwise backward* procedure (all variables are initially incorporated, followed by a one-by-one elimination of those variables not meeting a P value or other criterion for being retained), or permit a combination of the two. Operationally, some nonautomatic entry and exclusion of variables is often necessary (such as to investigate interactions among variables in a logical fashion), and most procedures permit variables to be "forced" into or out of the modeling process or to be incorporated in a selected sequence. Thus, in the analytic process, numerous computer runs are required gradually to eliminate from further consideration some variables while identifying others that are to be retained permanently in the model. Careful attention to groups of interrelated variables aids in the decision process to eliminate or retain variables.

Periodically the analytic progress should be reviewed by the surgical and statistical investigators for clinical relevance of the analyses. The review of analyses at that time may suggest that a variable not originally gathered should be incorporated (for example, if several variables have increased left ventricular wall thickness as a common denominator, an index of left ventricular hypertrophy noted in the operation report or on preoperative study might be gathered); or that a variable is truly spurious because of extreme *influential* values; or that specific interactions between variables should be examined; or that several working models should be developed along different lines for different inferential purposes. Not infrequently, we have found it important to restart an analysis from the beginning in light of new data or better insight. The ultimate quality of the final model is probably directly proportional to the intensity of interaction between the surgical and statistical investigators during the model development process.

While multivariate analysis is considered a sophisticated tool, one of its chief virtues is that it simplifies the study. It focuses attention on a small subset of variables that contain the major information content of the study as regards the event under consideration. These variables can be further studied in greater detail than is possible if all variables gathered had to be thoroughly examined and presented. Thus, the multivariate analysis is a major tool for synthesis of information. This is why we recommend its use early in the analytic process rather than later, as it immediately provides the investigators with an overview, extricating them from an overwhelming sea of information of very unequal value. For the same reason, we recommend that formal publication of a study emphasize the multivariate analysis and specific solutions of the resulting equation, rather than seemingly endless and boring tables of the results of univariate analysis.

The Analytic Tools

To perform the multivariate analysis, an underlying structure of the time-related risk of the event is required as well as some form of regression equation consisting of the sum of regression coefficients multiplied by their corresponding variables. The most widely employed regression model for time-related events is the proportional hazards model (Cox regression model) (4). This model makes no assumption about the structure of the underlying hazard function; rather, it estimates regression coefficients that shift the underlying hazard curve upward or downward in a proportionate fashion (eg., *yes* for a variable that multiplies risk by a constant over a value of *no*). The properties of this model have been well studied. Its disadvantages in the study of valve replacement devices are several: (1) it has no underlying hazard structure, so no direct numerical predictions are made; rather the nonparametric actuarial curve is simply shifted up or down (some of the newer methods already described will provide a more stable hazard estimate to be manipulated); (2) graphic display of the influence of risk factors is limited, which in our experience is a considerable limitation to the forming of inferences; (3) only one set of risk factors over all time is identified, whereas for some events, such as death after valve replacement, risk factors may change over time; and (4) the proportional hazards assumption (which has a distinct computational advantage of guaranteeing that the hazard function will not be negative) may not be correct.

These are among the reasons that methods have been developed to overcome some or all of these limitations (see, for example, Ref. 11). Almost any method to obtain a smooth underlying hazard function will permit graphic display of relationships in the hazard domain. Various ways to "break up" time into phases, with separate analysis of risk factors for each, have been proposed. If one has only Cox regression procedures available, then a separate analysis of 30-day survival (or logistic analysis of hospital death) and of late survival may be an appropriate strategy, and we have used this in the past. The newer parametric method developed by us generates a number of phases appropriate to the data and the most parsimonious equation for each based upon the data, and then permits a risk factor analysis to be performed simultaneously for all the phases identified (38). Within each phase, we also assume proportional hazards, but variables can exhibit complex interrelationships between phases that partially remove the limitations imposed by an overall proportional hazards model. Although the structure of the underlying hazard function must be ascertained explicitly with this model, the regression procedure for finding incremental risk factors for the event is no more difficult than Cox regression.

Limitations

There are both absolute and relative limitations of a multivariate risk factor analysis. If the number of events is small, no matter how large the total number of patients, the risk factor model can accommodate *at most* the number of parameters and risk factor coefficients equal to the number of events. If a multiple phase model is being employed, the number of events associated with that phase places an upper limit on the number of risk factors that can be accommodated. Particularly in the early phase of hazard, a variable (usually defining a rare subgroup) that is associated with either no events at all or one that identifies a subgroup of patients that all experienced the event poses computational difficulties (generally an infinitely large or infinitely small coefficient). In late hazard phases, these difficulties should not be encountered. The analysis is also limited by the extent of the follow-up; if it is short, only early-phase risk factors can be found.

A relative limitation in our experience has been the analysis of a clinical entity with generally poor results. Under this circumstance (for example, with event prevalences in the early phase of 30% or more), one often identifies no risk factors at all! Under these circumstances inferences for improving results must be drawn from intuition or from some other basis. It is when the results become generally good, but not yet perfect, that risk factor analysis is particularly valuable in identifying those factors still in need of neutralization. Of course, if the results are perfect, no analysis is possible; rather, one might wish to interpret this result in the light of its confidence limits to avoid being led astray in euphoria.

Another limitation is that risk factor analyses generally require the use of sophisticated computer hardware and carefully constructed software, coupled with a sophisticated familiarity with multiple regression in general, probably nonlinear regression, and, before embarking on the newer methods, logistic and Cox regression. Many, perhaps most, statisticians have had limited exposure to time-related events and to logistic or Cox regression, so finding a knowledgeable colleague may be difficult in some settings.

Predicting

The purpose of clinical studies was described in the beginning of this chapter as being "to develop inferences. These inferences relate to . . . predicting and comparing." It is often forgotten that the recording of achievements, meritorious as it may be in its own right, is not a basis for scientific inferences relating to predicting and comparing. Proper nonparametric and parametric depictions of the estimated freedom from an event, which include estimates of the degree of uncertainty, are predictions based upon the sample of patients being studied. They are intended to portray (1) the anticipated freedom at a future time in that specific group of patients to compare with the information available at that time, and (2) the anticipated freedom in similar patients both at that institution and in general. This is why it is important to state in a quantitative fashion the uncertainty associated with the estimates such as by confidence limits. The uncertainty does not arise (or should not arise) from uncertainty about the data. Rather, it arises from the initial size of the sample as representing patients with valve disease in general (and *future* patients specifically), even if the sample is one's complete series of patients, and the incomplete information arising from limited follow-up (censoring).

Extrapolation or projection of survival or freedom from any other event beyond the last observed event requires that assumptions be made about the structure of the time-related distribution of events. The easiest way to do this is to describe the distribution by a parsimonious equation. The equation can be solved for times beyond that of the last event to provide an estimate of the future behavior of the same or other patients as regards the event. The width of the confidence limits of the predictions will of necessity widen, usually dramatically, as the prediction extends in time beyond the data, but under some circumstances this may represent the best information available for decision making (64). Also, the distribution of events might be such that a certain amount of erratic behavior is apparent in the nonparametric estimates, but in general the trends are simple and well behaved. These are reasons why methods for obtaining stable estimates of the hazard function are important, particularly those that estimate parameters of an equation that can be manipulated easily.

The precision of prediction can be increased by an analysis of risk factors such as just discussed, particularly using completely parametric methods. After establishing a risk factor equation, survival or freedom from an event, or the hazard function, can be predicted for a specific set of risk factors pertinent to a given patient (see examples such as Fig. 4 of Ref. 12). A limitation of the analysis is that the prediction of the exact moment when an event will occur, even taking into account risk factors, is associated with rather great uncertainty. Incorporating time-varying covariates into the model can reduce this uncertainty.

Comparing

A fundamental concept underlying the comparison of results of valve replacement (or any other intervention) is that the patients being studied represent a *sample* from which inferences are drawn with a specific degree of uncertainty concerning the results that might be expected in similarly treated patients, including future patients. Acceptance of this concept has many implications. First, the group of patients, even if it is the entire experience of an institution, is not considered *the population*. As such, observed quantitative information, such as mortality, is not treated as a record of achievement, but as a vehicle for estimating outcome in other patients. Descriptive statistics and even nonparametric methods of estimation that describe in faithful detail the observations in the study patients are considered to be of less value than more general derived quantities, such as equations consisting of a few parameters, that may better portray underlying trends and better predict results in other (and future) patients. The presentation of even the simplest information concerning the study group is also accompanied by presentation of confidence limits to permit comparison and prediction. These may appear to some to be an unnecessary complexity, since there is nothing uncertain about the data themselves. Indeed, they would be unnecessary were not the purpose of the study to draw inferences from comparisons and predictions, both of which are associated with increasing uncertainty as the size of the study group sample decreases.

Informal comparisons may be made by examining point estimates and the degree of overlap of their confidence limits. Generally, if 70% confidence limits do not overlap (corresponding to ± 1 SD of the estimate), the difference is only possibly due to chance ($P < .15$, often $<.1$), and if 90% confidence limits do not overlap, the difference is unlikely to be due to chance ($P < .05$, often $<.01$) (1).

Formal methods of comparison provide more rigorous inferences. They include (1) randomized clinical trials, (2) analyses of combined series, and (3) application of equations from one experience to another to generate an expected event distribution (adjusted for possibly differing prevalences of risk factors) and expected number of events (18).

Relatively few *randomized trials* of valve replacement devices have been performed. Such trials should provide, in theory, the most direct and controlled comparisons (although if not multiinstitutional studies, they may not be a representative sample of all patients with valve disease). Randomized trials will be limited in sensitivity, however, by the observation that some events of interest in such studies may be determined more by patient-related characteristics and the structural and functional reserves of the heart than by differences in prosthetic heart valve type and structure. Those differences that are large and clearly evident (such as bioprosthesis degeneration) are probably quite well characterized by observational clinical studies. A further limitation is that events over even a 5-year period of time may be insufficient in number for any but a large study group to provide detectable and clinically meaningful differences; longer follow-up may provide more discriminating differences.

If a randomized trial is not available, then the next most direct method of comparison is performed using a *combined data* set with a specific analysis of the comparison variable (for example, mechanical versus biological valve prostheses, institution 1 versus institution 2, earlier and later time epochs). The overall distribution of events is first analyzed, if using parametric methods, and then the comparison variable is forced into the model as a risk factor (quite possibly with extensive formulation of interaction variables with other variables being considered), so that an "adjusted" evaluation of the comparison variable for other risk factors and for differences in risk factor prevalences is available.

An equation generated from a parametric risk factor analysis of an experience can also be *applied to another experience* as a way of making a valid comparison of outcome events that takes into account varying prevalence of risk factors (18). To do so requires that common risk factor variables and their definitions be available in both data sets. To obtain the expected number of outcome events in the second experience, were the quality of therapy the same as in the first experience, given the time frame for each patient's follow-up, the equation is solved for cumulative hazard and survivorship at the end of each patient's follow-up period. Either the sum of all probabilities of events so obtained, or the sum of the cumulative hazards, provide an estimate of the expected number of events:

$$\text{Events expected} = \sum_{i=1}^{n} [1 - S(\tau_i, \hat{\theta}_i)] \tag{17-37}$$

or

$$\text{Events expected} = \sum_{i=1}^{n} \Lambda(\tau_i, \hat{\theta}_i) \tag{17-38}$$

where n is the number of patients, τ_i is each patient's duration of follow-up, and $\hat{\theta}_i$ represents the model parameters, including risk factors specific to each patient. In theory, the sum of the cumulative hazards (Eq. 17-38) is the most appropriate of the two measures (64), but it may be biased by a few unusual patients who have cumulative hazard values greater than 1.0. A chi-square goodness of fit test yields a P value for the difference between observed and expected deaths (51) (for an example related to mitral valve replacement, see Ref. 18).

The equation from one experience can be used to generate an expected survivorship curve (were the quality of therapy the same) and compared with the observed one in the second experience. This is accomplished by solving the equation for each patient at a number of time intervals. The average survivorship curve from these individual ones is then obtained for comparison (illustrated in Ref. 18).

These latter two techniques, involving use of an equation established by a center that may be considered one of excellence, are particularly valuable because they demand a minimum of data collection (only the variables in the model), no data analysis (only application to the data of the equation), and minimal computer and software resources. They may, then, represent an approach that could be taken to the development of standards of quality.

INFERENCE

What is to be learned from the follow-up assessment of cardiac valve replacement? In common with the purpose of any seriously conceived and conducted clinical study, forming opinions, reaching decisions, and gaining insight from the data themselves, all in the context of the available knowledge in the field of valvular surgery, are accomplished in the process of developing inferences. Inferences are not a summarization of the results of a clinical study; they are statements that, to the best of one's scientific ability, represent the truths gleaned from the study; they are the answers to the broad questions that initially stimulated the study.

The inferential process just described should be differentiated from the narrower domain that statistical inference has come to occupy. Statisticians, in dealing with the very real problem of drawing a direct inference about a sample of data (for example, is NYHA functional class a risk factor in the early hazard phase for death?), use numerical models and tests from which inferential statements are made with a specified degree of uncertainty. Their investigations are often translated by investigators into statements that this or that variable is or is not a risk factor. While the activity of processing data to extract from them specific inferences about risk factors, or about whether an observed difference is more or less likely to be due to chance alone, is an essential step, it is only preparatory to the task of developing clinically relevant scientific inferences that relate specifically to valvular surgery and events more generally.

As an example in a field of concern to those interested in valvular surgery, one may test hypotheses about myocardial protective strategies in isolated rat hearts. The statistical testing of those data is one level of inference; formulating statements about the results of the experiment is yet another; inferring about better protecting the heart during cardiac surgery of patients with valvular heart disease is yet another; and inferring about the nature of global myocardial ischemia and the neutralization of its effects still another. For some reason, cardiac surgeons are more comfortable with the direct and narrow inferences from statistical tests than with heeding the admonition of the great statistician Sir Ronald Fisher (who entitled his statistical monograph *Statistical Methods and Scientific Inference* (65)), who emphasized that scientific inference is a means of understanding the real world.

The Process of Developing Inferences

The process of developing inferences is a completely intellectual one and cannot be done by a calculator or a computer. It is a step beyond assembling and analyzing the data, a step that unfortunately is often not taken. Although based on the data, the process of developing inferences also draws upon the investigator's prior knowledge and imagination. It should be apparent that the inferential process is closely related to the concept of obtaining an *overview* of the subject under inquiry. Indeed, at each stage of analysis, attempts must be made to step back and achieve a synthesis or overview of the whole. Without this, the analysis is fragmented and superficial, never achieving the satisfying depth that leads to the most relevant inferences.

Thus, inferences can be developed during the simple assembly stages of data. For example, assignment of the cause of death as being either from lack of scientific knowledge or from human error in the application or execution of knowledge can lead to inferences about the general direction of research to be taken or institutional protocols to be put into place to decrease the risks for future patients. Inferences can also be developed from the simple time-related depiction of events that occur after valve replacement. For example, a peaking early-risk phase for endocarditis does not appear to exist for allograft valves but does for mechanical prostheses, leading to inferences concerning the most appropriate device to use for valve replacement in the face of native valve endocarditis (1, 66).

More often, useful inferences are derived from analyses of correlates of an event. Grouping of risk factors into inferential clusters is an important step: what variables relate to the morphology of the valve lesion, to the function of left and right ventricles, to the systemic influence of the disease, to unsolved problems of myocardial protection?

The nature of interrelations among risk factors from which inferences are to be formulated may be appreciated best by construction of nomograms from the risk factor equation. From these nomograms strengths of relationships become apparent, evident differences may be ascertained (1) (such as the circumstances under which one type of cardiac valve replacement device might be recommended over another), and inferences derived about the optimal timing of operation.

Inferences can be developed from comparisons. The comparison of contrasts found within the data set being studied may lead to inferences. Inferences may be derived from randomized comparisons, from a combined data set with other institutions identifying both common factors and differences, from application of representative equations from one or several experiences to one's personal or institutional series and examining any discrepancies, from comparisons with information available in the literature, and from comparisons with natural history data or data representing the general population. These inferences arise from the synthesis of the comparative statistics into a few sentences that appear to best represent the truth derived from the findings.

Consequences of Focusing on Development of Inferences

This chapter began with the statement that clinical studies are performed so as to develop inferences. If the drawing of inferences is the focus of a study, then the study will be a serious scientific inquiry, not a record of personal or institutional achievement. To be able to work with reliable data, the basic clinical documents, such as the operative note, must have been structured so as to be useful sources of clinical variables. When embarking on the study, the investigator will define the study group carefully to encompass all pertinent patients, will compile and organize the data accurately, will thoughtfully select pertinent variables for analysis, and will work in close collaboration with those directly analyzing the data. When analyses (and often *re*analyses) are completed, relevant surgical inferences will be drawn together by the surgical investigator and the statistical investigator and will be committed to writing as a contribution to patients, to one's colleagues, and to the scientific community in general.

In this way, despite imperfect tools with their present limitations, the results of clinical research will have a positive impact on the lives of patients with valvular heart disease.

REFERENCES

1. Kirklin JW, Barratt-Boyes BG: Cardiac Surgery, New York, John Wiley & Sons, 1985, pp 177–204.
2. Walker SH, Duncan DB: Estimation of the probability of an event as a function of several independent variables. Biometrika 1967;54:167–179.
3. Kaplan EL, Meier P: Non-parametric estimation from incomplete observations. Am Stat Assoc J 1958;53:457–481.
4. Cox DR: Regression models and life tables. J R Stat Soc, 1972;34:187–220.
5. Grunkemeier GL, Thomas BR, Starr A: Statistical considerations in the analysis and reporting of time-related events: Application to analysis of prosthetic valve-related thromboembolism and pacemaker failure. Am J Cardiol, 1977;39:257–258.
6. Ascher H, Feingold H: Repairable Systems Reliability, New York, Marcel Dekker, 1984, pp 133–168.
7. Berkson J, Gage RP: Calculation of survival rates for cancer. Staff Meetings of the Mayo Clinic, 24 May 1950, pp 270–286.
8. Kay R: Proportional hazard regression models and the analysis of censored survival data. Appl Stat, 1977;26:227–237.
9. Edmunds LH Jr, Clark RE, Cohn LH, Miller DC, Weisel RD: Guidelines for reporting morbidity and mortality after cardiac valvular operations. J Thorac Cardiovasc Surg 1988;96:351–353.
10. Blackstone EH, Kirklin JW: Rational decision-making in paediatric cardiac surgery. In Godman MJ (ed): Pediatric Cardiology. Edinburgh, Churchill Livingstone, 1981, vol 4, pp 334–344.

11. Blackstone EH, Naftel DC, Turner ME Jr: The decomposition of time-varying hazard into phases, each incorporating a separate stream of concomitant information. J Am Stat Assoc 1986;81:615–624.
12. Blackstone EH, Kirklin JW: Death and other time-related events after valve replacement. Circulation 1985;72:753–767.
13. Wigglesworth EC: A teaching model of injury causation and a guide for selecting countermeasures. Occup Psychol 1972;46:69–78.
14. Hadon W: The prevention of accidents. In Clark DW, McMahon B (eds): The Textbook of Preventive Medicine. Boston, Little, Brown, 1967, pp 591–621.
15. Lawrence AC: Human error as a cause of accidents in gold mining. J Safety Res 1974;6:78–88.
16. Kirklin JK, Naftel DC, McGiffin DC, McVay RF, Blackstone EH, Karp RB: Analysis of morbid events and risk factors for death after cardiac transplantation. J Am Coll Cardiol 1988;11:917–924.
17. Feinstein AR: Clinical biostatistics: XX. The epidemiologic trohoc, the ablative risk ratio, and "retrospective" research. Clin Pharmacol Ther 1973;14:291–307.
18. Ferrazzi P, McGiffin DC, Kirklin JW, Blackstone EH, Bourge RC: Have the results of mitral valve replacement improved? J Thorac Cardiovasc Surg 1986;92:186–197.
19. Ascher H, Feingold H: Repairable Systems Reliability, New York, Marcel Decker, 1984, pp 7–46.
20. Aalen O: Nonparametric inference for a family of counting processes. Ann Stat 1978;6:701–726.
21. Gill RD: Understanding Cox's regression model: A martingale approach. J Am Stat Assoc, 1984;79:441–447.
22. Chiang CL: An Introduction to Stochastic Processes and Their Applications. Huntington, NY, Robert E Krieger Publishing, 1980, pp 300–476.
23. Clayton D: The analysis of event history data: A review of progress and outstanding problems. Stat Med 1988;7:819–841.
24. Voelkel JG, Crowley J: Nonparametric inference for a class of semi-Markov processes with censored observations. Ann Stat 1984;12:142–160.
25. Hazelrig JB, Turner ME Jr, Blackstone EH: Parametric survival analysis combining longitudinal and cross-sectional-censored and interval-censored data with concomitant information. Biometrics 1982;38:1–15.
26. Chiang CL: The Life Table and Its Applications, Malabar, Fla, Robert E Krieger Publishing, 1984, pp 221–243.
27. Benjamin B: Graunt, John. In Kruskal WH, Tanur JM (eds): International Encyclopedia of Statistics. New York, The Free Press, 1978, vol 1, pp 435–437.
28. David FN: Bills of mortality. In Games, Gods and Gambling. A History of Probability and Statistical Ideas. London, Griffin and Company, 1962, pp 98–109.
29. Elandt-Johnson RC, Johnson NL: Survival Models and Data Analysis, New York, John Wiley & Sons, 1980, pp 9–49.
30. Nelson W: Hazard plotting for incomplete failure data. J Qual Technol 1969;1:27–52.
31. Nelson W: Theory and applications of hazard plotting for censored failure data. Technometrics 1972;14:945–966.
32. Nelson W: Applied Life Data Analysis. New York, John Wiley & Sons, 1982, pp 103–161.
33. Greenwood M: The natural duration of cancer. Rep Public Health Med Subjects 1926;33:1–26.
34. Buckland WR: Statistical Assessment of the Life Characteristic. London, Charles Griffin & Co., 1964, pp 11–35.
35. Gross AJ, Clark VA: Survival Distributions: Reliability Applications in the Biochemical Sciences. New York, John Wiley & Sons, 1975, pp 49–96.
36. Cox DR, Oakes D: Analysis of Survival Data. London, Chapman and Hall, 1984, pp 32–47.
37. SAS Institute Inc: SAS User's Guide: Statistics, Version 5 Edition. Cary, NC, SAS Institute, 1985, pp 507–528.
38. SAS Institute Inc: Changes and Enhancements to the SAS System, Release 5.18, under OS and CMS. SAS Technical Report P-175. Cary, NC, SAS Institute, 1988, pp 192–265.
39. BMDP Statistical Software 1981. Los Angeles, University of California Press, 1981, pp 557–575.
40. Whittemore AS, Keller JB: Survival estimation using splines. Biometrics 1986;42:495–506.
41. Jarjoura D: Smoothing hazard rates with cubic splines. Commun Stat Simula 1988;17:377–392.
42. Efron B: Logistic regression, survival analysis, and the Kaplan-Meier curve. J Am Stat Assoc 1988;83:414–425.
43. Taulbee JD: A general model for the hazard rate with covariate. Biometrics 1979;35:439–450.
44. Herndon JE: A parametric survival model which generates monotonic and non-monotonic hazard functions and incorporates time-dependent covariables. Mimeo Series No. 1851T. Chapel Hill, NC, The Institute of Statistics, The University of North Carolina, 1988, pp 1–261.
45. Nelson W: Graphical analysis of system repair data. J Qual Technol 1969;1:27–52.
46. Turner ME Jr, Hazelrig JB, Blackstone EH: Bounded survival. Math Biosci 1982;59:33–46.
47. Prentice RL, Williams BJ, Peterson AL: On the regression analysis of multivariate failure time data. Biometrika 1981;68:373–379.
48. BMDP Statistical Software 1981, Los Angeles, University of California Press, 1981, pp 576–594.
49. SAS Institute Inc: SUGI Supplemental Library User's Guide, Version 5 Edition. Cary, NC, SAS Institute, 1986, pp 269–293.

50. Lagakos SW: General right censoring and its impact on the analysis of survival data. Biometrics 1979;35:139–156.
51. Blackstone EH: Analysis of death (survival analysis) and other time-related events. In Current Status of Clinical Cardiology. Hingham, Mass, MTP Press, 1986, pp 55–101.
52. Austin MA, Berreyesa S, Elliott JL, Wallace RB, Barrett-Connor E, Criqui MH: Methods for determining long-term survival in a population based study. Am J Epidemiol 1979;110:747–752.
53. David HA, Moeschberger ML: In Stuart A (ed): The Theory of Competing Risks. London, Charles Griffin, 1978, pp 1–85.
54. Porschan F: Theoretical explanation of observed decreasing failure rate. Technometrics 1963;5:375–383.
55. Vaupel JW, Yashin AI: Heterogeneity's ruses: Some surprising effects of selection on population dynamics. Am Statistician 1985;39:176–185.
56. Elveback L: Estimation of survivorship in chronic disease: The "actuarial" method. J Am Stat Assoc 1958;53:420–440.
57. Tallis GM, Leppard P, O'Neill TJ: The analysis of survival data from a central cancer registry with passive follow-up. Stat Med 1988;7:483–490.
58. Harrell FE, Lee KL, Califf RM, Pryor DB, Rosati RA: Regression modeling strategies for improved prognostic prediction. Stat Med 1984;3:143–152.
59. Meier P: Anatomy and interpretation of the Cox regression model. ASAIO J 1985;8:3–12.
60. Lew RA, Day CL Jr, Harrist TJ, Wood W, Mihm MC Jr: Multivariate analysis: Some guidelines for physicians. JAMA 1983;249:641–643.
61. Kirklin JK, Blackstone EH, Kirklin JW, McKay R, Pacifico AD, Bargeron LM Jr: Intracardiac surgery in infants under age 3 months: Incremental risk factors for hospital mortality. Am J Cardiol 1981;48:500–506.
62. Katz NM, Blackstone EH, Kirklin JW, Karp RB: Incremental risk factors for spinal cord injury following operation for acute traumatic aortic transection. J Thorac Cardiovasc Surg 1981;81:669–674.
63. Blackstone EH, Kirklin JW, Pluth JR, Turner JE Jr, Parr GVS: The performance of the Braunwald-Cutter aortic prosthetic valve. Ann Thorac Surg 1977;23:319–322.
64. Berry G: The analysis of mortality by the subject-years method. Biometrics 1983;39:173–184.
65. Fisher RA: Statistical Methods and Scientific Inference. New York, Hafner Press, 1973, pp 1–7.
66. Ivert TSA, Dismukes WE, Cobbs CG, Blackstone EH, Kirklin JW, Bergdahl LAL: Prosthetic valve endocarditis. Circulation 1984;69:223–232.

Bodnar, E. and Frater, R. W. M., editors
(1991) *Replacement Cardiac Valves,*
Pergamon Press, Inc. (New York), pp. 435–468
Printed in the United States of America

CHAPTER 18

CARDIAC VALVE PROSTHESES AND THE LAW

FRANCIS ROBICSEK AND SUSANNE ROBICSEK

Society is not tolerant of medical device mishaps, even when the potential for healing grossly outweighs the potential for harm.

Jayne A. Kykemo

In recent years we have witnessed a dramatic increase in product liability litigation (awards totaled $50 billion in 1975 alone) (1) (Figs. 18–1 and 18–2), and we have also seen the emergence of a new legal entity of government standards regulating various health products. Although the biomedical industry is one of the fastest growing industries in the United States, product litigation has grown faster. In this process, it is not only the medical technology industry but also the health providers who apply their products that have become prime targets for tort litigation. In this process, the legal trend seems to be moving toward absolute consumer protection (2), despite the fact that from a technological and clinical viewpoint there is no implantable medical device that is without some degree of risk or side effects, and prosthetic valves are no exception. In the year 1985 alone, about 30,000 charges of medical malpractice were made (3). This plethora of medical product and malpractice litigation may be attributed to several factors, including increasing consumer awareness, changing consumer attitudes, changes in the law (4), and the movement of the federal regulatory system into the medical device area (5). Additionally, the courts are drifting further away from a fault-based system in determining malpractice damages and have almost adopted the measure of strict liability, a standard by which the plaintiff is compensated for any injury resulting from medical treatment, regardless of whether negligence by either the manufacturer or the doctor was involved (6).

Another factor toward mushrooming medical liability is the rapid growth of an increasingly aggressive plaintiff's bar. With the emergence of new client-recruiting techniques, which include advertisements in the yellow pages, newspapers, radio, and television, and solicitation (7), attorneys specializing in malpractice can now locate prospective litigants rather than wait until traditionally contacted (Figs. 18–3 and 18–4). While this "specialization" of lawyers in medical and medical product litigation is well publicized, what has received scant attention is that, likewise, physician services as consultants and expert witnesses in court cases involving medical products and malpractice has also become a specialty. Now physicians compete aggressively for the "expert witness" business, and recent advertisements of organizations, such as the "American Board of Medico-Legal Consultants" and the FD-MD, Inc., boast large numbers of "certified medical specialists with impeccable credentials" willing to testify for the plaintiff (8). These factors, coupled with the liberal ruling of juries and permissive attitude of the courts, also contribute to the tremendous increase in medical device and malpractice litigation.

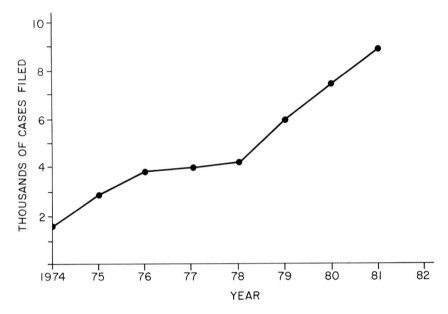

FIG. 18-1. Product liability cases filed each year in federal courts. (Federal Judicial System Data. After Piehler HR.: Clinical environment and the law: Product liability. In Medical Devices: Measurements, Quality Assurance: and Standards. American Society for Testing and Materials, 1983, p 246.

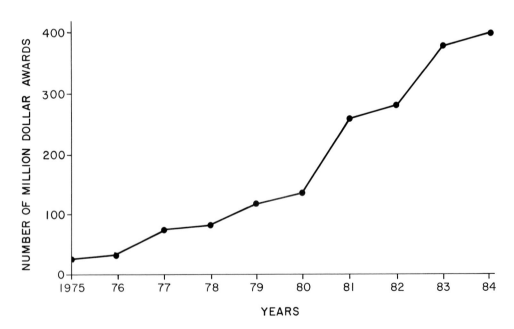

FIG. 18-2. Number of million dollar awards in product litigation cases. After Starr A: The thoracic surgical industrial complex. Ann Thorac Surg 1986;49:124–133.

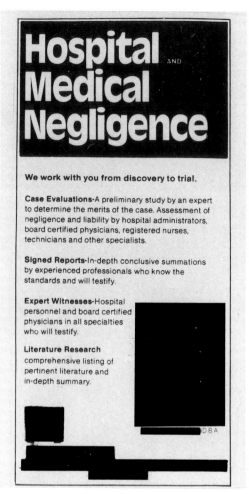

a

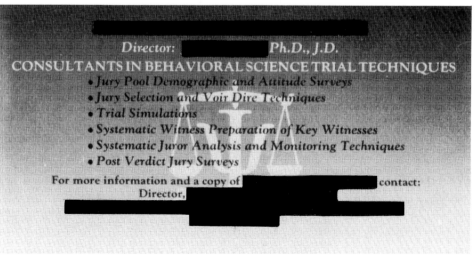

b

Fɪɢ. 18–3. Examples of legal service and expert witness advertisements. Trial, May 1986.

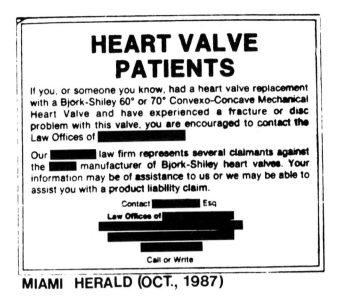

FIG. 18–4. Legal firm advertisement in the Miami Herald, October 1987.

In contrast to usual malpractice litigation, which pits a patient against his or her physician, legal actions involving medical devices, hence cardiac valve prostheses, are quadripartite. The initiator of the action is the plaintiff, who is naturally the patient, while the manufacturer, hospital, and surgeon occupy the seat of the defendant either together or alternately. This process involves complex issues of law, medicine, and technology (9). Even when a claim is raised against the manufacturer on the basis of failure to warn, negligent design and/or manufacture, breach of warranty, or strict liability (10), typically the implanting surgeon as well as other attending physicians are also sued on alleged medical malpractice in order to expand the scope of liability (11). To add to the complexity of the matter, there are recent legal precedents in which hospitals were held liable for all actions of the physician, thus putting them into the same category of liability as the physician. Also, in some cases both the hospital and the physician were held liable as implied sellers of the product instead of merely users, thus exposing them to all the liability responsibilities of a manufacturer, that is, product liability. The dispositions of the cases are about equally split between plaintiffs and defendants (12).

Legal actions arising from prosthetic heart valve–related injuries may fall into several categories, the main categories being failure to comply with government regulations, personal injuries, and direct economic loss resulting from the same. Therefore, prosthetic valve litigation involves three relevant areas of law. The first is government regulation special to medical devices. The other two are of tort law: product liability and negligence (which includes medical malpractice). One does not necessarily exclude the other. More often than not, litigation involving the manufacturer of medical devices is coupled with medical malpractice cases against the doctor and/or the hospital (13).

GOVERNMENT REGULATIONS INVOLVING THE MANUFACTURE AND SALE OF VALVE PROSTHESES

Over several years, scores of state and federal statutes directed at standard setting, product liability, medical malpractice, insurance or tort reform were enacted.

Standard setting and litigation both involve the assessment of risks and the acceptance of the responsibility for minimizing and warning of unavoidable hazards. While litigation is retrospective with the aim of determining whether the plaintiff did or did not receive a proper product and/or care, standard setting is a prospective process (13). Despite the fact that federal regulations are uniform by nature, there is a lack of uniformity in laws at the state level that makes it very difficult for the manufacturer to conform to such diverse standards (14).

No mention was made of medical devices in the Food and Drugs Act of 1976 (15). The first major intervention of the federal government into regulation of medical devices was the *Federal Food, Drug, and Cosmetic Act of 1938 (FFDCA)* (16), which required manufacturers to substantiate claims that their products are safe. This act provided very limited statutory powers, and even those could be exerted only *after* the fact; thus the federal Food and Drug Administration (FDA) could act only after collecting enough data to institute court action against manufacturers, who were not even obliged to maintain adequate reports or to report mishaps. The concept of effectiveness in addition to safety was introduced into drug regulation by the Kefauver-Harris Amendments of 1962, but medical devices were not mentioned.

The Consumer Product Safety Act (CPSA) was put into effect in 1972 and then revised in 1983 (17) with the aim of protecting the public from "unreasonable risks" associated with marketed products. It also established a Consumer Product Safety Commission, which was charged with creating standards of product safety to which the manufacturer was obliged to adhere. Human injuries resulting in failure to comply with these standards were regarded as a conclusive basis for the manufacturer's liability, that is, strict liability.

The true era of strict government regulation of medical devices began in 1976, when the federal government passed the *Medical Device Amendment (MDA) of 1976* (18), which gave the FDA broad authority over medical devices already in use at that time and also over those to be marketed in the future. It now appears that other countries will also enact regulations; on July 25, 1985, the Council of European Community issued a directive that took effect in August 1988, which required all member states to establish strict liability laws that are in many respects similar to those in the United States.

The *MDA of 1976* classifies medical devices into three categories:

Class I: Medical devices that are considered to represent the least risk of human injury. Marketing of class I devices requires only proof of general controls, such as compliance with the regulatory requirements of manufacturing, record keeping, and quality control.

Class II: Medical devices that are regarded as representing hazards of medium severity. In addition to the class I controls, class II requires adherence to established performance "standards" to ensure that the device is indeed effective and safe.

Class III: Medical devices that have a greater probability of causing disease and injury and are considered to represent high risks to the sustenance of human life. Besides the general controls and standards, these devices must have premarket approval of their performance and safety by the FDA. The manufacturer is required to present both experimental and limited clinical test data to prove that the product is safe, after which broader clinical testing is to be done according to specific FDA protocol. Finally, all results are reviewed by FDA specialists who judge not only product safety, but also approve labeling and protective advertisements (19).

Another significant development in medical device regulations was the enactment of the *Medical Device Reporting Regulation (MDRR),* put into effect December 13, 1984 (Federal Register 49:36347), which requires that the manufacturer report to the FDA within 5 calendar days by telephone, and within 15 working days in writing, any information referring to any marketed medical device that has "either caused or contributed to death or serious injury or has malfunctioned in such a way that death or serious injury would likely develop if the malfunction were to recur" (20).

The term *serious injury* is defined as an injury that (a) causes death or permanent functional impairment, (b) leads to medical or surgical intervention to preclude the same, or (c) may cause unanticipated damage of any sort. The term *unanticipated* is interpreted as an event generally unexpected (or which is not expected) to occur at all or at that particular time; and reference to such is either not made in the labeling of the device or the event occurs with greater frequency or severity than is reasonably expected and/or stated in the labeling.

When the *MDRR* established government standards for all implantable devices, it was received with absolute horror by the manufacturers and with a mixed reaction by the surgical profession. Some surgeons, and certainly most manufacturers, believed (1) that voluntary adherence to industry standards had already proved to be an adequate mechanism to ensure product safety, (2) that the cost of administering involuntary regulations would be high, and (3) that stringent regulation would hinder the development of new products. Albert Starr, one of the key personalities of prosthetic valve development, stated in his presidential address at the 1986 meeting of the Society of Thoracic Surgeons that the FDA approval process is both time-consuming and costly, diverting considerable capital from higher-risk implantable devices such as heart valves toward lower-risk non-implantable devices such as catheters. Starr felt that the regulations also discouraged efforts to improve upon already-FDA-approved valves because of the additional time and cost needed to repeat the approval process (14). Others, however, regard government regulations as a welcome protection against untested devices. The latter stance received strong support after the serial failure of a particular modularity of disk valve in Europe that had not been approved, and thus not used, in the United States.

Before the *MDA* was enacted, the only forum where the matter of surgical implant failure could be addressed was indeed tort litigation. While the enactment of government-established standards may have forced firms producing low-quality devices either to leave the market or to improve the quality of products, it did not eliminate litigation against the manufacturer. As a matter of fact, the act explicitly preserved the right of the injured to bring a suit against the manufacturer even if the manufacturer complied with the rules of the regulatory agency. As it stands today, the fact that the manufacturer complies with government standards in both the design and the manufacturing of the heart valves makes the case of the plaintiff certainly weaker, but does not destroy it. On the other hand, if in the process of discovery it is shown that the design or production of the valve prosthesis was not in compliance with required standards, the manufacturer's liability is almost ensured, even if the failure of the device was in fact caused by factors other than those noncompliant with government regulations. That is, the manufacturer is held strictly liable.

The amendments contain two provisions authorizing exemptions of class III devices from mandatory premarket approval: custom devices and those of investigational use.

1. *Custom devices* are intended to be used exclusively to meet the special needs of an individual patient. They are usually made in a specific form for the particular patient named in the order, and they should not be generally available in finished form for purchase.

2. Persons who wish to obtain exemption for a device for intended *investigational use* must
   a. Promptly notify the Secretary of Health for approval of the local institutional review committee of the clinical testing plan and request an exemption for investigational use. The manufacturer must also submit a plan for clinical testing of the valve and attach a report to the secretary of any prior investigation of the device, including tests on animals. A copy of the report should also be forwarded to and approved by the institutional review committee that has been established in accordance with these regulations.
   b. Obtain a signed agreement from each participating investigator that states that any testing on human subjects will be under that investigator's direct and close supervision.
   c. Obtain informed consent from each human subject unless a life-threatening situation makes it infeasible and there is no time to obtain such a consent from him or her or his or her representative (18). The consent must be given in writing without any form of duress or coercion. It should include (1) an explanation of all procedures to be applied, including the identification of any that are experimental, (2) a description of discomforts and risks, (3) an explanation of the likely outcome if the procedure fails, (4) a description of any benefits expected, (5) a disclosure of alternative procedures, (6) a statement that the subject is free to decline or discontinue participation, and (7) an offer to answer any inquiries. The consent agreement should not contain any statement that is made to waive any legal rights of the patient to release the institution, the investigator, or its agents from liability or negligence.

On November 28, 1990 the *Safe Medical Devices Act of 1990* was enacted. These 1990 Amendments made further revisions to the *FFDCA* that either impose or will impose significant new burdens on manufacturers, importers, or distributors of devices. In addition, device-use facilities are specifically identified; and, for the first time in the history of the FDA, users of products subject to regulation by the FDA are explicitly subject to restrictions and penalties:

Whenever a device-user facility receives or otherwise becomes aware of information that reasonably suggests that there is a probability that a device has caused or contributed to the death of a patient of the facility, the facility shall, as soon as practicable but not later than 10 working days after becoming aware of the information, report the information to the Secretary and, if the identity of the manufacturer is known, to the manufacturer of the device.

The 1990 Amendment also requires postmarket surveillance by the manufacturer, but users will be affected by the process because a principal investigator who will implement the protocol must be identified to the FDA. Further, the FDA will determine whether the principal investigator has sufficient qualification and experience to conduct the post-market surveillance.

The FDA may also order that health professionals and device-use facilities cease use of such devices. Such a notice could give rise to liability issues relating to use of devices by professionals after a notice has been given.

One cannot say how government standards and regulations may have changed the number and outcome of suits because of the presence of other events that have also influenced the medicolegal arena of litigation. It is likely, though, that the mere presence of established government standards may make winning a case either easier (if the product was not in compliance with those standards) or more difficult (if the product indeed was in compliance) (13).

PROSTHETIC VALVE FAILURE AS A POSSIBLE CAUSE OF LEGAL LIABILITY

It is estimated that approximately 33,000 prostheses are implanted each year in the United States alone (21). Since the first biological heart valve was transplanted experimentally by one of the authors (FR) in 1952 in the anatomic position (22), more than 60 different heart valve prostheses have been designed and used in various clinical situations. By 1986, a total of over 500,000 patients had undergone valve replacement of one or more diseased heart valves since prostheses were invented. In the mid-1980s the yearly sales of artificial heart valves were about $147 million (14). While most of these valves were regarded as acceptable when introduced into the world market, for various reasons of design, manufacture, and economics, only about 12 models are still used. These prostheses usually performed satisfactorily and markedly improved the quality and length of life in literally hundreds of thousands of patients with valvular disease (23), but they are still plagued with basic problems that have been only partially eliminated: (1) mechanical failure due to fatigue and/or chemical changes in valve materials, (2) thrombus formation and thromboembolism, (3) damage to blood elements, (4) tissue tearing, and (5) infections. In 1970, a federal survey of the preceding 10-year period revealed 10,000 injuries from medical devices including 731 deaths, with 512 deaths due to defective heart valves (24). According to data from the American Trial Bar Association (13), a survey revealed that artificial heart valves are reported second only to breast implants as sources of medical device failure, and in that particular survey, 20 out of 59 legal inquiries and 23 out of 75 alleged medical device failures involved heart valve prostheses. To this, the last decade brought a significant additional complication that involved both the manufacturer and the health provider: litigation (Table 18–1).

From a medicolegal viewpoint, prosthetic valve malfunctions are either *implant failures* or *clinical failures.*

Implant failures are caused by flaws in either design, construction, or manufacturing. Because of the intimate interaction with the human system, normal standards of wear and tear are inadequate to cover this unique situation. Application of true strict liability in tort standards would require the device manufacturer to design and assemble prosthetic valves so durable that normal use would never cause defective function. In practice, however, this avenue of legal recovery is successful only if the plaintiff can prove that the development of valve failure was in fact traceable to negligent design, structur-

TABLE 18-1. *Sources of Failure in Medical Device Reported Cases and Inquiries*

Device	Number of reported cases	Number of inquiries	Number of alleged device-caused failures	Number of clinical failures
Orthopedic implants	18	0	7	11
Catheters	15	6	1	20
Heart valves	4	20	23	1
Intraocular lens implants	0	19	15	4
Breast implants and silicone injections	5	24	29	0

ATLA data. From Medical Devices: Measurements, Quality Assurance: Standards. American Society for Testing and Materials, 1983, p 247.

ally inferior component materials, or improper assembly (25). In such cases, occurrence and success of litigation is usually inversely proportional to the length of time after insertion, that is, early structural failures constitute a much higher risk for litigation than failures occurring several years or even decades later.

Material degeneration occurred frequently in the earlier series of *mechanical valves.* Some of these early models were regarded as clinical experiments and were expected to disintegrate sooner or later, as many of them did. Justification for their use was simply that we did not have anything better and that they appeared preferable to the patient's own diseased heart valve. Silicone elastomeric ball occluders in the early models of caged-ball prostheses were especially prone to lipid infiltration and subsequent swelling as well as to distortion, grooving, cracking, embolization of poppet material, and abnormal movement of the poppet due to sticking—a spectrum known as *ball variance* (26). Other causes of prosthetic valve failure were frailing of strut fabric on the cloth-covered caged-ball Starr-Edwards valve (27) and wear of the disk occluder in caged-disk mitral prostheses (28).

Most mechanical valve prostheses currently in use have pyrolytic carbon occluders; some have both carbon occluders and carbon cage components. The use of pyrolytic carbon in general appears to have eliminated abrasive wear as a long-term complication of cardiac valve replacement (29).

By and large, it is now reasonable to expect that cardiac valve prostheses manufactured after 1975 will structurally outlast the patient's forseeable lifetime. For example, Schoen found no structural failure of contemporary mechanical prostheses of any type in his study of 33 mechanical valves explanted (29). Mechanical valves of relatively recent manufacture show no significant difference in durability and clinical performance (30), and therefore it would not make much sense either legally or medically to discuss the matter of choice of models with the patient.

The above statement is certainly not applicable to *bioprosthetic heart valves,* as the functional integrity of the devices even today is relatively short. The principal advantage of the tissue-derived prosthetic valve is its relatively low thrombogenicity compared with mechanical prostheses. Because patients with bioprosthetic valves usually don't need to be anticoagulated, the valves are attractive alternatives to mechanical prostheses, especially for patients with lifestyles and/or diseases in which anticoagulants are contraindicated or undesirable. Bioprosthetic valves also have better flow characteristics. A special, however relative, indication to choose a bioprosthetic instead of a mechanical valve exists for women who are of childbearing age and wish to become pregnant. The review of the literature indicates that (1) fetal complications among patients with mechanical valves are much higher compared with patients with bioprosthetic valves, and (2) maternal thrombotic and hemorrhagic events in patients with bioprosthetic valves who were not on Coumadin are very rare (31).

It needs to be reemphasized that bioprosthetic valves are nonviable, nonrenewing, subject to progressive degenerative changes, and, therefore, late deterioration of these valves with or without thrombosis or calcification is relatively frequent, especially after the first 6 years of implantation. The failure rate 7 to 10 years after implantation is 15 to 25% per patient year (29). Primary tissue failure of newer bioprosthetic valves such as the Carpentier-Edwards bioprosthesis is now reported as 3.4% per year, with 0.3% having fatal consequences, and freedom from treatment failure was about 85% after 9 years (32). Despite this recent improvement in results, it still appears that if the patient lives long enough, sooner or later any bioprosthetic valve will eventually fail. This fact should certainly be weighed against the known advantages of these particular prostheses. This process of bioprosthetic valve failure is especially accelerated in younger patients; therefore, their usage should be avoided, whenever possible, in individuals less than 35 years old. It seems proper, not only from a medicolegal but also from a medicoethical viewpoint, that the patient should be made aware of these facts and given an explanation why the bioprosthetic valve is the surgeon's general choice or choice in this particular case. The surgeon should provide sufficient general information to the patient to allow him or her to weigh the advantages and disadvantages of bioprosthetic versus mechanical valves, and to let the patient express his or her own preference. Because the final decision as to the type of prosthesis concerned may also be influenced by individual anatomic features discoverable only during surgery, the surgeon should have an absolutely free hand to make the final choice of valve type during surgery.

The surgeon should be aware of all the particular facets of the patient's history that may indicate that he or she would be less tolerant to one particular type of valve prosthesis than another, such as a history establishing an absolute or relative contraindication to the administration of anticoagulants and/or antiplatelet agents. Generally, if the patient has a history, especially a recent history, of a gastric or duodenal ulcer, renal calculi, or any other condition in which anticoagulants may create a high risk of bleeding complications, preference should be given to the use of a bioprosthetic rather than a mechanical prosthesis. Similarly, if the patient's socioeconomic situation or general attitude suggests that he or she is either unwilling or unable to follow an appropriate anticoagulant management, a bioprosthetic rather than a mechanical valve should be applied. In the choice of selecting a bioprosthetic valve versus a mechanical prosthesis, the patient's wishes should also be taken into serious consideration—such as whether or not she intends to bear children, will be engaged in athletic activities, would be annoyed by the noise of the mechanical prosthesis, and so forth. However, the surgeon should make it clear that he or she is willing to perform the operation only with a *carte blanche* from the patient, and if the operative situation and the anatomy found make it necessary, the surgeon should have a free hand to change the operative plan and choose the prosthesis he or she thinks would be in the patient's best interest. Otherwise surgeons leave themselves wide open to litigation. As has been mentioned in cases involving prosthetic heart valves, because of the sophisticated nature of the procedure the surgeon is held to national—even international—standards of care rather than to local standards. These standards are established by the specialty organizations, such as the American Association for Thoracic Surgery and the Society of Thoracic Surgeons, as well as by professional publications, and are usually presented to the jury by expert testimony.

The surgeon bears primary responsibility for his or her patient and thus is expressly liable for the *handling of the valve prosthesis* after it is removed from its original package. This responsibility is spelled out in the *Second Restatement of Torts,* which holds that the manufacturer is (and the surgeon is not) liable for the use of a damaged valve only if the product reaches the user "without substantial change in the condition in which it is sold" (33). Damage to the prosthesis, such as bent struts, scratched poppets, and so forth, will be constructed as prima facie evidence against the surgeon. The manufacturer's instructions on the proper handling of prosthetic valves usually include directions to: (1) handle the prosthesis in a specially designed holder supplied by the manufacturer, (2) avoid direct contact with the poppet, or in case of a bioprosthetic valve, with the leaflets, (3) test the function of the poppet using a cotton swab rather than metal instruments, and (4) rinse bioprosthetic valves in an atraumatic fashion for a time period specified by the manufacturer. The latter may be best accomplished by using a special rinsing device (34).

While implant failures of prosthetic valves, especially mechanical valves, are decreasing in number, *clinical failures* still occur frequently. The implanting surgeon may be held liable for malpractice in any of the many clinical and technical aspects of patient care that lead to clinical failure. The fact that prosthetic valve implantation is a complicated and delicate procedure, the outcome of which is influenced by the individual pathologic condition of the patient, does not relieve the surgeon of the responsibility of adhering to specific basic standards, such as an acceptable perfusion time, appropriate myocardial protection, sufficient number of sutures to hold the prosthesis, and assurances that the prosthesis is indeed functional after implantation.

The technical points most often raised in litigation against surgeons in connection with heart valve implantation are as follows:

1. The surgeon had chosen too large a prosthesis for the size of the valve annulus, and that has caused rupture of the left ventricle.

2. The surgeon had chosen too small a prosthesis, which led to decreased exercise tolerance of the patient and impediment of sexual activity.

3. The sutures used in fixation of the prosthesis were left in too long, and they encroached upon and impeded the function of the poppet.

4. The polyethylene tubing inserted during surgery to monitor left atrial pressure inadvertently slipped through the orifice of the prosthetic valve and caused malfunction of the poppet.

5. The sutures holding the prosthesis were improperly inserted, which led to the development of a paravalvular leak, or they were inserted too deeply, which led to obstruction of the coronary flow, causing massive myocardial infarction and death.

6. The surgeon did not follow the appropriate rules of sterility, and therefore the prosthesis became infected.

7. The surgeon selected a valve prosthesis that was incompatible with the patient's internal environment and daily activities.

8. The surgeon's inexperience, or any other inappropriate surgical technique, caused injury to the patient.

Schoen found through anatomic analysis of removed prosthetic heart valves that the causes of valve failure included paravalvular leak (15%), thrombosis (7%), tissue overgrowth (8%), degenerative malfunction in bioprosthetic valves (43%), and endocarditis (19%) (29).

From the manufacturer's viewpoint the most important types of valve problems are associated with material degeneration and valve durability, while medicolegal problems involving hospital and surgeon are usually caused by the clinical aspects of valve implantation. Often these two groups of problems cannot be separated because events associated with material degeneration and valve durability are complexly interwoven with clinical factors. For example, statistics have shown that identical batches of valves implanted in the mitral and aortic positions have shown different failure rates; 6% for the mitral and 4% for the aortic positions (29). The reason for this difference is not clear.

Other predictors of valve failure include younger age at operation, more severe functional disability, and earlier operative years (35) (Fig. 18–5). Additionally, patients with aortic regurgitation (vs. aortic stenosis), atrial fibrillation, diabetes, and hepatic or renal dysfunction all had decreased life expectancy following prosthetic valve implantation. Similarly, if the type of valve lesion is insufficiency rather than stenosis also has a marked negative influence on later survival for patients with prosthetic valves. These patient-related factors need to be considered when anybody tries to evaluate the long-term performance characteristics of a particular prosthetic valve and analyze the causes of valve failure. Therefore, it should not be forgotton that a proper patient selection with a "poor" valve substitute may yield good clinical results, whereas a "good" (or better) valve implanted in a population of higher-risk patients may just as easily yield poor clinical results (35).

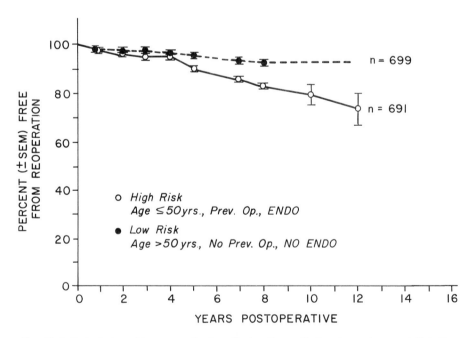

FIG. 18–5. Projected need for reoperation in patients with prosthetic valve replacement. Note the difference between patients younger than 50 years of age or who had a history of reoperation or endocarditis (high-risk) and those older than 50 years of age with no history of reoperation or endocarditis (low-risk). Modified after Ref 35.

Legal Obligations During Follow-Up

It is an open question what responsibilities the surgeon may have after the patient is discharged from the hospital with a seemingly well-functioning valve prosthesis. Beyond the usual one or two "postoperative visits," only a few centers will follow and take care of their patients indefinitely. Most surgeons refer the patient with the implanted heart valve back to the care of the primary physician, who is expected to bear the clinical, as well as the legal, obligations from there on regarding future care and monitoring of the patient. However, this "transfer of responsibility" presumes that

1. The patient has been informed of the necessity of follow-up and the importance of special measures, such as anticoagulation.
2. The primary physician is willing to accept the responsibility of further care.
3. The surgeon remains available to the patient in case his or her special services are required.

Recent cases of product litigation suggest there is a continuing legal responsibility by the surgeon to inform the patient either of newly discovered risks or of significant increases of risks previously known about the implanted device (36). Such an implied obligation makes it desirable for both the manufacturer and the hospital to maintain an *implant registry*, which would allow the ready indentification of either patients bearing valves of batches later recognized to be defective or those with prostheses of earlier manufacture that have shown a high failure rate at particular periods. Cases so identified should receive individual scrutiny, and the risks of acute failure of that particular device should be weighed against the hazards of reoperation.

An undecided issue is what to do with earlier models that are still going strong and apparently functioning flawlessly. Some of them, such as the Starr-Edwards silastic ball valves or the Smeloff-Sutter prosthesis, still have an enviable track record, and unless there are clinical signs of malfunction, they are better left alone. Others, like the Wada prosthesis, the Kay-Cross valve, and the metal-ball Starr-Edwards valve, which were acceptable at the time of their implantation but failed later in large numbers, should be exchanged for newer models unless either clinical contraindication exists or the patient refuses surgery even after being properly informed. The legal obligation to relay the information rests with the physician who regularly follows the patient; therefore, it is mandatory that physicians who are involved with valve implantation should be reasonably well informed on all major news concerning prosthetic valve failure. It should be noted that while recall notices have been sent out on automobiles that are apt to fail, they are seldom issued on early heart valve prostheses, and even if they are sent it is not ensured that the "owner," that is, the patient, gets them. The implanting surgeon, who is usually the best informed, may totally lose track of the patient or may be dead himself or herself. Evidently the system needs a radical overhaul.

In recent years there were several instances when valve manufacturers recalled a specific model of heart valve or a particular size of that specific model. The "recall" (using the terminology applied particularly by the automobile industry) usually meant that (1) the manufacturer discontinued, or modified significantly, the production of that specific model or a particular size of that model, and (2) it issued a statement notifying the surgeons of the failure rate that had occurred or was expected of that particular device. If such a recall occurs (37), the courts state that the physician who is following a patient with an implanted device (in that case a pacemaker) has a duty to advise the patient of a manufacturer's recall of the implanted device.

A so-called class I recall may be issued by the FDA, as was the case when 5700 Björk-Shiley heart valves were recalled (38). Because of the reported strut fractures of Björk-Shiley 60-degree convexoconcave valves in the sizes 29 to 33 produced in 1983, the manufacturer, Shiley, Inc., notified all cardiovascular surgeons on February 18, 1985, requesting them to closely monitor patients with these valves, to report any failures to the manufacturer, and to return any unused valves of that particular model and size. A more recent voluntary recall was issued on the Edwards Duromedics bileaflet prosthetic valve (32). On May 19, 1988, Edwards CVS Division suspended the marketing of bileaflet valves models 310 and 920 because of several cases in which the pyrolytic carbon leaflet "escaped" from the valve. According to the manufacturer, "Scientific investigation and monitoring of existing implants yielded no definite results regarding the mechanism and risk of leaflet escape" (32). If either voluntary or involuntary recall occurs, it is recommended that the surgeon immediately return to the manufacturer all unused recalled valves in his or her hospital's possession. The surgeon should then notify either personally or by correspondence all the patients in whom he or she has already implanted such a device as well as the patient's personal physician, and convey the facts related to the surgeon by the manufacturer. The surgeon should make it clear to the patient what the risks involved by the presence of the valve are and match those risks against those of a possible operation to exchange the valve for another type. Thus informed, the patient should have the final word whether or not to go ahead with such a reoperation. The surgeon may follow a similar course even if the valve has not been recalled by the manufacturer if he or she has found that according to the data in medical literature or to the surgeon's own experience, the valve has outlived the expected average duration.

THEORIES OF RECOVERY

The marketing of an artificial heart valve with even the slightest defect can result in hundreds of serious injuries. A patient injured by such a defective heart valve may sue the manufacturer or seller under three theories of recovery:

1. *Strict liability:* The prosthesis was defective and unreasonably dangerous when implanted.
2. *Negligence:* The manufacturer failed to exercise proper care in the production and marketing of the device.
3. *Breach of warranty:* The manufacturer breached an expressed or implied promise on the performance and hazards connected with the use of the product.

The same theories may apply to the hospital and/or surgeon as follows:

1. *Strict liability:* The proof of harm to the patient.
2. *Negligence:* The failure to exercise proper care in judgment of operative indication, in handling and implanting the valve, or in the general care of the patient.
3. *Breach of warranty:* The breach of either implied or express promises to the patient.

Additional theories under which health providers may be found liable include:

4. *Duty to warn:* Known hazards associated with the valve.
5. *Technical battery:* For the administration of treatment that went beyond that which had been consented to by the patient.

6. *Lack of informed consent:* By instituting therapy, especially surgical or experimental procedures, without fully explaining to the patient the potential risks and expected benefits.

Strict Liability

The significant increase in medical device litigation has coincided with some major changes in product liability law. In the past, the plaintiff had to prove that the manufacturer of heart valves was legally negligent in either the design or the production of the product, and that his conduct was substandard. Today, though, most states allow the plaintiff to act freely under the strict liability doctrine: the plaintiff needs but to prove that the product was unreasonably dangerous, that is, that a defect existed at the time the product was marketed, and that the defect in the product caused the harm to the user. Thus, even the best design and manufacturing techniques do not release the manufacturer from recovery if the jury or the judge decides that the product is "unreasonably dangerous."

The terms *unreasonably dangerous* and *unreasonably unsafe* are quite vague. At least one court has found that it simply means "not reasonably safe" (39) that is, it is up to the jury to decide. Another definition of an unreasonably unsafe product is "one which does not meet the reasonable expectations of the ordinary consumer" (33). To determine this, the *utility test* (40) bears utmost importance. Under this approach, the product is regarded as defective if the "magnitude of the injury outweighs the utility of the product." This theory underlines the approach that virtually all products have both risks and benefits and that there is no way to evaluate design hazards intelligently without weighing the danger against the utility.

Under this concept, the product becomes unreasonably dangerous only if (1) a reasonable person would conclude that the danger, whether foreseeable or not, outweighs the utility of the product, (2) there were other products available to serve the same needs but with less risk of harm, or (3) there was a feasible way to design the product with less potential for harmful consequences (41). Certainly a product that deviates from the manufacturer's own standards is unreasonably unsafe. If such standards are not set, facts are usually judged by the courts on a risk–benefit analysis in which a construction defect is defined as an inadvertent deviation in the manufacturing process.

Strict liability is based upon product performance, unlike negligence or warranty, which both depend on the manufacturer's behavior. The concept of strict liability is that the law holds the manufacturer liable if its product creates a risk that is unreasonably high to society. Proof of strict liability is usually established by expert testimony showing fault in either the design or the manufacture of the valve prosthesis. The generally accepted formulation of this doctrine of strict liability regarding medical devices is found in the Second Restatement of Torts §402A (4):

1. One who sells any product in a *defective* condition *unreasonably dangerous* to the user . . . is subject to liability for physical harm to the *ultimate* user . . . if
   a. the seller is engaged in the business of selling such a product, and
   b. it is expected to and does reach the user . . . without substantial change in the condition in which it is sold.

2. The rule stated in subsection (1) applies even though:
    a. the user . . . has not bought the product from or entered into any contractual relation with the seller.
    b. the seller has exercised all possible care in the preparation and sale of his product.

Thus, the question of liability may arise even if the device is properly made without defects, because it may be only partially effective in its use. In other words: there may be liability involved even with properly manufactured valves since they are imperfect at best (33).

On October 13, 1979, the Department of Commerce issued the Model Uniform Product Liability Act (MUPLA). Its primary aim was to eliminate the uncertainties of tort litigation. The act rejected the all-purpose definition of defectiveness found in the Second Restatement of Torts §402A and set forth new criteria as follows: (a) unreasonably unsafe in design, (b) unreasonably unsafe in construction, (c) inadequate warnings or instructions, and (d) failure to conform with the seller's explicit warranty. According to the above, the MUPLA thus places fault upon the production of an unreasonably dangerous product rather than upon the manufacturing of a product that causes injury.

Originally, strict liability was applied only against assembler-manufacturers or the company that assembled the heart valve in its final state. During the past decade, however, strict liability laws have been extended to include all parties involved in the production of the product. If the failure of the entire device is due to a flaw in a particular component part, then the component part itself is considered to be defective and is regarded as the cause for the defectiveness of the entire assembled product. The seller of the component part thus is also subject to the laws of strict liability.

A strict liability suit may also be brought against the manufacturer and its agents at any time when a patient suffers harm that is remotely connected to the implantation of a prosthetic valve, regardless that all possible care had been exercised in the manufacturing, sale, shipment, storage, and implantation of the product. The fact that the plaintiff suffered bodily harm *alone* may be satisfactory to establish the existence of a defect, either in design, manufacturing, or implantation, thus rendering the valve *unreasonably dangerous.* From there on there is only one small step to establishing liability: a direct or even causative connection between the defect and injury.

Unfortunately, the courts continue to remain vague on the definition of the term *unreasonably dangerous.* As a matter of fact, there is not even a generally accepted definition as to what a defect is in a product (42), and various courts have offered widely different definitions as to what the term *unreasonably dangerous* really means (43, 37). Some judges postulate that the mere *presence of* a defect may render a medical device to be unreasonably dangerous (44). Others regard the product to be defective only if it is in a state "not contemplated by the consumer, which will be unreasonably dangerous to him" (4). This led to different interpretations and variable outcomes in practically identical cases of medical product liability.

While most medical device litigations based on strict liability are directed against manufacturers, there are legal precedents in which doctors and/or hospitals were also held liable on the basis of strict liability (45–48). At the present time, there is a strong drive by the trial bar and various consumer groups to extend the concept of strict liability to both hospitals and physicians because (a) the hospitals are thought to be able to absorb the cost of injuries caused by defective devices, (b) the hospitals and physicians are in the best position to discover defective products and keep them out of public use, and (c) the hospitals are in the optimal position to identify other parties, if any, who may also be held responsible (11).

Restating the entire line of reasoning: theoretically, if an injury may be traced to a device, such as an implanted heart valve, it may be automatically regarded as defective, *ergo propter* unreasonably dangerous; thus there is justification for claim for damages. With all fairness toward our courts though, it also needs to be noted that the number of cases where proven negligence was absent and where manufacturers and sellers of medical devices or implanting surgeons were held liable on a strict liability theory alone is relatively low (11, 49, 50).

Negligence

The earliest cases of medical malpractice were treated as liability for battery. Beginning around 1960, however, the emphasis changed to regard the matter as really one of professional conduct, and so now negligence has generally replaced battery as the most commonly used basis of liability.

Prosser set out the four necessary elements for a cause of action sounding in negligence (40):

1. The existence of a duty or obligation, recognized by law, to conform to certain standards of conduct.

2. A breach of that duty.

3. A causative connection between the breach and the resulting injury.

4. Actual damages resulting from the injury.

The evidence against a valve manufacturer must show that a negligent act occurred among the multiplicity of events necessary to produce a valve prosthesis. To establish fault against the valve manufacturer, the plaintiff must either show that the particular valve prosthesis was of inferior quality by industry standards in design, production, assembly, testing, or packaging, or that the state of the art of the available techniques *at the time* of production would have allowed a better design or production. To prove that such events occurred is usually quite difficult, and the product may have to be traced through the entire process of manufacturing and distribution (11). Negligence in the case of the manufacturer may occur not only in the creation of the product but also in the *failure to discover* a particular flaw. Both of these may result in "negligence in selling the product with a flaw" (51).

As franchises have become an increasingly popular means of marketing products, the judicial trend has been to treat the franchiser as if it were a seller, at least in those cases in which the general public would believe that the franchiser was either the manufacturer or had substantial control over the franchise process (52). Therefore, if heart valves are sold by secondary firms instead of the manufacturer, those firms bear the full responsibility for product defects. This is clearly spelled out in the Second Restatement of Torts. "It can be said that all those who participate in the process of making products available to users for profit or financial gain are subject to liability on the negligence theory" (40).

Most lawyers agree that negligence as the cause of action is the most acceptable theory to the jury. Also, strict liability is time-barred (53) while other actions may not be as limited by the statute of limitations. Thus, the common strategy by the plaintiff's counsel is to file claims against the valve manufacturer, the hospital, and the surgeon under strict liability, negligence, and warranty simultaneously. This gives the counsel a free hand to argue that the valve was ill-designed, mismanufactured, posed an unreasonably high risk, and performed below expectation, and that the clinical care of the patient was substandard. Product liability laws vary from state to state. For example, Michigan recognizes only two theories of recovery, negligence and breach of warranty, but not strict liability. Other jurisdictions only allow strict liability in actions against the manufacturer (54).

Until 1965, *hospitals* were relatively immune from patient injuries arising from actions of physicians practicing within their walls. The courts viewed the hospital as an innkeeper—someone who provided space where the patient received care from a physician of his or her own choice. Now the hospitals may be held liable on the basis of two different doctrines: (1) As a *supervisor of quality care,* and (2) as the *seller* of devices. In the former doctrine, the landmark case was *Darling v. Charleston Community Hospital* (55), in which the Illinois Supreme Court held that the hospital owed an independent duty of care to the patient—an obligation that was breached by the hospital's failure to provide proper supervision for the doctor and the quality of his work. Hospitals are less likely to be held liable for the acts of private practitioners operating at the hospital (independent contractors) than for the acts of a surgeon employed directly by the institution. As far as the health provider's role as *seller* is concerned, the subject will be discussed later in this chapter.

Action against the *hospital* may be brought for failure to inspect a valve for defects, for the negligent storing or handling of a valve, for the supply of a defective valve, for granting staff privileges to an incompetent surgeon, or for the negligent operation of its facilities. The presence of negligence of either the doctor or the hospital is proved by the use of expert testimony (56–58), usually a surgeon who must be recognized by the court as qualified by reason of training and experience. While in the past it was quite difficult, and sometimes impossible, for plaintiff's attorneys to obtain medical experts because of the reluctance of physicians to testify against each other, this problem has eased considerably. Some surgeon-defendants now complain bitterly of the easy flip-of-the-fingers availability of so-called hired gun professionals whose moral integrity and professional standing are often questioned.

Against the *physician,* the patient may bring legal action on the basis of negligence; though not an exhaustive list, the patient may allege any or all of the following: (1) failure to reach a decision whether or not an artificial heart valve should be implanted, (2) improper selection of the type or size of the cardiac valve prosthesis, (3) failure to warn the patient of potential risks, side effects, or complications of artificial heart valves, (4) negligence in the general conduct of the surgery itself, and (5) negligence in postimplantation care.

For a malpractice claim to be successful against the physician, the plaintiff must first demonstrate that (1) a duty existed to treat the injured party, (2) the physician was derelict or negligent in performing the duty owed, and (3) this negligence was the cause of the harm to the patient.

Negligence in warning may occur in many ways: no warning at all was given as to particular risks related to the use of the valve, warning was given but it was inadequate (i.e., it was not as specific as it could have been), or warning was given but the means used were inadequate to reach all those to whom harm was reasonably foreseeable (for further discussion, see the discussion of warranty).

Besides the ease of obtaining expert testimony against physicians, the amount of factual proof needed to proceed in a malpractice suit has also decreased. The courts allow a prima facie case to be based solely upon information obtained from the defendant's testimony, or, in the absence of any evidence, many states allow the plaintiff to proceed on the legal theory of *res ipsa loquitur*. The concept of *res ipsa loquitur,* or "the thing speaks for itself," originated in early English common law and may be relied upon by the jury to infer the negligence of the physician. The application of this doctrine in medical malpractice cases varies greatly in different states but is basically a showing of a breach of duty by the use of circumstantial evidence (59, 38). The theory assumes that had negligence not been present the injury would not have happened. The plaintiff must first establish that the event was of a kind that ordinarily does not occur in the absence of negligence, and second that the occurrence was within the exclusive control of the defendant (40).

Examples of cases where *res ipsa loquitor* may be applied were reported in March 1988 in the Edwards Laboratory's *Clinical Letter.* Six incidents were described involving the inadvertent implantation of the cotton packaging from Carpentier-Edwards bioprosthetic valves (32). Occurrences in which heart valve prostheses were inserted in reverse would also fit into the category that may be accepted by the court as a *res ipsa loquitor.* In such cases, no expert witness is required to present complex arguments or facts to prove guilt, and in reality the burden is effectively shifted to the surgeon to prove that he or she had not misused the valve prosthesis. Some consider this an implication of guilt, unless proved innocent. The *res ipsa loquitur* doctrine was originally designed to save the courts from lengthy deliberations and the plaintiff from obtaining expert testimony. However, putting the burden of proof on the defendant leaves him or her without the basic rights assumption applied in criminal cases, that is, the defendant is always innocent until *proved* guilty.

Breach of Warranty

While formal contractual agreements between the patient and the heart valve manufacturer are unheard of, the claim for breach of warranty may be invoked by the plaintiff if he or she can show that the valve failed to function as stated in either *an expressed or an implied warranty.*

A particularly sensitive area regarding product liability of the heart valve manufacturer is the behavior of its sales and marketing personnel. They often exaggerate the safety and other advantages of a particular product, provide technical information they are not qualified to provide, offer obsolete advertising or scientific literature, verbally downplay an otherwise adequately written warning, or use flowery adjectives in describing the use and safety performance of the product. This could bind the manufacturer to an express warranty it did not intend to give. Such practices may transform a clinically safe and legally sound device into a legally hazardous and defective one (20). The warranty concept for the manufacturer underwrites the expense of a physician who propagates, or even discusses the manufacturer's product in his lectures. This may itself be regarded as an express warranty.

The manufacturer of most medical devices is required by law to provide *express warranties,* that is, a written promise or affirmation of fact that becomes part of the bargain of sale to a user. The implantation of heart valves, as well as other devices that are implanted, is controlled to a large degree by the surgeon; therefore, the term *user* refers to the surgeon as well as the patient.

The surgeon seldom, if ever, gives a written or even oral warranty or guarantee that the valve prosthesis is going to last for a particular period, or even that the operation will succeed for certain; thus, he or she does not provide *expressed* warranty. However, the surgeon's behavior could still be interpreted as an *implied* warranty (40).

To recover under these theories of implied warranty, the plaintiff need not prove fault, only that (1) the product was defective when the plaintiff received it, (2) because of this defect that heart valve did not conform to implied warranty, and (3) the defect was the direct cause of injury. Statements of suggested uses of the device, descriptions of characteristics (33), even attached relevant literature that implies that the valve prosthesis is free of mechanical failure that later occurs in the plaintiff (32) will constitute implied warranty.

Duty to Warn

Five relevant standards concerning the adequacy of such warnings have been identified (38):

1. The warning should adequately indicate the scope of danger.
2. The warning should reasonably communicate the extent or seriousness of the harm that could result.
3. The physical aspects of the warning must be adequate to alert a reasonably prudent person.
4. The warning should state the consequence that might result from failure to follow it.
5. The means of conveying the warning must be adequate.

The transfer of information referring to nonspecific risks associated with the general use of prosthetic valves is not the duty of the manufacturer. The manufacturer should take it for granted that they are known to the surgeon engaged in valve implantation. The manufacturer should, however, forward any data it may have available regarding any precautions that may minimize or eliminate risks during preimplantation handling, during surgery, and during the postimplantation follow-up period *specific for that particular model* of valve.

Opinion differs as to whom the manufacturer has a duty to warn. Most jurisdictions adopted the *learned intermediary doctrine,* which places the duty to warn the physican on the manufacturer, while placing the duty to warn the patient of hazards upon the physician (60). However, there are court decisions that extend the obligation of the manufacturer of medical devices to warn the patient (61, 19). To our knowledge, this matter has not been raised in any case of litigation involving heart prostheses, but there is a definite possibility that the time is not too far off when a heart valve manufacturer will be held liable on the basis that it (the seller) did not warn the patient (the ultimate user) directly.

The regulations are also unclear as to the importance of the past track record of a particular valve prosthesis, or how much follow-up data the manufacturer must provide to the surgeon *after* the device has been implanted. While the manufacturer is obliged to disclose faults if the product causes death or serious injury, especially if it leads to discontinuation or recall of the product, manufacturers seldom, if ever, provide information that may indicate that their product may be inferior in one or more aspects to similar products of other companies. This places a strong moral, rather than a legal, obligation on the surgeon to stay abreast of relevant professional literature. This endeavor is usually facilitated by the fact that scientific literature and industrial testing data that are uncomplimentary to a particular valve prosthesis are usually readily supplied by competing firms.

It is not spelled out explicitly, but the courts also expect that after a full disclosure of such product use and associated dangers is given to the surgeon, he or she is to transfer some but certainly not all of this technical information to the patient. To this the surgeon should add relevant clinical information and instruction which in his or her opinion fulfills the requirements of both sound legal and medical practices. Naturally, the information a surgeon may be able to provide about a prosthetic valve is virtually endless. Therefore, a number of recent cases have defined the surgeon's duty to disclose arising when a reasonable person in the patient's position would attach significance to that particular information (40).

The fact that the doctor had failed to provide all the available information is not sufficient for him or her to be held liable without additional elements. The plaintiff must also establish a direct link between the nondisclosure and harm suffered, and prove that he or she would not have undergone the treatment had he or she known of the risk of the harm that did in fact occur (62). Because of the patient's obvious bias in testimony, the courts usually consider not only the amount of information a reasonably prudent medical practitioner should have revealed, but also whether a reasonable layperson in the patient's position knowing the information would have withheld consent to the treatment or procedure if the risk had been disclosed.

The *duty to warn* of the inherent hazards of artificial heart valves is not a one-time obligation but is a continuing process; therefore, the manufacturer has a duty to periodically provide physicians with updated information, whether favorable or unfavorable, on the performance and on recently discovered faults of the device. If there are several cases of litigation involving the same device, the courts may turn to consolidation. While this may result in judicial economy, it may also have profound effects on the outcome of the case itself by being enormously prejudicial to the defendant manufacturer. On the other hand it may result in the dismissal of punitive damages and an equal distribution of funds available among several plaintiffs (63).

As far as notification of newly discovered defects, the U.S.C. House Amendments state that all "health professionals who prescribed or used the device presenting the risk were required to be notified, and all persons exposed to the risk were to be notified unless the Secretary (of Health) determines that notification by the Secretary, manufacturer, importer, distributor, or retailer presented a greater danger to the health of such persons than no such notice. In such instances, the Secretary is to require health professionals who prescribed or used the device to notify the persons whom they treated with the device of the risk it presented and of action which could be taken to reduce or eliminate such risk" (64).

Assault and Battery

Legal action based on assault and battery stands on the principle of individual integrity, that is, the premise that every person has the right to determine what shall or shall not be done to his or her own body. Action may be instigated against the health provider on the basis of technical battery if the patient can prove that, while the patient was in an incoherent state of mind, he or she was either confined to the hospital against his or her own will, while a procedure was performed on him or her without his or her consent, or a different procedure had been done than the patient consented to. The most common mistakes the surgeon may make in exposing himself or herself to battery charges are

1. Failure to obtain a broad written consent for admission to the health facility and for the performance of whatever procedures, including operations, the surgeon deemed to be necessary.
2. Failure to obtain permission for surgery before the patient is placed under the influence of drugs that could significantly impair his or her ability to judge the necessity of the procedure proposed.
3. Extending the scope of a relatively minor planned procedure without commanding reason to a major one that the patient did not agree to.

In emergency situations the patient may not need to give permission if he or she is unconscious or incoherent. Based on expert testimony, or on testimony from the defendant surgeon, the court may presume that had the patient been conscious and capable of giving consent he or she would have consented to the operation (38). However, if the situation is short of the acute need of intervention it is advisable either to wait until the patient is in control of his or her mental capacities or to obtain the permission of his or her legal representative, usually the closest kin.

Lack of Informed Consent or Informal Refusal

According to the informed consent doctrine, the surgeon is required by law to provide the information that would be given by a reasonably prudent practitioner that would enable a patient to render an intelligent decision whether or not to submit to the proposed course of treatment. The disclosure should include the nature of the underlying valve disease, the proposed treatment with its major risks, any alternative method of treatment if there is any, and the risks of failing to undergo any treatment at all. The burden of providing this information is on the surgeon, because even if he or she performs the procedure skillfully and successfully, the surgeon may still be liable for adverse consequences if the patient was not properly informed. If such a refusal occurs, the physician must explain the consequences to the patient and advise him or her of the material risks of his or her decision to refuse the recommended treatment.

The patient should be made to realize that even after successful implantation of a prosthetic heart valve, his or her clinical status certainly cannot be considered normal but only an improvement over his or her preexisting situation. The patient should know that the durability of a heart valve prosthesis may have a time limitation so that he or she may need additional surgery in the future, that he or she will require regular care in a physician's office, that according to the valve prosthesis's type and possible associated clinical condition he or she must remain on an anticoagulant regimen, and that antibiotic coverage may become necessary for different medical treatments, such as tooth pulling, and so forth. The patient should also be informed of principal symptoms that may indicate impending or occurred failure of the prosthesis.

It is advisable that hospitals prepare an information booklet to be given to every prosthetic valve patient, and a notation should be included in the patient's records that the patient received the booklet. It needs to be realized, however, that such a booklet *alone* is not enough to personalize the patient's particular problem; thus it is not enough to give the patient a brochure and tell him or her to read it. A minimum part of the information needs to be relayed by a trained health professional, preferably by the surgeon himself or herself. Most, if not all, health institutions also require that the patient or his or her legal representative sign some type of consent form prior to undergoing major surgery, or even before being admitted to the hospital. While the absence of such a written consent could certainly be used against the defendant surgeon and/or hospital, neither the manufacturer nor the health provider should have the misconception that any document intended to hold either a manufacturer or a physician harmless in the event of malpractice is likely to survive judicial scrutiny. Even contracts that merely limit a doctor's or manufacturer's liability are likely to get shot down in court.

The problem becomes even more complex when more than one doctor is involved in a patient's care. Typically, when a primary care physician refers a patient to a surgeon, the surgeon is responsible for obtaining informed consent. But the Maine Supreme Court recently held that a general practitioner could be held liable for failing to advise a patient about the risks and alternatives of an open heart operation during which serious complications developed. The issue was whether the general practitioner sent his patient to the surgeon as a referrel or a consultation. If a referral, the general practitioner had no responsibility of obtaining informed consent for surgery, the court held, but if it was a consultation, he was obliged to discuss the surgeon-consultant's recommendations with the patient! In the court's view, whether or not the general practitioner had primary responsibility was a proper question to the jury (65). Cases have also been recorded when an internist was held liable for complications that arose after cardiac surgery because he had resumed control of the patient postoperatively (65).

THEORIES OF DEFENSE IN LEGAL ACTIONS INVOLVING HEART VALVE PROSTHESES

Punitive Damages

The concept of punitive damages in malpractice litigation is in reality a legal paradox. It came about as a punitive device in cases of *criminal* negligence, that is, when criminal charges are filed along with a malpractice claim. However, one may argue that punishment has no place in *civil* suits; if the negligence is judged to be criminal, the case should be removed from civil court and declared to be criminal; or civil defendants should be afforded the same protective rights regarding self-incrimination, discovery, the necessity of being proved guilty beyond a reasonable doubt, and so forth, all of which are provided to protect those accused of crimes. There are two types of implied warranties in product liability law. The first is the implied warranty of merchantability. This means that the valves are of an equal quality generally acceptable to others who deal in similar heart valves. The second is the implied warranty of fitness for a particular purpose. This arises when the seller knows that the product is required for a particular purpose and that the buyer is relying upon the seller's skill or judgment to select the goods. The risk of a heart valve manufacturer being assessed with punitives is especially high if it can be proved to the jury that there was gross negligence in the manufacture or design of the prosthesis, or if it is shown that after the defect was discovered the manufacturer had continued to sell that particular valve without correcting the fault and had taken no action to prevent the injury suffered by the plaintiff. In mass product liability cases based upon strict liability, federal courts are generally reluctant to permit awards for punitive damages (63).

The issue of punitive damage in claims involving prosthetic heart valves is particular to product liability litigation in the United States and is absent in similar regulations recently advanced by the Council of European Common Market Countries (the laws of some individual European countries, however, do not exclude punitive damages).

Claims for punitive damages are often brought against the implanting surgeon but not frequently awarded. The demand for punitive damages is a tactic often used by plaintiff attorneys primarily to intimidate the physician, because malpractice insurance policies seldom, if ever, cover punitive damages. Thus, the threat tends to make the physician more apt to testify against codefendants as well as soften his or her resistance to pretrial settlement.

The Manufacturer

The best approach for a heart valve manufacturer to prevent the occurrence of, and to defend itself in, a liability action is to improve the quality of its product. It is especially important that a manufacturer of heart valves continues to monitor the performance of the heart valve prosthesis after it reaches the market, keeps updated regarding scientific publications referring to its product, and immediately investigates and reports to the FDA any adverse results discovered after placing the product on the market. Additionally, the manufacturer should continue to test the valve and to warn the users, both physicians and patients, of dangers subsequently discovered (20).

Besides adhering to the above rules of good manufacturing, the manufacturer may be in a position to apply one or more of the following defenses if legal action is taken against it:

1. *Proving that the failure of the prosthesis was due to clinical factors rather than to faults in design or manufacture:* In medical device litigation cases, it is customary for the manufacturer to assert as the primary factual defense that the symptoms alleged to device failure are not causatively related to the product. This may be the case if, for example, a bearer of an apparently well functioning prosthesis suffers a heart attack or dies of cardiomyopathy. Evidently, in such a situation, the manufacturer has no liability and may file a *demurrer,* a declaration that even if the facts alleged made were all true, there would still be no basis for liability.

The situation is similar but not as clear-cut if the injury to the plaintiff occurs because of a prosthetic valve malfunction that is not caused by structural failure, but rather because of thrombosis, infection, tissue ingrowth, and so forth, factors that are at a minimum partially attributable to the patient's individual biological response and behavioral patterns. If adequate warnings have been given by the manufacturer, plaintiff's litigation is usually unsuccessful.

2. *Statute of limitation:* The statute of limitation is the period after which the law does not allow the plaintiff to bring legal action. Most states have established statutes of limitation, although the limitation periods differ according to each state's statutes. In most states, medical device litigation that is based on breach of warranty is subject to a statute of limitation that runs for 2 to 5 years after the *sale* of the device (66). However, if the same case is based on strict liability, it will be governed by tort statutes which have widely varying periods. The Kentucky liability law, for example, states that the product is not defective if injury occurs more than 5 years after the sale or more than 8 years after the manufacture of the product. Other states link the rules of statutes of limitation with the time of discovery of the injury. In those states, the statute of limitation period runs from

the time the claimant discovers the causal connection between his or her injury and the use of the product, in some instances creating a practically indefinite exposure time to liability.

3. *Useful life:* If the manufacturer can prove to the jury that the failure of the product was caused by expected wear and tear rather than by a defect existing at sale, it is usually found to be not liable.

4. *State of the art:* Manufacturers who are concerned that their product may be judged by hindsight and found defective in light of current technological information, may argue that they should not be held accountable for standards of design that were not available at the time of manufacture (67). This *state of the art principle* bears utmost importance in medical device, as well as in surgical malpractice, litigation. It is generally agreed that a heart valve cannot be regarded as defectively designed when sold simply because after the sale, but prior to the trial or the time of a claimant injury, there was a technological breakthrough that made it possible to eliminate or lower the risk of harm. The courts used to hold almost universally that the feasibility of manufacturing a safer product must be determined as of *the time that particular product was designed* (68). It should be noted, however, that this important defense tool, *the state of the art defense,* has eroded over the years, primarily due to the legal argument that while the breakthrough in manufacturing was not made, the technology for the breakthrough was already available, and thus it *could have been made* (14).

5. *Compliance with safety standards:* Most states have held that a manufacturer's compliance with mandatory government or voluntary industry standards is admissible as evidence toward showing that the product was not defectively designed. However, these standards are now being considered by some courts to be minimal and not optimal; therefore, compliance with them is not a conclusive defense. On the other hand, noncompliance with such standards in most cases conclusively establishes negligence.

6. *Unforeseeable alteration:* In general, the seller is not liable for unforeseeable alterations after the sale, or unforeseeable misuse of the product.

7. *Unavoidably unsafe products:* A defense strategy introduced during the past decades into product liability litigation is the theory of unavoidably unsafe products. This doctrine was developed because the courts recognized that according to the classic definition of tort (40), most, if not all, medical devices, and certainly all prosthetic valves, are unsafe, simply because they carry *some* unavoidable risk. Therefore, the courts in their wisdom may choose to accept the fact that some products cannot be dissociated from inherent risks and they accept them as not unavoidably unsafe nor as unreasonably dangerous, given that appropriate warnings and instructions accompany their sale. Thus, it is "the warning or the lack of warning which determine if the product is unreasonably dangerous or not" (45). Considering that all the presently sold prosthetic valves are products whose probable benefits outweigh potential risks, unless negligent design or faulty production is proved, and that adequate information has been provided on their potential risks, their failure per se should not be considered a fault (62, 33).

The problem is that it is hard to explain to a lay jury what an unavoidably dangerous product really is. Juries are conditioned to reject nonfunctioning lawnmowers, automobiles with failing brakes, broken-down refrigerators, and so forth. It is therefore difficult to convince them of the concept of *statistically acceptable risks* connected with prosthetic valves. They are not easily persuaded by the fact that only a fraction of the valves produce side effects when they are faced with the catastrophy of a particular individual. As Joseph M. Price, trial attorney, so eloquently stated: "Physicians and other health care providers are willing to accept a reasonable degree of risk associated with the use of a medical product when compared to the benefit to be achieved by that product, but lay juries are less likely to tolerate the concept of an acceptable failure rate" (20).

To be able to apply the doctrine of the unavoidably unsafe product in its defense, the manufacturer has to prove that it carried out sufficient experimentation, ran all the necessary tests, and inspected the product at all stages of the development and manufacturing process; in other words, that it did everything possible to see that the unavoidable risk of causing injury to the patient had been decreased to the minimum (33). In cases involving prosthetic heart valves, the tests generally recognized as necessary include in vitro and in vivo durability studies, as well as the study of hemodynamic characteristics and thrombogenicity.

8. *Jurisdictional barriers:* Litigation may fail because of the suits being filed in a court that does not have jurisdiction over the defendant (11).

9. *Medical error:* In past trials involving medical devices, especially implantable surgical devices such as heart valves, there has been a tendency among defendant-manufacturers to imply *medical error* as a part, and often the strongest part, of their defense (13). Therefore, discovery, and eventually the trial process, always includes critical examination of the surgeon's actions, even in the rare case when the plaintiff's attorney has not named him or her as a codefendant in the litigation.

The Surgeon

Just as good production and sales practices are the best defense for the manufacturer, the most appropriate measure that the surgeon can use as his or her shield to prevent and cope with prosthetic valve–related legal litigation is the continued practice of high-quality surgical care. Again, there are also some legal devices that he or she may apply if suits are filed against him or her.

1. *Statute of limitation:* The doctrine of the statute of limitation applies to the actions of the surgeon just as it does to the actions of the manufacturer.

2. *Strict locality rule:* The strict locality rule in the past allowed the surgeon's performance to be judged by often lower local, rather than by higher, national standards. This rule, which first appeared in court decisions in the 1870s, came under sharp attack recently. In the landmark case of *Shilkret v. Annapolis Emergency Hospital,* the Maryland Court of Appeals reversed the strict locality rule (69), noting that it effectively immunized any sole practicing specialist in his or her community and also that a plaintiff may have great difficulty in obtaining local expert medical testimony. Many courts have adopted the *modified locality rule* that the physician's actions may be compared not only with the standards of care of his or her own but also to those of *similar* localities (8). The trend, however, especially in cardiac surgery, continues to drift away from standards based solely on geography. Because of the sophisticated nature of valve implantation, now the cardiac surgeon under legal fire is expected to be held responsible for conforming to national, or even worldwide, rather than to local standards.

3. *Contributory negligence:* In general, prosthetic malfunctions caused by the patient's reluctance to follow instructions are regarded as his or her own fault and should not constitute a case for litigation. Each state, however, varies in its contributory negligence laws. Contributory negligence by the patient is when he or she fails to follow medical advice such as taking anticoagulants or refuses to take antibiotics before unrelated surgical and dental procedures despite instructions to the contrary, and so forth. Some states

provide that any amount of contributory negligence acts as a *complete* bar to recovery; others have comparative negligence statutes that allow the plaintiff to recover a percentage of his or her damages. A *partial* comparative statute allows recovery only if the defendant was more than a specific percentage at fault, usually 50%. A *pure* comparative statute allows the plaintiff to recover no matter how much he or she contributed to his or her own injury, again a partial recovery based upon the percentage fault of the defendant.

4. *Error in judgment:* Contrary to general belief, both among the lay public and also among the medical profession, if the physican has exercised due care of informing himself or herself of the patient's condition and his or her behavior in the course of the operation conformed with the standards of his or her profession, the commitment of error, either in patient care or in a surgical technique in an area in which different medical practitioners may have made different judgments, does not make him or her legally liable. Such errors are not regarded by the courts as negligence but are judged in the mirror of general professional standards of care.

5. *Acts of God:* The failure of a properly selected, flawlessly implanted, and structurally intact prosthetic valve that is due to the progression of the patient's underlying disease or development of new diseases, such as superimposed infection, tissue ingrowth, thrombosis despite proper anticoagulant management, or other presently uncontrollable factors, is to be regarded as nobody's fault—acts of God. Most clinical failures of prosthetic valves fall into this category.

The Health Provider as Codefendant and a Possible Adversary of the Manufacturer

In product litigation trials involving heart valve prostheses, the physician may become a codefendant as either an *inventor-physician* or as a *treating physician.* In either case, he or she may find himself or herself in an adversary position, not only with the patient-plaintiff, but also with the codefendant valve manufacturer.

The decision to include the physician as codefendant may have direct impacts upon the trial strategy. For example, in states where mandatory health claim arbitration exists, the treating physician may request that the claim against him or her be considered as malpractice litigation and be separated from actions against the manufacturer (70). In some cases, such separation of claims may be favorable to the physician by inducing the plaintiff to abandon the health claim action. In other instances it may benefit the manufacturer-defendant by eliminating prejudicial evidence admissible due to the conduct of the physician (63).

As has been stated, there have also been several instances in which a manufacturer has implied (6) that defects occurred not during manufacture but in the course of implantation of the prosthetic valve and has effectively tried to shift the blame for the defect to the surgeon. The implanting surgeon may also become an adversary to the manufacturer by the doctrine of learned adversary. Because the surgeon has a duty to warn the patient, if a valve prosthesis is supplied with defects that are unknown to him or her and that are the basis for which the surgeon is held legally responsible, there may be no other recourse left to him or her but to sue the manufacturer (60). Thus, the surgeon may be thrust into a position of attacking the manufacturer as a defense against a patient who was inadequately warned (63).

All valve prostheses are sold with detailed instructions on how they should be removed from their original package, how they should be handled afterward, what instruments should be used in their orientation and handling, and so forth. Beware the surgeon who does not follow these guidelines, however unnecessary they may appear to him or her! The first thing the manufacturer (and often the plaintiff) will investigate is whether or not the surgeon handled the prosthesis properly, that is, according to the instructions. To protect himself or herself, it is very important that the surgeon do everything possible to preserve technical and clinical evidence, because any damage to the prosthetic valve during explantation and handling may be attributed to faulty techniques during implantation. The valve that is explanted during surgery, or removed in the course of autopsy, should preferably be first photographed *in loco* and its function tested. After it has been explanted, it should be handled with care and protected from injury as much as possible. Whenever the valve is removed in the course of an autopsy, it should preferably be removed by, or at least in the presence of, the implanting surgeon. The photographs taken and the valve itself should be preserved as potential evidence. The operative records or autopsy descriptions should be exact and meticulous. If the prosthesis was inadvertently damaged during explantation, this fact should be carefully documented.

While the courts attempt to allow all parties equal access to look at and to use all the material obtained as evidence, the manufacturer is not required to restrict the initial exploratory testing to nondestructive methods (13). Because of the potential conflict between the manufacturer and the surgeon, who may both be held liable, it is wise for the latter to submit the explanted valve to an independent testing laboratory before he or she surrenders it to the manufacturer. If the tests reveal that the prosthesis is indeed physically damaged and the damage did not occur during explantation, the test results may be used to find the surgeon guilty of negligence and to exonerate the manufacturer.

Another area of possible conflict of legal responsibility between the manufacturer and the health provider may lie in the legal theory of *privity.* By the classic rules of law, to obtain recovery of damages for a product one may need a *privity of contract,* or a direct contractual link, between the two parties. In most cases of medical device use, and certainly in all sales involving heart valves, the ultimate consumer, the patient, has no direct dealing with the manufacturer; therefore, no privity of contract exists between the two. In the past this fact often hindered suits directed by the patient against the manufacturer because the valve was purchased from the manufacturer, not by the patient but by the hospital (usually at the surgeon's recommendation), which in turn "sold" it to the patient. By the original rules requiring privity of contract, the course of recovery for damages would involve a suit by the patient against the hospital and/or the physician, who in turn could sue the manufacturer (33).

It has now been established that in product liability cases no privity of contract is required for recovery, and the avenue to direct recovery of the customer from the manufacturer is open. The first case so holding was *Baxter v. Ford Motor Co.* (71) in 1932. The courts have restated on several occasions that they are willing to disregard privity in suits based on either tort or warranty because this saves a multiplicity of litigation in which the manufacturer will be held liable at the end anyway. In the case of *Randy Knitwear v. American Cyanamid Co.,* the court explicitly stated that the manufacturer may finally be obliged to "shoulder the responsibility which should have been his in the first instance" (72).

The position of the courts has not been completely uniform in this matter. Under U.C.C. §2-315, some courts have held that the physician and hospital alike may indeed be held liable for medical products manufactured by others (56, 45) because the patient relies on their "expertise, skill, and judgment in the selection of the device" (63), a precedent that may take on special significance if a hospital supplies, and a surgeon implants, a valve prosthesis that has been recalled or even if it has not been recalled but has a track record inferior to those of other devices available. The exposure of the hospital to liability as a seller of cardiac valves is further accentuated if

1. The hospital bills for the valve in an itemized statement.
2. There is a surcharge on the same.
3. The hospital or physician makes warranty representations.
4. The hospital inspects the device before it is inserted into the patient and fails to recognize identifiable faults (73).

In regard to the application of privity as a defense by the health provider, court rulings differ and are highly controversial. By and large, the courts usually refuse to rule that physicians and hospitals are *sellers of goods,* a condition that would make them liable under certain warranty theories (74, 75). Hospitals and physicians are regarded as being principally engaged in providing services, and are therefore purchasers and users of prosthetic valves and other medical devices rather than sellers or merchants (76–79). In other words, physicians provide a service and not products, and medical devices, such as heart valves, that are charged to the patient are merely incidental to these services (76, 80–84). Some courts, in their quest for manufacturer liability where traditional privity did not exist, declared the physician or the hospital to be an agent of the patient for the purposes of reliance (5, 47) and definitely not a seller of the medical devices. This view has been emphasized in the *Second Restatement of Torts,* which states: "One who sells any product in a dangerous condition unreasonably dangerous to the user or consumer or to his property is subject to liability for physical harm thereby caused to the *ultimate* user or consumer" (33). This direct liability of the manufacturer of health products to the patients is further expanded in the case of *Tinnerholm v. Parke Davis,* where the court stated that "the real purchaser is the patient as he is the one who receives the benefit of the product and pays the bill. Therefore, the fact that the physician or hospital is performing a service with the use of the product is of no consequence when the manufacturer's relation to the patient alone is considered. The real sale is from the manufacturer to the patient and not to the doctor or hospital" (85).

The above precedent in substance should effectively neutralize the privity defense and subject the manufacturer of heart valves to direct liability to the recipient patient, despite the fact that the patient did not buy the product directly from it. This view has been widely accepted in cases involving medical products (45, 85, 86).

This abandonment of the principles of privity in product liability in general may get both physician and hospital off the hook, because the patient is allowed to sue the manufacturer directly rather than naming the doctor and/or hospital as the defendant. Naturally the plaintiff may still consider filing suits against the surgeon and hospital directly for other reasons, unless he or she wants to enlist them as allies in his or her suit against the manufacturer.

In *Truly v. Providence Hospital* (87), the court held that the hospital acted as a seller of products that were provided incidental to services; thus it was liable for breach of implied warranty. Furthermore, the U.C.C. §2-315, as adopted by most states, indicates that the implied warranty of fitness for a particular purpose, that is, a valve prosthesis for implantation, arises "where the buyer is relying on the seller's skill and judgment to select and furnish suitable goods."

There have been several other controversial rulings, especially in connection with hospitals "reselling" blood obtained from blood banks. Some of the rulings held the hospital immune (88, 74). Others held that it does not matter that the hospital is not primarily in the business of selling the product, but that "ancillary selling in connection with other services was sufficient to bring the strict liability rule into action" (45). Similar decisions were made regarding not only blood, but also blood products. In a somewhat surprising move, some courts have removed blood and tissue from the definition of merchandise and legally relabeled them as medical services, making the liability of hospitals and physicians even more expressed. U.C.C. §3-316 states: "The implied warranties of merchantability and fitness shall not be applicable to furnishing of human blood, human blood plasma or *other human tissue or organs* . . . such blood, plasma, tissue or organs . . . shall be considered as *medical services*." This statement, especially the portion referring to tissues, is of great concern to cardiac surgeons because it may open an entirely new field of litigation regarding blood used routinely in the course of heart operations. It also may well be interpreted to remove litigation concerning homologous heart valve transplants from the area of warranty and toss it into the arena of negligence and strict liability. This relatively recent development situation has left both surgeons and hospitals in legal limbo concerning the implied warranties of fitness for a particular purpose and merchantability. The issue of merchantability of human tissue is further complicated by a recent lawsuit, John Moore versus his physician, the University of California at Los Angeles, and many others. The case, which involves commercial use of splenic tissue removed from the patient, revolves around the subject of whether a patient should or should not benefit if a product that derives from his body parts is manufactured and sold. While the lawsuit was dismissed three times by the state court, it was reinstated by the 2nd District Court of Appeals, which stated: "The patient must have the power to control what becomes of his or her tissue." While this theory has not yet been introduced into the field of cardiac valve and artery homografts, it may open up a new area of litigation when the patient or his or her heirs may demand a share of the tissue if it was processed and sold commercially (89).

The Health Provider as Inventor of the Device

Another conflict of interest between the physician and the manufacturer is if the former is sued not as the alleged prescriber-seller but the *inventor of the device,* that is, a participant in the process of design and manufacture. Examples of this have repeatedly occurred in litigation involving cardiac valve prostheses (VO Björk, personal communication, 1988). Because the allegations against the doctor are usually made on a breach of warranty basis, the best defense may be for the physician to emphasize that the design has been sold to the manufacturer (63). Courts generally accept that in most instances the public is not relying upon the licensure; therefore, the patent holder is usually not involved in medicolegal procedures. Again, to make this position safer it is highly advisable that the inventor, in his or her contract with a production firm, make it absolutely clear that he or she sold his idea to the manufacturer and does not participate in or warrant the manufacturing process (63).

According to Albert Starr, there are six basic forces that shape the thoracic industrial complex, three acting in the positive direction: technological innovation, enterpreneural activity, and flow of capital into the system; while an equal number work in the negative direction: government regulation, cost containment, and product liability litigation (14).

As we examine the effect of the problem of medicolegal litigation connected with prosthetic heart valve implantation, it certainly appears to have reached a crisis level in the United States and seems to be spreading to other countries as well. While attention is presently focused on professional liability (negligence), product liability is coming more and more into the foreground. As a report prepared by the AMA board of trustees points out, both professional and product liability are having a profound impact on the practice of the individual physician and on the marketing and development of new medical technology. The number of cases in federal court involving professional liability has increased at a compounded annual rate of more than 17% during the past 4 years, and during the past decade, the average jury award rose from $495,580 to $1,850,452 (90). The result of the combination of these events is that while the biomedical market shows a steady growth, the number of new implantable products is dropping, not only in that there are no longer newer-model heart valves but also in that manufacturers are reluctant to introduce even minor modifications to their products for fear of the legal implications. Increases in the cost of product liability insurance, or total inability to get it, have become a major deterrent to medical product manufacturers, some of whom reported staggering increases in their insurance rate of 2500 to 4000% (20). In the course of this process, not only were hospitals and surgeons intimidated, but several smaller companies were forced out of the market because of unexpected lawsuits that were not covered, or only partially covered, by insurance. We have also seen major companies become disinterested in prosthetic heart valve manufacturing for the same reasons, and watched as they turned toward the manufacture of products less likely to expose them to suits. A recent example of this is the complete withdrawal of the Shiley Company from the American heart valve market.

There is no question that the current legal interpretations of both professional and product liability laws diminish incentives for the design and manufacture of new medical devices, especially implantable devices. The result is that health care has been inhibited and valuable tools have been denied to the physician that could save lives and alleviate suffering. It is ironic that rules, laws, and regulations that were designed with the best intentions of protecting the public occasionally have the effect of slowing progress and denying accessibility to valuable technology to the very individuals they are meant to protect.

What changes can be made to improve this certainly less-than-desirable situation?

First of all, there is a definite and urgent need to reform and streamline the existing Federal Medical Device Regulations so that the process of compliance and approval becomes shorter and less bureaucratic without sacrificing the desirable level and quality of standards. In this process, the original role of different panels of professional experts should be restored from their present position of serving merely as consultants of secondary importance to authoritative advisors whose opinion is decisive, whose views may or may not be respected by clerical personnel.

Secondly, the manufacturers' presently existing double exposure to legal liability should be eliminated, that is, being exposed to product litigation even if in absolute compliance with government standards. Initially the courts regarded any medical device that met FDA standards as nondefective. This concept has been challenged repeatedly by the plaintiff's bar alleging that meeting "FDA standards for medical devices does not preclude recovery since they are so ineffectual as to be virtually meaningless" (19). Plaintiff's attorneys who were previously hesitant to dispute government standards on various products are now readily challenging them, implying that they represent rules of nonacceptable minimum with ample room for improvement, rather than the desirable optimum. This effectively shifts the burden of setting acceptable medical standards from the government to the court (13). This situation is counterproductive and serves neither justice nor public interest.

Finally, there is a long overdue need to reform the medical liability situation that, as it exists today in the United States, is unique in its complexity and controversy. Of the many recommendations made, the following are heard most often:

1. Implement uniform medical device liability law.

2. Put limits on compensation.

3. Eliminate punitive damages in the absence of criminal negligence and/or grant them to recipients other than the plaintiff.

4. Allow more pretrial elimination of cases to the discretion of the judge and/or by the use of mediation panels.

5. Make the contingency fee system in litigation illegal.

While it is the duty of the health care profession to protect individuals from as much harm as possible, this is feasible only if the medical profession is protected from *unjust* liability action. The physician should do his or her utmost to provide services of high clinical quality, and the manufacturer should use every effort to make an unavoidably unsafe product as safe as humanly possible. In addition to the obvious and well-documented need to modify and improve the tort system, creative solutions and reforms must be developed and put in place in order to prevent professional malpractice and product liability litigation from stalling the development and use of services and technologies that have the potential to benefit millions, not only in the United States but also in the entire world.

REFERENCES

1. Galante JO, Rostoker W, Doyle JM: Failed femoral stems in total hip prostheses. J Bone Joint Surg 1975;57A:230–236.
2. Rubin R: Manufacturer and professional user's liability for defective medical equipment. Akron Law Rev 1974;8:100–110.
3. Fish RM, Ehrhardt ME, Fish B (eds): Malpractice: Managing Your Defense. Oradell, NJ, Medical Economic Books, 1985.
4. Second Restatement of Torts §402A (1965).
5. Food, Drug and Cosmetic Act. 21 USC §360 (1976).
6. Anderson BJ. Cited by Holoweiko M: Watch out for these new liability risks. Medical Economics 1988;65(8):66–87.
7. Bates v State Bar of Arizona. 43 US 350, 1977.
8. Hirsh BD: "Professional" medical experts compete to testify for malpractice plaintiff. Group Practice News, June/July 1988.
9. Rosenn G: Litigation involving manufacturer's liability for defective medical products. Judicial Perspectives. 2 Am J L Med 1977;2:145.
10. Overview of litigation concerning products liability and medical devices. Am J Trial Advoc 1977;5:319–321.
11. Caldwell AM: Product liability and medical devices: diagnosis and care.
12. Corporate Research Group Staff, Gingerich D (eds): Medical Product Liability: A Comprehensive Guide and Sourcebook. New York, Frost and Sullivan, 1981, pp 5–6.
13. Piehler HR: Clinical environment and the law: Product liability. In Medical Devices: Measurements, Quality Assurance, and Standards. ASTM special technical publication 800. Philadelphia, American Society for Testing and Materials, 1983, pp 244–268.
14. Starr A: The thoracic surgical industrial complex. Ann Thorac Surg 1986;49:124–133.
15. Beall AC Jr: The medical device amendment of 1976 (Public Law 94-295) MS.
16. Federal Food, Drug and Cosmetic Act. Ch 675, 52 Stat 1040 (1938) (codified as amended at 21 USC §§301–92 (1972 suppl 1985).

17. Consumer Product Safety Act 15 USC §§2051–2081.
18. Medical Device Amendment of 1976. Pub L No 94-295, 90 Stat 539 (codified at 21 USCA §350c–360k (West suppl 1981).
19. Ramey MB: Medical device defects. Trial, May 1986:39–42.
20. Price JM: The liabilities and consequences of medical device development. J Biomed Mater Res 1987;21:35–58.
21. American Heart Association: Heart Facts. Dallas, AHA Publishers, 1982.
22. Robicsek F: Cardiac valve transplantation. Acta Medica, 1954;5:1–2.
23. Hwang NHC, Nan XZ, Gross DR: Prosthetic heart valve replacements. CRC Crit Rev Biomed Eng 1983;9:99–132.
24. Rooney FB: Statement of Representative Fred B. Rooney at hearings on HR 5545, HR 974, and S 510 before the Subcommittee of Health and Environment on Interstate and Foreign Commerce, 94th Congress, 1st Session, 1975.
25. Frumer L, Friedman M: Products Liability, 1960.
26. Hylen JC, Hodam RP, Kloster FE: Changes in the durability of silicone rubber in ball-valve prostheses. Ann Thorac Surg 1972;13:324–329.
27. Shah A, Dolgin M, Tice DA, Trehan N: Complications due to cloth wear in cloth-covered Starr-Edwards aortic and mitral valve prostheses—and their management. Am Heart J 1978;96:407–414.
28. Silver MD, Wilson GJ: The pathology of wear in the Beall model 104 heart valve prosthesis. Circulation 1977;56:617–622.
29. Schoen FJ, Titus JL, Lowrie GM: Bioengineering aspects of heart valve replacement. Ann Biomed Eng 1982;10:97–128.
30. Douglas PS, Hirshfeld JW, Edie RN, Harken AH, Stephenson LW, Edmunds LH, Jr: Clinical comparison of St. Jude and porcine valve prostheses. Circulation 1985;72(suppl II):135–139.
31. Deviri E, Levinsky L, Yechezkel M, Levy MJ: Pregnancy after valve replacement with porcine Xenograft prosthesis. Surg Gyn Obstet 1985;160:437–443.
32. Baxter Health Care Corporation, Edwards CVS Division: Suspension of Marketing of Edwards-Duromedica Bi-Leaflet Valves Models 316 and 920, All Sizes. May 19, 1988.
33. Metcalf LC: Legal problems in medical device development. Insurance Counsel Journal, July 1977;408–415.
34. Robicsek F: Cleansing of bioprosthetic valves. Thor Cardiovasc Surg 1983;31:187–188.
35. Mitchell RS, Miller DC, Stinson EB, Oyer PE, Jamieson SW, Baldwin JC, Shumway NE: Significant patient-related determinants of prosthetic valve performance. J Thorac Cardiovasc Surg 1986;91:807–817.
36. Sponagle v Pre-Term Inc. A 2d 366, 368 (DC 1980).
37. Reyes v Anka Research Ltd, New York (1981).
38. Sanbar SS: Implantable cardiovascular devices: Medico-legal aspects, 1986.
39. Gottsdanker v Cutter Laboratories. 183 Cal App 2d 602, 6 Cal Rptr 320 (1960).
40. Prosser WL: Handbook of the Law of Tort, ed 4. St. Paul, West Publishing, 1971.
41. Turner v General Motors Corp. Tex 584 SW 2d 844, 850–851 (1979).
42. Hursh and Bailey: American Law and Products Liability. 2d 4:12, 1974.
43. Pyatt v Engel Equipment Inc. 17 Ill App 3d 1070, 209 NE 2d 225 (1974).
44. Cronin v FBE Olsen Inc. 8 Cal 3d 121, 501 P2d 1153, 104 Cal Rptr 433 (1972).
45. Cunningham v McNeal Memorial Hospital. 47 112d 443 266 NE2d 897 (1970).
46. Grubb v Albert Einstein Medical Center. 255 Pa Super 387 A2d 480 (1978).
47. Hoffman v Misericordia Hospital of Philadelphia. 439 Pa 501, 267 A2d 867 (1970).
48. Jackson v Muhlenberg Hospital. 96 NF Super 314, 232 A2d 879 (1967).
49. Ethicon Inc v Parten. 520 SW 2d Tex Civ App (1975).
50. McKasson v Zimmer Mfg Co. 12 Ill App 3d 429, 299 NE 2d 38 (1973).
51. NcPherson v Buick Motor Co. 217 NY 382, 111 NE 1050 (1916).
52. Clark v Bendix Corp. 42 AD 2d 727, 345 NYS 2d.
53. Thornton GR: Intrauterine devices. Trial, Nov. 1986;42–49.
54. Lemire v Garrand Drugs. 95 Mich App 520, 291 NW 2d 103 (1985).
55. Crane M: Hospital role. Medical Economics, April 18, 1988:88–120.
56. Beane v Perley. 99 NH 309, 100, A2d 848 (1954).
57. Morris: The role of expert testimony in the trial of negligence issues. 26 Tex L Rev 1 (1947).
58. Shen v Phillips. 213 Ga 269, 98 SE 2d 552 (1957).
59. Dykema JA: Medical devices: Cure the harm or harm the care, 1986.
60. Terhune v AH Robbins Co. 577/P2d 975, 978, Wash (1978).
61. Lukassevick v Ortho Pharmaceutical Corp. 510 F Suppl 961 (ED Wis 1978).
62. Sard v Hardy. 281 Md 432, 379 A2d 1014, 1024 (1977).
63. Jennings DE: Litigating medical device product liability claims. The Forum 1984;11:141–151.
64. USC vol 3, 1976.
65. Crane M: Informed consent mistakes. Medical Economics, August 15, 1988:87–96.
66. UCC §2-725.

67. Keeton WP, Owen DG, Montgomery JE: Products Liability and Safety. New York, The Foundation Press, 1980.
68. Catepillar Tractor v Beck Alaska. 593 P2d 871 (1979).
69. Shilkrest v Annapolis Emergency Hospital. 349 A 2d 245 (Md 1975).
70. Cannon v Fox. 296 Md 21, 38 at n4 (1963).
71. Baxter v Ford Motor Co. 168 Wash 456, 12 P2d 409 (1932).
72. Randy Knitwear Inc v American Cyanamid Co. 11 NY 2d, 181 NE 2d, 399 (1962).
73. Providence Hospital. 611 SW 2d 121 131 Tec Circ App (1981).
74. Perimutter v Beth David Hospital. 308 NY 100, 123 NE 2d 792 (1954).
75. Russell v Community Blood Bank, Inc. 185 So 2d 749 Fla (1916).
76. Cheshire v Southampton Hospital Assn. Misc 2d 355 278 NYS 2d 531 (1967).
77. Cutler v General Electric Co. 4 UCCRS 300 NY (1967).
78. Fisher v Sibley Memorial Hospital. 403 A2d 1130 DC (1979).
79. Preston v Thomason. 280 SE 2d 780 NC App (1981).
80. Geotz v Wadley Institute and Blood Bank. 350 SW 2d 573 Tex Civ App (1961).
81. Magrine v Krasmica. 94 NJ Super 228, 227 A2d 539 (1967).
82. Potts v W Q Richards Memorial Hospital. 558 SW 2d 939. Tex Civ App (1977).
83. Shepherd v Alexion Bros. Hospital. 33 Cal App 3d 606. 109 Cal Rptr 132 (1973).
84. Silverhort v Mount Zion Hospital. 20 Cal App 3d 1022, 98 Cal Rptr 187 (1971).
85. Tinnerholm v Parke-Davis Co. 285 F2d 432 SDNY (1968).
86. Putensen v Clay Adams Inc. 12 Cal App 3d 1062, 91 Cal Rptr 319 (1970).
87. Truly v Providence Hospital. 611 SW 2d 127. Tex Civ App (1980).
88. Carter v Inter-Faith Hospital. 60 Misc 2d 733, 304 NYS2d 97 (1969).
89. Who owns human tissue? Am Med Assoc News, August 5, 1988.
90. Product liability suits hamper advances. Am Med Assoc News, June 3, 1988.

INDEX